Congenital Anomalies of the Upper Extremity

Donald R. Laub Jr.
Editor

Congenital Anomalies of the Upper Extremity

Etiology and Management

Springer

Editor
Donald R. Laub Jr., MS, MD, FACS
Fletcher Allen Health Care and Vermont Children's Hospital
Departments of Surgery and Pediatrics
University of Vermont School of Medicine
Burlington, VT, USA

ISBN 978-1-4899-7863-9 ISBN 978-1-4899-7504-1 (eBook)
DOI 10.1007/978-1-4899-7504-1
Springer New York Heidelberg Dordrecht London

Printed on acid-free paper

Springer is part of Springer Science+Business Media (www.springer.com)

To Don Sr., Judy, Susan, Dylan, Genevieve, Sharon, Jack, and Erik, with love and gratitude.

Preface

Hominem ad deos nulla re propius accedunt quam salutem hominibus dando.
In nothing do men more nearly approach the gods, than in giving health to men.

—Marcus Tullius Cicero

How much more do we approach divinity when we help a child to health?

I am very honored to be in the company of all of the authors of this text. Not only have they collaborated on this book you now hold in your hands but also we share one of the finest activities in the world: we have been trusted by parents to care for their children's limbs and health.

This text, like all texts, will become dated and be superseded by new knowledge. However, it stands as a milestone of where we are now in our knowledge and also as a direction sign of where our knowledge is heading.

It is my hope that readers of this text will join us in the care of children with congenital anomalies of the upper extremity and will be inspired to further advance our knowledge in this field.

Burlington, VT, USA

Donald R. Laub Jr.

Contents

Contributors

Hisham Abdel-Ghani, MD Department of Orthopedics, Kasr Al Ainy University Hospital, Cairo University, Cairo, Egypt

Shady Abdel-Rehim, MBChB, MSc, MRCS (Ed) Department of Plastic Surgery, University of Michigan Healthcare System, Ann Arbor, MI, USA

Mohammad M. Al-Qattan, MBBS Department of Surgery, King Saud University, Riyadh, Saudi Arabia

Goo Hyun Baek, MD, PhD Department of Orthopedic Surgery, Seoul National University Hospital, Seoul, South Korea

Andrea S. Bauer, MD Department of Orthopaedic Surgery, Shriners Hospital for Children Northern California, Sacramento, CA, USA

Michael S. Bednar, MD Department of Orthopedic Surgery and Rehabilitation, Loyola University Medical Center, Maywood, IL, USA

Scott E. Benjamin, MD Department of Orthopaedics and Rehabilitation, University of Vermont College of Medicine, Fletcher Allen Health Care, Colchester, VT, USA

Department of Pediatrics, University of Vermont College of Medicine, Fletcher Allen Health Care, Colchester, VT, USA

Leah W. Burke, MAT, MD, FAAP, FABMG Department of Pediatrics, Fletcher Allen Health Care, University of Vermont College of Medicine, Burlington, VT, USA

Jennifer M. Chan, OTR, CHT Rehabilitation Services, Lucile Packard Children's Hospital at Stanford, Menlo Park, CA, USA

James Chang, MD Division of Plastic and Reconstructive Surgery, Stanford University Medical Center, Palo Alto, CA, USA

Arhana Chattopadhyay, BA Division of Plastic and Reconstructive Surgery, Stanford University Medical Center, Palo Alto, CA, USA

Kevin Chung, MD, MS Department of Plastic Surgery, University of Michigan Healthcare System, Ann Arbor, MI, USA

William J. Dahl, MD Department of Orthopaedic Surgery, University of California, Irvine, Orange, CA, USA

Roberto Diaz, MD Department of Orthopaedic Surgery, Stanford University Medical Center, Redwood City, CA, USA

Borzoo Farhang, DO Department of Anesthesiology, The University of Vermont College of Medicine/Fletcher Allen Health Care, Burlington, VT, USA

Lauren E. Fonseca, BA Department of Medicine, Fletcher Allen Health Care, Burlington, VT, USA

Ginny Gibson, OTD, OTR/L, CHT Pediatric Rehabilitation, UCSF Benioff Children's Hospital Oakland, Oakland, CA, USA

Department of Occupational Therapy, Samuel Merritt University, Oakland, CA, USA

Hilton Phillip Gottschalk, MD Department of Pediatric Orthopaedics, Dell Children's Medical Center, Austin, TX, USA

Joseph Hardwicke, PhD, MBChB, FRCS (Plast) College of Medical and Dental Sciences, University of Birmingham, Edgbaston, Birmingham, West Midlands, UK

Ann E. Van Heest, MD Department of Orthopaedic Surgery, University of Minnesota, Minneapolis, MN, USA

Carlos Garrido-Allepuz Herrera, PhD Department of Molecular and Cellular Anatomy, Instituto de Biomedicina y Biotecnologia de Cantabria (IBBTEC), CSIC-SODERCAN-Universidad de Cantabria, Santander, Spain

Sandip Hindocha, MD, MBChB, MPhil, MRCS Plastic Surgery, Whiston Hospital, Liverpool, UK

Matthew E. Hiro, MD Department of Orthopaedic Surgery and Rehabilitation, Stritch School of Medicine, Loyola University Chicago, Maywood, IL, USA

Neil F. Jones, MD, FRCS Department of Orthopedic Surgery, University of California Irvine Medical Center and Shriners Hospital Los Angeles, Orange, CA, USA

Daniel J. Jordan, MBChB Plastic Surgery, Whiston Hospital, Liverpool, UK

Amy L. Ladd, MD Department of Orthopaedic Surgery, Stanford University Medical Center, Redwood City, CA, USA

Donald R. Laub Jr., MS, MD, FACS Fletcher Allen Health Care and Vermont Children's Hospital, Departments of Surgery and Pediatrics, University of Vermont School of Medicine, Burlington, VT, USA

Ann F.T. Lawrence, DO Department of Anesthesiology, The University of Vermont College of Medicine/Fletcher Allen Health Care, Burlington, VT, USA

Alex C. Lesiak, MS, MD Department of Orthopaedics and Rehabilitation, Fletcher Allen Health Care, University of Vermont College of Medicine, Burlington, VT, USA

Ruth Lester, MBChB, DObstRCOG, DCH, FRCS Department of Plastic Surgery, Birmingham Children's Hospital NHS Foundation Trust, Birmingham, West Midlands, UK

Terry R. Light, MD Department of Orthopaedic Surgery and Rehabilitation, Loyola University Stritch School of Medicine, Maywood, IL, USA

Jennifer W. Lisle, MD Department of Orthopedics and Rehabilitation, University of Vermont/ Fletcher Allen Health Care, South Burlington, VT, USA

Karin Ljungquist, MD Bone and Joint Center, Department of Orthopaedics and Sports Medicine, University of Washington Medical Center, Seattle, WA, USA

Mostafa Mahmoud, MD Department of Orthopedics, Kasr Al Ainy University Hospital, Cairo University, Cairo, Egypt

H. Relton McCarroll, MD Department of Orthopaedic Surgery, Shriners Hospital for Children Northern California, Sacramento, CA, USA

Kerby C. Oberg, MD, PhD Department of Pathology and Human Anatomy, Loma Linda University Medical Center, Molecular Embryopathy Laboratory, Loma Linda, CA, USA

Toshihiko Ogino, MD, PhD Hokushin-Higashi Hospital, Sapporo Hand Surgery and Congenital Hand Differences Center, Sapporo, Hokkaido, Japan

Scott Oishi, MD Hand Service, Texas Scottish Rite Hospital for Children, Dallas, TX, USA

Brian C. Pridgen, MD Division of Plastic and Reconstructive Surgery, Stanford University Medical Center, Palo Alto, CA, USA

Manoj Ramachandran, BSc, MBBS, FRCS (Orth) Center for Orthopaedics, The Royal London and Barts & The London Children's Hospitals, London, UK

Sarah E. Sibbel, MD Department of Orthopaedic Surgery, Shriners Hospital for Children Northern California, Sacramento, CA, USA

Emma Snashall, MBChB Burns and Plastic Reconstruction Unit, Whiston Hospital, Liverpool, UK

Sondra Elice Solomon, PhD College of Arts and Science, Department of Psychology Science, University of Vermont, Burlington, VT, USA

College of Medicine, Department of Psychiatry, University of Vermont, Burlington, VT, USA

Emily L.A. Stebbins, MD Department of Anesthesiology, The University of Vermont College of Medicine/Fletcher Allen Health Care, Burlington, VT, USA

Chris Stutz, MD Department of Orthopaedics, Monroe Carell Jr. Children's Hospital, Vanderbilt University Medical Center, Nashville, TN, USA

Tarun Taneja, MBBS, MS, FRCS (Orth) Center for Orthopaedics, The Royal London and Barts & The London Children's Hospitals, London, UK

Michael A. Tonkin, MBBS, MD, FRACS, FRCS (Ed Orth) Department of Hand Surgery and Peripheral Nerve Surgery, Royal North Shore Hospital, The Children's Hospital at Westmead, University of Sydney, Sydney, Australia

Raymond Tse, MD, FRCS(C) Pediatric Plastic Surgery, University of Washington, Seattle Children's Hospital, Seattle, WA, USA

Part I

General Considerations

Embryology and Classification of Congenital Upper Limb Anomalies

1

Carlos Garrido-Allepuz Herrera, Michael A. Tonkin, and Kerby C. Oberg

Morphological Overview

In vertebrates, the limb bud starts as an accumulation of cells within the lateral plate mesoderm (LPM) forming an oblong ventrolateral bulge on the body wall. The limb is a composite structure of cells from the LPM (precursors of limb-associated skeletal tissues) and associated somites (muscle and vascular precursors). In humans, the upper limb bud appears during the fourth week of development around day 26 (Carnegie stage 12) and is located between somites 9 and 12 (Fig. 1.1a) [1, 2]. The limb emerges only in certain zones of the body known as limb fields. The position of limb fields are thought to be specified by a quantitative and/or qualitative combination of Hox transcription factors (see Fig. 1.1b) [3, 4].

By day 37 of development (Carnegie stage 16), the distal portion of the limb can be recognized as a handplate. At the same time there is progressive mesodermal condensation along the proximodistal axis forming the skeletal elements of the limb. By day 56 the major morphologic features of the limb are complete.

C.G.-A. Herrera, Ph.D.
Department of Molecular and Cellular Anatomy, Instituto de Biomedicina y Biotecnologia de Cantabria (IBBTEC), CSIC-SODERCAN-Universidad de Cantabria C/Albert Einstein, 22. 39011 (PTCAN), Santander, Cantabria 39, Spain
e-mail: arcanumes@hotmail.com

M.A. Tonkin, M.B.B.S., M.D., F.R.A.C.S., F.R.C.S. (Ed Orth)
Department of Hand Surgery and Peripheral Nerve Surgery, Royal North Shore Hospital, The Children's Hospital at Westmead, University of Sydney, Sydney, NSW 2065, Australia
e-mail: mtonkin@med.usyd.edu.au

K.C. Oberg, M.D., Ph.D. (✉)
Department of Pathology and Human Anatomy, Loma Linda University Medical Center, Molecular Embryopathy Laboratory, 24785 Stewart St., Loma Linda, CA 92354, USA
e-mail: koberg@llu.edu

Limb Initiation

After the upper limb fields have been specified, induction of the limb bud occurs. The cells of the LPM located within the limb fields maintain active proliferation, while non-limb field LPM begins to divide more slowly [5]. Initially *Fgf10* is expressed broadly along the LPM, but just before the limb emerges, the domain of *Fgf10* expression becomes restricted to the limb fields. In chicken, the expression of *Tbx5* and *Wnt2b* in the LPM cells of the limb field are responsible for the induction of *Fgf10* in the presumptive limb (Fig. 1.2) [6–8]. Recent studies suggest that *Tbx5* expression can be induced and regulated by Hox transcription factors, suggesting a role for Hox genes in both positioning limb fields and initiating limb outgrowth [9]. Fgf10 through its receptor FgfrIIa has been shown to induce *Wnt3* and *Wnt3a* in prospective mouse and chick limb ectoderm, respectively. Concurrently, Bone Morphogenetic Protein (Bmp) signaling in the ventral ectoderm induces β-catenin competency in cells of the presumptive apical ectodermal ridge (AER) at the dorsal–ventral boundary [10, 11]. In turn, Wnt3 or Wnt3a induces *Fgf8* in a Wnt/β-catenin-dependent manner in the precursor cells of the AER [6, 12]. Fgf8 secreted from the recently formed AER maintains the expression of *Fgf10* in the mesoderm, establishing a positive regulatory loop that maintains proximal–distal growth [6, 12].

Another signaling molecule that is fundamental to the induction of the limb bud appears to be retinoic acid (RA), the active metabolite of vitamin A. This molecule is produced in the somites of the embryo by the enzyme Raldh2 [13–15]. RA restricts the early expression of Fgf8 within the heart field, which, in turn, permits the expression of *Tbx5* in the limb field to initiate forelimb development [16, 17]. Furthermore, RA has been shown to regulate the expression of *Hox* genes both in vitro and in vivo, which may contribute to limb field induction and/or positioning (see Fig. 1.2) [18, 19].

D.R. Laub Jr. (ed.), *Congenital Anomalies of the Upper Extremity: Etiology and Management*, DOI 10.1007/978-1-4899-7504-1_1, © Springer Science+Business Media New York 2015

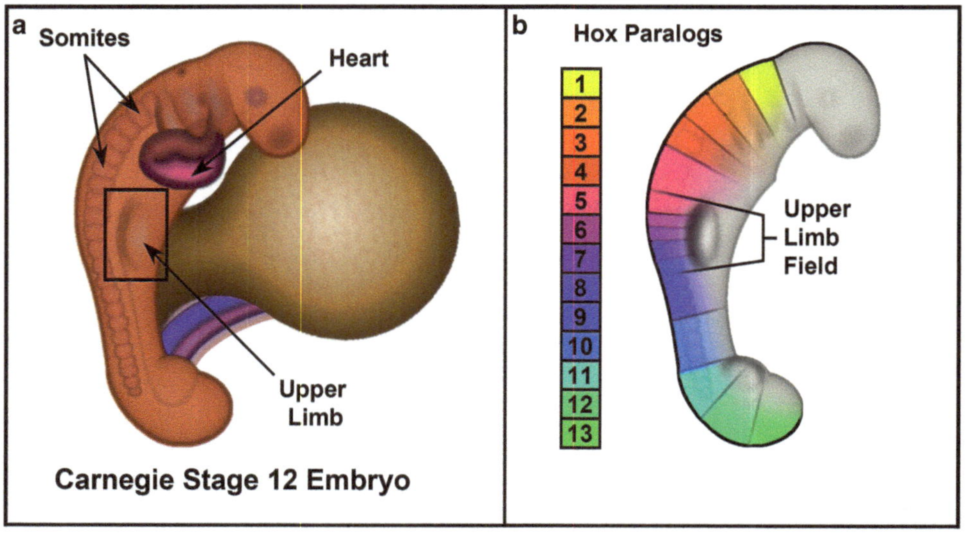

Fig. 1.1 Human embryo at stage of limb initiation and presumed Hox positioning. (**a**) Depiction of an emerging upper limb bud (boxed) in Carnegie stage 12 embryo. (**b**) Hox genes establish upper limb position and polarity. Courtesy of K.C. Oberg and Loma Linda University

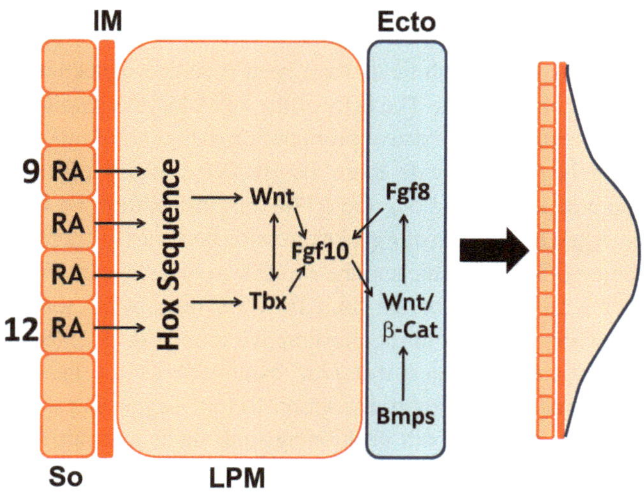

Fig. 1.2 Molecular pathways involved in limb induction. Depiction of the tissues involved in the initiation of the right upper limb bud emerging from lateral plate mesoderm (LPM) at somite (So) levels 9-12. Molecular interactions between LPM and ectoderm (Ecto) are also illustrated. IM-intermediate mesoderm. Courtesy of K.C. Oberg and Loma Linda University

Signaling Centers

Between the fourth and eighth weeks of development, the limb bud undergoes growth and differentiation to transform it into a fully patterned limb. This process can be described in terms of three coordinate axes: proximal–distal (P–D), anterior–posterior or radial–ulnar (A–P/R–U), and dorsal–ventral (D–V) modulated by three signaling centers [20].

Along the P–D axis, the AER appears as thickened ectoderm overlying the distal edge of the limb bud [21]. The AER is the signaling center that regulates the P–D growth and Fgfs are the signaling molecules that accomplish its function. Excision of the AER in chicken embryos at different stages of limb development results in limb truncations in a progressive fashion; the later the AER removal, the more distal the resulting truncation [22].

The signaling center for the A–P/R–U axis is the zone of polarizing activity (ZPA), a cluster of mesodermal cells located at the distal posterior (ulnar) margin. The ZPA directs A–P/R–U patterning and Shh is the signaling molecule that mediates its function. Both mice (*Shh* knock-out) that lack Shh function or mutant chickens (Oligozeugodactyly—*Ozd* mutants) that fail to have limb-specific Shh expression show marked loss of posterior (ulnar) elements [23, 24].

Dorsal non-AER ectoderm directs D–V patterning with Wnt7a as the signaling molecule that promotes dorsalization. Excision and rotation of the dorsal ectoderm results in the formation of dorsal structures within the ventral aspect of the limb [25].

Patterned Development Along Coordinate Axes

Pattern formation is a process by which the cells are sequentially specified, determined, and then differentiated to form the morphological structures of the limb. In this section we will focus on how the process of patterning is accomplished along each axis as directed by the signaling centers and the associated molecular pathways, recognizing that the molecular cascades of these three axes are operating concurrently and integrated together like a fine-tuned instrument.

Proximal–Distal Patterning (P–D)

The upper limb can be divided into three different segments along the P–D axis (Fig. 1.3): (1) the proximal segment or

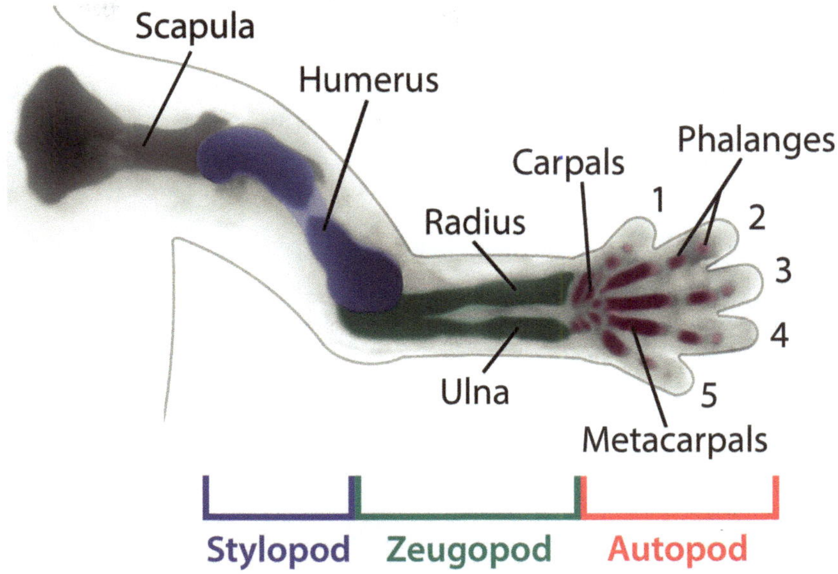

Fig. 1.3 Limb elements. The upper limb consists of a limb girdle or shoulder, and three limb segments known as the stylopod (humerus - colored blue), the zeugopod, which includes the radius and ulna (colored green) and the autopod or handplate (colored magenta). Courtesy of K.C. Oberg and Loma Linda University

stylopod where the skeletal elements of the humerus develop; (2) the intermediate segment or zeugopod where the radius and ulna form; and (3) the distal segment or autopod where the carpals, metacarpals, and digits form.

Patterning along the P–D axis begins during limb initiation with the formation of the AER, stratified ectoderm at the distal dorsal–ventral boundary of the developing limb bud. The AER secretes fibroblasts growth factors (Fgfs), the molecules primarily responsible for P–D patterning. Fgf8 is the first and functionally most important Fgf secreted from the AER during induction and maintained until the AER regresses, when the drafts of the last phalanges are formed. *Fgf4*, *Fgf9*, and *Fgf17* are activated sequentially in the posterior AER and expand to the anterior aspect as the limb develops [26, 27]. Classical experiments in chick embryos showed that AER removal abated distal limb outgrowth and resulted in truncations that corresponded to the timing of AER removal; in other words, the later the AER removal, the more distal the structures that were present [22]. Moreover, FGF-soaked beads were able to restore limb bud outgrowth and patterning after AER removal, indicating that Fgfs were the functional signaling factors of the AER [28, 29].

Among the different *Fgfs* expressed, *Fgf8* is thought to be the main AER signal, while *Fgf4*, *Fgf9*, or *Fgf17* are considered secondary or redundant [30, 31]. This concept is supported from experiments with *Fgf8* knock-out mice that showed smaller AERs, delayed limb bud outgrowth, and loss of some skeletal elements [26, 32]. In contrast, knock-out mice for *Fgf4*, *Fgf9*, and/or *Fgf17* did not develop limb anomalies. Interestingly, *Fgf4* expression in *Fgf8* knock-out mice was up-regulated, suggesting that redundant expression may have lessened the phenotype of these mutants. This was confirmed by the removal of both *Fgf4* and *Fgf8* that resulted in a worse phenotype with notably smaller limb buds [32, 33].

Several models have been proposed for P–D patterning. The progress zone model proposes that mesenchymal cell fate is determined by the length of time spent under the direct influence of the AER in a proliferative region called the progress zone (PZ) [34, 35]. The early specification model [36] postulates that the P–D identities are specified early and the different progenitor pools expand sequentially as the limb grows. The differentiation front model suggests that the AER maintains mesenchymal cells in an undifferentiated state; as the limb expands, the cells that are no longer under the influence of the AER differentiate [37].

However, the accumulating evidence supports an alternative model. The two signal model [30] proposes that two opposing signals pattern the limb along the P–D axis: RA emanating from the flank will specify a proximal fate, while Fgfs from the AER will specify a distal fate (Fig. 1.4a) [38, 39]. In somites, Raldh2 oxidizes Retinol to form RA which can act locally in the proximal limb buds to promote the expression of *Meis1* and *Meis2*. The expression of *Meis1/2* defines the proximal limb segment and where the humerus (stylopod) will develop. Distally, Fgf signaling induces 5′*Hoxa* genes (*Hoxa11*, *Hoxa13*) and limits distal *Meis1/2* expression. Although the mechanism for this repression is not fully understood, it is known that Fgf8 signaling induces the expression of *Cyp26b1* in the distal mesenchyme of the limb bud; the product of this gene oxidizes RA into a non-active form, thus clearing the distal region of active RA (see Fig. 1.4c) [40]. Some have questioned RA role as a proximalizing agent [16], and further investigations are warranted to clarify whether RA or another factor influenced by RA is the proximalizing signal.

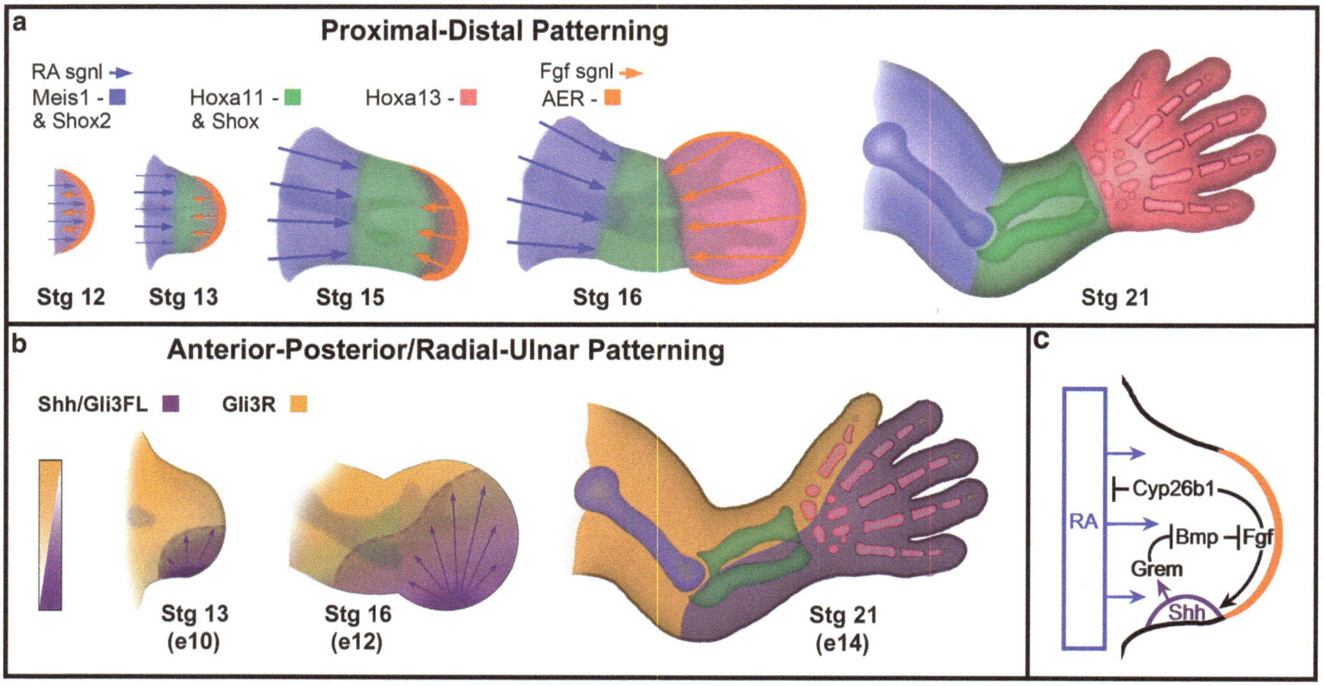

Fig. 1.4 Molecular pathways regulating proximal-distal & anterior-posterior/radial-ulnar axes. (**a**) Progressive segment specification along the proximal-distal axis based on the two signal model with RA-related proximalizing signals countered by distalizing Fgf signals. Outgrowth separates the signals and an intermediate zone is formed. Mies1 and Shox2 are restricted to the stylopod, Hoxa11 and Shox are markers for the zeugopod, and Hoxa13 delimits the handplate boundaries. (**b**) Opposing gradients of Gli3 repressor (Gli3R) and Shh-maintained full length Gli3 activator (Gli3FL) establish boundaries between the radius and ulna in the zeugopod and the thumb and ulnar digits in the autopod or hand. c) Some of the molecular interactions that maintain and terminate Shh expression in the ZPA (→ indicates positive regulation, while ⊣ indicates inhibition). Courtesy of K.C. Oberg and Loma Linda University

Anterior–Posterior/Radial–Ulnar Patterning (A–P/R–U)

The limb along the A–P/R–U axis is divided into two segments: the anterior (radial), comprises the thumb and radius, and the posterior (ulnar) with the ulna and ulnar digits (digits two through five) [41].

Patterned development along the A–P/R–U axis is controlled by the zone of polarizing activity (ZPA), a cluster of mesenchymal cells maintained in the distal posterior/ulnar aspect of the developing limb (see Fig. 1.4b). The ZPA was discovered in 1968 through grafting experiments in chick limb buds [42]. In these experiments, grafts from the distal posterior/ulnar mesenchyme were excised from one group of chicks and then inserted into the distal anterior/radial aspect of another group of chicks. The limbs that developed from these grafts demonstrated mirror image duplication of structures [42–44]. RA was found to be the first molecule that mimicked ZPA grafts when applied to the distal anterior/radial aspect of the limb bud [45–48]. Later it was shown that Shh was the molecule responsible for the phenotype induced by RA [49].

Shh is critical to the correct developmental pattern of the limb, particularly for the forearm (zeugopod) and hand (autopod). This is demonstrated in *Shh* knock-out mice, which have a correctly developed stylopod, a single skeletal element (radius) for the zeugopod, and a minimal autopod. In the upper limb, the autopod forms as a small cartilage condensation [23, 50], while in the lower limb, the autopod consists of a single digit with two phalanges [23, 50].

A–P/R–U polarity and subsequent Shh expression is initiated by axial Hox gene segmentation [51] followed by several other factors that contribute to Shh induction and the establishment of the ZPA. Hand2, expressed in the posterior/ulnar half of the limb bud, is required for Shh induction [52, 53] and has been shown to directly interact with limb-specific Shh regulatory region [54]. Similarly, distal Hoxd (Hoxd10-13) transcription factors also interact with the limb-specific Shh regulatory region, and evidence suggests that their initial phase of limb bud expression helps to localize Shh expression (Fig. 1.5) [55].

The first or initial phase of distal Hoxd expression in the limb bud occurs in a nested collinear (corresponding to their gene order) fashion along the anterior–posterior axis, with Hoxd10 exhibiting the broadest initial expression domain. The expression of each successively more distal Hoxd gene is nested within the previous gene's expression domain (see Fig. 1.5). Hoxd13, the terminal transcription factor in the Hoxd cluster, has the most restricted expression domain within the distal posterior or ulnar aspect of the limb bud overlapping the ZPA. This first phase of distal Hoxd expression plays a role in localizing Shh expression and temporally corresponds to specification of the forearm or zeugopod.

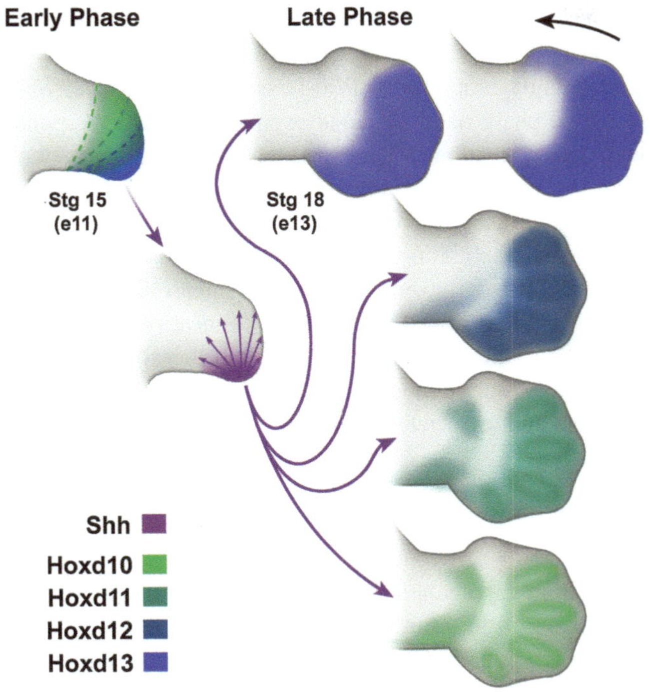

Fig. 1.5 Distal Hoxd genes are expressed in the limb bud in two phases. In the early phase, there is a nested collinear expression pattern. Dotted lines highlight the boundaries of expression, from broadest expression of Hoxd10 (green) to the most restricted of Hoxd13 (blue). In the late phase, Hoxd expressioin demonstrates quantitative colinearity with progressively more robust expression. Courtesy of K.C. Oberg and Loma Linda University

The role of Shh in A–P/R–U axis patterning has been characterized largely through knock-out mice for members of the Gli protein family of transcription factors (Gli1, Gli2, and Gli3). *Gli3* mutant mice are polydactylous without digit identity while the zeugopod is perfectly formed [56, 57]. Remarkably, the limbs of the double knock-out mice for both *Gli3* and *Shh* were indistinguishable from the *Gli3* mutant alone [58, 59], suggesting that the principal function of Shh is mediated through Gli3. Molecular studies demonstrated that Shh signaling prevents the posttranslational processing of full-length Gli3 protein into a short form, which functions as a strong repressor of Shh target genes.

Secreted Shh diffusing from the ZPA establishes a posterior to anterior concentration gradient. A complementary gradient of Gli3R forms with high levels of Gli3R in the anterior zone where Shh signaling is minimal (see Fig. 1.4b) [59]. In the absence of *Shh*, the level of Gli3R is uniform along the A–P/R–U axis and the elevated levels of Gli3R, unopposed by Shh, are accompanied by an increase in the apoptotic rate of the limb mesenchyme [58, 60]. Thus, the A–P/R–U gradient of Gli3R and its reciprocal full length Gli3 activator are responsible for conveying pattern information along this axis. However, it remains unclear whether the critical patterning signal is the absolute level of GLi3R or the relative levels between the repressor and the activator forms [58, 59]. Collectively, these data help to characterize the role of Shh in A–P/R–U patterning which, at least, in part, is to regulate the form and function of its transcription factor, Gli3.

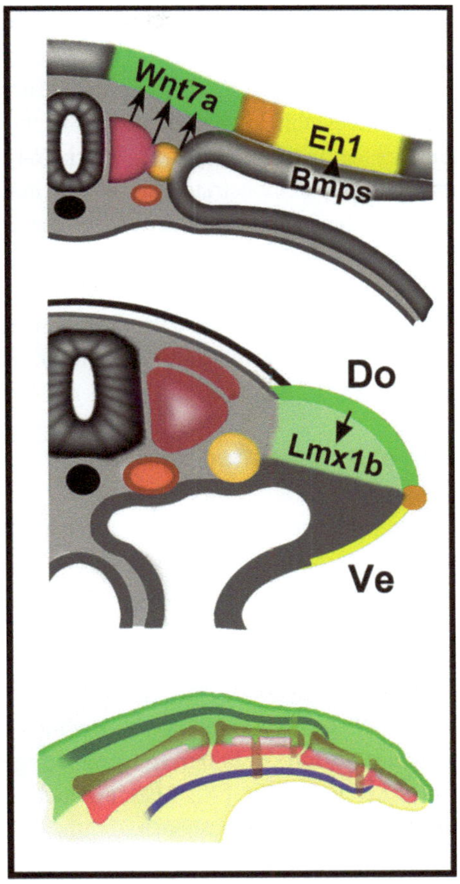

Fig. 1.6 Molecular pathways regulating the dorsal-ventral axis. From top to bottom, unknown factors in somites and/or intermediate mesoderm initiate Wnt7a expression in medial dorsal ectoderm. Bmps induce the expression of En1 in what will become the ventral ectoderm establishing the dorsal ventral boundary where the AER will form (orange). Wnt7a will induce Lmx1b in the underlying mesoderm to dorsalize developing tendons, joints and soft tissues. Courtesy of K.C. Oberg and Loma Linda University

Dorsal–Ventral Patterning (D–V)

Patterning along this axis is regulated by signals from the non-AER ectoderm that surrounds the limb mesenchyme. The dorsal and ventral areas are defined by the expression of two different genes: *Wnt7a* in the dorsal ectoderm and *En-1* in the ventral ectoderm (Fig. 1.6). *Wnt7a* signaling defines the dorsal fate of the limb structures [61], while *En-1* restricts *Wnt7a* expression to the dorsal ectoderm, preventing the dorsalization of ventral limb tissues [62, 63]. It is not yet known how *Wnt7a* is induced in the presumptive limb ectoderm; however, there is evidence that BMP and WNT canonical signaling are responsible for the induction of *En-1* in the ventral ectoderm. Knock-out mice have further elaborated their functional roles. *Wnt7a* mutants have biventral limbs, while

En-1 mutants have bi-dorsal limbs [64, 65]. Interestingly, double compound mutant mice for *En-1* and *Wnt7a* display a biventral phenotype, suggesting that the default limb phenotype is ventral and establishing Wnt7a's role as the dorsalizing signaling molecule of the limb's D–V axis [64].

Additional studies demonstrate that *Wnt7a* manifests its function through the induction of *Lmx1b* in the underlying dorsal mesoderm. Lmx1b function is both sufficient and necessary for the induction of dorsal fates. In chicken and mice, ventral *Lmx1b* expression led to bi-dorsal limbs, whereas its inactivation resulted in biventral limbs [61, 64, 66, 67].

Integration of Axis-Related Signaling

The three signaling centers coordinate patterned limb development through interactions between their molecular signaling cascades. One of the most studied interactions is the interaction between the ZPA and the AER. Shh signaling from the ZPA induces the expression of *Gremlin* in the adjacent mesenchyme that underlies the AER [26]. Gremlin is an antagonist of BMP signaling, repressing *Bmp* expression in the mesenchyme [68, 69]. Although Bmp signaling is needed in limb and AER induction [70, 71], mesenchymal BMP inhibits the expression of AER-associated Fgfs and increases mesenchymal cell death [70, 71]. Thus, Shh through Gremlin prevents these BMP-associated functions thereby maintaining Fgf expression. Correspondingly, Fgf8 secretion into the mesenchyme maintains Shh expression in the ZPA (through pathways that are not yet characterized) forming a positive feedback loop that supports continued limb growth and patterning. Termination of this reciprocal loop has been proposed as the mechanism that stops limb outgrowth once the appropriate size has been achieved [72].

Integration also occurs between other axes. *Wnt7a* knockout mice shows a reduction in *Shh* expression [61] with a loss of the posterior digits (corresponding to the little finger). In chickens, elimination of the dorsal ectoderm of the limb showed similar results [73, 74]. These findings suggest that Wnt7a signaling from the dorsal ectoderm is capable of inducing or maintaining Shh expression in the ZPA [61]. Although the characterization of pathways that interconnect these three signaling centers is incomplete, it is intuitive that interaction between them is crucial for the proper development of a patterned limb.

Handplate Patterning

The handplate or autopod is the distal-most element of the limb and the last to form. It is composed of digits (fingers) and wrist bones. The axes-related pathways converge to form the most complicated, pattern-rich structures of limb development. Hoxa13, the terminal transcription factor of the Hoxa cluster, is confined to the handplate, demarcating its proximal boundary along the P–D axis (see Fig. 1.4a) [75, 76]. Concurrently, along the A–P/R–U axis, a second "late" Shh-regulated phase of distal Hoxd expression (that corresponds with digit formation) is generated that partially reverses their expression domains, i.e., reverse colinearity (see Fig. 1.5) [77]. More importantly, there is progressive expression intensity, with Hoxd13 exhibiting the most robust expression within the digits and Hoxd10 exhibiting the least intense expression, in what has been termed quantitative colinearity [78]. Along the D–V axis, expression of Lmx1b, the dorsalizing Wnt7a-mediated transcription factor, becomes restricted to dorsal tendons and joint-associated tissues (see Fig. 1.6) [79].

Establishing Digit Number

In addition to regulating the second phase of Hoxd gene expression in the limb bud, Shh-expressing ZPA cells also make a direct contribution to digit development. Fate mapping studies have demonstrated that descendants from Shh-expressing cells of the ZPA populate digit 5, 4 and half of digit 3. The cells of digit 5 have had the longest exposure to Shh and at higher levels, while the cells of the digit 2 are only affected by diffusion of Shh [80, 81]. Moreover, premature arrest in *Shh* expression causes a reduction in the number of digits corresponding to the stage and duration of arrest. With normal Shh levels, the order of condensation is d4, d2, d5, and d3, and with the premature arrest in shh, the loss follows a predictable order, where digit 3 is lost first, followed by d5, d2, and d4 [82]. Studies of digit duplication in chicken wings by *Shh* misexpression show that the most posterior/ulnar digits need higher Shh concentrations and longer exposure times than the more anterior digits [83].

Recent experiments in chicken show that Shh integrates both proliferation and specification of digit precursors and that Shh expression is controlled by cell proliferation [82, 84]. These data prompted two models to explain how digit morphology and number are achieved. The biphasic model suggests that an early phase specifies digit number and potential morphology and a second proliferative phase allows for digit growth and final morphologic determination [82]. The growth-morphogen model posits that both Shh concentration and exposure duration progressively expands the limb to specify digit number and morphology [84].

Although a Shh concentration gradient can account for some features of digit morphogenesis, it does not fully explain the repeating digit/interdigit pattern. Experiments out of Marian Ros' laboratory found that compound gene deletions of *Hoxa13* (the terminal *Hoxa* gene demarcating the handplate), *Hoxd11-13* (the Shh-dependent *Hox* genes of the A–P/R–U axis), and *Gli3* (the gene mediating Shh activity along the A–P/R–U axis) exposed an intrinsic self-organizing mechanism in mice involved in digit patterning

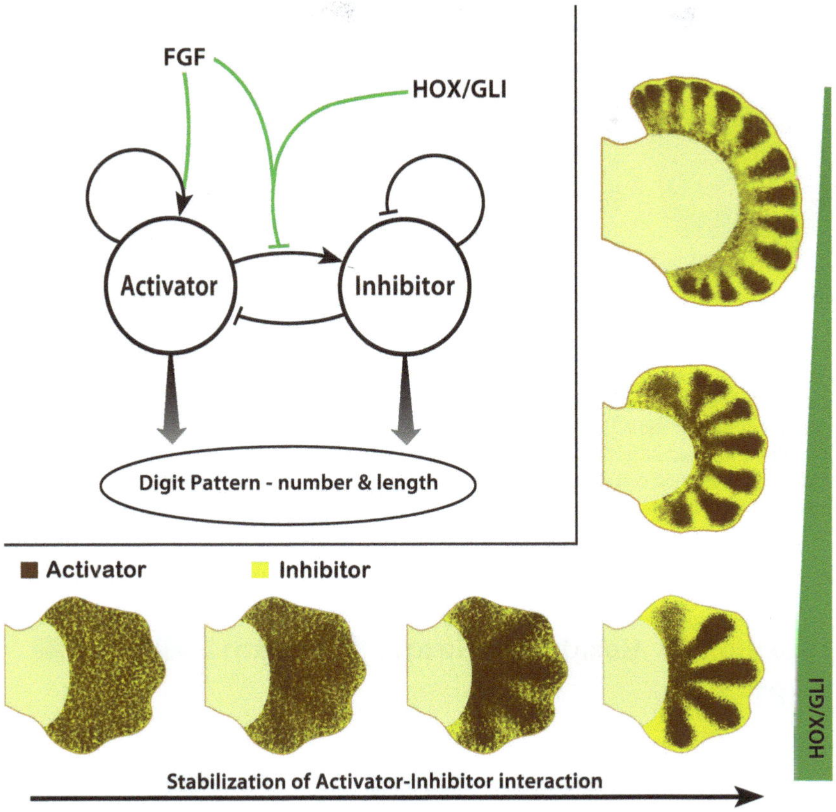

Fig. 1.7 Turing-like patterning in limbs. In the upper left-hand corner is a diagram of the diffusion-driven instability model with an activator and inhibitor modulated by FGF and HOX/GLI. In the model described by Sheth et al. (2012), FGF from the apical ectodermal ridge (AER) promotes a radial stripe pattern from this intrinsic self-organizing mechanism (ISOM) and ultimately regulates digit length, while FGF in concert with distal HOX and GLI transcription factors limit the number of digits. The bottom of the illustration has a series of handplates that show the rapid progression from fluctuating activator-inhibitor interaction (noise) to a stabilized 5-digit pattern. On the right, progressive loss of digit suppressing HOX/GLI transcription factors (green bar) causes an increase in the number of digits patterned by the ISOM. Courtesy of K.C. Oberg and Loma Linda University

[85]. Progressive reduction of the *Hox* gene dosage in the absence of Gli3 progressively increased digit numbers (up to 14 digits) that was not accompanied by a corresponding increase in handplate size; thus, the digits were increasingly thinner and shorter.

Alan Turing developed a mathematical diffusion-reaction model to account for repetitive self-organizing patterns, such as stripes or spots in animal skin and fur [86]. This model considers two molecules, an activator and inhibitor, which diffuse into a field of cells. The activator auto-up-regulates itself and up-regulates its own inhibitor. In contrast, the model's inhibitor suppresses the activator and auto-inhibits its own expression (Fig. 1.7).

Small random molecular variations of activator and inhibitor eventually lead to a stable pattern, typically spots or stripes. The pattern is dependent upon the level of activator and inhibitor as well as their diffusion rates. The evidence suggests that an intrinsic self-organizing or Turing mechanism establishes the initial alternating digit/non-digit pattern in the handplate. Although the identity of the activator and inhibitor are not yet known, the compound *Hox/Gli3* experiments indicate that the terminal Hoxa/d transcription factors involved in the P–D and A–P/R–U axes, in concert with Shh/Gli3 regulation, modulate the intrinsic self-organizing mechanism and are critical in establishing the common digit/interdigit pattern of pentadactyly.

Defining Digit-Specific Morphology

Once the number of digits has been established, each digit must then acquire its specific morphology, i.e., thumb and index finger. At the distal end of each digit is a cluster of cells called the phalanx forming region (PFR) or digital crescent that, with progressive digital outgrowth, regulates *Sox9* expression and chondrogenesis, thereby shaping phalangeal morphology (Fig. 1.8) [87–89]. The PFR also maintains digit-associated Fgf expression in the overlying AER during digit outgrowth [87].

Although the mechanisms are not fully characterized, evidence suggests that Shh plays a pivotal role in defining digit-specific morphology for digits 2–5 (the Shh-dependent digits). Three Shh-regulated gradients converge to define the appropriate size and number of phalanges. The Shh-dependent

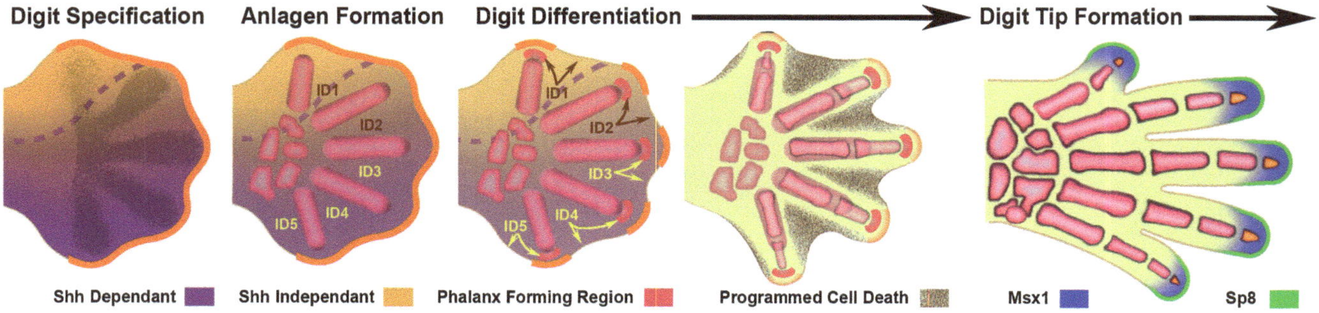

Fig. 1.8 Molecular pathways regulating digit development. After establishing digit number and the Shh dependant/independent domains (boundaries indicated by dashed line), digit morphologies are specified. Interdigital mesoderm as illustrated (ID1–ID5) regulates regression of the overlying AER (orange) and digit morphologies of the adjacent anterior condensing digit via the phalanx forming region (PFR—magenta) capping the distal tip of each anlagen. The PFR, in concert with the AER, determines phalanx size, length and joint position. The interdigital tissue subsequently undergoes Bmp mediated programmed cell death (speckled regions). As the AER overlying the digit regresses the distal or ungual phalanx begins to form and is demarcated by expression of mesodermal Msx1 (blue) and ectodermal Sp8 (green) (Image adapted from Oberg et al., 2010) [209]. Courtesy of K.C. Oberg and Loma Linda University

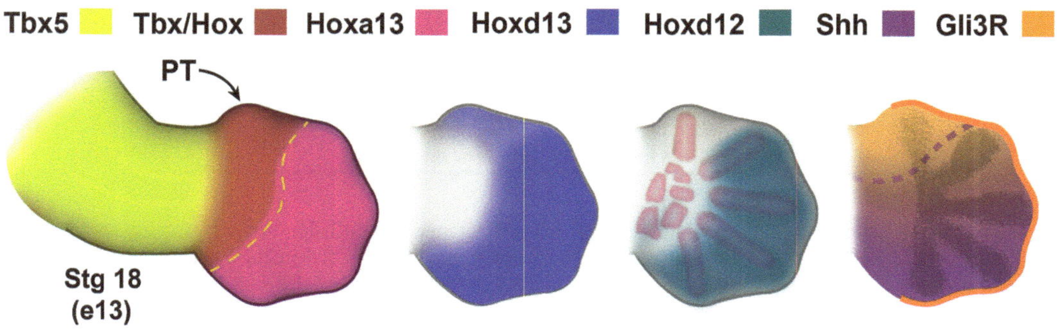

Fig. 1.9 Molecular regulation of thumb patterning. The presumptive thumb domain (PT) is defined by the overlapping expression of Tbx5, Gli3R, Hoxa13, and Hoxd13. The other Hoxd transcription factors (10-12) have overlapping expression domains in presumptive digits 2-5, but are restricted from the thumb domain. Note that the Hoxd genes are also restricted from the developing carpal region (Image modified from Oberg, 2014) [97]. Courtesy of K.C. Oberg and Loma Linda University

Hoxd10-13 transcription factors within the developing digits interact directly with Gli3 [90]. However, the form of Gli3 present at each digit varies based on the Shh-regulated Gli3R/Gli3 activator counter gradients [91]. In addition, Shh induces a Bmp gradient that is also known to regulate digit morphology [89, 92]. The signals that determine digit morphology are conveyed to the PFR through the adjacent posterior interdigital tissue [87, 89] and through Fgf and Wnt proteins secreted from the overlying AER [88, 93–96]. Changes in the interdigital BMP levels or swapping interdigital mesenchyme can transform digit morphology [87, 89].

The thumb is a distinctly different digit in its shape, position, and structure [97]. It is Shh-independent and has a compilation of genes expressed within its domain that is dissimilar from other digits (Fig. 1.9). *Hoxa13* is expressed within the entire handplate [75, 76] and overlaps the expression of *Tbx5*, which extends into the carpal and thumb domains but not into the domains of the ulnar digits (digits 2–5) [98]. Moreover, the thumb domain is accentuated by the lack of Shh-regulated *Hoxd10-12* expression [99]. The absence of distal *Hoxd* gene expression has been used as a marker of "thumbness" across species [100, 101]. Interestingly, the wrist is also a zone with limited Hox protein expression (see the illustration in Fig. 1.9 associated with Hoxd12 expression). Recent experiments with mouse mutants that express low levels of Hox proteins showed transformations of metacarpal bones to carpal-like elements [102]. Thus, Tbx5 and low levels of Hox transcription factors may limit the size of the thumb and carpal bones, while the distal Hoxd transcription factors are thought to elongate digits [75, 98, 103].

The terminal phalanges differ structurally from other phalanges: they are cone shaped and associated with a surface modification at the dorsal tip called the unguis or nail, which is dense keratinized epithelium that protects the tip of the digit. Terminal phalanges also differ in their development, with ossification beginning at the distal tapered tip of the cartilage model rather than forming a collar around the midshaft [104]. As the AER regresses, the terminal phalanges begin to form [94, 105]. Sp8, a specificity protein transcription factor that mediates Wnt signaling, is expressed in the distal tip ectoderm [104, 106] and appears to direct dorsal signals to form the nail. In mice with a reduction in Sp8 levels, dorsal dimelia forms (Haro et al., [107]). The distal tip mesoderm also expresses Bambi, a Bmp inhibitor, and Msx1, a transcription factor that is thought to provide regenerative competency to fingertips [104, 108, 109].

Interdigital Cell Death

In the interdigit mesenchyme, BMP signaling also induces cell apoptosis, in part, by repressing Fgf expression in the overlying ectoderm [110]. RA also appears to play a principal role in regulating interdigital cell death. *Rdh10* knockout mice, which fail to convert precursors to RA, show interdigital webbing and a reduction in the expression of *Bmp7* [111]. RA beads are capable of inducing *Bmp* expression and cell death when implanted in the interdigit regions [112]. Weatherbee and coworkers have also suggested that levels of Gremlin, an Shh-regulated factor that inhibits Bmps, correlates with the degree of webbing across species [113]. Thus, Shh and RA signals may work in concert in the interdigital regions to signal digit morphology and interdigital cell death.

Limb Differentiation

While the limb is growing and acquiring its overall shape, cells from both ectoderm and mesoderm begin to differentiate into the various tissues required for limb function. The differentiation process is tightly regulated by signaling molecules of the three axes. Although we will discuss the different tissues separately (vessels, muscle, bone, cartilage, and nervous tissue), these processes are occurring concurrently, with several signaling molecules shared across tissues.

Limb Vasculogenesis

Vascularization begins with the transformation of mesenchymal cells into hemangioblasts [114]. Bmp4 signaling induces the expression of *Flk1* (also known as Vegf-receptor 2) [115], the functional marker of hemangioblasts that confers the capacity to respond to vascular endothelial growth factor (Vegf) [116]. Embryos that lack *Flk1* die around day 9 without any vascular development [117, 118]. Hypoxia-inducible factor 1 (HIF1alpha), sensing the local demands for oxygen in the growing tissue, induces *Vegf* [119]. Bmp4 conjointly with Vegf differentiates hemangioblasts into angioblasts (CD31, CD34, Flk1-positive cells), the precursors of vascular tissue [120, 121].

Angioblasts within the developing limb bud are derived from limb mesenchyme and cells that migrate from adjacent somites [122]. In the emerging limb bud, angioblasts aggregate and differentiate into vascular channels to form the primitive capillary plexuses [121, 123, 124] This process, known as vasculogenesis, is under the control of Vegf [125]. New vessels will sprout from these rudimentary vessels in response to local environmental and chemotactic factors, in a process termed angiogenesis. During angiogenesis, Notch-Delta signaling limits the number of sprouting "tip" cells to support directional outgrowth and remodeling [126, 127]. Interestingly, many of the molecules directing angiogenesis are also involved in axonal guidance (Ephrins/Eph receptors, Slit/Robo signaling, Netrins, Semiphorins, etc.) [128]. This may, in part, explain the parallel pathways taken by these tissues to form neurovascular bundles.

Angiogenesis progressively remodels limb vessels from proximal to distal. In addition to Vegf and Notch signaling, Angiopoietin/Tie signaling is involved in this second stage of vessel formation/remodeling [129, 130]. Around Carnegie stage 13 (day 28 post fertilization), remodeling forms a central limb artery (the primitive subclavian artery) that connects with the dorsal aorta (Fig. 1.10a); concurrently, two peripheral veins form to drain into the posterior cardinal system [123, 131]. The endothelial cells from these remodeled vessels secrete platelet-derived growth factor (Pdgf), which recruits smooth muscle cells and pericytes to surround the growing vessels [132]. Arteries and veins differ in the thickness of surrounding smooth muscle and pericytes. In addition, arteries express Ephrin B2, while veins express Eph-B4 receptors [119].

RA plays an inhibitor role in the angiogenesis process [133, 134]. Experiments with mice lacking Cyp26, an RA degrading enzyme, showed an underdeveloped vasculature that did not progress beyond primitive plexuses [133, 134]. The data suggests that RA can have an inhibitory function on the expression of *Flk1* thus halting the development of vessels [133, 134]. Endothelium expresses Cyp26 and may function to limit the presence of RA [Unpublished data, 132] thereby promoting angiogenesis. Alternatively, these early vessels may limit the level of RA accessible to the developing tissues they supply.

Progressive proximal-to-distal remodeling of limb vessels continues as the limb develops with primitive capillary plexuses persisting in the distal limb until about Carnegie stage 19 (post fertilization day 48). By Carnegie stage 21 (post fertilization day 52), the major vessels and general architecture is completed [135, 136]. The vascular network develops arteries, capillaries, and veins. The low pressure venous sys-

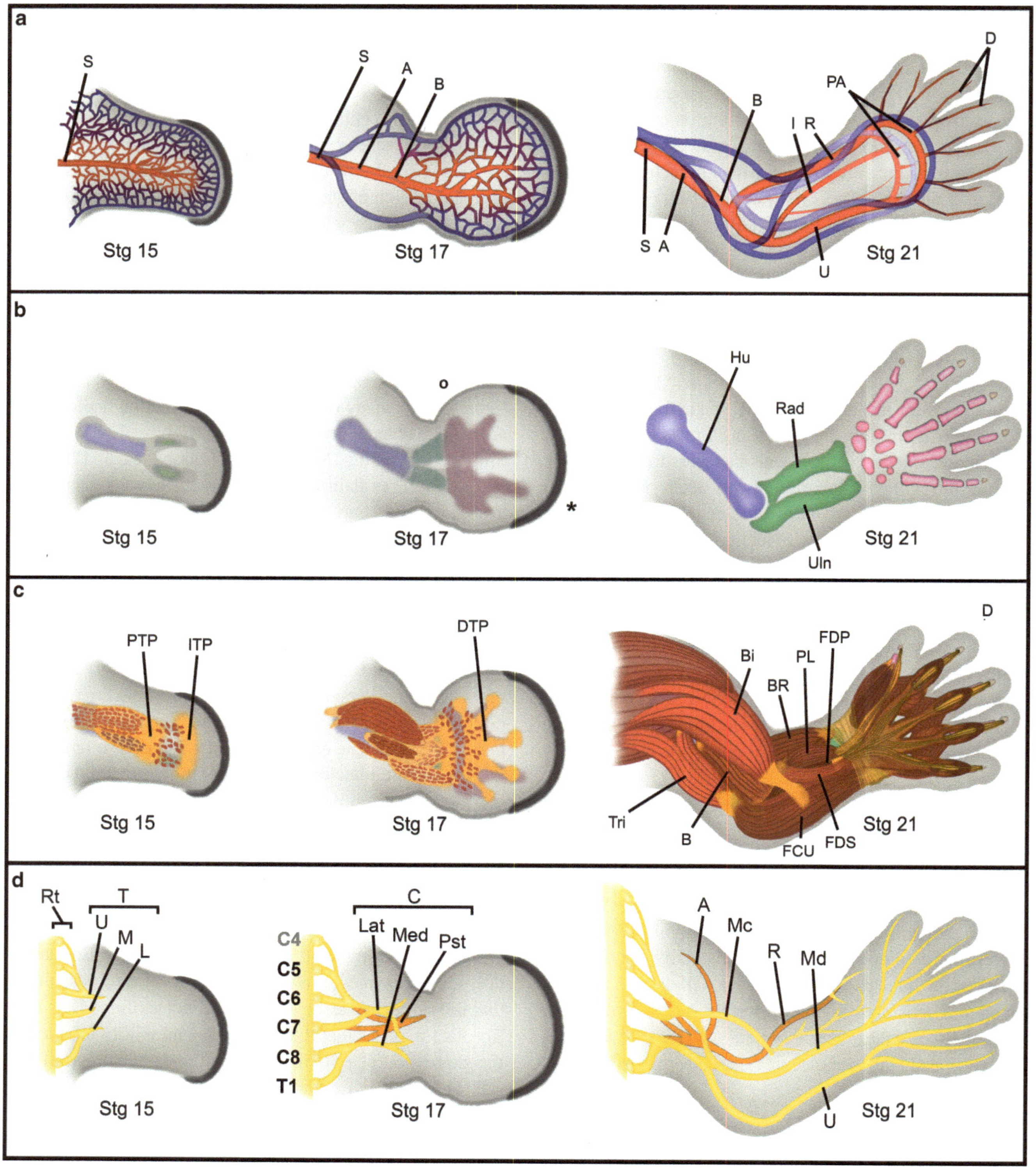

Fig. 1.10 Differentiation of limb tissues. Progressive differentiation of limb tissues from Stage 15 (post fertilization day 35) to stage 21 (day 52 near the end of the embryonic period). (**a**) Vascular differentiation showing the formation and remodeling of the subclavian (S), the axillary (A), the brachial (B), interosseous (I), radial (R), ulnar (U), palmar arch (PA) and digital (D) arteries. (**b**) Progressive skeletal differentiation showing anlagen condensation and definition for the humerus (Hu), radius (Rad), ulna (Uln), carpi and digits. (**c**) Progressive muscle differentiation. Myocyte migration is guided by tendon primoria: First the proximal tendon primordium (PTP) then the intermediate tendon primordium (IPT) and finally the distal tendon primordium (DTP). Secondary myocyte migration and subsequent proliferation within the fascicles defines muscle groups. Triceps (Tri), biceps (Bi), brachialis (B), brachioradialis (BR), flexor carpi ulnaris (FCU), palmaris longus (PL), flexor digitorum superficialis (FDS), and flexor digitorum profundus (FDP). d) Progressive differentiation of limb nerves. The nerve roots (Rt) from cranial 4 through thoracic nerve 1 coalesce to form the upper (U), the middle (M) and lower (L) nerve trunks (T) as they enter the limb bud. Further rearrangements define the lateral (Lat), median (Med), and posterior (Pst) cords (C). As the muscles differentiate and require innervation, major nerves are formed – axillary (A), musclulocutaneous (Mc), radial (R), median (Md) and ulnar (U). (Modified from Tonkin and Oberg, 2012) [198]. Courtesy of K.C. Oberg and Loma Linda University

tem is not able to collect all of the fluid distributed to the tissues by the higher pressured arterial system; therefore, a second low pressure vascular system, the lymphatics, forms. The lymphatic vessels also arise from angioblasts that are derived from LPM and somites [122]. Although a unique homeodomain transcription factor, Prox1, distinguishes lymphatics from arterial or venous vessels, the same signaling molecules that direct artery and vein formation likewise appear to control lymphatic vascular development [119].

Limb Skeletogenesis

The limb skeleton is derived from LPM and its development can be described in two steps: (1) chondrogenesis, the process of mesenchymal condensation and chondrocyte differentiation to form endochondral anlagen; and (2) endochondral ossification, the progressive transformation of the cartilage anlagen into the bones of the growing limb. The formation of joints is a related but separate process.

The first indication of chondrogenesis is the up-regulation of Sox9, a high-mobility group transcription factor, in chondrogenic precursors [137]. Sox9 is necessary for skeletogenesis; the lack of Sox9 in animal models results in the complete absence of cartilage and bone, culminating in limb regression [138]. However, Sox9 alone is not sufficient for chondrocyte differentiation. Additional Sox transcription factors (Sox5 and Sox6) are also needed for chondrocyte maturation, i.e., type II collagen production and chondrocyte hypertrophy [139, 140].

Bmp signaling also plays a role in the condensation of cartilaginous anlagen. Studies using constitutively activated and dominant-negative constructs in chicks show that signaling through Bmp receptor 1B (BMPR-1B) is necessary and sufficient to induce cartilage condensation [141]. The induction of Noggin, a potent inhibitor of BMPs, in the limb bud results in the complete absence of mesenchymal condensation [142]. Similarly in mice, knock-out of Bmp receptors 1a and 1b (*BmpR1a*, *BmpR1b*) impairs chondrocyte differentiation and Sox5/6/9 expression [143].

The ablation of individual Bmp proteins instead of their receptors does not prevent chondrogenesis in mice but rather delays the process [70]. This finding suggests that Bmps have a redundant function in chondrogenesis and that a threshold level of Bmp is needed to trigger the induction of Sox 5/6/9 and promote anlagen condensation. Despite the delay in cartilage condensation, individual Bmp knock-out mice exhibit normal endochondral ossification [70] (for a full review of the role of Bmp in skeletogenesis and embryonic development see [144]).

In contrast to Bmp, RA limits the expression and activity of *Sox9* [145, 146]. Experiments with *Cyp26b1* knock-out mice demonstrate impaired RA clearance. The elevated level of RA in the limb arrests or restricts cells to a pre-chondrocytic state and aborts cartilage formation and skeletal progression [147]. Interestingly, Bmp signaling counters this activity by inhibiting *Raldh2*, a gene that encodes for an RA synthesizing enzyme [148]. Thus, Bmps utilize direct and indirect pathways to promote chondrogenesis.

As with other aspects of limb development, chondrogenesis also progresses in a proximal-to-distal fashion. By Carnegie stage 15 (35 days post fertilization), the humerus, radius, and ulna anlagen are evident as a "Y"-shaped condensation (see Fig. 1.10b) [149]. During the next week of gestation (post fertilization days 36–42), condensations form within the handplate. A consistent order of digital condensations in vertebrates has been demonstrated with digit 4 forming first [150, 151] followed by digit 2, digit 5, digit 3, and finally the thumb or digit 1 [82]. Forming last appears to have put the thumb at increased risk, being the most common digit disrupted in malformation syndromes [97]. By Carnegie stage 21, the cartilaginous pattern is established.

Endochondral ossification is mediated in large part by the Runx2 transcription factor that differentiates precursors into osteoblasts and promotes chondrocyte hypertrophy [152]. In addition, Sp7 (also called Osterix), another specificity protein transcription factor, mediates osteocyte maturation, collagen I production and bone matrix deposition [153]. Sp7 works in concert with another transcription factor, ATF4, to maintain osteocyte function [154]. The ossification of long bones is also characterized by an epiphyseal plate that forms between the diaphysis (shaft) and epiphysis (ends). The epiphyseal plate is a growth center responsible for longitudinal growth. At the epiphyseal plate, cartilage proliferation forms regular columns of chondrocytes. These chondrocytes undergo hypertrophy, maturation, and apoptosis with subsequent ossification. These steps are tightly regulated by Runx2, Twist1, Ihh (and Gli3), Vegf, BMP, and FGF signaling [155].

Endochondral ossification transforms the cartilage models into bone. Primary ossification begins as a collar around the diaphyses of all limb long bones except the distal phalanges. Ossification in distal phalanges starts at the distal tip then progresses proximally over the cartilaginous model [104]. There is a consistent sequence to the formation of primary ossification centers in the upper limb. The first anlagen to begin ossification is the humerus (Carnegie stage 23, post fertilization day 56 or 8 weeks gestation), followed by the radius, ulna, distal phalanges, metacarpals, proximal phalanges, and finally middle phalanges by 10 weeks post fertilization [156]. Notably, George L. Steeter, the embryologist entrusted with characterizing the Carnegie collection of human gestations in the 1940s, regarded humeral ossification as the *sine qua non* of the beginning of the fetal period. Thus, the initiation of limb long bone ossification with the formation of primary ossification centers is a fetal endeavor.

Ossification of carpal bones does not start until around the time of birth [157]. The initiation of carpal ossification also follows a typical sequence beginning with the capitate and

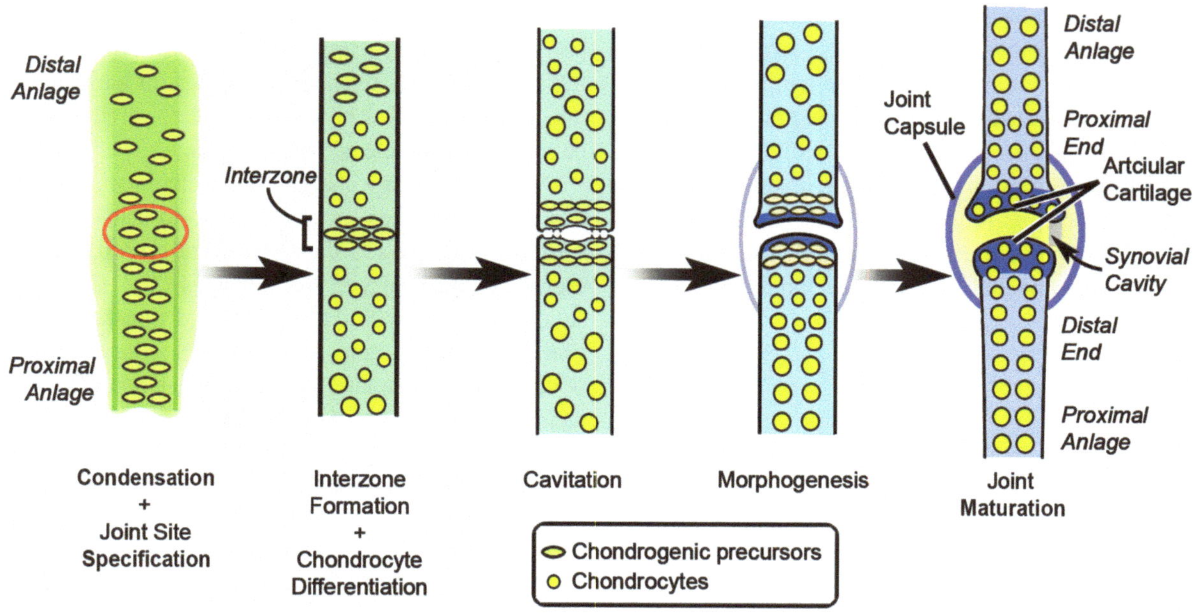

Fig. 1.11 Joint formation. Transformation of a presumptive joint in cartilage anlagen to a joint with synovial cavity and capsule (Image adapted from Pacifici et al., 2005) [164]. Courtesy of K.C. Oberg and Loma Linda University

hamate (the ulnar aspect of the distal row) and ending with the trapezium, trapezoid (the radial aspect of the distal row), and the scaphoid (the radial aspect of the proximal row) [157]. Formation of secondary ossification centers within the epiphyses of the long bones also occurs postnatally. The characteristic pattern of hand and wrist ossification is a useful tool in assessing skeletal maturity in children. Prior to puberty, a sex-related difference is evident in hand and wrist ossification; in girls, formation of primary ossification centers is completed at around 6 years of age, whereas in boys, it is completed around 8 years of age [157].

The expression of the distal Hoxa transcription factors, Hoxa10, Hoxa11, and Hoxa13, correlates with the stylopod (arm), the zeugopod (forearm), and autopod (hand), respectively [76]. Synovial joints form within the developing skeletal anlagen at the boundaries between these three skeletal segments. Morphologically, a joint passes through three stages (Fig. 1.11): (1) interzone formation, with condensation of a cell dense region of flattened cells called the interzone; (2) cavitation, the formation of a gap separating the two skeletal elements; and (3) morphogenesis, the process of forming complementary articular cartilage-lined surfaces to facilitate movement. Wnt14 is expressed in the presumptive joint and up-regulates Gdf5 prior to interzone formation [158]. Gdf5 becomes tightly restricted to the interzone as it forms and promotes subsequent joint formation [159]. Centrally the interzone begins to cavitate, becomes hypocellular, and accumulates hyaluronan [160, 161]. Although joint-related muscular contractions are not needed for interzone formation, they are essential for proper cavitation to occur [162]. Integrated axis-related patterning pathways and cell movement work together to form complementary cartilage-lined surfaces on the opposing skeletal ends for appropriate articulation [163, 164]. Concurrently, mesoderm surrounding the developing joint condenses, forming fortifying ligaments and the joint capsule [165, 166].

Limb Myogenesis

Formation of the upper limb musculature is an integrated process involving tendons, myocytes, and nerves. Disruption of any one of these structures results in muscle abnormalities [167]. The arrangement of tendons and their sites of bony attachment establish the framework within which muscles will develop (see Fig. 1.10c). The tendon primordia develop from limb mesenchyme. The first indication of tendon formation is the expression of Scleraxis (Scx), a tendon-specific transcription factor in precursor tenocytes [168]. Subsequently, the cells express the extracellular matrix protein tenascin [169].

Three dorsal–ventral pairs of tendon primordia progressively develop within each limb segment [170]. The tendon primordia, which includes connective tissue cells that will encase and direct the developing myocytes, forms under the influence of axis-related signals and initially is independent from the influence of migrating myocytes [171]. For example, Wnt7a from the dorsal ectoderm regulates dorsal tendon formation and mice that lack *En-1*, the transcription factor that limits Wnt7a expression to the dorsal ectoderm, develop a symmetrical bi-dorsal phenotype, i.e., dorsal or extensor tendons for both the dorsal and "ventral" aspects of the limb [62, 65]. However, muscle interaction is an absolute requirement for maintenance of the tendon primordia and the final muscle arrangement; in muscle deficient limbs, the tendons form but then degenerate [170].

Muscle undergoes progressive and somewhat overlapping phases of development [172]: (1) an embryonic phase with development of primary mononuclear fibers from migrating myoblasts; (2) a fetal/neonatal phase generating secondary multinucleate fibers from migrating myoblasts; and (3) an adult phase that contributes multinucleated fibers derived from satellite cells.

The first marker of limb-related myocyte differentiation during the embryonic phase of myogenesis is the expression of Pax3, a pair-ruled homeodomain transcription factor, in the dorsolateral cells of the dermomyotome in limb-associated somites [173–175]. Subsequently, the Pax3-positive cells will delaminate and migrate into the developing limb bud. *Pax3* knock-out mice show a loss of limb musculature and a loss of cell movements away from the somite [173, 176].

Delamination and migration are also dependent upon scatter factor/hepatocyte growth factor (Sf/Hgf) secreted from the developing limb bud mesenchyme and the corresponding expression of the Sf/Hgf receptor (c-met) in the myocyte precursors [177–180]. Pax3 regulates the expression of *c-met* in myocytes [181], while AER-associated Fgfs via Fgfr4 signaling control *Sf/Hgf* expression and thus the migratory routes of myocytes [180]. Mice deficient in *c-met* or *Hgf* expression lack migration and show a complete absence of limb musculature [178, 182].

As the myocyte precursors migrate into the limb bud, they split into dorsal and ventral precursors. Lbx1, a homeodomain transcription factor expressed in dorsal myocyte precursors, mediates this segregation. Disruption of *Lbx1* disrupts dorsal muscle migration without significantly affecting the migration of ventral myocytes [183].

AER-related Fgfs regulate the expression of SF/Hgf within the limb mesoderm thereby controlling the migration of myocytes as they infiltrate tendon primordia to arrive at their final destination [180]. Within the limb bud, myocyte precursors begin to express *MyoD* and *Myf5*, committing them to a myocyte fate [184]. Activation of these myocyte-specific genes is also thought to depend on axis-related signal molecules, such as Wnt7a and Shh [174, 180]. The myocytes elongate and form primary mononuclear muscle fibers.

Progressive proximal-to-distal differentiation also occurs during myogenesis (see Fig. 1.10c). As myocyte precursors extend into the distal primordial tendons, a second wave of myocyte precursors migrates into the proximal limb. These myocyte precursors express Pax7 in addition to Pax3. Some of these precursors will coalesce around primary myofibers and fuse to form secondary multinucleated myofibers [185]. In addition, a population will remain in a precursor state at the periphery as a satellite cell [186]. Adult multinucleated muscle fibers are derived from satellite cells. It is during secondary or fetal myogenesis that motor endplates form and neuromuscular communication begins.

Limb Innervation

Innervation of the limb follows myocyte migration (see Fig. 1.10d). The axons of both motor and sensory neurons from the limb-associated spinal cord aggregate at the proximal limb boundary, forming several thick fascicles. These fascicles differentiate into the upper, middle, and lower trunks of the brachial plexus [187]. The nerve fascicles enter the limb then subdivide into dorsal and ventral branches. The dorsal branches coalesce to form the posterior cord. The upper and middle regions of the ventral branches join to form the lateral cord and the lower branch continues as medial cord. The cords then divide into the terminal branches of mixed motor and sensory axons. These branches follow a predictable pattern within the limb bud that appear to be controlled by variations in the extracellular matrix [188–190]. The initial entrance and distribution of the terminal branches within the limb do not appear to require signals from the final target tissue. However, for terminal sensory branching, the presence of skin is required [191]. Similarly, for fine targeted branching of motor nerves, differentiating muscle bundles are required [192].

The molecular control of axonal guidance and tissue targeting begins prior to axonal outgrowth during motor neuron differentiation. Shh secreted from the notochord and the floor plate of the spinal cord induces motor neuron and pancreas *homeobox1* (*Mnx1*, previously called *Hb9*), which encodes a transcription factor that transforms the neuroepithelium into motor neurons [193]. Hox transcription factors expressed within the spinal cord organize motor neurons destined for the upper limb into the lateral motor column (LMC), which is also demarcated by the expression of Islet1 and Islet2 (Isl1/Isl2) lim homeodomain transcription factors. The expression of *Raldh2*, and thus the production of RA, within the lateral LMC induces the expression of lim homeodomain 1 (Lhx1) transcription factor and inhibits the expression of Isl1, further subdividing the LMC into medial Isl1/Isl2-positive neurons that will project into the ventral limb and lateral Lhx1/Isl2-positive neurons that extend into the dorsal limb [194].

A second phase of complex Hox transcription factor expression coupled with the expression of forkhead box P1 (FoxP1) transcription factor is thought to convey axon targeting information to specific partner muscles within the limb defined by axis-related cues [195]. A complex interplay of Ephrins and Eph receptors is involved in the regulation of branching and axonal guidance (see Kao et al. [195] for a comprehensive review). Finally, at the target site, Etv4

Table 1.1 Comparison of the Swanson's and OMT classification schemes

I. Failure of formation of parts/arrest of development	I. Malformations
– Transverse deficiencies	A. Abnormal axis formation/differentiation—entire upper limb
– Longitudinal deficiencies	1. Proximal–distal axis
II. Failure of separation or differentiation of parts	2. Radial–ulnar (anterior-posterior) axis
– Soft tissue deficiency	3. Dorsal–ventral axis
– Skeletal deficiency	4. Unspecified axis
III. Duplication	B. Abnormal axis formation/differentiation—hand plate
– Radial polydactyly	1. Proximal–distal axis
– Central polydactyly	2. Radial–ulnar (anterior-posterior) axis
– Ulnar polydactyly	3. Dorsal–ventral axis
– Mirror hand/Ulnar dimelia	4. Unspecified axis
IV. Overgrowth	II. Deformations
– Hemihypertrophy	A. Constriction ring sequence
– Macrodactyly	B. Trigger digits
V. Undergrowth	C. Not otherwise specified
– Hypoplastic hand	III. Dysplasias
– Brachymetacarpia	A. Hypertrophy
– Brachydactyly	1. Whole limb
VI. Constriction band syndrome	2. Partial limb
VII. Generalized skeletal disorder	B. Tumorous conditions
	1. Vascular
	2. Neurological
	3. Connective tissue
	4. Skeletal
	IV. Syndromes

transcription factors are required to promote the axonal arborization needed for terminal neuromuscular innervation [196].

Dysmorphogenesis and Classification

Congenital upper limb anomaly designations are typically based on appearance. We readily understand the terms such as polydactyly, syndactyly, or radial club hand. However, these terms often fail to inform us of the prognosis, approach to treatment, or the etiology. Many equate congenital upper limb malformations with abnormalities of the skeleton, but disruption of any aspect of limb development can lead to dysmorphology including vascular and neuromuscular differentiation. Classification provides a mechanism to organize dysmorphologies into categories that describe one or more aspects of these anomalies. Ideally, a classification for upper limb anomalies would incorporate the etiologic basis, provide insight into prognosis, and guide treatment [197]. Furthermore, it should provide a universal language for discussion across disciplines regarding epidemiology, treatment, and research [198].

A number of classification schemes have been proposed to organize the known spectrum of upper limb anomalies. Probably the earliest recorded classification system was in 1829 by Isidore Saint-Hilaire who initially described anomalies simply as mild or severe [199]. He subsequently focused on what was missing, coining the terms ectromelia (limb absence), phocomelia (missing limb segments), and hemimelia (missing limb parts) [200]. In 1895, Kümmel described upper limb anomalies in terms of defects (deficiencies), adhesions (fusions), or superior numbers (duplications).

Swanson proposed a new classification scheme in 1964 [201]. Swanson's scheme was geared to hand surgeons and was considered to be an anatomic and clinical classification that indicated the type of primary embryonic damage [202]. While in the emerging field of clinical genetics, Temtamy had proposed a classification that focused on the genetic basis of malformation [202–204]. A modified version of Swanson's classification, subsequently adopted by the International Federation of Societies for Surgery of the Hand (IFSSH) in 1974, categorized limb anomalies based on failed formation, failed differentiation, duplication, overgrowth, undergrowth, constriction bands, and generalized skeletal anomalies (Table 1.1) [205]. This same year, Kelikian reviewed a number of the classifications schemes that had been proposed and insightfully concluded that our knowledge was still insufficient to formulate a "comprehensive classification" [206].

Nevertheless, the modified Swanson's classification served as the primary basis for scientific communication and discussion for upper limb anomalies among hand surgeons for more than 40 years [197]. With time it was recognized that complex disorders were difficult or impossible to classify within this scheme, prompting a number of authors to suggest modifications [207, 208].

Increased knowledge of the molecular basis of limb development from clinical genetics and developmental biology has also challenged the utility of many of the categories in indicating the underlying etiology. For example, altered Shh expression along the radial–ulnar axis can cause ulnar deficiency, triphalangeal thumb, and ulnar dimelia, but these three conditions are listed separately in different categories with no mechanism to demonstrate that all three conditions are part of the same molecular pathway [197, 208, 209]. Mounting evidence regarding the etiology of cleft hand prompted the Japanese Society for Surgery of the Hand to add two additional groups: Group IV, abnormal induction of digital rays (thereby shifting the subsequent groups to V through VIII) and Group IX, unclassifiable cases [210]. However, this modification does not address the need to incorporate genetic etiologic information into other conditions. Our increased knowledge requires a more comprehensive classification system.

In 2010, a new classification scheme was proposed that combined anatomic and genetic information [209] (see Table 1.1). To facilitate communication, the authors, Drs Oberg, Manske, and Tonkin, used the general headings "Malformation, Deformation and Dysplasia," terms well established and used by dysmorphologists, clinical geneticists, and developmental biologists. The headings and sub-

Table 1.2 The new IFSSH (OMT) extended classification of congenital hand and upper limb anomalies

I. Malformations
A. Abnormal axis formation/differentiation—entire upper limb
1. Proximal–distal axis
(i) Brachymelia with brachydactyly
(ii) Symbrachydactyly
(a) Poland syndrome
(b) Whole limb excluding Poland syndrome
(iii) Transverse deficiency
(a) Amelia
(b) Clavicular/scapular
(c) Humeral (above elbow)
(d) Forearm (below elbow)
(e) Wrist (carpals absent/at level of proximal carpals/at level of distal carpals) (with forearm/arm involvement)
(f) Metacarpal (with forearm/arm involvement)
(g) Phalangeal (proximal/middle/distal) (with forearm/arm involvement)
(iv) Intersegmental deficiency
(a) Proximal (humeral—rhizomelic)
(b) Distal (forearm—mesomelic)
(c) Total (Phocomelia)
(v) Whole limb duplication/triplication
2. Radial–ulnar (anterior-posterior) axis
(i) Radial longitudinal deficiency—Thumb hypoplasia (with proximal limb involvement)
(ii) Ulnar longitudinal deficiency
(iii) Ulnar dimelia
(iv) Radioulnar synostosis
(v) Congenital dislocation of the radial head
(vi) Humeroradial synostosis—Elbow ankyloses
3. Dorsal–ventral axis
(i) Ventral dimelia
(a) Fuhrmann/Al-Awadi/Raas-Rothschild syndromes
(b) Nail–Patella syndrome
(ii) Absent/hypoplastic extensor/flexor muscles
4. Unspecified axis
(i) Shoulder
(a) Undescended (Sprengel)
(b) Abnormal shoulder muscles
(c) Not otherwise specified
(ii) Arthrogryposis

(continued)

Table 1.2 (continued)

B. Abnormal axis formation/differentiation—hand plate
1. Proximal–distal axis
(i) Brachydactyly (no forearm/arm involvement)
(ii) Symbrachydactyly (no forearm/arm involvement)
(iii) Transverse deficiency (no forearm/arm involvement)
(a) Wrist (carpals absent/at level of proximal carpals/at level of distal carpals)
(b) Metacarpal
(c) Phalangeal (proximal/middle/distal)
2. Radial–ulnar (anterior-posterior) axis
(i) Radial deficiency (thumb—no forearm/arm involvement)
(ii) Ulnar deficiency (no forearm/arm involvement)
(iii) Radial polydactyly
(iv) Triphalangeal thumb
(v) Ulnar dimelia (mirror hand—no forearm/arm involvement)
(vi) Ulnar polydactyly
3. Dorsal–ventral axis
(i) Dorsal dimelia (palmar nail)
(ii) Ventral (palmar) dimelia (including hypoplastic/aplastic nail)
4. Unspecified axis
(i) Soft tissue
(a) Syndactyly
(b) Camptodactyly
(c) Thumb in palm deformity
(d) Distal arthrogryposis
(ii) Skeletal deficiency
(a) Clinodactyly
(b) Kirner's deformity
(c) Synostosis/symphalangism (carpal/metacarpal/phalangeal)
(iii) Complex
(a) Complex syndactyly
(b) Synpolydactyly—central
(c) Cleft hand
(d) Apert hand
(e) Not otherwise specified
II. Deformations
A. Constriction ring sequence
B. Trigger digits
C. Not otherwise specified
III. Dysplasias
A. Hypertrophy
1. Whole limb
(i) Hemihypertrophy
(ii) Aberrant flexor/extensor/intrinsic muscle
2. Partial limb
(i) Macrodactyly
(ii) Aberrant intrinsic muscles of hand
B. Tumorous conditions
1. Vascular
(i) Hemangioma
(ii) Malformation
(iii) Others
2. Neurological
(i) Neurofibromatosis
(ii) Others

(continued)

Table 1.2 (continued)

3. Connective tissue
(i) Juvenile aponeurotic fibroma
(ii) Infantile digital fibroma
(iii) Others
4. Skeletal
(i) Osteochondromatosis
(ii) Enchondromatosis
(iii) Fibrous dysplasia
(iv) Epiphyseal abnormalities
(v) Others
IV. Syndromes[a]
A. Specified
1. Acrofacial Dysostosis 1 (Nager type)
2. Apert
3. Al-Awadi/Raas-Rothschild/Schinzel phocomelia
4. Baller-Gerold
5. Bardet-Biedl Carpenter
6. Catel-Manzke
7. Constriction band (Amniotic Band Sequence)
8. Cornelia de Lange (types 1-5)
9. Crouzon
10. Down
11. Ectrodactyly-Ectodermal Dysplasia-Clefting
12. Fanconi Pancytopenia
13. Fuhrmann
14. Goltz
15. Gorlin
16. Greig Cephalopolysyndactyly
17. Hajdu-Cheney
18. Hemifacial Microsomia (Goldenhar syndrome)
19. Holt-Oram
20. Lacrimoauriculodentodigital (Levy-Hollister)
21. Larsen
22. Leri-Weill Dyschondrosteosis
23. Moebius sequence
24. Multiple Synostoses
25. Nail-Patella
26. Noonan
27. Oculodentodigital dysplasia
28. Orofacialdigital
29. Otopalataldigital
30. Pallister-Hall
31. Pfeiffer
32. Poland
33. Proteus
34. Roberts-SC Phocomelia
35. Rothmund-Thomson
36. Rubinstein-Taybi
37. Saethre-Chotzen
38. Thrombocytopenia Absent Radius
39. Townes-Brock
40. Trichorhinophalangeal (types 1-3)
41. Ulnar-Mammary
42. VACTERLS association
B. Others

[a]The specified list of syndromes are those considered most relevant; however, many other syndromes have a limb component and are "B. Others"

headings indicate not only the altered morphology but also the disrupted molecular pathways identified by clinical genetics. The "OMT" classification scheme has undergone critical evaluation by a group of international hand surgeons (the Congenital Hand Anomalies Study Group, or CHASG) and its capacity/utility to classify upper limb malformations demonstrated [211]. In February of 2014, the OMT classification was adopted by the IFSSH as the recommended classification scheme [212].

Malformations

Malformations are failures of normal development and/or differentiation and are, by far, the most common form of upper limb anomaly [213]. Malformations are subdivided into "Entire upper limb" and "Handplate" based on basic limb development and evolutionary patterning. Although the three basic axes of development are in play for the handplate as well as the entire limb, the handplate recruits a number of additional molecules/molecular cascades to pattern the increased complexity of the hand. Correspondingly, the handplate has more evolutionary variation and more targets for dysmorphogenesis [97]. This has been corroborated by a recent epidemiological study of congenital hand anomalies in Stockholm, Sweden, using this new classification scheme, with 356 of the 429 malformations being classified as handplate anomalies (and only 73 as entire upper limb) [213].

Malformations are further subdivided by the primary axis disrupted (Table 1.2). Using the example above, ulnar longitudinal deficiency (ULD), ulnar dimelia, and triphalangeal thumb are all subclassified as disorders of the radial–ulnar axis. ULD and ulnar dimelia are both disorders of the entire upper limb, while triphalangeal thumb is a disorder limited to the handplate. A category entitled "Unspecified axis" is included for entities that do not have a known axis-related nature (e.g., syndactyly) or the suspected axis-related nature is not yet characterized (e.g., clinodactyly).

Deformations

Deformations occur after normal development and differentiation; from an intervention standpoint, there is a better chance that normal structures will still be present. Dysmorphologists also speak of disruption, which is a breakdown of normal tissues, often vascular. For the purposes of congenital upper limb anomalies, both disruption and deformation are changes that occur after development so are collectively included under the heading "Deformation." The classic example is constriction ring sequence (also called amniotic band sequence), which can result in deformed or disrupted tissues. No axis-related subclassification is used because deformations occur after and exogenous to patterned development.

Dysplasias

Dysplasias are abnormalities of development and/or differentiation of isolated tissues common to the limb such as vascular, neural, or skeletal. Dysplasias can disrupt normal development (malformation) and/or cause progressive deformation.

Syndromes

It is not possible to list all of the syndromes that have a limb anomaly as a component. For example, there are over 110 syndromes with thumb hypoplasia or aplasia as a feature [97]. In the following chapter (Chap. 2), Drs. Laub and Burke will review syndromes that have an upper limb anomaly as a primary feature.

In summary, this new classification scheme combining anatomic and genetic information about congenital anomalies has been introduced to the IFSSH member societies by the IFSSH Congenital Committee [214]. Although our knowledge is still insufficient, hopefully we are a step closer to a comprehensive classification system.

Acknowledgements The authors would like to thank Charmaine Pira for suggestions, insight, and careful review of this manuscript.

References

1. O'Rahilly R, Muller F. Developmental stages in human embryos. Washington, DC: Carnegie Institution of Washington; 1987.
2. Tickle C. Embryology. In: AKS Gupta (Ed.), *The growing hand: diagnosis and management of the upper extremity in children*. Sheker LR. London: CV Mosby; 2000;25–32.
3. Cohn MJ, Tickle C. Developmental basis of limblessness and axial patterning in snakes. Nature. 1999;399(6735):474–9.
4. Burke AC, Nelson CE, Morgan BA, Tabin C. Hox genes and the evolution of vertebrate axial morphology. Development. 1995;121(2):333–46.
5. Searls RL, Janners MY. The initiation of limb bud outgrowth in the embryonic chick. Dev Biol. 1971;24(2):198–213.
6. Kawakami Y, Capdevila J, Buscher D, Itoh T, Rodriguez Esteban C, Izpisua Belmonte JC. WNT signals control FGF-dependent limb initiation and AER induction in the chick embryo. Cell. 2001;104(6):891–900.
7. Ohuchi H, Nakagawa T, Yamamoto A, Araga A, Ohata T, Ishimaru Y, Yoshioka H, Kuwana T, Nohno T, Yamasaki M, et al. The mesenchymal factor, FGF10, initiates and maintains the outgrowth of the chick limb bud through interaction with FGF8, an apical ectodermal factor. Development. 1997;124(11):2235–44.
8. Minguillon C, Del Buono J, Logan MP. Tbx5 and Tbx4 are not sufficient to determine limb-specific morphologies but have com-

mon roles in initiating limb outgrowth. Dev Cell. 2005;8(1):75–84.
9. Minguillon C, Nishimoto S, Wood S, Vendrell E, Gibson-Brown JJ, Logan MP. Hox genes regulate the onset of Tbx5 expression in the forelimb. Development. 2012;139(17):3180–8.
10. Pizette S, Abate-Shen C, Niswander L. BMP controls proximodistal outgrowth, via induction of the apical ectodermal ridge, and dorsoventral patterning in the vertebrate limb. Development. 2001;128(22):4463–74.
11. Soshnikova N, Zechner D, Huelsken J, Mishina Y, Behringer RR, Taketo MM, Crenshaw III EB, Birchmeier W. Genetic interaction between Wnt/beta-catenin and BMP receptor signaling during formation of the AER and the dorsal-ventral axis in the limb. Genes Dev. 2003;17(16):1963–8.
12. Barrow JR, Thomas KR, Boussadia-Zahui O, Moore R, Kemler R, Capecchi MR, McMahon AP. Ectodermal Wnt3/beta-catenin signaling is required for the establishment and maintenance of the apical ectodermal ridge. Genes Dev. 2003;17(3):394–409.
13. Abu-Abed S, Dolle P, Metzger D, Beckett B, Chambon P, Petkovich M. The retinoic acid-metabolizing enzyme, CYP26A1, is essential for normal hindbrain patterning, vertebral identity, and development of posterior structures. Genes Dev. 2001;15(2):226–40.
14. Hogan BL, Thaller C, Eichele G. Evidence that Hensen's node is a site of retinoic acid synthesis. Nature. 1992;359(6392):237–41.
15. Niederreither K, McCaffery P, Drager UC, Chambon P, Dolle P. Restricted expression and retinoic acid-induced downregulation of the retinaldehyde dehydrogenase type 2 (RALDH-2) gene during mouse development. Mech Dev. 1997;62(1):67–78.
16. Cunningham TJ, Zhao X, Sandell LL, Evans SM, Trainor PA, Duester G. Antagonism between retinoic acid and fibroblast growth factor signaling during limb development. Cell Rep. 2013;3(5):1503–11.
17. Zhao X, Sirbu IO, Mic FA, Molotkova N, Molotkov A, Kumar S, Duester G. Retinoic acid promotes limb induction through effects on body axis extension but is unnecessary for limb patterning. Curr Biol. 2009;19(12):1050–7.
18. Kessel M, Gruss P. Homeotic transformations of murine vertebrae and concomitant alteration of Hox codes induced by retinoic acid. Cell. 1991;67(1):89–104.
19. Deschamps J. Ancestral and recently recruited global control of the Hox genes in development. Curr Opin Genet Dev. 2007;17(5):422–7.
20. Wolpert L. Positional information and the spatial pattern of cellular differentiation. J Theor Biol. 1969;25(1):1–47.
21. Fallon JF, Kelley RO. Ultrastruct analysis of the apical ectodermal ridge during vertebrate limb morphogenesis. II. Gap junctions as distinctive ridge structures common to birds and mammals. J Embryol Exp Morphol. 1977;41:223–32.
22. Summerbell D, Lewis JH. Time, place and positional value in the chick limb-bud. J Embryol Exp Morphol. 1975;33(3):621–43.
23. Chiang C, Litingtung Y, Harris MP, Simandl BK, Li Y, Beachy PA, Fallon JF. Manifestation of the limb prepattern: limb development in the absence of sonic hedgehog function. Dev Biol. 2001;236(2):421–35.
24. Ros MA, Dahn RD, Fernandez-Teran M, Rashka K, Caruccio NC, Hasso SM, Bitgood JJ, Lancman JJ, Fallon JF. The chick oligozeugodactyly (ozd) mutant lacks sonic hedgehog function in the limb. Development. 2003;130(3):527–37.
25. MacCabe JA, Errick J, Saunders Jr JW. Ectodermal control of the dorsoventral axis in the leg bud of the chick embryo. Dev Biol. 1974;39(1):69–82.
26. Lewandoski M, Sun X, Martin GR. Fgf8 signalling from the AER is essential for normal limb development. Nat Genet. 2000;26(4):460–3.
27. Fernandez-Teran M, Ros MA. The Apical Ectodermal Ridge: morphological aspects and signaling pathways. Int J Dev Biol. 2008;52(7):857–71.
28. Niswander L, Tickle C, Vogel A, Booth I, Martin GR. FGF-4 replaces the apical ectodermal ridge and directs outgrowth and patterning of the limb. Cell. 1993;75(3):579–87.
29. Fallon JF, Lopez A, Ros MA, Savage MP, Olwin BB, Simandl BK. FGF-2: apical ectodermal ridge growth signal for chick limb development. Science. 1994;264(5155):104–7.
30. Mariani FV, Ahn CP, Martin GR. Genetic evidence that FGFs have an instructive role in limb proximal-distal patterning. Nature. 2008;453(7193):401–5.
31. Sun X, Lewandoski M, Meyers EN, Liu YH, Maxson Jr RE, Martin GR. Conditional inactivation of Fgf4 reveals complexity of signalling during limb bud development. Nat Genet. 2000;25(1):83–6.
32. Sun X, Mariani FV, Martin GR. Functions of FGF signalling from the apical ectodermal ridge in limb development. Nature. 2002;418(6897):501–8.
33. Boulet AM, Moon AM, Arenkiel BR, Capecchi MR. The roles of Fgf4 and Fgf8 in limb bud initiation and outgrowth. Dev Biol. 2004;273(2):361–72.
34. Summerbell D, Lewis JH, Wolpert L. Positional information in chick limb morphogenesis. Nature. 1973;244(5417):492–6.
35. Summerbell D, Wolpert L. Precision of development in chick limb morphogenesis. Nature. 1973;244(5413):228–30.
36. Dudley AT, Ros MA, Tabin CJ. A re-examination of proximodistal patterning during vertebrate limb development. Nature. 2002;418(6897):539–44.
37. Tabin C, Wolpert L. Rethinking the proximodistal axis of the vertebrate limb in the molecular era. Genes Dev. 2007;21(12):1433–42.
38. Rosello-Diez A, Ros MA, Torres M. Diffusible signals, not autonomous mechanisms, determine the main proximodistal limb subdivision. Science. 2011;332(6033):1086–8.
39. Rosello-Diez A, Torres M. Regulative patterning in limb bud transplants is induced by distalizing activity of apical ectodermal ridge signals on host limb cells. Dev Dyn. 2011;240(5):1203–11.
40. Yashiro K, Zhao X, Uehara M, Yamashita K, Nishijima M, Nishino J, Saijoh Y, Sakai Y, Hamada H. Regulation of retinoic acid distribution is required for proximodistal patterning and outgrowth of the developing mouse limb. Dev Cell. 2004;6(3):411–22.
41. Knezevic V, De Santo R, Schughart K, Huffstadt U, Chiang C, Mahon KA, Mackem S. Hoxd-12 differentially affects preaxial and postaxial chondrogenic branches in the limb and regulates Sonic hedgehog in a positive feedback loop. Development. 1997;124(22):4523–36.
42. Saunders JW, Gasseling MT. Ectodermal-mesenchymal interactions in the origin of limb symmetry. In: Fleischmajer R, Billingham RE, editors. Epithelial-mesenchymal interactions. Baltimore: William and Wilkins; 1968. p. 78–97.
43. Tickle C, Summerbell D, Wolpert L. Positional signalling and specification of digits in chick limb morphogenesis. Nature. 1975;254(5497):199–202.
44. Tickle C. Limb regeneration. Am Sci. 1981;69(6):639–46.
45. Tickle C, Lee J, Eichele G. A quantitative analysis of the effect of all-trans-retinoic acid on the pattern of chick wing development. Dev Biol. 1985;109(1):82–95.
46. Tickle C, Crawley A, Farrar J. Retinoic acid application to chick wing buds leads to a dose-dependent reorganization of the apical ectodermal ridge that is mediated by the mesenchyme. Development. 1989;106(4):691–705.
47. Tickle C. Retinoic acid and chick limb bud development. Dev Suppl. 1991;1:113–21.
48. Wanek N, Gardiner DM, Muneoka K, Bryant SV. Conversion by retinoic acid of anterior cells into ZPA cells in the chick wing bud. Nature. 1991;350(6313):81–3.

49. Riddle RD, Johnson RL, Laufer E, Tabin C. Sonic hedgehog mediates the polarizing activity of the ZPA. Cell. 1993;75(7): 1401–16.
50. Kraus P, Fraidenraich D, Loomis CA. Some distal limb structures develop in mice lacking Sonic hedgehog signaling. Mech Dev. 2001;100(1):45–58.
51. Xu B, Wellik DM. Axial Hox9 activity establishes the posterior field in the developing forelimb. Proc Natl Acad Sci U S A. 2011;108(12):4888–91.
52. Zeller R, Lopez-Rios J, Zuniga A. Vertebrate limb bud development: moving towards integrative analysis of organogenesis. Nat Rev Genet. 2009;10(12):845–58.
53. Charitè J, McFadden DG, Olson EN. The bHLH transcription factor dHAND controls Sonic hedgehog expression and establishment of the zone of polarizing activity during limb development. Development. 2000;127(11):2461–70.
54. Capellini TD, Di GG, Salsi V, Brendolan A, Ferretti E, Srivastava D, Zappavigna V, Selleri L. Pbx1/Pbx2 requirement for distal limb patterning is mediated by the hierarchical control of Hox gene spatial distribution and Shh expression. Development. 2006;133(11):2263–73.
55. Zakany J, Kmita M, Duboule D. A dual role for Hox genes in limb anterior-posterior asymmetry. Science. 2004;304(5677):1669–72.
56. Schimmang T, Lemaistre M, Vortkamp A, Ruther U. Expression of the zinc finger gene Gli3 is affected in the morphogenetic mouse mutant extra-toes (Xt). Development. 1992;116(3): 799–804.
57. Hui CC, Joyner AL. A mouse model of greig cephalopolysyndactyly syndrome: the extra-toesJ mutation contains an intragenic deletion of the Gli3 gene. Nat Genet. 1993;3(3):241–6.
58. Litingtung Y, Dahn RD, Li Y, Fallon JF, Chiang C. Shh and Gli3 are dispensable for limb skeleton formation but regulate digit number and identity. Nature. 2002;418(6901):979–83.
59. te Welscher P, Zuniga A, Kuijper S, Drenth T, Goedemans HJ, Meijlink F, Zeller R. Progression of vertebrate limb development through SHH-mediated counteraction of GLI3. Science. 2002;298(5594):827–30.
60. McGlinn E, van Bueren KL, Fiorenza S, Mo R, Poh AM, Forrest A, Soares MB, Bonaldo Mde F, Grimmond S, Hui CC, et al. Pax9 and Jagged1 act downstream of Gli3 in vertebrate limb development. Mech Dev. 2005;122(11):1218–33.
61. Parr BA, McMahon AP. Dorsalizing signal Wnt-7a required for normal polarity of D-V and A-P axes of mouse limb. Nature. 1995;374(6520):350–3.
62. Loomis CA, Harris E, Michaud J, Wurst W, Hanks M, Joyner AL. The mouse Engrailed-1 gene and ventral limb patterning. Nature. 1996;382(6589):360–3.
63. Logan C, Hornbruch A, Campbell I, Lumsden A. The role of Engrailed in establishing the dorsoventral axis of the chick limb. Development. 1997;124(12):2317–24.
64. Cygan JA, Johnson RL, McMahon AP. Novel regulatory interactions revealed by studies of murine limb pattern in Wnt-7a and En-1 mutants. Development. 1997;124(24):5021–32.
65. Loomis CA, Kimmel RA, Tong CX, Michaud J, Joyner AL. Analysis of the genetic pathway leading to formation of ectopic apical ectodermal ridges in mouse Engrailed-1 mutant limbs. Development. 1998;125(6):1137–48.
66. Riddle RD, Ensini M, Nelson C, Tsuchida T, Jessell TM, Tabin C. Induction of the LIM homeobox gene Lmx1 by WNT7a establishes dorsoventral pattern in the vertebrate limb. Cell. 1995;83(4): 631–40.
67. Vogel A, Rodriguez C, Warnken W, Izpisua Belmonte JC. Dorsal cell fate specified by chick Lmx1 during vertebrate limb development. Nature. 1995;378(6558):716–20.
68. Zuniga A, Haramis AP, McMahon AP, Zeller R. Signal relay by BMP antagonism controls the SHH/FGF4 feedback loop in vertebrate limb buds. Nature. 1999;401(6753):598–602.
69. Michos O, Panman L, Vintersten K, Beier K, Zeller R, Zuniga A. Gremlin-mediated BMP antagonism induces the epithelial-mesenchymal feedback signaling controlling metanephric kidney and limb organogenesis. Development. 2004;131(14):3401–10.
70. Bandyopadhyay A, Tsuji K, Cox K, Harfe BD, Rosen V, Tabin CJ. Genetic analysis of the roles of BMP2, BMP4, and BMP7 in limb patterning and skeletogenesis. PLoS Genet. 2006;2(12):e216.
71. Benazet JD, Bischofberger M, Tiecke E, Goncalves A, Martin JF, Zuniga A, Naef F, Zeller R. A self-regulatory system of interlinked signaling feedback loops controls mouse limb patterning. Science. 2009;323(5917):1050–3.
72. Verheyden JM, Sun X. An Fgf/Gremlin inhibitory feedback loop triggers termination of limb bud outgrowth. Nature. 2008; 454(7204):638–41.
73. Yang Y, Niswander L. Interaction between the signaling molecules WNT7a and SHH during vertebrate limb development: dorsal signals regulate anteroposterior patterning. Cell. 1995;80(6):939–47.
74. Fernandez-Teran M, Ros MA, Mariani FV. Evidence that the limb bud ectoderm is required for survival of the underlying mesoderm. Dev Biol. 2013;381(2):11.
75. Woltering JM, Duboule D. The origin of digits: expression patterns versus regulatory mechanisms. Dev Cell. 2010;18(4):526–32.
76. Yokouchi Y, Sasaki H, Kuroiwa A. Homeobox gene expression correlated with the bifurcation process of limb cartilage development. Nature. 1991;353(6343):443–5.
77. Nelson CE, Morgan BA, Burke AC, Laufer E, DiMambro E, Murtaugh LC, Gonzales E, Tessarollo L, Parada LF, Tabin C. Analysis of Hox gene expression in the chick limb bud. Development. 1996;122(5):1449–66.
78. Kmita M, Fraudeau N, Herault Y, Duboule D. Serial deletions and duplications suggest a mechanism for the collinearity of Hoxd genes in limbs. Nature. 2002;420(6912):145–50.
79. Dreyer SD, Naruse T, Morello R, Zabel B, Winterpacht A, Johnson RL, Lee B, Oberg KC. Lmx1b expression during joint and tendon formation: localization and evaluation of potential downstream targets. Gene Expr Patterns. 2004;4(4):397–405.
80. Zeller R. It takes time to make a pinky: unexpected insights into how SHH patterns vertebrate digits. Sci STKE. 2004;2004(259):e53.
81. Harfe BD, Scherz PJ, Nissim S, Tian H, McMahon AP, Tabin CJ. Evidence for an expansion-based temporal Shh gradient in specifying vertebrate digit identities. Cell. 2004;118(4):517–28.
82. Zhu J, Nakamura E, Nguyen MT, Bao X, Akiyama H, Mackem S. Uncoupling Sonic hedgehog control of pattern and expansion of the developing limb bud. Dev Cell. 2008;14(4):624–32.
83. Yang Y, Drossopoulou G, Chuang PT, Duprez D, Marti E, Bumcrot D, Vargesson N, Clarke J, Niswander L, McMahon A, et al. Relationship between dose, distance and time in Sonic Hedgehog-mediated regulation of anteroposterior polarity in the chick limb. Development. 1997;124(21):4393–404.
84. Towers M, Mahood R, Yin Y, Tickle C. Integration of growth and specification in chick wing digit-patterning. Nature. 2008; 452(7189):882–6.
85. Sheth R, Marcon L, Bastida MF, Junco M, Quintana L, Dahn R, Kmita M, Sharpe J, Ros MA. Hox genes regulate digit patterning by controlling the wavelength of a Turing-type mechanism. Science. 2012;338(6113):1476–80.
86. Turing AM. The chemical basis of morphogenesis. 1953. Bull Math Biol. 1990;52(1–2):153–97.
87. Suzuki T, Hasso SM, Fallon JF. Unique SMAD1/5/8 activity at the phalanx-forming region determines digit identity. Proc Natl Acad Sci U S A. 2008;105(11):4185–90.
88. Montero JA, Lorda-Diez CI, Ganan Y, Macias D, Hurle JM. Activin/TGFbeta and BMP crosstalk determines digit chondrogenesis. Dev Biol. 2008;321(2):343–56.
89. Dahn RD, Fallon JF. Interdigital regulation of digit identity and homeotic transformation by modulated BMP signaling. Science. 2000;289(5478):438–41.

90. Chen Y, Knezevic V, Ervin V, Hutson R, Ward Y, Mackem S. Direct interaction with Hoxd proteins reverses Gli3-repressor function to promote digit formation downstream of Shh. Development. 2004;131(10):2339–47.
91. Wang B, Fallon JF, Beachy PA. Hedgehog-regulated processing of Gli3 produces an anterior/posterior repressor gradient in the developing vertebrate limb. Cell. 2000;100(4):423–34.
92. Drossopoulou G, Lewis KE, Sanz-Ezquerro JJ, Nikbakht N, McMahon AP, Hofmann C, Tickle C. A model for anteroposterior patterning of the vertebrate limb based on sequential long- and short-range Shh signalling and Bmp signalling. Development. 2000;127(7):1337–48.
93. Rowe DA, Cairns JM, Fallon JF. Spatial and temporal patterns of cell death in limb bud mesoderm after apical ectodermal ridge removal. Dev Biol. 1982;93(1):83–91.
94. Sanz-Ezquerro JJ, Tickle C. Fgf signaling controls the number of phalanges and tip formation in developing digits. Curr Biol. 2003;13(20):1830–6.
95. Winkel A, Stricker S, Tylzanowski P, Seiffart V, Mundlos S, Gross G, Hoffmann A. Wnt-ligand-dependent interaction of TAK1 (TGF-beta-activated kinase-1) with the receptor tyrosine kinase Ror2 modulates canonical Wnt-signalling. Cell Signal. 2008; 20(11):2134–44.
96. Witte F, Chan D, Economides AN, Mundlos S, Stricker S. Receptor tyrosine kinase-like orphan receptor 2 (ROR2) and Indian hedgehog regulate digit outgrowth mediated by the phalanx-forming region. Proc Natl Acad Sci U S A. 2010;107(32):14211–6.
97. Oberg KC. Review of the molecular development of the thumb: digit primera. Clin Orthop Relat Res. 2014;472(4):1101–5.
98. Koshiba-Takeuchi K, Takeuchi JK, Arruda EP, Kathiriya IS, Mo R, Hui CC, Srivastava D, Bruneau BG. Cooperative and antagonistic interactions between Sall4 and Tbx5 pattern the mouse limb and heart. Nat Genet. 2006;38(2):175–83.
99. Saint-Hilaire IG: Histoire g´en´erale et particuli `ere des anomalies de l'organisation chez l'homme et les animaux. Paris: J.B. Baillière; 1932.
100. Vargas AO, Fallon JF. Birds have dinosaur wings: the molecular evidence. J Exp Zool B Mol Dev Evol. 2005;304(1):86–90.
101. Vargas AO, Kohlsdorf T, Fallon JF, Vandenbrooks J, Wagner GP. The evolution of HoxD-11 expression in the bird wing: insights from Alligator mississippiensis. PLoS One. 2008;3(10): e3325.
102. Villavicencio-Lorini P, Kuss P, Friedrich J, Haupt J, Farooq M, Turkmen S, Duboule D, Hecht J, Mundlos S. Homeobox genes d11-d13 and a13 control mouse autopod cortical bone and joint formation. J Clin Invest. 2010;120(6):1994–2004.
103. Hasson P, DeLaurier A, Bennett M, Grigorieva E, Naiche LA, Papaioannou VE, Mohun TJ, Logan MP. Tbx4 and tbx5 acting in connective tissue are required for limb muscle and tendon patterning. Dev Cell. 2010;18(1):148–56.
104. Casanova JC, Badia-Careaga C, Uribe V, Sanz-Ezquerro JJ. Bambi and Sp8 expression mark digit tips and their absence shows that chick wing digits 2 and 3 are truncated. PLoS One. 2012;7(12): e52781.
105. Casanova JC, Sanz-Ezquerro JJ. Digit morphogenesis: is the tip different? Dev Growth Differ. 2007;49(6):479–91.
106. Kawakami Y, Esteban CR, Matsui T, Rodriguez-Leon J, Kato S, Izpisua Belmonte JC. Sp8 and Sp9, two closely related buttonhead-like transcription factors, regulate Fgf8 expression and limb outgrowth in vertebrate embryos. Development. 2004;131(19):4763–74.
107. Haro E, Delgado I, Hunco M, Yamada Y, Mansouri A, Oberg KC, Ros MA: Sp6 and Sp8 transcription factors control AER formation and Dorsoventral Patterning in Limb Development. PLoS genetics. 2014;In Press.
108. Allan CH, Fleckman P, Fernandes RJ, Hager B, James J, Wisecarver Z, Satterstrom FK, Gutierrez A, Norman A, Pirrone A, et al. Tissue response and Msx1 expression after human fetal digit tip amputation in vitro. Wound Repair Regen. 2006;14(4): 398–404.
109. Han M, Yang X, Farrington JE, Muneoka K. Digit regeneration is regulated by Msx1 and BMP4 in fetal mice. Development. 2003;130(21):5123–32.
110. Yoon BS, Pogue R, Ovchinnikov DA, Yoshii I, Mishina Y, Behringer RR, Lyons KM. BMPs regulate multiple aspects of growth-plate chondrogenesis through opposing actions on FGF pathways. Development. 2006;133(23):4667–78.
111. Cunningham TJ, Chatzi C, Sandell LL, Trainor PA, Duester G. Rdh10 mutants deficient in limb field retinoic acid signaling exhibit normal limb patterning but display interdigital webbing. Dev Dyn. 2011;240(5):1142–50.
112. Rodriguez-Leon J, Merino R, Macias D, Ganan Y, Santesteban E, Hurle JM. Retinoic acid regulates programmed cell death through BMP signalling. Nat Cell Biol. 1999;1(2):125–6.
113. Weatherbee SD, Behringer RR, Rasweiler JJ, Niswander LA. Interdigital webbing retention in bat wings illustrates genetic changes underlying amniote limb diversification. Proc Natl Acad Sci U S A. 2006;103(41):15103–7.
114. Choi K. Hemangioblast development and regulation. Biochem Cell Biol. 1998;76(6):947–56.
115. Nimmagadda S, Geetha Loganathan P, Huang R, Scaal M, Schmidt C, Christ B. BMP4 and noggin control embryonic blood vessel formation by antagonistic regulation of VEGFR-2 (Quek1) expression. Dev Biol. 2005;280(1):100–10.
116. Park C, Afrikanova I, Chung YS, Zhang WJ, Arentson E, Fong Gh G, Rosendahl A, Choi K. A hierarchical order of factors in the generation of FLK1- and SCL-expressing hematopoietic and endothelial progenitors from embryonic stem cells. Development. 2004;131(11):2749–62.
117. Shalaby F, Rossant J, Yamaguchi TP, Gertsenstein M, Wu XF, Breitman ML, Schuh AC. Failure of blood-island formation and vasculogenesis in Flk-1-deficient mice. Nature. 1995;376(6535): 62–6.
118. Shalaby F, Ho J, Stanford WL, Fischer KD, Schuh AC, Schwartz L, Bernstein A, Rossant J. A requirement for Flk1 in primitive and definitive hematopoiesis and vasculogenesis. Cell. 1997;89(6): 981–90.
119. Ferguson M, Byrnes C, Sun L, Marti G, Bonde P, Duncan M, Harmon JW. Wound healing enhancement: electroporation to address a classic problem of military medicine. World J Surg. 2005;29 Suppl 1:S55–9.
120. Drake CJ. Embryonic and adult vasculogenesis. Birth Defects Res C Embryo Today. 2003;69(1):73–82.
121. Moser M, Patterson C. Bone morphogenetic proteins and vascular differentiation: BMPing up vasculogenesis. Thromb Haemost. 2005;94(4):713–8.
122. He L, Papoutsi M, Huang R, Tomarev SI, Christ B, Kurz H, Wilting J. Three different fates of cells migrating from somites into the limb bud. Anat Embryol (Berl). 2003;207(1):29–34.
123. Caplan AI. The vasculature and limb development. Cell Differ. 1985;16(1):1–11.
124. Vargesson N. Vascularization of the developing chick limb bud: role of the TGFbeta signalling pathway. J Anat. 2003;202(1):93–103.
125. Deckers MM, van Bezooijen RL, van der Horst G, Hoogendam J, van Der Bent C, Papapoulos SE, Lowik CW. Bone morphogenetic proteins stimulate angiogenesis through osteoblast-derived vascular endothelial growth factor A. Endocrinology. 2002;143(4): 1545–53.
126. Hellstrom M, Phng LK, Hofmann JJ, Wallgard E, Coultas L, Lindblom P, Alva J, Nilsson AK, Karlsson L, Gaiano N, et al. Dll4 signalling through Notch1 regulates formation of tip cells during angiogenesis. Nature. 2007;445(7129):776–80.
127. Siekmann AF, Lawson ND. Notch signalling limits angiogenic cell behaviour in developing zebrafish arteries. Nature. 2007;445(7129):781–4.
128. Jones CA, Li DY. Common cues regulate neural and vascular patterning. Curr Opin Genet Dev. 2007;17(4):332–6.

129. Thurston G. Role of Angiopoietins and Tie receptor tyrosine kinases in angiogenesis and lymphangiogenesis. Cell Tissue Res. 2003;314(1):61–8.
130. Krebs LT, Xue Y, Norton CR, Shutter JR, Maguire M, Sundberg JP, Gallahan D, Closson V, Kitajewski J, Callahan R, et al. Notch signaling is essential for vascular morphogenesis in mice. Genes Dev. 2000;14(11):1343–52.
131. Tamura K, Amano T, Satoh T, Saito D, Yonei-Tamura S, Yajima H. Expression of rigf, a member of avian VEGF family, correlates with vascular patterning in the developing chick limb bud. Mech Dev. 2003;120(2):199–209.
132. Betsholtz C, Lindblom P, Gerhardt H. Role of pericytes in vascular morphogenesis. EXS. 2005;94:115–25.
133. Ribes V, Otto DM, Dickmann L, Schmidt K, Schuhbaur B, Henderson C, Blomhoff R, Wolf CR, Tickle C, Dolle P. Rescue of cytochrome P450 oxidoreductase (Por) mouse mutants reveals functions in vasculogenesis, brain and limb patterning linked to retinoic acid homeostasis. Dev Biol. 2007;303(1):66–81.
134. Ribes V, Fraulob V, Petkovich M, Dolle P. The oxidizing enzyme CYP26a1 tightly regulates the availability of retinoic acid in the gastrulating mouse embryo to ensure proper head development and vasculogenesis. Dev Dyn. 2007;236(3):644–53.
135. Rodriguez-Niedenfuhr M, Burton GJ, Deu J, Sanudo JR. Development of the arterial pattern in the upper limb of staged human embryos: normal development and anatomic variations. J Anat. 2001;199(Pt 4):407–17.
136. Mrazkova O. Ontogenesis of arterial trunks in the human forearm. Folia Morphol (Praha). 1973;21(2):193–6.
137. Kawakami Y, Rodriguez-Leon J, Belmonte JC. The role of TGFbetas and Sox9 during limb chondrogenesis. Curr Opin Cell Biol. 2006;18(6):723–9.
138. Akiyama H, Chaboissier MC, Martin JF, Schedl A, de Crombrugghe B. The transcription factor Sox9 has essential roles in successive steps of the chondrocyte differentiation pathway and is required for expression of Sox5 and Sox6. Genes Dev. 2002;16(21):2813–28.
139. Lefebvre V, Li P, de Crombrugghe B. A new long form of Sox5 (L-Sox5), Sox6 and Sox9 are coexpressed in chondrogenesis and cooperatively activate the type II collagen gene. EMBO J. 1998;17(19):5718–33.
140. Karsenty G. Transcriptional control of skeletogenesis. Annu Rev Genomics Hum Genet. 2008;9:183–96.
141. Zou H, Wieser R, Massague J, Niswander L. Distinct roles of type I bone morphogenetic protein receptors in the formation and differentiation of cartilage. Genes Dev. 1997;11(17):2191–203.
142. Pizette S, Niswander L. BMPs are required at two steps of limb chondrogenesis: formation of prechondrogenic condensations and their differentiation into chondrocytes. Dev Biol. 2000;219(2): 237–49.
143. Yoon BS, Ovchinnikov DA, Yoshii I, Mishina Y, Behringer RR, Lyons KM. Bmpr1a and Bmpr1b have overlapping functions and are essential for chondrogenesis in vivo. Proc Natl Acad Sci U S A. 2005;102(14):5062–7.
144. Bandyopadhyay A, Yadav PS, Prashar P. BMP signaling in development and diseases: a pharmacological perspective. Biochem Pharmacol. 2013;85(7):857–64.
145. Weston AD, Rosen V, Chandraratna RA, Underhill TM. Regulation of skeletal progenitor differentiation by the BMP and retinoid signaling pathways. J Cell Biol. 2000;148(4):679–90.
146. Weston AD, Chandraratna RA, Torchia J, Underhill TM. Requirement for RAR-mediated gene repression in skeletal progenitor differentiation. J Cell Biol. 2002;158(1):39–51.
147. Dranse HJ, Sampaio AV, Petkovich M, Underhill TM. Genetic deletion of Cyp26b1 negatively impacts limb skeletogenesis by inhibiting chondrogenesis. J Cell Sci. 2011;124(Pt 16):2723–34.
148. Hoffman LM, Garcha K, Karamboulas K, Cowan MF, Drysdale LM, Horton WA, Underhill TM. BMP action in skeletogenesis involves attenuation of retinoid signaling. J Cell Biol. 2006;174(1): 101–13.
149. Gray DJ, Gardner E, O'Rahilly R. The prenatal development of the skeleton and joints of the human hand. Am J Anat. 1957;101(2):169–223.
150. Shubin NH, Alberch P. A morphogenetic approach to the origin and basic organization of the tetrapod limb. In: Evolutionary Biology. New York: Plenum Press; 1986. p. 319–87.
151. Hinchliffe JR, Johnson DR. The development of the vertebrate limb. Oxford: Clarendon; 1980.
152. Kim IS, Otto F, Zabel B, Mundlos S. Regulation of chondrocyte differentiation by Cbfa1. Mech Dev. 1999;80(2):159–70.
153. Nakashima K, Zhou X, Kunkel G, Zhang Z, Deng JM, Behringer RR, de Crombrugghe B. The novel zinc finger-containing transcription factor osterix is required for osteoblast differentiation and bone formation. Cell. 2002;108(1):17–29.
154. Yang X, Matsuda K, Bialek P, Jacquot S, Masuoka HC, Schinke T, Li L, Brancorsini S, Sassone-Corsi P, Townes TM, et al. ATF4 is a substrate of RSK2 and an essential regulator of osteoblast biology; implication for Coffin-Lowry Syndrome. Cell. 2004; 117(3): 387–98.
155. Mackie EJ, Ahmed YA, Tatarczuch L, Chen KS, Mirams M. Endochondral ossification: how cartilage is converted into bone in the developing skeleton. Int J Biochem Cell Biol. 2008; 40(1):46–62.
156. Noback CR, Robertson GG. Sequences of appearance of ossification centers in the human skeleton during the first five prenatal months. Am J Anat. 1951;89(1):1–28.
157. Stuart HC, Pyle SI, Cornoni J, Reed RB. Onsets, completions and spans of ossification in the 29 bone growth centers of the hand and wrist. Pediatrics. 1962;29:237–49.
158. Hartmann C, Tabin CJ. Wnt-14 plays a pivotal role in inducing synovial joint formation in the developing appendicular skeleton. Cell. 2001;104(3):341–51.
159. Storm EE, Kingsley DM. GDF5 coordinates bone and joint formation during digit development. Dev Biol. 1999;209(1):11–27.
160. Dalgleish AE. Development of the limbs of the mouse. Stanford: Stanford University; 1964.
161. Craig FM, Bayliss MT, Bentley G, Archer CW. A role for hyaluronan in joint development. J Anat. 1990;171(4):17–23.
162. Nowlan NC, Sharpe J, Roddy KA, Prendergast PJ, Murphy P. Mechanobiology of embryonic skeletal development: Insights from animal models. Birth Defects Res C Embryo Today. 2010;90(3):203–13.
163. Khan IM, Redman SN, Williams R, Dowthwaite GP, Oldfield SF, Archer CW. The development of synovial joints. Curr Top Dev Biol. 2007;79:1–36.
164. Pacifici M, Koyama E, Iwamoto M. Mechanisms of synovial joint and articular cartilage formation: recent advances, but many lingering mysteries. Birth Defects Res C Embryo Today. 2005;75(3):237–48.
165. Tozer S, Duprez D. Tendon and ligament: development, repair and disease. Birth Defects Res C Embryo Today. 2005;75(3):226–36.
166. Mitrovic D. Development of the diarthrodial joints in the rat embryo. Am J Anat. 1978;151(4):475–85.
167. Sharma K, Izpisua Belmonte JC. Development of the limb neuromuscular system. Curr Opin Cell Biol. 2001;13(2):204–10.
168. Schweitzer R, Chyung JH, Murtaugh LC, Brent AE, Rosen V, Olson EN, Lassar A, Tabin CJ. Analysis of the tendon cell fate using Scleraxis, a specific marker for tendons and ligaments. Development. 2001;128(19):3855–66.
169. Ros MA, Rivero FB, Hinchliffe JR, Hurle JM. Immunohistological and ultrastructural study of the developing tendons of the avian foot. Anat Embryol (Berl). 1995;192(6):483–96.
170. Kardon G. Muscle and tendon morphogenesis in the avian hind limb. Development. 1998;125(20):4019–32.

171. Edom-Vovard F, Duprez D. Signals regulating tendon formation during chick embryonic development. Dev Dyn. 2004;229(3):449–57.
172. Murphy M, Kardon G. Origin of vertebrate limb muscle: the role of progenitor and myoblast populations. Curr Top Dev Biol. 2011;96:1–32.
173. Williams BA, Ordahl CP. Pax-3 expression in segmental mesoderm marks early stages in myogenic cell specification. Development. 1994;120(4):785–96.
174. Buckingham M, Bajard L, Chang T, Daubas P, Hadchouel J, Meilhac S, Montarras D, Rocancourt D, Relaix F. The formation of skeletal muscle: from somite to limb. J Anat. 2003;202(1): 59–68.
175. Sze LY, Lee KK, Webb SE, Li Z, Paulin D. Migration of myogenic cells from the somites to the fore-limb buds of developing mouse embryos. Dev Dyn. 1995;203(3):324–36.
176. Bober E, Franz T, Arnold HH, Gruss P, Tremblay P. Pax-3 is required for the development of limb muscles: a possible role for the migration of dermomyotomal muscle progenitor cells. Development. 1994;120(3):603–12.
177. Dietrich S, Abou-Rebyeh F, Brohmann H, Bladt F, Sonnenberg-Riethmacher E, Yamaai T, Lumsden A, Brand-Saberi B, Birchmeier C. The role of SF/HGF and c-Met in the development of skeletal muscle. Development. 1999;126(8):1621–9.
178. Bladt F, Riethmacher D, Isenmann S, Aguzzi A, Birchmeier C. Essential role for the c-met receptor in the migration of myogenic precursor cells into the limb bud. Nature. 1995;376(6543):768–71.
179. Brand-Saberi B, Muller TS, Wilting J, Christ B, Birchmeier C. Scatter factor/hepatocyte growth factor (SF/HGF) induces emigration of myogenic cells at interlimb level in vivo. Dev Biol. 1996;179(1):303–8.
180. Scaal M, Bonafede A, Dathe V, Sachs M, Cann G, Christ B, Brand-Saberi B. SF/HGF is a mediator between limb patterning and muscle development. Development. 1999;126(21):4885–93.
181. Epstein JA, Shapiro DN, Cheng J, Lam PY, Maas RL. Pax3 modulates expression of the c-Met receptor during limb muscle development. Proc Natl Acad Sci U S A. 1996;93(9):4213–8.
182. Schmidt C, Bladt F, Goedecke S, Brinkmann V, Zschiesche W, Sharpe M, Gherardi E, Birchmeier C. Scatter factor/hepatocyte growth factor is essential for liver development. Nature. 1995;373(6516):699–702.
183. Schafer K, Braun T. Early specification of limb muscle precursor cells by the homeobox gene Lbx1h. Nat Genet. 1999;23(2):213–6.
184. Tajbakhsh S, Buckingham ME. Mouse limb muscle is determined in the absence of the earliest myogenic factor myf-5. Proc Natl Acad Sci U S A. 1994;91(2):747–51.
185. Ontell M, Kozeka K. The organogenesis of murine striated muscle: a cytoarchitectural study. Am J Anat. 1984;171(2):133–48.
186. Otto A, Collins-Hooper H, Patel K. The origin, molecular regulation and therapeutic potential of myogenic stem cell populations. J Anat. 2009;215(5):477–97.
187. Dieu T, Newgreen D. Chicken wings and the brachial plexus. Neurol Res. 2007;29(3):225–30.
188. Wehrle-Haller B, Koch M, Baumgartner S, Spring J, Chiquet M. Nerve-dependent and -independent tenascin expression in the developing chick limb bud. Development. 1991;112(2):627–37.
189. Swanson GJ, Lewis J. Sensory nerve routes in chick wing buds deprived of motor innervation. J Embryol Exp Morphol. 1986;95:37–52.
190. Swanson GJ. Paths taken sensory nerve fibres in aneural chick wing buds. J Embryol Exp Morphol. 1985;86:109–24.
191. Martin P, Khan A, Lewis J. Cutaneous nerves of the embryonic chick wing do not develop in regions denuded of ectoderm. Development. 1989;106(2):335–46.
192. Lewis J, Chevallier A, Kieny M, Wolpert L. Muscle nerve branches do not develop in chick wings devoid of muscle. J Embryol Exp Morphol. 1981;64:211–32.
193. Polleux F, Ince-Dunn G, Ghosh A. Transcriptional regulation of vertebrate axon guidance and synapse formation. Nat Rev Neurosci. 2007;8(5):331–40.
194. Dasen JS, Jessell TM. Hox networks and the origins of motor neuron diversity. Curr Top Dev Biol. 2009;88:169–200.
195. Kao TJ, Law C, Kania A. Eph and ephrin signaling: lessons learned from spinal motor neurons. Semin Cell Dev Biol. 2012;23(1):83–91.
196. Dasen JS. Transcriptional networks in the early development of sensory-motor circuits. Curr Top Dev Biol. 2009;87:119–48.
197. Manske PR, Oberg KC. Classification and developmental biology of congenital anomalies of the hand and upper extremity. J Bone Joint Surg Am. 2009;91 Suppl 4:3–18.
198. Tonkin MA, Oberg KC. Congenital hand I—embryology, classification, and principles. In: Cheng J, Neligan PC, editors. Plastic surgery, vol 6: hand and upper extremity. 3rd ed. New York: Elsevier; 2012. p. 526–47.
199. Saint-Hilaire IG. Propositions sur la monstruosité. Paris: Imp. Didot le Jeune; 1829.
200. Saint-Hilaire IG. Histoire générale et particuli ère des anomalies de l'organisation chez l'homme et les animaux. Paris: J.B. Baillière; 1932.
201. Swanson AB. A classification for congenital malformations of the hand. N J Bull Acad Med. 1964;10:166–9.
202. Lösch GM, Buck-Gramcko D, Cihak R, Sharader M, Seichert V. An attempt to classify the malformations of the hand based on morphogenetic criteria. Chir Plastica. 1984;8(1):18.
203. Temtamy SA. Genetic factors in hand malformations. Baltimore: Johns Hopkins University; 1966.
204. Temtamy SA, McKusick VA. The genetics of hand malformations. Birth Defects Orig Artic Ser. 1978;14(3):i–619.
205. Kay H. A proposed international terminology for the classification of congenital limb deficiencies. ICIB/JACPOC. 1974;13(7):1–16.
206. Kelikian H. Congenital deformities of the hand and forearm. Philadelphia: WB Saunders Company; 1974.
207. Knight SL, Kay SPJ. Classification of congenital anomalies. In: Gupta A, Kay SPJ, Scheker LR, editors. The growing hand. London: Harcourt; 2000. p. 125–35.
208. Tonkin MA. Description of congenital hand anomalies: a personal view. J Hand Surg Br. 2006;31(5):489–97.
209. Oberg KC, Feenstra JM, Manske PR, Tonkin MA. Developmental biology and classification of congenital anomalies of the hand and upper extremity. J Hand Surg Am. 2010;35(12):2066–76.
210. Ogino T. JSSH CHCot: modified IFSSH classification. J Jpn Soc Surg Hand. 2000;17:353–65.
211. Tonkin MA, Tolerton SK, Quick TJ, Harvey I, Lawson RD, Smith NC, Oberg KC. Classification of congenital anomalies of the hand and upper limb: development and assessment of a new system. J Hand Surg Am. 2013;13:10.
212. Ezaki M, Baek GH, Horii E, Hovius SE. Classification of congenital hand and upper limb anomalies. In: Ezaki M, editor. Scientific committee on congenital conditions, vol. 14. IFSSH Ezine; 2014. p. 4.
213. Ekblom AG, Laurell T, Arner M. Epidemiology of congenital upper limb anomalies in Stockholm, Sweden, 1997 to 2007: application of the Oberg, Manske, and Tonkin classification. J Hand Surg. 2014;39(2):237–48.
214. Oberg KC, Feenstra JM, Manske PR, Tonkin MA. A new classification of congenital anomalies of the hand and upper limb. IFSSH Ezine. 2011;1(2):3.

Incidence and Syndromes Associated with Congenital Anomalies of the Upper Limb

2

Leah W. Burke and Donald R. Laub Jr.

Incidence

The best epidemiological studies of incidence of congenital anomalies are total population studies; there are four total population studies of congenital anomalies of the upper extremity (CAUE) in the literature (Table 2.1). A 5-year birth registry study of Edinburgh, Scotland by Rogala et al. found the prevalence of babies born with any limb anomalies to be 30 out of 10,000 live births, and the incidence of upper limb anomalies to be 22.5 out of 10,000 live births [1]. Of those with upper limb anomalies, 35 % had another non-upper limb anomaly. They used an older classification, that of Temtamy and McKusick [2], so direct comparisons to more recent studies are difficult. One striking finding in this study is the complete lack of isolated simple syndactyly, which in other studies was found to be relatively common.

An 11-year total population study of Western Australia found the prevalence of babies born with upper limb anomalies to be 19.76 in 10,000 live births [3]. Forty-six percent of those affected had another non-hand congenital anomaly. Fifty-one percent had bilateral hand anomalies, and 17 % had multiple different hand anomalies. The most common anomalies were failures of differentiation (35 %), duplications (33 %), and failures of formation (15 %). Congenital upper limb anomalies were more common in boys; preterm, post-term, and multiple births; and older mothers. No significant differences in prevalence or frequency of anomalies were found between whites and nonwhites, left and right sides, and in babies that survived and those who died shortly after birth.

L.W. Burke, M.A.T., M.D., F.A.A.P., F.A.B.M.G.
Department of Pediatrics, Fletcher Allen Health Care, University of Vermont College of Medicine, Burlington, VT, USA

D.R. Laub Jr., M.S., M.D., F.A.C.S. (✉)
Fletcher Allen Health Care and Vermont Children's Hospital, Departments of Surgery and Pediatrics, University of Vermont School of Medicine, Burlington, VT, USA
e-mail: dlaub@uvm.edu

Similarly, an 11-year total population study of the Stockholm region of Sweden found a recorded incidence of congenital anomalies of the upper limb of 21.5 per 10,000 live births [4]. Fifty-four percent of the children with congenital anomalies of the upper limb were boys. The anomalies affected the right side only in 30 %, the left side only in 33 %, and both sides in 37 %. Non-hand anomalies were recorded in 23 % of the children with congenital anomalies of the upper limb, most commonly in the lower limbs. In 17 % of the affected children, there was a known occurrence among relatives. Failure of differentiation was the most common category (47 %) followed by duplication (26 %), failure of formation (18 %), undergrowth (3 %), generalized abnormalities and syndromes (2.4 %), overgrowth (1.7 %), and constriction ring syndrome (1.5 %).

There are more total population studies of limb deficiency anomalies, for example: a 9-year total population study of the national incidence of upper limb deficiencies in Finland found an incidence of congenital deficiency anomalies of the upper limb of 5.26 per 10,000 live births [5]. These studies approximate the "failure of formation" category of complete CAUE population studies (Table 2.2).

Incidence figures derived by extrapolation from surveys of patients presenting for treatment show slightly lower incidence: an estimated 16–18 per 10,000 births [9–11]. It is thought that these population studies may underestimate incidence, as the milder deformities may never present for treatment. A comparison of a population-based study and clinic registry of Swedish children with CAUE showed an underestimation of incidence by 6 % in the clinic registry, and a low degree of correlation of classification of anomalies [12].

The IFSSH classification is a useful tool for classifying most CAUE and enables comparison between studies, but is based on theories of embryological failure and is subject to some differences of interpretation. Ambiguities in the categorization of anomalies may then lead to differences of incidence of certain classifications [13]. For instance, the IFSSH classification could classify polydactyly with complex syndactylies as duplication, but for clinical purposes it fits better

D.R. Laub Jr. (ed.), *Congenital Anomalies of the Upper Extremity: Etiology and Management*,
DOI 10.1007/978-1-4899-7504-1_2, © Springer Science+Business Media New York 2015

into the category of failure of differentiation. Miura et al. [14] and Ogino [15, 16] suggested that a common teratological mechanism causes cleft hand, syndactyly, and polydactyly and that they should be put into a new category: failure of induction of digital rays. Classifying congenital absence of digits is also ambiguous; the distinctions between brachysyndactyly, symbrachydactyly (atypical cleft hand), and transverse arrest are not clearly defined.

In the Stockholm study thumb hypoplasia was categorized as failure of formation, longitudinal arrest, and radial ray deficiency, whereas in the study from Western Australia, thumb hypoplasia was categorized as undergrowth. The Stockholm study showed a much lower frequency of undergrowth as a result. There was also a surprisingly large disparity between the categories of transverse arrest and symbrachydactyly regarding associated non-hand anomalies. Other differences in relative frequencies are also likely caused by other differences of interpretation of classification strategies.

Epidemiologic studies are important for health care planning, detecting changes in incidence over time, and comparing differences among regions. These two total population studies of CAUE agree on total incidence figures. These population studies are slightly higher than the estimated 0.16–0.18 % incidence for CAUE of in surveys of patients presenting for treatment (Table 2.3) [9, 10, 17–19]. It is assumed that this is due to the fact that milder deformities may never present for treatment.

These studies do, however, reveal the difficulties in comparing studies owing to different classification strategies and weaknesses within the IFSSH classification. For example, two studies of CAUE in Edinburgh, UK [2, 10] and two studies from Japan [17, 18] show markedly different relative frequency of incidence of duplication; presumably such a finding in ethnically similar populations is due to differences in classification (see Table 2.3). We hope that the ongoing discussion of classification systems for CAUE (see Chap. 1) will inspire improvements in registration and population studies.

Table 2.1 Incidence and classification of congenital anomalies of the upper extremity (CAUE) in total population studies

Study	Ekblom et al. [4]	Giele et al. [3]	Rogala et al. [1]
Country	Sweden	Australia	Scotland
Years of survey	1997–2007	1980–1990	1964–1968
Incidence (per 10,000 live births)	21.50	19.76	16.00
Non-hand anomaly present (%)	23	46	15[a]
Failure of formation (%)	18	15	35
Duplication (%)	26	33	38[a]
Overgrowth (%)	2	1	35[a]
Undergrowth (%)	3	10	1[a]
Constriction ring (%)	1	3	2[a]
Generalized (%)	2	3	2[a]

[a]Author's interpretation: classification system differs

Associated Conditions

The genetics of hand formation have already been reviewed (Chap. 1). The genetic pathways were originally elucidated through chick and mouse studies. Genetic studies of human malformations and malformation syndromes have provided further insight. Congenital hand malformations can be categorized using a number of different criteria. A common classification scheme uses the broad designations of polydactyly, syndactyly, brachydactyly, and oligodactyly or reduction defects. Hand malformations can occur in isolation or as a part of a larger pattern of malformation. Although there are over a hundred recognized syndromes with hand anomalies as a part of their expression, this review will concentrate on only those syndromes for which the hand malformation is a cardinal or defining feature.

1. Syndromes with polydactyly
2. Syndromes with syndactyly
3. Syndromes with brachydactyly
4. Syndromes with oligodactyly
5. Syndromes with reduction defects

Syndromes with Polydactyly

Polydactyly was classified in 1978 by Temtamy and McKusick [20] into the following categories:

Postaxial type A—Postaxial extra digits that are well developed

Table 2.2 Incidence of upper limb deficiency anomalies in total population studies

Study	Koskimies et al. [5]	Giele et al. [3]	Kallen et al. [6]	Rogala et al. [1]	Aro et al. [7]	Froster and Baird [8]
Country	Finland	Australia	Sweden	Scotland	Finland	Canada
Years of survey	1993–2005	1980–1990	1965–1979	1964–1968	1964–1077	1952–1984
Incidence (per 10,000 live births)	5.25	5.12	4.00	6.70	4.00	3.40

Table 2.3 Comparison of classification of relative frequency of CAUE in population studies and large case series

Study	Ekblom et al. [4]	Giele et al. [3]	Flatt [9]	Ogino et al. [18]	Cheng et al. [19]	Lamb et al. [10]	Rogala et al. [2]	Yamaguchi et al. [17]
Country	Sweden	Australia	USA	Japan	China	UK	UK	Japan
Years of compilation	1997–2007	1980–1990	1960–1994	1968–1984	1976–1986	1976–1978	1964–1968	1961–1972
Failure of formation (%)	21.50	15	15	11	11	18	28	16
Failure of differentiation (%)	23	32	41	52	30	41	21	28
Duplication (%)	18	38	15	19	40	20	40	26
Overgrowth (%)	26	1	1	1	1	1	–	1
Undergrowth (%)	2	8	9	9	2	14	8	14
Constriction ring (%)	3	3	2	5	5	4	3	1
Generalized (%)	1	3	4	3	4	–	–	–
Unclassified (%)	2	–	13	1	3	–	–	14

Table 2.4 Primarily craniofacial syndromes associated with postaxial polydactyly

Syndrome	Other cardinal features	Inheritance/OMIM Gene/locus
Oral-facial-digital II, Mohr (OFD II)	Preaxial polysyndactyly of the feet, cleft tongue, midline partial cleft lip, hypertrophic frenulae, hamartomas of the tongue, conductive deafness	AR/252100
Oral-facial-digital III (OFD III)	See-saw winking of eyelids, oral frenulas, hamartomas of the tongue, supernumerary teeth, intellectual disability	AR/258850
Oral-facial-digital V (OFD V)	Hypertelorism, midline cleft of the upper lip, lobulated tongue, intellectual disability	AR/174300 DDX59/1q32.1
Oto-palato-digital, type II	Hypertelorism, micrognathia, cleft palate, overlapping fingers, dense bones	XLR/304120 FLNA/Xq28

Postaxial type B—Pedunculated postminimus
Preaxial type I—Duplication of thumbs/great toes
Preaxial type II—Triphalangeal thumbs/duplication of great toes
Preaxial type III—Absent thumbs, one or two extra preaxial digits
Preaxial type IV—Broad thumbs, preaxial polysyndactyly, postaxial postminimus

In 1998, Castilla reported on the congenital hand malformations using a study of Latin American Collaborative Study of Congenital Malformations [20]. He reviewed 5,927 consecutively born polydactyly cases. Castilla divided the polydactylies into *postaxial*, *preaxial*, and *rare*, a group in which he included *mesoaxial* and combinations of digits. These groups were then further subdivided into *isolated* or *associated*, depending upon whether there were other anomalies present. The *associated* category was then further subdivided into *combined*, if the other anomaly was a limb anomaly, *syndromic*, if the polydactyly occurred in a combination of anomalies representing a syndrome, and *MCA*, or multiple congenital anomalies, if the anomalies did not fit a recognizable pattern or syndrome.

From Castilla's study, several patterns emerged. Postaxial is the most common type of polydactyly and the most likely to be isolated. The rare polydactylies, that is, not clearly only postaxial or only preaxial, are the most likely to be associated with an underlying syndrome. Trisomy 13, Meckel syndrome, and Down syndrome accounted for 75 % of the syndromic polydactyly cases in this study. In both Meckel and Trisomy 13 syndromes, postaxial polydactyly is a cardinal feature of the syndrome. For Down syndrome, although preaxial polydactyly can be seen in Down syndrome with a higher frequency than in the general population, it would not be considered a cardinal feature of Down syndrome. For the purposes of this chapter, only the syndromic category will be included, as the isolated forms are reviewed in other chapters.

Syndromes in which polydactyly is a cardinal feature can be subdivided using the classification of postaxial, preaxial, mesoaxial and combined, and further subdivided by the other common findings or by a common aspect of development.

Syndromes with Postaxial Polydactyly: Craniofacial Anomalies as a Primary Feature

Polydactyly is a cardinal feature for a group of syndromes in which the major or defining features are craniofacial abnormalities (Table 2.4). These include the various types of oral-facial-digital (OFD) syndrome. Various reviewers have described the different types of OFD syndromes on their various oral, facial, and digital abnormalities, and many are now known to be genetically distinct. The primary findings of the OFD syndromes are polydactyly and a combination of oral anomalies, most prominently, abnormalities of the tongue and frenula.

Postaxial Polydactyly as a Feature in Ciliopathies

Ciliopathies are a group of conditions in which the genes code for proteins that are important in the cilium-centrosome complex (CCC). The function of the CCC is to sense a wide variety of intracellular signals that affect polarity, proliferation, differentiation, and tissue maintenance. Many of the syndromes in which postaxial polydactyly is a cardinal feature belong to a group of conditions known as the single-gene ciliopathies [21] and are in Table 2.5.

The single-gene ciliopathies with postaxial polydactyly include a group of skeletal dysplasias characterized by their narrow thoraces and short ribs: short rib polydactyly Types I, II, and IV, Ellis van–Creveld, and Jeune asphyxiating thoracic dysplasia, Type 1 and 2. The short rib polydactylies are characterized by early respiratory distress related to very small thoracic cages resulting in lung hypoplasia, and often, early infant death. Ellis–van Creveld, and Jeune Thoracic Dystrophy, also include short ribs as a defining feature, but have other distinctive features that separate them from the short rib polydactyly group. The configuration of the ribs is different in these last two conditions as well.

Ciliopathies also include Bardet–Biedl syndrome and Meckel–Gruber syndrome. Both of these syndromes can be caused by one of multiple genes, but all of the genes share the property that they encode proteins important in the CCC [21].

Bardet–Biedl is a multisystem disorder in which the primary features are retinal degeneration, cystic kidney disease or urinary tract malformation, intellectual disability, diabetes mellitus, obesity, infertility, and postaxial polydactyly. The delineation of the genetics of Bardet–Biedl syndrome helped establish ciliopathies as an important disease entity when it was shown that many of the proteins formed by genes responsible for BBS were expressed in the ciliated sensory neurons of the nematode *C. elegans* [22]. The polarization of cells required for the formation of the tubules in the kidney represent the action of these ciliary proteins that are affected by BBS gene mutations [21].

Both McKusick–Kaufman syndrome and Bardet–Biedl 6 (BBS6) are caused by mutations in the MKKS gene. McKusick–Kaufman is an autosomal recessive, multisystem condition with polydactyly, heart defects, and genital abnormalities, and is most common in the Old Order Amish community. MKKS codes for a protein important in centrosomal function, possibly acting as a chaperonin. Silencing of the transcript of that gene leads to multinucleate and multicentrosomal cells with cytokinesis defects [5].

Meckel–Gruber is a recessively inherited condition in which the cardinal features include central nervous system malformations, particularly occipital encephalocele, Arnold–Chiari malformation, absence of midline structures such as the corpus callosum and septum pellucidum, and cerebellar malformations. Other major findings include cystic changes in the kidneys and liver. The genes that cause Meckel–Gruber code for proteins that localize to the centrosome, pericentriolar region or to the cilium itself.

Oral-facial-digital syndrome, type 1 (OFD1) is an X-linked disorder in which the gene product has been shown to localize in the renal epithelial cells in the polarized region. Expression of OFD1 is necessary for primary cilia formation and left–right axis specification [21, 24], making OFD1 a ciliopathy syndrome as well. The hand findings in OFD1 are variable and primarily involve asymmetric shortening of the digits in the hands with variable syndactyly and preaxial polydactyly of the feet. However, postaxial and preaxial polydactyly of the hands has also been reported.

Other Syndromes with Polydactyly of Varying Types

Table 2.6 lists some of the many other syndromes associated with polydactyly. Grebe chondrodysplasia is a dwarfing condition in which all of the long bones are severely shortened, particularly the distal portions and is associated with postaxial polydactyly of the hands. Grebe chondrodysplasia is caused by mutations in the growth differentiation factor 5 (GDF5) gene, also known as the cartilage-derived morphogenetic protein 1 (CDMP1) gene. This gene has been found to be responsible for other types of chondrodysplasias including acromesomelic dysplasia, Hunter–Thompson type, Du Pan syndrome (fibular hypoplasia and complex brachydactyly), Multiple synostosis syndrome 2, as well as isolated heritable hand malformations including brachydactyly types A1, A2, and C and proximal symphalangism type 1B (OMIM gene 601146).

Greig cephalopolysyndactyly is a multiple malformation syndrome that is usually ascertained through the limb abnormalities, but includes craniofacial findings such as macrocephaly with an unusual head shape. In Greig, the hand and foot abnormalities are quite variable and include a combination of polydactyly and syndactyly. The polydactyly can be postaxial, preaxial, mesoaxial, or a mixture of all three, and can vary from limb to limb in the same individual. Greig is caused by mutations in the Gli-Kruppel Family member 3 (GLI3) gene on 7p13. GLI3 is a gene in the zinc finger gene family and is also the gene responsible for Pallister–Hall syndrome, a syndrome in which the polydactyly can be postaxial or mesoaxial and other cardinal features include hypothalamic hamartoma, pituitary dysfunction, and visceral malformations. Mutations in GLI3 are also found in some of the isolated heritable forms of polydactyly, including postaxial polydactyly types A1 and B, and preaxial polydactyly type IV [25, 26].

Table 2.5 Ciliopathy syndromes associated with postaxial polydactyly

Syndrome	Other cardinal features	Inheritance/OMIM Gene/locus
Acrocallosal	Hypoplastic or absent corpus callosum, other brain abnormalities, preaxial polydactyly/syndactyly of the feet	AR/200990
		KIF7/15q26.1
Bardet–Biedl	Obesity, intellectual disability, retinal dystrophy, renal anomalies, male hypogonadotrophic hypogonadism, complex female genitourinary malformations	AR
BBS1		BBS1/11q13.2
BBS2		BBS2/16q12.2
BBS3		ARL6/3q11.2
BBS4		BBS4/15q24.1
BBS5		BBS5/2q31.1
BBS6		MKKS/20p12.2
BBS7		BBS7/4q27
BBS8		TTC8/14q31.3
BBS9		BBS9/7p14.3
BBS10		BBS10/12q21.2
BBS11		TRIM32/9q33.1
BBS12		BBS12/4q27
BBS13		MKS1/17q22
BBS14		CEP290/12q21.32
BBS15		WDPCP/2p15
BBS16		SDCCAG8/1q43
Ellis–van Creveld	Atrial septal defect, short ribs, acromesomelic limb shortening, oral frenulae	AR/225500
		EVC/4p16
		EVC2, 4p16
Jeune asphyxiating thoracic dystrophy	Short ribs, brachydactyly, short stature, renal failure, hepatic and pancreatic fibrosis, retinal degeneration	AR/208500
ATD1		ATD1
Asphyxiating thoracic dystrophy 2	Narrow thorax, brachydactyly, short stature, shortened and bowed femora	AR/611263
(ATD2)		IFT80/3q25.33
McKusick–Kaufman	Mesoaxial polydactly, congenital heart disease, and hydrometrocolpos in females and genital malformations in males (most commonly hypospadias, cryptorchidism, and chordee)	AR/236700
		MKKS/20p12.2
Meckel–Gruber	Encephalocele, cystic kidneys, microphthalmia, cleft lip/palate, hepatic fibrosis	AR/249000
MKS1		MKS1/17q22
MKS2		TMEM216/11q12.2
MKS3		TMEM67/8q22.1
MKS4		CEP290/12q21.32
MKS5		RPGRIP1L/16q12.2
MKS6		CC2D2A/4p15.32
MKS7		NPHP3/3q22.1
MKS8		TCTN2/12q24.31
MKS9		B9D1/17p11.2
MKS10		B9D2/19q13.2
Oral-facial-digital, type I (OFD I)	Syndactyly and asymmetric brachydactyly of hands with occasional pre- and postaxial polydactyly of hands, preaxial polydactyly of feet, midline cleft lip, cleft tongue, hamartomas of the tongue, hyperplastic frenulae, intellectual disability, polycystic kidneys	XLR/311200
		OFD1/Xp22.2
Short rib polydactyly Type I	Short ribs, imperforate anus, urogenital abnormalities, congenital heart anomalies	AR/263530
Short rib polydactyly Type II	Short ribs, midline cleft of the upper lip, ovoid tibia	AR/263520
		NEK1/4q32.3
Short rib polydactyly Type III	Short ribs, craniofacial abnormalities	AR/263510
		DYNC2H1/11q21.22.1
Short rib polydactyly Type V	Short ribs, acromesomelic hypomineralization and campomelia, laterality defects, and cystic kidneys	AR/614091
		WDR35/2p24.3

Table 2.6 Other selected syndromes associated with polydactyly

Syndrome	Type	Other cardinal features	Inheritance/OMIM Gene/locus
Carpenter syndrome	Postaxial	Brachydactyly with clinodactyly and syndactyly, broad bifid thumbs, brachycephaly, craniosynostosis, intellectual disability	AR/201000 RAB23/6p11.2
Chondrodysplasia, Grebe type	Postaxial	Hypoplastic digits, severe shortening of long bones	AR/200700 CDMP1/GDF5/20q11.2
Greig cephalopolysyndactyly	Preaxial/postaxial	Preaxial polydactyly of feet, syndactyly, craniosynostosis, macrocephaly with frontal bossing, absence of corpus callosum	AD/175700 GLI3/7p14.1
Laurin–Sandrow	Preaxial/postaxial Mirror	Mirror polysyndactyly of hands and feet, ulnar and fibular dimelia, dysplasia or absence of the radius and tibia, cleft nares	AD/135750 14q13
Pallister–Hall	Postaxial/mesoaxial	Hypothalamic hamartoblastoma, hypopituitarism, imperforate anus, abnormal or absent epiglottis, early death	AD/146510 GLI3/7p14.1
Simpson-Golabi-Behmel	Postaxial	Brachydactyly, syndactyly, overgrowth, coarse facial features, intellectual disability	XL/312870 GPC3, GPC4/Xq26.2
Smith–Lemli–Opitz	Postaxial	2–3 syndactyly of toes, microcephaly, intellectual disability, hypospadias, cryptorchidism	AR/270400 DHCR7/11q13.4
Townes–Brocks	Preaxial	Distal deviation of thumbs, hypoplastic thumbs, microcephaly, ear anomalies and hearing loss, anal and intestinal atresias, genital anomalies, renal anomalies and kidney disease	AD/107480 SALL1/16q21.1
Ulnar–mammary	U	Postaxial polydactyly, apocrine abnormalities, hypopigmentation and hypoplasia of areola, nipple and breast, genital anomalies in males, delayed puberty	AD/181450 TBX3/12q24.21

Syndromes with Syndactyly

Syndactyly is harder to accurately study as mild cutaneous syndactyly is often not reported as a congenital anomaly. Significant cutaneous syndactyly and bony syndactyly is associated with a number of underlying syndromes. Complete syndactyly of the third and fourth digits of the hands, also called zygodactyly can be seen in fetuses with triploidy (karyotype with three copies of every chromosome) but can also occur as an isolated finding.

Syndactyly can be found as a defining feature in a group of syndromes with craniosynostosis as a major feature, often called acrocephalosyndactylies (Table 2.7). Syndactyly of all the fingers into a mitten like extremity occurs in Apert syndrome, an MCA syndrome in which there is significant craniosynostosis involving multiple sutures.

Syndactyly is also seen in a number of other syndromes. It is a defining characteristic in only some of these, which are listed in Table 2.8.

Syndromes with Brachydactyly

Isolated Brachydactyly

Brachydactyly of the hands or shortened digits can be due to absent, underdeveloped, or abnormally shaped phalanges (brachyphalangy), or metacarpals (brachymetacarpia), or a combination of these. Brachydactyly can involve all of the digits or only some of the digits. Bell classified isolated brachydactyly in 1951 [2, 27] into Types A through E with subtypes.

Type A: Brachymesophalangy

Type A-1: Brachymesophalangy II–V; brachyphalangy I

Type A-2: Brachymesophalangy II

Type A-3: Brachymesophalangy V

Type B

Aplasia terminal phalanges, II–V

Hypoplasia middle phalanges, II–V

Broad distal phalanges, I

Type C

Brachymesophalangy II, III, V

Hypersegmentation, proximal phalanges, II, III

Type D

Short, broad thumb distal phalanx

Type E

Brachymetacarpia

Brachymetatarsia

Brachydactyly of one or all the digits can also be found as a feature of multiple syndromes (Table 2.9).

Brachydactyly is a common finding in more than 50 different skeletal dysplasias, but rarely is the defining characteristic. Chapter 26 reviews many of these, and Table 2.10 lists many of these skeletal dysplasias as well.

Table 2.7 Craniosynostosis syndromes associated with syndactyly

Syndrome	Digits involved on the hand	Other cardinal features	Inheritance/OMIM Gene/locus
Apert	1–5; can be osseous or cutaneous, often resulting in a "mitten" hand	Midface hypoplasia, cleft palate, hypertelorism, hyperhidrosis, variety of brain malformations, fusion of cervical vertebrae, intellectual disability, hearing loss	AD/101200 FGFR2/10q26.13
Carpenter syndrome	2–5	Postaxial polydactyly, brachydactyly with clinodactyly, broad bifid thumbs, brachycephaly, intellectual disability	AR/201000 RAB23/6p11.2
Pfeiffer	2–3	Syndactyly of toes, broad and medially deviated distal phalanges of thumb and great toe, brachymesophalangy hypertelorism, brachycephaly	AD/101600 FGFR1/8p11.23-p11.22 FGFR2/10q26.13
Saethre–Chotzen	2–3	3–4 syndactyly of toes, brachydactyly and clinodactyly, ossification defects and hyperostosis of skull, short clavicles, facial asymmetry	AD/101400 TWIST/7p21 FGFR2/10q26.13 FGFR3/4p16.3

Table 2.8 Other syndromes associated with syndactyly as a defining or significant feature

Syndrome	Digits involved	Other cardinal features	Inheritance/OMIM Gene/locus
Focal dermal hypoplasia (Goltz)	Primarily 3–4 but can include others	Ectrodactyly, oligodactyly, dermal hypoplasia, microphthalmia, other eye abnormalities, facial asymmetry, cleft palate	XL/305600 PORCN/Xp11.23
Fraser	1–5; can be osseous or cutaneous, often resulting in a "mitten" hand	Midface hypoplasia, cleft palate, hypertelorism, hyperhidrosis, variety of brain malformations, fusion of cervical vertebrae, intellectual disability, hearing loss	AD/101200 FGFR2/10q26.13
Greig cephalopolysyndactyly	1–5, variable	Preaxial polydactyly of feet, syndactyly of toes, macrocephaly with frontal bossing, absence of corpus callosum	AD/175700 GLI3/7p14.1
Laurin-Sandrow	1–5	Mirror polysyndactyly of hands and feet, ulnar and fibular dimelia, dysplasia or absence of the radius and tibia, cleft nares	AD/135750 14q13
Oculodentodigital (ODD)	4–5	Syndactyly of third and fourth toes, microcephaly, intellectual disability, hearing loss, brain abnormalities abnormalities, microphthalmia, cleft lip/palate, microdontia, enamel hypoplasia, hyperostosis of skull and vertebrae, palmoplantar keratoderma	AD/164200 GJA1/6p22.31
Oral-facial-digital II, Mohr (OFD II)	1–5	Preaxial polysyndactyly of the feet, cleft tongue, midline partial cleft lip, hypertrophic frenulae, hamartomas of the tongue, conductive deafness	AR/252100
Pallister–Hall	4–5	Postaxial/mesoaxial polydactyly, hypothalamic hamartoblastoma, hypopituitarism, imperforate anus, abnormal or absent epiglottis, early death	AD/146510 GLI3/7p14.1
Poland	Unilateral brachydactyly, syndactyly, oligodactyly	Aplasia of the pectoralis major, cardiac defects, rib anomalies, can be seen with Moebius	AD or sporadic/173800 Unknown

There are single reports of families in which brachydactyly occurs as a dominant trait with one or two other features, but the genetics of these conditions is not well defined. These single-family reports will not be included in this review. Numerous multiple malformation syndromes have brachydactyly as a prominent or cardinal feature. Some of the more common of these are listed in Table 2.11.

Cornelia de Lange, or Brachman de Lange, syndrome is a multiple malformation syndrome that was first described in severely affected cases in which there was moderate to severe intellectual disability and severely affected upper limbs with oligodactyly and ulnar deficiency. Short stature and microcephaly were often severe. The facial appearance was also striking, with high arched eyebrows and synophrys, a small upturned nose, and a long philtrum with thin lips and a crescent-shaped mouth with downturned edges. Most cases were sporadic. When the first gene was identified, NIPBL, the phenotype was found to be much more variable in

Table 2.9 Genetics of isolated brachydactyly

Classification	Description	Genetics OMIM
Type A1	Brachymesophalangy II–V; brachyphalangy I	AD/112500 IHH/2q35 BDA1B/5p13.3-p13.2
Type A2	Brachymesophalangy II	AD/112600 BMPR1B/4q22.3 BMP2/20p12.3 GDF5/20q11.22
Type A3	Brachymesophalangy V	AD/112700
Type B	Aplasia terminal phalanges, II–V, hypoplasia middle phalanges, II–V, broad distal phalanges, I, symphalangism, syndactyly	AD/113000 ROR2/9q22.31
Type C	Hypersegmentation of proximal and middle phalanges, II, III, brachymesophalangy II and III, ulnar deviation II and III	AD/113100 GDF5/20q11.22
Type D	Stub thumb; short, broad thumb distal phalanx	AD/113200 HOXD13/2q31.1
Type E	Brachymetacarpia, variable	AD/113300 HOXD13/2q31.1
Sugarman	Brachydactyly with major proximal phalangeal shortening, duplicated first metacarpals	AR/272150
Temtamy type (Type A4, not classified by Bell)	Brachymesophalangy II and V	AD/112800

Table 2.10 Skeletal dysplasias with brachydactyly[a]

Achondrogenesis	Lenz–Majewski hyperostotic dwarfism
Achondroplasia	Metaphyseal chondrodysplasia (McKusick)
Acrodysostosis	Metaphyseal dysplasia with exocrine pancreatic
Acrodysplasia with retinitis pigmentosa and nephropathy	insufficiency and cyclic neutropenia metatropic dysplasia
Acromesomelic dysplasia, Campailla-Martielli	Moerman lethal short limb dwarfism with brain abnormalities
Acromesomelic dysplasia, Maroteaux	Multiple epiphyseal dysplasia
Acromicric dysplasia	Nance–Sweeney dwarfism
Asphyxiating thoracic dystrophy	Opsismodysplasia
Atelosteogenesis	Osebold–Remondini
Campomelic dysplasia	Osteoglophonic dwarfism
Cephaloskeletal dysplasia	Osteosclerosis, Stanescu
Chondrodysplasia punctata	Oto-palato-digital
Chondrodysplasia, Grebe type	Pseudoachondrodysplasia
Chondrodysplasia, Hunter–Thompson type	Pycnodysostosis
Cleidocranial dysplasia	Robinow
Cranioectodermal dysplasia	Ruvalcava
Deafness and metaphyseal dysplasia	Short rib-polydactyly
Dyggve–Melchior–Clausen	Spondyloepimetaphyseal dysplasia, Irapa type
Dyschonrosteosis	Spondyloepiphyseal dysplasia congenital
Dyssegmental dysplasia	Spondylometaphyseal dysplasia, Kozlowski
Ellis–van Creveld	Spondyloperipheral dysostosis
Enchondromatosis	Thanatophoric-clover leaf skull
Fibrochondrogenesis	Thanatophoric dysplasia
Geleophysic dysplasia	Thricho-rhino-phalangeal
Hypochondroplasia	Weill–Marchesani
Larsen	

[a]Adapted from Everman DB. Hands and feet. In: Stevenson RE, Hall JG, eds. Human malformations and related anomalies, 2nd edition. New York: Oxford University Press; 2006. By permission of Oxford University Press, USA

Table 2.11 Syndromes with brachydactyly as a major feature

Syndrome	Hand features	Other cardinal features	Inheritance/OMIM Gene/locus
Aarskog	Brachydactyly of all fingers with clinodactyly of fifth, unusual positioning of fingers on extension	Short stature, hypertelorism, shawl scrotum	XL/305400 FGD1/Xp11.21
Acrodysostosis	Brachyphalangia and brachymetacarpia	Brachymetatarsia Brachymelic short stature, saddle nose, intellectual disability	AD/101800 PRKARIA/17q24.2 PDE4D, 5q11.2-12.1
Adams–Oliver	Digits may be short or have terminal transverse defects	Cutis aplasia, terminal transverse defects of limbs, intellectual disability in recessive form	AD/100300 ARHGAP31, 3q13.33 AR/614219 DOCK6/19p13.2
Albright hereditary osteodystrophy	Short distal phalanx of thumb, brachymetacarpia (4 and 5)	Short stature, intellectual disability, obesity, round face, resistance to PTH, TSH, and GHRH, hypogonadism	AD/103580 GNAS1/20q13.2
Brachydactyly–ectrodactyly-fibular aplasia (Genuardi)	Brachydactyly, ectrodactyly	Fibular aplasia or hypoplasia	AD/113310
Brachydactyly-hallux varus-thumb abduction (Christian)	Brachymetacarpia (1), broad abducted thumbs	Hallux varus	AD/112450
Brachydactyly-hypertension	Brachyphalangy, brachymetacarpia	Hypertension	AD/112410 12p12.2-p11.2
Carpenter syndrome	Brachydactyly with clinodactyly, postaxial polydactyly, broad bifid thumbs, syndactyly (2–5)	Brachycephaly, craniosynostosis, intellectual disability	AR/201000 RAB23/6p11.2
Coffin–Lowry	Brachydactyly with tapering fingers, tufted drumstick appearance to distal phalanges on X-ray, small fingernails	Short stature, short bifid sternum with pectus deformities, coarse facial features, hypertelorism, scoliosis, hypodontia, rectal/uterine prolapse	XL/303600 RPS6KA3/Xp22.12
Coffin–Siris	Hypoplasia of 5th fingers (particularly distal phalanx), absence of 5th fingernail	Hypoplastic or absent toenails, short stature, sparse scalp hair, intellectual disability, coarse facial features, wide mouth with full lips, feeding difficulties, frequent infections	AR/135900 7q32-q34
Cohen	Brachymetacarpia, narrow hands	Short stature, obesity, prominent upper central incisors, intellectual disability	AR/2165500 COH1/8q22.2
Cornelia de Lange	Brachymetacarpia (1), clinodactyly (5), oligodactyly, ulnar deficiency	Short stature, microcephaly, intellectual disability, characteristic face with arched eyebrows, synophrys, down turned mouth and upturned nose, hirsuitism, variable phenotype	AD/122470+ NIPBL/5p13.2 RAD21/8q24.11 CSPG6/10q25.2 XL/300040+ SMC1A/Xp11.22 HDAC8/Xq13.1
Cranioectodermal dysplasia	Brachydactyly, single transverse palmar creases, clinodactyly (5) short, broad distal phalanges	Short stature, sagittal craniosynostosis, skeletal dysplasia, fine, sparse hair, lax skin, dental abnormalities, liver and kidney failure	AR/218330+ IFT122/3q21.3-q22.1 WDR35/2p24.1 IFT43/14q24.3 WDR19/4p14
DOOR	Hypoplastic or absent distal phalanges, triphalangeal thumbs	Sensorineural deafness, onychodystrophy, osteodystrophy, intellectual disability, seizures, visual impairment, microcephaly	AR/220500 TBC1D24/16p13.3
Floating Harbor	Brachydactyly, clinodactyly (5), broad thumbs	Short stature, severe speech and language delay, deep set eyes, bulbous nose, behavioral problems	AD/136140 SRCAP/16p11.2
Hand–foot–genital	Short, proximally placed thumbs, brachydactyly (5), ulnar deviation (2), clinodactyly (5), hypoplastic middle phalanges, delayed ossification of carpals, short 1st metacarpals, pseudoepiphyses	Absent/short halluces with medial deviation, brachydactyly, delayed ossification of tarsals, short first metatarsal, hypoplastic distal and middle phalanges of feet, genital defects (internal—female, external—male)	AD/140000 HOXA13/7p15.2

(continued)

Table 2.11 (continued)

Syndrome	Hand features	Other cardinal features	Inheritance/OMIM Gene/locus
Holt–Oram	Spectrum of upper limb defects, primarily involving the radial ray but can include the ulna, humerus, and the shoulder girdle; brachydactyly, oligodactyly, syndactyly	Cardiac defects include ventricular septal defect, atrial septal defect, and others	AD/142900 TBX5/12q24.1
Kabuki	Brachydactyly, short middle phalanges, short metacarpals (4 and 5), clinodactyly (5), prominent fingertip pads	Distinctive facial features with long palpebral fissures and lateral ectropion, ptosis, cleft palate, cardiac defects, hyperextensible joints, intellectual disability	AD/147920 MLL2/12q13.12 XL/300867 KDM6A/Xp11.3
Moebius	Brachydactyly, oligodactyly	Sixth and seventh nerve palsy, absent pectoral muscles, Klippel–Feil anomaly	AD/157900 Linked to several loci
Pfeiffer	Brachymesophalangy, syndactyly, broad and medially deviated distal phalanx of thumb	Syndactyly of toes, broad and medially deviated distal phalanges of great toe, craniosynostosis, hypertelorism, brachycephaly	AD/101600 FGFR1/8p11.23-p11.22 FGFR2/10q26.13
Poland	Unilateral brachydactyly, syndactyly, oligodactyly	Aplasia of the pectoralis major, cardiac defects, rib anomalies, can be seen with Moebius	AD or sporadic/173800 Unknown
Robinow	Brachydactyly, brachymetacarpia, bifid terminal phalanges, clinodactyly (5), hypoplastic/absent thumbs	Short stature, hypertelorism, costovertebral abnormalities, "fetal face"	AD/180700 WNT5A/3p14.3 AR/268130 ROR2/9q22.31
Rubinstein–Taybi	Brachydactyly, broad thumbs with radial deviation, clinodactyly (5)	Broad great toes, short stature, intellectual disability, microcephaly, downslanting palpebral fissures, narrow palate, beaked nose, grimacing smile	AD/180849 CREBBP/16p13.3 Deletion 16p13.3
Saethre–Chotzen	Brachydactyly, clinodactyly, 2–3 syndactyly	3–4 syndactyly of toes, craniosynostosis, ossification defects and hyperostosis of skull, short clavicles, facial asymmetry	AD/101400 TWIST/7p21 FGFR2/10q26.13 FGFR3/4p16.3
Schinzel–Giedion	Brachydactyly, brachymetacarpia (1), hypoplastic distal phalanges	Severe pes planus, short stature, intellectual disability, seizures, sclerotic skull and long bones, skeletal abnormalities, renal and genital anomalies	AD/269150 SETBP1/18q12.3
Smith–Magenis	Brachydactyly, broad hands	Brachycephaly, broad, flat midface, intellectual disability, sleep disturbance, characteristic behavior	AD/182290 RAI1/17p11.2 Deletion 17p11.2
Townes–Brocks	Distal deviation of thumbs, hypoplastic thumbs, preaxial polydactyly	Microcephaly, ear anomalies and hearing loss, anal and intestinal atresias, genital anomalies, renal anomalies and kidney disease	AD/107480 SALL1/16q21.1
Turner	Brachymetacarpia (4 and 5)	Short stature, webbed neck, ovarian failure, horseshoe kidney, coarctation of the aorta	Monosomy X

affected individuals. In particular the upper limb defects ranged from the classical findings of ulnar ray deficiency, to individuals with small hands, and individuals with brachydactyly. Following that, several more genes were identified that caused the same phenotype, confirming the inheritance as both autosomal dominant and X-linked.

Syndromes with Oligodactyly/Reduction Defects

The final category of syndromes with hand defects involves a group of syndromes in which the hands have reduction defects, resulting in either oligodactyly or adactyly (Table 2.12). Reduction defects are usually divided into those with radial ray defects and those with ulnar ray defects, and then a third category for conditions in which either or both rays might be involved. The reduction defects may just involve the digits, leading to oligodactyly, or may involve whole parts of the hand and/or upper extremity. They can be classified by the part of the hand structure that is involved.

Hand malformations are an important feature of many multiple malformation syndromes, and the genes involved give clues to the morphogenesis of the limbs as well as many other areas of development.

Table 2.12 Syndromes with oligodactyly or adactyly

Syndrome	Segment involved Radial (R), Ulnar (U), Middle (M), All (A)	Other cardinal features	Inheritance/OMIM Gene/locus
Adams–Oliver	R, M, U	Brachydactyly, cutis aplasia, intellectual disability in recessive form	AD/100300 ARHGAP31, 3q13.33 AR/614219 DOCK6/19p13.2
Brachydactyly–ectrodactyly-fibular aplasia (Genuardi)	M	Brachydactyly, fibular aplasia or hypoplasia	AD/113310
CHILD	M, U		XL/308050 NSDHL/Xq28
Cornelia de Lange	U, M	Short stature, microcephaly, intellectual disability, characteristic face with arched eyebrows, synophrys, down turned mouth and upturned nose, hirsuitism, variable phenotype	AD/122470+ NIPBL/5p13.2 RAD21/8q24.11 CSPG6/10q25.2 XL/300040+ SMC1A/Xp11.22 HDAC8/Xq13.1
Ectrodactyly–ectodermal dysplasia-clefting	M	Ectrodactyly of the feet, cleft lip/palate, light-colored and sparse hair, anodotia or oligodontia, tear duct anomalies, urinary tract abnormalities	AD/ TP63/
Fanconi anemia	R	Short stature, intellectual diability, renal anomalies, genital abnormalities, microcephaly, café au lait spots, deafness, cardiac defects, chromosomal breakage	AR/227650 PHF9/2p16.1 FANCD2/3p25.3 FANCE/6p21.31 XRCC9/9p13.3 FANCC/9q22.32 FANCF/11p14.3 BRCA2/13q13.1 FANCM/14q21.2 FANCI/15q26.1 SLX4/16p13.3 ERCC4/16p13.12 PALB2/16p12.2 FANCA/16q24.3 RAD51C/17q22 BRIP1/17q23.2 FAAP95/Xp22.2
Hand–foot–genital	R	Brachydactyly, clinodactyly (5), and ulnar deviation (2), abnormalities of the toes and metatarsals, primarily the great toe, brachydactyly of toes, genital defects (internal—female, external—male)	AD/140000 HOXA13/7p15.2
Holt–Oram	R	Brachydactyly, syndactyly, occasional involvement of shoulder girdle, cardiac defects include ventricular septal defect, atrial septal defect, and others	AD?142900 TBX5/12q24.1
Nager	R	Malar hypoplasia, downslanting palpebral fissures, partial absence of lower eyelashes, high nasal bridge, micrognathia, cleft palate, abnormal ears, radioulnar synostosis	AD/154400 SF3B4/1q21.2
Poland	Unilateral R	Unilateral aplasia of the pectoralis major with ipsilateral brachydactyly and syndactyly, cardiac defects, rib anomalies, can be seen with Moebius	AD or sporadic/173800 Unknown
Postaxial acrofacial dysostosis (POADS)—also known as Miller	U	Malar hypoplasia, downslanting palpebral fissures, eyelid coloboma, micrognathia, cleft lip/palate, abnormal ears, accessory nipples	AR/263750 DHODH/16q22.2

(continued)

Table 2.12 (continued)

Syndrome	Segment involved Radial (R), Ulnar (U), Middle (M), All (A)	Other cardinal features	Inheritance/OMIM Gene/locus
Roberts	U	Phocomelia, prenatal onset growth deficiency, microcephaly, ear, eye, heart and urogenital anomalies, intellectual disability	AR/268300 ESCO2/8p21.1
Robinow	R	Brachydactyly, short stature, hypertelorism, costovertebral abnormalities, "fetal face"	AD/180700 WNT5A/3p14.3 AR/268130 ROR2/9q22.31
Ulnar–mammary	U	Postaxial polydactyly, apocrine abnormalities, hypopigmentation and hypoplasia of areola, nipple and breast, genital anomalies in males, delayed puberty	AD/181450 TBX3/12q24.21
VACTERL	R	Vertebral defects, anal atresia, cardiac defects, renal defects, ear defects, tracheoesophageal atresia	

References

1. Rogala EJ, Wynne-Davies R, Littlejohn A, Gormley J. Congenital limb anomalies: frequency and aetiological factors. Data from the Edinburgh Register of the Newborn (1964-68). J Med Genet. 1974;11:221–33.
2. Temtamy SA, McKusick VA. The genetics of hand malformations. Birth Defects Orig Artic Ser. 1978;14(3):i–xviii, 1–619.
3. Giele H, Giele C, Bower C, Allison M. The incidence and epidemiology of congenital upper limb anomalies: a total population study. J Hand Surg Am. 2001;26(4):628–34.
4. Ekblom AG, Laurell T, Arner M. Epidemiology of congenital upper limb anomalies in 562 children born in 1997 to 2007: a total population study from Stockholm, Sweden. J Hand Surg Am. 2010;35(11):1742–54.
5. Koskimies E, Lindfors N, Gissler M, Peltonen J, Nietosvaara Y. Congenital upper limb deficiencies and associated malformations in Finland: a population-based study. J Hand Surg Am. 2011;36(6):1058–65.
6. Kallen B, Rahmani T, Winberg J. Infants with congenital limb reduction registered with the Swedish Register of Congenital Malformations. Teratology. 1984;29:73–85.
7. Aro T, Heinonen OP, Saxen L. Incidence and secular trends of congenital limb defects in Finland. Int J Epdemiol. 1982;3:239–44.
8. Froster U, Baird P. Upper limb deficiencies and associated malformations: a population-based study. Am J Med Genet. 1992;44:767–81.
9. Flatt AE. Classification and Incidence. In: The care of congenital hand anomalies. 2nd ed. St. Louis: Quality Medical Publishers; 1994. p. 47–63.
10. Lamb DW, Wynne-Davies R, Soto L. An estimate of the population frequency of congenital malformations of the upper limb. J Hand Surg Am. 1982;7(6):557–62.
11. Conway H, Bowe J. Congenital deformities of the hands. Plast Reconstr Surg. 1956;18:286–90.
12. Hermansson L, Bodin L, Wranne L. Upper Limb deficiencies in Swedish children—a comparison between a population-based and clinic-based register. Early Hum Dev. 2001;63:131–44.
13. Tonkin MA. Description of hand anomalies: a personal view. J Hand Surg Br. 2006;31B:489–97.
14. Miura T, Nakamura R, Horii E. The position of symbrachydactyly in the classification of congenital hand anomalies. J Hand Surg Br. 1994;19B:350–4.
15. Ogino T. Clinical and experimental studies on the teratogenic mechanisms of the cleft hand, polydactyly and syndactyly. J Jap Orthop Assoc. 1979;53:1753–60.
16. Ogino T. Teratogenic relationship between polydactyly, syndactyly and cleft hand. J Hand Surg Br. 1990;15B:201–9.
17. Yamaguchi S. Incidence of various congenital anomalies of the hand from 1961 to 1972. Japanese Society for Surgery of the Hand, Fukuoka, Japan, 1973, cited in: Flatt AE: The care of congenital hand anomalies. 2nd ed. St. Louis: Quality Medical Publishers; 1994. p. 62.
18. Ogino T, Minami A, Fukuda K, Kato H. Congenital anomalies of the upper limb among the Japanese in Sapporo. J Hand Surg Br. 1986;11B:364–71.
19. Cheng JCY, Chow SK, Leung PC. Classification of 578 cases of congenital upper limb anomalies with the IFSSH system—a 10 years' experience. J Hand Surg Am. 1987;12A(6):1055–60.
20. Castilla EE, Lugarinho R, da Graca Dutra M, Salgado LJ. Associated anomalies in individuals with polydactyly. Am J Med Genet. 1998;80(5):459–65.
21. Hildebrandt F, Benzing T, Katsanis N. Ciliopathies. N Engl J Med. 2011;364(16):1533–43.
22. Ansley SJ, Badano JL, Blacque OE, Hill J, Hoskins BE, Leitch CC, et al. Basal body dysfunction is a likely cause of pleiotropic Bardet-Biedl syndrome. Nature. 2003;425(6958):628–33.
23. Kim JC, Ou YY, Badano JL, Esmail MA, Leitch CC, Fiedrich E, et al. MKKS/BBS6, a divergent chaperonin-like protein linked to the obesity disorder Bardet-Biedl syndrome, is a novel centrosomal component required for cytokinesis. J Cell Sci. 2005;118(Pt 5):1007–20.
24. Romio L, Wright V, Price K, Winyard PJ, Donnai D, Porteous ME, et al. OFD1, the gene mutated in oral-facial-digital syndrome type 1, is expressed in the metanephros and in human embryonic renal mesenchymal cells. J Am Soc Nephrol. 2003;14(3):680–9.
25. Biesecker LG. What you can learn from one gene: GLI3. J Med Genet. 2006;43(6):465–9.
26. Johnston JJ, Sapp JC, Turner JT, Amor D, Aftimos S, Aleck KA, et al. Molecular analysis expands the spectrum of phenotypes associated with GLI3 mutations. Hum Mutat. 2010;31(10):1142–54.
27. Temtamy SA. Classification of hand malformations as isolated defects: an overview. J Genet Hum. 1982;30(4):281–90.
28. Everman DB. Hands and feet. In: Stevenson RE, Hall JG, editors. Human malformations and related anomalies. 2nd ed. New York: Oxford University Press; 2006.

Anesthesia Concerns in Congenital Anomalies of the Upper Extremity

3

Ann F.T. Lawrence, Emily L.A. Stebbins, and Borzoo Farhang

Introduction

Children with congenital anomalies of the upper extremity often have multiple congenital anomalies. These children have special needs, and every step requires specific planning and vigilance to ensure safe, effective, and exemplary delivery of anesthetic care. Preoperative discussions with surgeons, anesthesiologists, critical care physicians, pulmonologists, cardiologists, endocrinologists, geneticists, and/or nephrologists can turn what might have been a simple procedure into something more complex. These discussions should work toward a common goal of providing surgical care at the optimal time based on risk-assessment and clinical need.

Several issues that may be encountered preoperatively include anxiety, complex social situations, difficult intravenous access, an inability to tolerate safe fasting requirements, as well as common childhood problems such as upper respiratory infection (URI). Intraoperative considerations include difficult airway management, special positioning requirements, and systemic comorbidities. Extubation, disposition, and analgesia are only a few of the concerns and potential complications that can be encountered in the postoperative period. All of these considerations must be addressed to achieve the best possible outcome for patients undergoing surgery for congenital anomalies of the upper extremity. This chapter will address anesthetic concerns as they relate to the global patient population and several common congenital syndromes that present for surgical evaluation.

A.F.T. Lawrence, D.O. (✉) • E.L.A. Stebbins, M.D. • B. Farhang, D.O.
Department of Anesthesiology, The University of Vermont College of Medicine/Fletcher Allen Health Care, 111 Colchester Avenue, Burlington, VT 05401, USA
e-mail: ann.lawrence@vtmednet.org; Emily.Stebbins@vtmednet.org; Borzoo.Farhang@vtmednet.org

Anxiety

Preoperative anxiety is a significant problem that can add to delay and frustration on the day of surgery. All children should have some kind of psychological preparation for the hospital experience, particularly when accompanied by surgery [1]. In this regard patients with congenital anomalies present a unique population of children who often have had multiple previous exposures to hospitals and hospital staff. Although many of these encounters may seem benign, repetitive experiences, good or bad, can bias them for future hospital encounters [2]. In addition, situational anxiety of the parent, family composition, and the chronological or developmental age of the child can predispose a child to increased risk for anxiety [1, 3]. Postoperative implications of this preoperative anxiety can be profound. In young children, preoperative anxiety has been associated with a more painful postoperative recovery and higher incidence of nightmares, separation anxiety, eating problems, and an increased fear of physicians [1, 4]. The goal of the entire operating room team should be to make a child's preoperative experience as smooth as possible. Multiple modalities are available to provide anxiety relief to children undergoing upper extremity surgery. The most widely used modalities include preparation programs, parental presence, and premedication [2].

In many hospitals and medical centers, there is no formal preoperative preparation. Patient education in these hospitals is shared through printed materials and perhaps guided operating room tours [5]. Some programs are fortunate to have programs run by child life specialists. Studies have shown that these programs help reduce anxiety by enhancing the coping skills of children [6]. Many of these programs incorporate modeling, play therapy, printed and web site materials, operating room tours, and special coping techniques [6]. Unfortunately, studies have also found that children who have had prior surgeries or hospitalizations may react negatively when receiving a lot of new information prior to their procedure [7]. These children may benefit from a tailored preparation program, individualized to their specific learning

D.R. Laub Jr. (ed.), *Congenital Anomalies of the Upper Extremity: Etiology and Management*, DOI 10.1007/978-1-4899-7504-1_3, © Springer Science+Business Media New York 2015

and developmental delays and prior experiences. Such a program can make for a lengthy and labor-intensive process.

Another technique to address anxiety is parental presence in the operating room during induction. Purposed advantages are decreased need for preoperative sedatives, avoiding the fear that can occur on separation from a parent, smoother anesthetic induction, and decreased parental anxiety [8, 9]. One study showed an advantage to having maternal presence in the operating room, but emphasized the benefit is strongest in parents who are not anxious themselves [10]. Another study showed that premedication alone was more beneficial for preoperative anxiety in children, and parental presence offered no advantage. This study did, however, show that parents who accompany their child into the operating room had less anxiety and felt more satisfied with their overall anesthetic experience [11]. Possible disadvantages to parental presence include disruption of operating room routine and unpredictability of parental behavior [9]. It must also be noted that the practice of parental presence during induction of anesthesia is not allowed in all hospitals and therefore may not be an option.

Premedication is another option to address preoperative anxiety in children. In institutions with minimal resources for education or policies against parental presence for induction, premedication is widely available. Multiple medications have been used for preoperative sedation, including diazepam, ketamine, and clonidine; however, midazolam is the overwhelming choice among anesthesiologists [11].

Upper Respiratory Infection

Upper respiratory tract infection (URI) is a common childhood ailment that can affect children on the day of surgery. A child with a cold frequently presents the anesthesiologist with the dilemma of whether to proceed with the anesthetic or to postpone until the child is healthier [12]. Most agree that otherwise healthy children with mild uncomplicated URIs limited to the nose and upper parts of the throat, not involving airway instrumentation, can safely be anesthetized without any increased risk [13]. Factors that may increase risk of anesthesia in children with URIs include history of passive smoking, snoring, productive cough, production of sputum, fever, nasal congestion, lethargy, and wheezing [12, 13]. Type of surgery also increases the risk when a URI is present, with the highest risk in airway surgery. In one study, ENT surgery was shown to be up to nine times more likely than orthopedic surgery to have adverse respiratory events associated with a URI [14]. In some children with congenital anomalies even a mild, seemingly uncomplicated URI can cause problems. Children with Apert syndrome, for example, are already at increased risk for airway complications as many have obstructive sleep apnea (OSA) due to their nasopharyngeal malformation [15]. Adding a simple cold to this risk can severely complicate the anesthetic course. Decisions regarding the viability of proceeding with anesthesia must be made on an individualized basis. Identifying risk factors, the electiveness of surgery, and the anesthesiologist's experience and comfort anesthetizing the child, must all be taken into consideration before proceeding with surgery [14]. Once the decision to cancel the procedure is made, surgery should be postponed for a minimum of 4 weeks to optimally decrease the risk of any adverse respiratory events [13, 14].

Fasting Requirements

To minimize the risk of pulmonary aspiration of gastric contents, infants and children are fasted before sedation and anesthesia. The American Society of Anesthesiologists [ASA] has developed preoperative fasting guidelines, updated on a regular basis and found www.asahq.org. In healthy patients undergoing elective surgery, patients should fast for 2 h for clear liquids, 4 h for breast milk, 6 h for formula and non-human milk, 6 h for a light meal (plain toast and clear liquid), and 8 h or more for meals that include fried/fatty food or meat. It should be noted that these are just guidelines and in no way ensure that a patient will not aspirate. In addition, patients with syndromes such as arthrogryposis are at increased risk for aspiration due to poor airway reflexes and gastroesophageal reflux [16]. These patients may benefit from longer fasting periods and intravenous fluids prior to surgery. The ultimate decision to extend these fasting times should be based on the comorbidities of each individual patient.

Intravenous Catheters

In children, peripheral intravenous access can be obtained before or after induction of general anesthesia depending on the clinical situation. Intravenous access is ideally obtained in the nonoperative extremity and in a different extremity from the blood pressure cuff.

The appropriate catheter is chosen based on the patient's size and expected fluid requirement. In most cases a 24-gauge catheter is sufficient for infants and a 22-gauge catheter for children [17]. Should the patient require significant volume replacement, multiple catheters can be inserted [18]. Difficult intravenous access should be anticipated in patients with a history of multiple hospitalizations and procedures as well as dehydration.

When more than one extremity is prepped and draped for the planned procedure, such as harvesting donor nerves, limited availably of access sites makes intravenous access a challenge. Furthermore, patients between the ages of 9–12 months present an additional challenge due to distribution of subcutaneous fat [19]. In such cases, additional time to obtain intravenous access must be anticipated.

Antibiotic Prophylaxis

Although historically many patients with congenital heart disease (CHD) received antibiotic prophylaxis for endocarditis, recommendations have changed and were updated again in 2007. Currently, antibiotic prophylaxis is recommended in patients with specific cardiac lesions undergoing certain dental procedures, procedures on the respiratory tract involving incision or biopsy of the respiratory mucosa, and for surgical manipulation of infected areas of the skin, subcutaneous tissue, and musculoskeletal tissue. The specific cardiac conditions for antibiotic prophylaxis include children with a history of infective endocarditis, unrepaired cyanotic CHD, a completely repaired CHD with prosthetic material (within the first 6 months of surgery), and repaired CHD with residual defects at the site of the prosthetic material. Although prosthetic cardiac valve repair and cardiac transplantation with residual valvulopathy are less common in children, antibiotics are also recommended in patients with these conditions [20]. The pediatric cardiologist should be consulted prior to making a final decision regarding antibiotic prophylaxis in this patient population.

Thermoregulation

Thermoregulation during the operative period is critical. Delayed wound healing, coagulopathy, and infection are known complications of hypothermia. In addition, hypothermia can lead to pharmacologic inhibition of muscle activity and blunting of the thermoregulatory pathways. In newborns, inhalational anesthetics inhibit non-shivering thermogenesis from brown fat which further exposes them to risk of hypothermia [21]. Hypothermia, especially in neonates, delays metabolism and excretion of anesthetics and prolongs neuromuscular blockade [22]. Under anesthesia the most common types of heat loss are radiation and convection. Heat loss can be minimized most effectively by warming the operating room to 80 °F and using radiant heat lamps. Once the patient is draped, the operating room temperature may be decreased and forced air heating blankets used [23].

Positioning

Patients under general anesthesia are vulnerable to injury resulting from prolonged immobility, the inability to voluntarily change position, and/or improper positioning. Most vulnerable to injury are peripheral nerves (such as ulnar and peroneal), male genitalia, and nipples. In the prone position, the brachial plexus is vulnerable to stretch [24]. It is paramount to ensure adequate pressure-point padding (elbows, breasts, scrotum, and feet) to decrease the risk of peripheral nerve compression and soft tissue damage [24].

Regional Anesthesia with Upper Extremity Nerve Block

The mainstay of pain management traditionally has been opioid therapy for acute pain. However, a multimodal approach to pain management has been shown to provide superior results while minimizing side effects of opioids such as nausea, vomiting, pruritus, urinary retention, and constipation [25]. Use of regional techniques, either a single injection block or a continuous infusion catheter, can provide superior pain control, improve patient satisfaction, decrease discharge time from the post-anesthesia care unit, and decrease total cost [26, 27].

Upper extremity nerve blocks may be used for surgery of the shoulder, arm, and hand. Depending on the surgical site, the anesthesiologist may use one of several blocks of the brachial plexus. The interscalene block is useful for surgical procedures of the shoulder and upper arm and the supraclavicular can be used for surgery of upper and lower arm. The axillary block is best for analgesia and anesthesia of the lower arm and hand; however with this technique a second injection may be required to block the musculocutaneous nerve. The infraclavicular nerve block has been used as well, but is not often performed in children due to increased risk of pneumothorax.

Contraindications to regional anesthesia in pediatric population include the presence of a skin lesion at the site of injection, severe systemic infection, severe thrombocytopenia, and a history of previous nerve injury. Perhaps the most important contraindication to regional anesthesia is refusal by the parent or guardian. Placement of cast or brace on the operative limb is not a contraindication, but additional monitoring should be planned to assess perfusion [28].

In children, unlike adults, it is considered standard practice to perform most major regional blocks under general anesthesia or deep sedation. This is done to ensure the safety of a patient who could potentially move and cause unintentional injury. In recent history, ultrasound has been billed as a safer technique than the traditional nerve stimulator guided blocks. Some studies have shown the use of ultrasound provides a safe and effective block, with less local anesthetic in children as young as 6 months of age [29]. These studies however have been limited in size and therefore further studies, especially in the youngest patients, are needed to better evaluate the risks and benefits of this procedure.

Regional anesthesia can be performed safely in the hands of experienced anesthesiologists to patients of any age [28]; however, many institutions do not perform upper extremity nerve blocks in children under general anesthesia.

Tourniquets

Tourniquet application in orthopedic surgery is common to improve visualization of the operative field and limit blood loss. However, high tourniquet pressure and long tourniquet times lead to increased risk of neurologic complication [30, 31]. The most common complication of tourniquet use is nerve injury, likely due to mechanical compression and neural ischemia. The injury can be transient or irreversible [32]. There are no absolute rules for tourniquet time and pressure and there is minimal literature regarding the use of tourniquets in pediatric patients [31, 32]. Lynn et al. studied 15 healthy children to assess the effects of tourniquet release under general anesthesia. The operative extremity was exsanguinated and the tourniquet was inflated to ≥75 mmHg higher than the awake systolic blood pressure. With tourniquet deflation, there was a statistically significant respiratory and lactic acidosis [30]. If emergence and extubation immediately follow tourniquet release, this acidosis must be considered.

In a survey of 92 US and Canadian pediatric orthopedic surgeons, the most common complication in pediatric patients was skin damage. The selection of tourniquet pressure varies from using a standard pressure (100 mmHg over the systolic blood pressure or two times the systolic blood pressure); the age, extremity, and size of the patient; or the patient's blood pressure. With no standard recommendation, pressures used may be higher than necessary [31]. While complications rates are relatively low, longer tourniquet time increases the risk of neurologic complication, and tourniquet time should be kept to a minimum. As a general rule, tourniquet time should not exceed 3 h and ideally not exceed 2 h [33]. Tredwell et al. have made several recommendations for tourniquet use in the pediatric patient, including inflating the tourniquet in 25-mmHg increments until arterial flow has stopped, using protective padding and minimizing tourniquet time [31].

General Postoperative Care

Several complications can occur in the PACU. Inadequate pain control, respiratory depression, postoperative nausea and vomiting (PONV), and apnea are among the most common. Premature infants are at increased risk for developing apnea within the first 24–48 h after surgery. Apnea is a stress response in neonates, and inadequate analgesia is associated with increased apnea and respiratory complications in this age group. The risk of developing postoperative apnea in premature neonates is inversely proportional to post-conceptual age at the time of surgery and remains significant up to 60 weeks post-conceptual age (and 1 month in full-term infants). If surgery is required within this time period, overnight observation and monitoring are indicated [34].

Combining nonsteroidal anti-inflammatory drugs, acetaminophen, opioids, and regional analgesia have an invaluable role in postoperative pain management. Patient-controlled analgesia (PCA), nurse-controlled analgesia, and parent-controlled analgesia can all be used postoperatively depending on the accepted practice of the institution. PCA has been successfully used in children as young as 5 years [35]. A pain-free experience is an illusion. Nevertheless, practitioners should strive to achieve tolerable pain control in the perioperative setting.

Anesthesia Concerns of Specific Congenital Syndromes/Anomalies

Amniotic Band Syndrome

Amniotic band syndrome (ABS) results from premature intrauterine rupture of the amnion leading to oligohydramnios with fetal passage into the chorionic cavity. This leads to unpredictable anomalies of the fetus including extremity, thorax, and craniofacial skeletal and soft tissue changes [36]. This occurs in 1:2,000 to 1:15,000 live births and there is no predilection for race, ethnicity, or gender [37]. Potential causes include genetic mutation, teratogenicity (has occurred in twins), abnormal intrauterine environment (based on the presence of pseudosyndactyly and rare occurrences within families) and maternal factors [37].

Defects relate to timing of the amnion rupture during development [36]. Bands of the extremities are most common [37], including clubfoot and clubhand [38]. Craniofacial involvement occurs in about one-third of cases [36], with cleft lip and/or palate in up to 15 % of cases [37]. Cleft anomalies are thought to occur from fetal swallowing of amniotic bands at about 5 weeks gestation [36]. Recent literature suggests that the pattern of cleft lip and/or palate have a more typical pattern instead of random [39]. Banding can create a clinical presentation similar to Pierre Robin as the bands pull the head to the chest wall, compress the mandible and impair fusion of the palate [37].

Preoperative Preparation

Airway evaluation is critical, especially with craniofacial involvement. Old anesthetic records are helpful to determine previous airway management. If there are no prior records, the anesthesiologist should be prepared for a difficult airway. The decision to proceed with a mask versus intravenous induction should be made on an individual basis based on the perceived difficulty of mask ventilation and intubation as well as intravenous placement with extremity anomalies. In patients with severe scoliosis, there may be pulmonary or cardiac disease due to restricted thoracic size [40]. Preoperative assessment by cardiology and/or pulmonology should be considered to assess readiness for surgery and to optimize treatment for the underlying disease.

Induction and Maintenance of Anesthesia

Each patient with ABS will have a unique pattern of constrictions and contractures requiring an individualized anesthetic airway plan. Use of airway adjuncts such as laryngeal mask airways (LMAs) may not be feasible. In one case report, video laryngoscope was used successfully; however fiber optic intubation should also be considered [41]. Positioning of patients with abnormal extremity contractures can be difficult and care must be taken to support and pad pressure points appropriately prior to surgical incision.

Postoperative

Timing of extubation in patients with severe craniofacial anomalies should be determined on a case-by-case basis. Special mattresses or beds may be required based on the extent of the disease to ensure adequate padding and support. Routine postoperative pain management should be followed.

Apert Syndrome

Apert syndrome falls under the broad classification of craniofacial/limb anomalies. Apert's is an autosomal-dominant syndrome caused by one of two mutations on chromosome 10. Children with this syndrome exhibit irregular craniosynostosis associated with a tall brachycephalic skull, mid-face hypoplasia, and bilateral syndactyly of the hands and feet [42].

Associated anomalies include choanal stenosis, ventriculomegaly, hydrocephalous, developmental delay, congenital cardiac and renal defects, and fusion of the cervical spine [43, 44]. These children can have wide variations in learning abilities, from severe cognitive delays to normal intelligence [43, 45]. They can display expressive language difficulties as well as fine motor deficits due to hand anomalies [43]. Specific concerns when preparing for anesthesia include difficulty of airway management and predisposition to OSA. The potential for increased intracranial pressure (ICP) and difficulties with communication can also complicate the care of these children.

Patients with Apert's often have a difficult airway due to cervical fusion and structural abnormalities of the midface. Cervical fusion involving C5-C6 is present in 71 % of patients [44], which limits range of motion and can make airway instrumentation more difficult. Difficult mask fit secondary to hypertelorism and proptosis [46] can contribute to the dreaded scenario of "cannot ventilate, cannot intubate." In addition, patients have maxillary hypoplasia, a narrowed nasopharyngeal airway [46] and choanal stenosis [47], resulting in predominant mouth breathing. Obstruction of the oropharynx can lead to significant difficulty in ventilation [46]. A large percentage of patients also have OSA and are at risk for cognitive dysfunction, insulin resistance, hypertension, and cor pulmonale [43, 48–50] as well as airway obstruction.

In nearly half of children with Apert's, lower airway compromise can also be an issue due to complete or partial cartilage sleeve abnormalities of the trachea with fusion of the tracheal rings [15, 43]. Even a small decrease in cross-sectional area can significantly contribute to airway obstruction [46]. Although increased ICP is present in up to one-third of patients, and is borderline in another third, elevated ICP is usually not problematic in patients with Apert's undergoing upper limb surgery.

While communication with these patients can be difficult due to their expressive language difficulties and cognitive delays, nearly 50 % of patients with Apert syndrome do have normal or borderline IQs (IQ>70) [45]. In all children, communication with the parent or guardian is of the utmost importance. Assistance from a child life specialist, if available, may be helpful in helping the child's caregiver understand the process and ensure appropriate communication [51].

Preoperative Evaluation

Since patients with Apert syndrome are often exposed to multiple anesthetics, it is important to gather information pertaining to previous surgeries. On physical exam, the mobility of the head and neck should be evaluated in conjunction with obtaining a history of any prior difficult ventilation or intubation. The need to place an intravenous line (IV) prior to entering the operating room (OR) should be addressed. This decision must take into account the anxiety surrounding IV placement, as well as possible limited access due to the nature of the surgery. In children with a history of sleep apnea, a polysomnogram with room air arterial oxygen saturation and evaluation of any cardiac disturbances should be obtained [46]. Renal and cardiac defects are reported in some patients with Apert's and these should be clearly defined prior to surgery [43]. Any significant symptoms due to increased ICP must be evaluated and addressed. History of current or recent URI should be noted since there are increased respiratory complications in this patient population [15]. If adjunctive regional anesthesia is to be used, this will also need to be discussed, and a plan formulated. Finally a plan should be made for dealing with the potential anxiety of the patient and their family with the common goal of making the preoperative experience as smooth as possible.

Induction and Maintenance of Anesthesia

There is no preferred method of inducing and maintaining anesthesia. The decision is made based on the exact nature and length of the surgery [46]. All patients get standard monitors including ECG, pulse oximetry, and blood pressure monitoring. The decision to induce anesthesia with an IV or an inhalation induction should have been made prior to entering the OR and is usually based on the anesthesiologist's preference and difficulty of the airway. Proper sized oral airways, LMAs, endotracheal tubes, laryngoscopes, and fiberoptic tools should be readily available. After induction of general anesthesia, preparation should be made if a regional block is to be placed. Special attention should be given to protecting the eyes and proper padding and positioning of the body. The patient's temperature should be monitored, and appropriate warming should be instituted based on the length of the surgery and the size of the patient. A discussion of whether or not to use muscle relaxation should occur between the surgical and anesthesia teams as well as the need for preoperative antibiotics. Anesthesia may be maintained by volatile or intravenous agents, and narcotics and other analgesics are titrated to effect. Once the surgery has ended, the patient should be breathing spontaneously and fully awake prior to removing the endotracheal tube [46]. The patient should be placed in a position that allows for patency of the airway. If the lateral position proves to be best, care must be taken to place the surgical side up to avoid any extra pain or injury. The patient should be transported to the recovery room with careful monitoring of breathing and use of oxygen if need be.

Postoperative Concerns

Once in the post-anesthesia recovery unit, patients should be monitored for apnea, pain, and temperature, as well as observing for any complication from the surgery. Children with cardiac anomalies or cardiac manifestations of OSA should be monitored closely for additional hemodynamic changes including cardiac rhythm and blood pressure abnormalities. Children who have severe enough sleep apnea to require CPAP should have their machines readily available for use in the PACU.

Arthrogryposis

Arthrogryposis multiplex congenita (AMC) is an uncommon condition with multiple persistent joint contractures [16]. It results from neuropathic, myopathic, or connective tissue abnormalities, as well as maternal disorders and conditions that would lead to decreased limb movement in utero [52, 53]. There are over 300 conditions in which AMC may be present [53]. Children with this syndrome often need surgical intervention to correct contractures affecting mostly distal joints [54]. The various associated abnormalities more relevant to the anesthesiologist include scoliosis and resultant pulmonary dysfunction, hypoplasia of the lungs, tracheal stenosis, and structural abnormalities of the kidneys [55]. Gastroschisis, bowel atresia, and cleft palate may also be found in these patients [56, 57]. In some patients there is associated CHD, including patent ductus arteriosus, aortic stenosis, coarctation of the aorta, and various forms of cyanotic heart disease [58, 59]. Complications of CHD in these patients include pulmonary hypertension and cor pulmonale [52].

Difficulty of airway management is of grave concern in patients with arthrogryposis. These patients may present with severe micrognathia and a short, rigid neck. They may also have cleft palate, temporomandibular joint rigidity, limited mouth opening, and occasional fusion or underdevelopment of the first and second cervical vertebrae [55–57].

Patients with arthrogryposis have atrophic changes of skin and subcutaneous tissue and extensive contractures that can make IV placement extremely difficult [55, 57, 60]. The laterality of the surgery also limits sites for IV access. Despite potential difficult IV placement, some anesthesiologist will opt for IV access before induction of anesthesia to administer atropine and other emergency drugs [57].

Children should be carefully padded since they are at increased risk of injury due to their multiple joint contractures, minimal muscle mass, atrophic skin, and deficient subcutaneous tissue abnormalities [55, 56, 60].

These children are prone to unusual reactions to anesthetic drugs [54, 55, 58]. They are very sensitive to opioids and other anesthetics and are prone to hypotension due to their myopathy and skeletal deformities [55, 58, 60, 61]. They can have a hyperkalemic response to succinylcholine [55, 60]. In the myopathic form of arthrogryposis, patients can develop a hypermetabolic response to all types of anesthesia [58]. Case studies have reported hyperpyrexia in these children that responds well to cooling. This reaction is not associated with malignant hyperthermia (MH); however, it is possible for AMC and MH to present independently in the same patient [56, 62, 63].

Lastly, these patients have respiratory depression with alveolar hypoventilation, microatelectasis, and decreased ability to cough due to associated myopathy, pulmonary hypoplasia, and skeletal deformities [55, 58]. Respiratory issues can further be compromised by recurrent aspiration related to poor airway reflexes and gastroesophageal reflux [16].

Preoperative Evaluation

Patients with arthrogryposis often require multiple surgeries for correction of skeletal deformities and associated visceral anomalies. As with any patient with potential anesthetic concerns, all information regarding previous anesthetics should be obtained. History of difficult endotracheal intubation as well as steps to successful intubation should be noted.

A thorough evaluation of mouth opening, mandibular size, and neck mobility should be performed [60]. In older children with cervical spine symptoms, it may be advisable to obtain diagnostic neuroimaging of the craniocervical junction [16]. A plan for intubation should be formulated including the need for a backup surgical team with a rigid bronchoscope and a tracheostomy tray ready in the case of a failed airway [57]. Plans should be made for appropriate patient support, such as child life specialists and nursing for placement of an intravenous line. All previous unusual reactions to medication should be reviewed. Any comorbid conditions should be addressed and evaluations obtained from appropriate services such as cardiology, pulmonology, gastroenterology, and urology. Any history of current or recent URIs as well as history of pneumonia should also be obtained due to patients' compromised respiratory function. Fasting times should be carefully reviewed since aspiration related to poor airway reflexes and gastroesophageal reflux could cause prolonged intubation and an ICU stay [16]. Although the use of peripheral nerve blocks in these children may prove difficult, there have been case reports of delivering regional anesthesia as the primary anesthetic [55, 56, 60]. If chosen, this plan will need to be discussed with the family as well as the surgical team to decide if it is the best method for treatment of the child.

Induction and Maintenance of Anesthesia

Although there is no established method of anesthesia in these patients, when a difficult airway is suspected, an inhalation induction with spontaneous ventilation is often employed until the endotracheal tube is in place [54, 60]. All airway equipment for a difficult intubation should be close by including appropriate sized LMAs and fiberoptic scopes [16]. Case studies demonstrated the utility of using the LMA as a conduit for fiberoptic endotracheal tube placement in these patients, and the use of LMAs has since been described in current anesthesia textbooks [57]. As previously stated, even if an inhalation technique is chosen, it may be wise to place an IV prior to entering the OR for administration of atropine, and other emergency medications [57]. Placement of blood pressure cuff, pulse oximeter, and ECG should occur before induction if possible. Temperature monitoring and appropriate warming devices should be in place, as well as a means to cool the patient if they become hyperpyrexic. Special attention should be given to padding pressure points since these children are at increased risk of injury from malpositioning [55, 56, 60]. Anesthesia may be maintained by intravenous or inhalation agents and opioids must be titrated conservatively due to the potential for an exaggerated response [54, 55]. At the conclusion of the surgery, the patient should be breathing spontaneously and fully awake before removing the endotracheal tube. Transport to the recovery room should include blow by oxygen as well as careful observation of respirations.

Postoperative Concerns

Once in the PACU, patients should be monitored carefully. The potential for postoperative respiratory dysfunction and poor upper airway control may predispose these patients to respiratory failure in the recovery room [16]. Children should also be monitored for signs of hyperpyrexia. Lastly, pain control should be titrated carefully due to their exaggerated response to opioids [54, 55].

Brachial Plexopathies

Hereditary Brachial Plexopathy

Hereditary brachial plexopathy, also known as hereditary neuralgic amyotrophy, is a rare autosomal-dominant disorder characterized by recurrent painful brachial plexopathies and can present in childhood [64–66]. The course of the disease is characterized by a relapsing-remitting course with spontaneous resolution [65]. While any nerve in the brachial plexus can be involved, injury to the upper part of the brachial plexus is most frequent. Nerves outside the brachial plexus can also be involved, including the lumbosacral plexus, the phrenic nerve, and the recurrent laryngeal nerve [66]. Characteristically, these patients present with short stature, hypotelorism, a small face, unusual skin folds and creases on the neck [67].

Congenital Brachial Plexus Palsy

Risk factors for congenital brachial plexopathy include large maternal weight gain, maternal diabetes, multiparity, fetal macrosomia, and breech position [68, 69]. Iatrogenic lateral traction on the fetal head, typically when shoulder dystocia impedes delivery, is thought to be the etiology of congenital brachial plexus palsy [70].

Surgical intervention is indicated if the motor function does not improve after 3 months of age and is undertaken prior to 12 months of age since irreversible loss of the neuromotor end plate may occur [71, 72]. Current treatment includes microsurgical repair and involves resection of neuromas with interpositional nerve grafting [73].

Preoperative Evaluation

Preoperative assessment of any preexisting neurologic condition should be documented prior to induction and positioning. Obtain a complete blood count, serum electrolytes, and/or coagulation parameters preoperatively if indicated by significant coexisting disease states.

Induction and Maintenance of Anesthesia

Most infants who undergo brachial plexus reconstruction are generally healthy except for the nerve injury. Obtaining intravenous access and monitoring blood pressure and pulse oximetry may be challenging due to unavailability of operative extremities, especially when both lower extremities are prepped and draped for harvesting donor nerves. Difficult mask fit due to facial anomalies can be an issue with the hereditary form of this condition. Many of these operative interventions last several hours, making positioning very important. Additionally, paralytics are avoided to facilitate intraoperative electrophysiologic testing [74]. An indwelling urinary catheter is used to decompress the bladder. Maintenance of normothermia and prevention of fluid overload are important during this prolonged surgery. Maintenance fluid will usually suffice [74], since blood loss is often minimal.

Postoperative Concerns

Postoperative analgesia requirements are usually minimal and acetaminophen in combination with NSAIDs can provide excellent pain relief. Shoulder spica casts can be applied to avoid sudden neck movements postoperatively if the lower branches of the accessory nerve are used.

Epidermolysis Bullosa Dystrophica

Epidermolysis bullosa (EB) is a genetic condition with more than 20 subtypes. The three major subtypes are dystrophic EB (DEB) (blisters forming within the dermis), EB simplex (EBS) (blisters forming within the epidermis), and junctional EB (JEB) (blisters forming within the basement membrane) [75]. DEB is the most common type that requires surgery. Disease ranges from minor disability to death in early infancy.

Plastic surgery may involve intervention for joint contractures and correction of pseudosyndactyly. Other common reasons for surgery in this population include dressing changes, dental extraction, esophageal endoscopy and dilation, open gastrostomy, long-term intravenous access, ophthalmic surgery, skin biopsy, Nissen's fundoplication, and skin grafting [75].

Difficult airway is always a concern due to chronic oral scarring and mouth contraction, tongue fixation, limited mouth opening, and laryngeal obstruction [75, 76]. Significant comorbidities include malnutrition, anemia, electrolyte imbalances, renal failure, and amyloidosis with progressive disease. Patients are often on chronic steroid therapy [77].

Preoperative Preparation

Due to the extensive time required to safely place monitors, secure IV access, and position the patient, twice the standard OR time should be allowed and the case should be booked for first case of the day. Patients should be evaluated by an appropriate specialist if comorbid disease is new or has worsened. Appropriate methods to address anxiety should be discussed with the anesthesiologist and the family, since these patients are at risk for shearing of the skin if struggling occurs during induction. If intravenous placement prior to induction is indicated, topical local anesthetic agents can be used as long as they are covered with clear plastic wrap that does not contain an adhesive dressing [75].

Induction and Maintenance of Anesthesia

Intravenous induction is preferred if venous access is available. Intramuscular ketamine injection is an option and advantageous for maintaining spontaneous ventilation [78]. Inhalation induction is possible, however, care must be taken to use a soft mask covered in paraffin gauze to avoid sheering of skin. Hand placement for mask ventilation and cricoid pressure must be done carefully to avoid rupture of bullae or cause new bullae formation. All intubation equipment should be lubricated. Succinylcholine should be avoided since the muscle fasciculations can be associated with shearing of the skin, as well as hyperkalemia if malnutrition and muscle atrophy are present. One should always be prepared for a difficult airway. Oral-tracheal intubation with a tube one half size smaller than predicted can reduce the risk of tracheal bullae formation. The endotracheal tube can be secured by wiring it to a tooth or securing around the neck with a vaseline gauze. Bipolar cautery is preferred to eliminate the need for placement of a grounding pad. All monitors should be placed without adhesive and padded with gauze [75], including the EKG leads. Placement of the blood pressure cuff should be done carefully to avoid severe skin damage [78]. Regional anesthesia has also been used with excellent success [75].

In a study by Kelly et al., eight patients, ages 5–8 years, undergoing pseudosyndactyly repair for recessive dystrophic epidermolysis bullosa received an axillary block. Intramuscular ketamine was given, monitors were placed and the axillary block was performed. A tourniquet was used for hemostasis on the upper arm with gauze placed beneath. The surgical time was 90–120 min with adequate analgesia and without complications [78].

Postoperative

Pain management in this group can be difficult due to both acute and chronic pain, and psychological factors. In the postoperative period, pain control is essential. A child who is restless or tugging at their dressing in response to pain can cause substantial blister formation. If an IV is still present, this is the preferred route for analgesic administration. Otherwise, oral medications may be given if there is no oral swelling. The rectal route is relatively contraindicated due to risk of trauma and blister formation [75].

Even with careful preparation and gentle manipulation of the face, oral pharynx, trachea, and skin, new bullae formation is very possible. In centers that care for these patients regularly, the complication rate is low [75].

Holt–Oram Syndrome

Holt–Oram syndrome (HOS) is an autosomal-dominant malformation syndrome with 90–100 % penetrance, variable expression which is characterized by congenital upper limb malformations and atrial and ventricular septal defects (ASD, VSD) [79–82]. It is also known as atriodigital dysplasia, cardiac-limb syndrome, and heart-hand syndrome [83]. Different degrees of cardiac and forelimb anomalies have been associated with phenotypic variation [84]. ASD and VSD are the most common cardiac anomalies associated with this syndrome; however, patients may also have conduction defects and structural abnormalities [85–87].

Skeletal abnormalities affect the upper limbs exclusively. These abnormalities are always bilateral and usually asymmetric, predominantly involving the radial ray. The thumb is the most commonly affected structure and can be triphalangeal, hypoplastic, or completely absent [88]. HOS is usually diagnosed at birth or prenatally via ultrasound. Clinical presentation varies significantly with degree of cardiac involvement [83].

Preoperative Evaluation

Given the strong association of upper limb defect and cardiac disease in this syndrome, a cardiology evaluation is critical. Prior to surgical scheduling, the patient should undergo a detailed history and physical exam to elicit signs and symptoms suggestive of cardiac disease, ventricular failure, and cyanosis since many agents used during anesthesia are cardiac depressants. An electrocardiogram and echocardiography can help define cardiac anatomy. Based on the data obtained, cardiac catheterization may be indicated for complex lesions [83]. If the patient has an ASD or VSD that is large, results in right heart dilation or has significant right to left shunting, the patient should be evaluated for cardiac intervention prior to any elective procedure.

Induction and Maintenance of Anesthesia

The anesthetic technique is dictated by the presence of cardiac disease. In a patient with a small ASD or VSD, inhalation or intravenous induction are both options. Inhalation induction with a left to right cardiac shunt does not change speed of induction. When intravenous access is obtained, a filter should be placed at the end of the tubing to avoid introduction of air into the venous line which could cross into the arterial circulation.

Postoperative Concerns

Once in the recovery room, standard postoperative pain management and monitoring apply, especially for cardiac arrhythmia and cyanosis given common ASD and VSD pathology.

Poland Syndrome

Poland syndrome, also known as Poland sequence, Poland syndactyly, and Poland anomaly [89], is an uncommon form of congenital anterior chest wall deformity that has often been confused with unilateral pectus excavatum. Its pathophysiology remains unknown, however it is thought that there may be an interruption of early embryonic blood supply in the subclavian or vertebral arteries, resulting in unilateral upper limb anomalies and unilateral or, very rarely, bilateral chest wall deformities [83].

It is characterized by brachy syndactyly and hypoplasia or absence of the breast, nipple, subcutaneous tissue, costosternal portion of the pectoralis major muscle, pectoralis minor muscle or ribs 2–5. This chest wall defect can often be associated with lung herniation [90–93]. Its occurrence is sporadic [94]. The clinical manifestations of Poland syndrome are variable and are not often all seen in the same patient [95, 96].

Preoperative Evaluation

ECG and echocardiography is strongly recommended especially when there is concern for cardiac involvement. Additionally, a chest radiograph should be obtained to elucidate extent of any bony defect in chest wall. If there is renal involvement, blood urea nitrogen, creatinine, and electrolyte panel should be obtained [83]. In the presence of compromised respiratory function, administration of opioids and benzodiazepines for premedication should be done cautiously.

Induction and Maintenance of Anesthesia

The chest wall defect can lead to paradoxical chest movement during spontaneous ventilation and resultant inadequate ventilation; therefore, mechanical ventilation is recommended. If renal anomalies are present, fluid balance and administration of renally excreted drugs warrants special attention [83]. In the presence of renal disease, atracurium or *cis*-atracurium are acceptable muscle relaxants to improve mechanical ventilation. Succinylcholine should be avoided, especially if Poland syndrome is associated with degenerative diseases of cranial nerve motor nuclei [97].

Postoperative Concerns

If the patient has a significant chest wall deformity, the decision to extubate or leave the patient intubated with recover in the intensive care unit should be made on an individual basis.

VACTERL

VACTERL is an acronym representing the following association of conditions: vertebral anomalies (70 %), anal malformation (80 %), cardiovascular defects (53 %), tracheal and esophageal malformation (70 %), renal agenesis (53 %), and limb anomalies (65 %). This condition has a sporadic presentation [98]. Limb anomalies, including radial longitudinal deficiency are common in these patients [99]. Radial longitudinal deficiency involves dysplasia and hypoplasia of the thumb, wrist, and forearm.

Limb anomalies are of secondary concern in patients with VACTERL that also have tracheoesophageal (TE) fistula, esophageal atresia (EA), and CHD since mortality is high in these patients [100]. Radial longitudinal deficiency has also been associated with syndromes such as HOS (atrial septal defects and arrhythmias), Fanconi's anemia (pancytopenia developing between 5 and 10 years of age) and thrombocytopenia and absent radius (thrombocytopenia and anemia at birth which improves in the first year of life) [99]. Plastic and orthopedic surgical repair may be necessary; however, life-threatening comorbidities must be addressed first.

Preoperative Preparation

When a radial defect presents at birth, other more severe anomalies in this syndrome must be ruled out [98]. Any child presenting with a radial deficiency should have a thorough evaluation of cardiac, renal, gastrointestinal, and hematopoietic systems. This evaluation would include an echocardiogram, renal ultrasound, assessment of electrolytes, and complete blood count. Special attention should be paid to preoperative anxiety in patients and their families since many of these children have had previous operative and hospital experiences. IV access should be obtained in patients with significant comorbidities prior to induction of anesthesia.

Induction and Maintenance of Anesthesia

As with all anesthetics, standard monitors, airway equipment, and appropriate medications should be available. Patients who have had tracheoesophageal repair often have hyper-reactive airways and can have weakened tracheal musculature [98]. Ventilation may be difficult and IV access and monitor placement should be considered prior to induction. Induction and maintenance of anesthesia should take into consideration cardiac, renal, and pulmonary function and anatomy. Drug metabolism and dosage can be affected if renal disease exists. Patients with repair of TE fistula and EA repair may be more prone to reflux and fasting times may need to be adjusted accordingly. If the patient has other severe vertebral anomalies, positioning and padding are imperative to avoid pressure sores and nerve injury. At the conclusion of surgery, the patient should be monitored closely for respiratory and cardiovascular instability, due to the increased risks of associated comorbidities.

Postoperative

Postsurgical disposition is based on operative length, blood loss, hemodynamic status, and coexisting cardiac, pulmonary, and renal physiology. Pain control can be achieved with intravenous and oral methods.

Summary

A thorough preoperative evaluation begins with the decision to provide an operative intervention. It is important to recognize the significant comorbid diseases that accompany many of these upper extremity anomalies. Consultation with anesthesiologists and subspecialists should be done well ahead of time to avoid unnecessary delay or cancelation on the day of surgery. The goal of the anesthesiologist is to minimize anxiety for the patient and family, provide a safe and effective surgical field, and maintain hemodynamic stability. Communication between the surgeon, anesthesiologist, and all perioperative consultants is paramount to achieving this goal and delivering the best possible outcome for patients with upper extremity congenital anomalies.

References

1. McGraw T. Preparing children for the operating room: psychological issues. Can J Anaesth. 1994;41(11):1094–103.
2. Kain ZN, Mayes LC, Bell C, Weisman S, Hofstadter MB, Rimar S. Premedication in the United States: a status report. Anesth Analg. 1997;84:427–32.
3. Kain ZN, Mayes LC, O'Connor TZ, Cicchetti DV. Preoperative anxiety in children: predictors and outcomes. Arch Pediatr Adolesc Med. 1996;150(12):1238–45.
4. Kain ZN, Mayes LC, Caldwell-Andrews AA, Karas DE, McClain BC. Preoperative anxiety, postoperative pain, and behavioral recovery in young children undergoing surgery. Pediatrics. 2006;118(2):651–8.
5. O'Byrne K, Peterson L, Saldana L. Survey of pediatric hospitals' preparation programs: evidence of the impact of health psychology research. Health Psychol. 1997;16:147–54.
6. Saile H, Burgmeier R, Schmidt LR. A meta-analysis of studies on psychological preparation of children facing medical procedures. Psychol Health. 1988;2:107–32.
7. Kain ZN, Mayes LC, Caramico LA. Preoperative preparation in children: a cross-sectional study. J Clin Anesth. 1996;8:508–14.
8. McCann ME, Kain ZN. The management of preoperative anxiety in children: an update. Anesth Analg. 2001;93:98–105.
9. Gauderer MW, Lorig JL, Eastwood DW. Is there a place for parents in the operating room? J Pediatr Surg. 1989;24(7):705–6.
10. Messeri A, Caprilli S, Busoni P. Anaesthesia induction in children: a psychological evaluation of the efficiency of parents' presence. Paediatr Anaesth. 2004;14(7):551–6.
11. Kain Z, Mayes L, Wang S, Caramico LA, Hofstadter MB. Parental presence during induction of anesthesia vs. sedative premedication: which intervention is more effective? Anesthesiology. 1998;89:1147–56.
12. Parnis SJ, Barker DS, Van Der Walt JH. Clinical predictors of anaesthetic complications in children with respiratory tract infections. Paediatr Anaesth. 2001;11:29–40.
13. Tait AR, Malviya S. Anesthesia for the child with an upper respiratory tract infection: still a dilemma? Anesth Analg. 2005;100(1): 59–65.

14. Tait AR, Malviya S, Voepel-Lewis T, Munro HM, Seiwert M, Pandit UA. Risk factors for perioperative adverse respiratory events in children with upper respiratory tract infections. Anesthesiology. 2001;95(2):299–306.
15. Elwood T, Sarathy PV, Geiduschek JM, Ulma GA, Karl HW. Respiratory complications during anaesthesia in Apert syndrome. Pediatr Anesth. 2001;11:701–3.
16. Martin S, Tobias JD. Perioperative care of the child with arthrogryposis. Pediatr Anesth. 2006;16:31–7.
17. Hodge D, Fleisher G. Pediatric catheter flow rates. Am J Emerg Med. 1985;3(5):403.
18. Ramasethur J, Macdonald MG. Atlas of procedures in neonatology. 3rd ed. Philadelphia: Lippincott Williams & Wilkins; 2007.
19. Iovino F. Central venous catheterization: complications of different placements. Ann Chir. 2001;126(10):1001.
20. Wilson W, Taubert KA, Gerwitz M, Lockhart PB, Baddour LM, Levison M, et al. Prevention of infective endocarditis: guidelines from the American Heart Association. Circulation. 2007;116:1736.
21. Aono J, Mamiya K, Manabe M. Preoperative anxiety is associated with a high incidence of problematic behavior on emergence after halothane anesthesia in boys. Acta Anaesthesiol Scand. 1999;43: 542–4.
22. Maxwell LG, Yaster M. Perioperative management issues in pediatric patients. Anaesthesiol Clin North Am. 2000;18:601–32.
23. Davis PJ, Cladis FP, Motoyama EK, editors. Smith's anesthesia for infant and children. 8th ed. Philadelphia: Mosby Elsevier; 2011.
24. Martin JT, Warner MA. The ventral decubitus (prone) position. In: Martin JT, Warner MA, editors. Positioning in anesthesia and surgery. Philadelphia: WB Saunders; 1997. p. 155.
25. Hanna MN, Murphy JD, Kumar K, Wu CL. Regional anesthesia and outcome: what is the evidence. Curr Opin Anaesthesiol. 2009;22:672–7.
26. Hadzic A, Williams BA, Karaca PE, Hobeika P, Unis G, Dermksian J, et al. For outpatient rotator cuff surgery, nerve block anesthesia provides superior same-day recovery over general anesthesia. Anesthesiology. 2005;102:1001–107.
27. Pavlin DJ, Rapp SE, Polissar NL, Malmgren JA, Koerschgen M, Keyes H. Factors affecting discharge time in adult outpatients. Anesth Analg. 1998;87:816–26.
28. Markakis DA. Regional anesthesia in pediatrics. Anaesthesiol Clin North Am. 2000;18:355–81.
29. Misamore G, Webb B, McMurray S, Sallay P. A prospective analysis of interscalen brachial blocks performed under general anesthesia. J Shoulder Elbow Surg. 2011;20:308–14.
30. Lynn AM, Fischer T, Brandford HG, Pendergrass TW. Systemic responses to tourniquet release in children. Anesth Analg. 1986;65: 865–72.
31. Tredwell SJ, Wilmink M, Inkpen K, McEwen JA. Pediatric tourniquets: analysis of cuff and limb interface, current practice, and guidelines for use. J Pediatr Orthop. 2001;21:671–6.
32. Sharma JP, Salhotra R. Tourniquets in orthopedic surgery. Indian J Orthop. 2012;46(4):377–83.
33. Kutty S, McElwain JP. Padding under tourniquets in tourniquet controlled surgery: Bruner's ten rules revisited. Injury. 2002;33:75.
34. Sale SM. Neonatal apnoea. Best Pract Res Clin Anaesthesiol. 2010;24(3):323–36.
35. Chidambaran V, Sadhasivam S. Pediatric acute and surgical pain management: recent advances and future perspectives. Int Anesthesiol Clin. 2012;50(4):66–82.
36. Bagatin M, Der Sarkissian R, Larrabee Jr WF. Craniofacial manifestations of the amniotic band syndrome. Otolaryngol Head Neck Surg. 1997;116:525–8.
37. Coyle S, Karp JM, Shirakura A. Oral rehabilitation of a child with amniotic band syndrome. J Dent Child. 2008;75:74–9.
38. Taub PJ, Lin H, Silber L. Mandibular distraction for amniotic band syndrome in the neonate. Ann Plast Surg. 2007;59:334–7.
39. Taub PJ, Bradley JP, Setoguchi Y, Schimmenti L, Kawamoto Jr HK. Typical facial clefting and constriction band anomalies: an unusual association in three unrelated patients. Am J Med Genet. 2003;120A:256–60.
40. Nargozian C. The airway in patients with craniofacial abnormalities. Paediatr Anaesth. 2004;14:53–9.
41. Verchere S, Khalil B, Maddukuri V, Hagberg CA. Use of the DCI video laryngoscope system in a pediatric patient with amniotic band syndrome and craniofacial abnormalities affecting the airway. J Clin Anesth. 2012;24:151–4.
42. Shipster C, Hearst D, Dockrell JE, Kilby E, Hayward R. Speech and language skills and cognitive functioning in children with Apert syndrome: a pilot study. Int J Lang Commun Disord. 2002;37:325–43.
43. Barnett S, Moloney C, Bingham R. Perioperative complications in children with Apert syndrome: a review of 509 anesthetics. Pediatr Anesth. 2011;21:72–7.
44. Hemmer KM, McAlister WH, Marsh JL. Cervical spine anomalies in the craniosynostosis syndromes. Cleft Palate J. 1987;24(4): 328–33.
45. Sarimski K. Children with Apert syndrome: behavioural problems and family stress. Dev Med Child Neurol. 1998;40:44–9.
46. Nargozian C. Apert syndrome. Anesthetic management. Clin Plast Surg. 1991;18(2):227–30.
47. Lowe LH, Booth TN, Joglar JM, Rollins NK. Midface anomalies in children. Radiographics. 2000;20:907–22.
48. Kasai T, Bradley TD. Obstructive sleep apnea and heart failure pathophysiologic and therapeutic implications. J Am Coll Cardiol. 2011;57(2):119–27.
49. Ip MS, Lam B, Ng MM, Lam WK, Tsang KW, Lam KS. Obstructive sleep apnea is independently associated with insulin resistance. Am J Respir Crit Care Med. 2002;165(5):670–6.
50. Findley LJ, Barth JT, Powers DC, Wilhoit SC, Boyd DG, Suratt PM. Cognitive impairment in patients with obstructive sleep apnea and associated hypoxemia. Chest. 1986;90(5):686–90.
51. Koh JGH. Perioperative management of pediatric patients with craniosynostosis. Anesthesiol Clin. 2007;25(3):465–81.
52. Zuckerberg AL, Yaster M. Anesthesia for orthopedic surgery. In: Davis PJ, editor. Smith's anesthesia for infants and children. 8th ed. Philadelphia: Elsevier Mosby; 2011.
53. Bamshad M, Van Heest AE, Pleasure D. Arthrogryposis: a review and update. J Bone Joint Surg Am. 2009;91 Suppl 4:40–6.
54. Gornik-Wlaszczuk E, Majewski J, Szczygiel R, Kurak J. Anaesthesia in patients with arthrogryposis. Anestezjol Intens Ter. 2011;43(2):90–2.
55. Sreevastava D, Trikha A, Sehgal L, Arora MK. Interscalene brachial plexus block for shoulder surgery in a patient with arthrogryposis multiplex congenita. Anaesth Intensive Care. 2002;30: 495–8.
56. Ion T, Cook-Sather D, Finkel S, Cucchiaro G. Fascia iliaca block for an infant with arthrogryposis multiplex congenita undergoing muscle biopsy. Anesth Analg. 2005;100:82–4.
57. Nguyen NH, Morvant EM, Mayhew JF. Anesthetic management for patients with arthrgryposis multiplex congenita and severe micrognathia: case reports. J Clin Anesth. 2000;12:227–30.
58. Oberoi GS, Kaul HL, Gill IS, Batra RK. Anaesthesia in arthrogryposis multiplex congenita: case report. Can J Anaesth. 1986;34(3):288–90.
59. Lammers C, Wyckaert C. Anesthesia for orthopedic surgery. In: Gregory GA, Andropoulos DB, editors. Gregory's pediatric anesthesia. 5th ed. Oxford: Wiley-Blackwell; 2012.
60. Zamudio IA, Brown TCK. Arthrogryposis multiplex congenita (AMC). A review of 32 years' experience. Paediatr Anaesth. 1993;3:101–6.
61. Oda Y, Yukioka H, Fujimori M. Anesthesia for arthrogryposis multiplex congenita. J Anesth. 1990;4(3):275–8.

62. Hopkins PM, Ellis FR, Halsall PJ. Hypermetabolism in arthrogryposis multiplex congenita. Anaesthesia. 1991;46:374–5.
63. Benca J, Hogan K. Malignant hyperthermia, coexisting disorders, and enzymopathies: risks and management options. Anesth Analg. 2009;109(4):1049–53.
64. Dunn HG, Daube JR, Gomez MR. Heredofamilial branchial plexus neuropathy (hereditary neuralgic amyotrophy with branchial predilection) in childhood. Dev Med Child Neurol. 1978;20:28.
65. Klein CJ, Barbara DW, Sprung J, Dyck PJ, Weingarten TN. Surgical and postpartum hereditary brachial plexus attacks and prophylactic immunotherapy. Muscle Nerve. 2013;47:23.
66. van Alfen N, van Engelen BG. The clinical spectrum of neuralgic amyotrophy in 246 cases. Brain. 2006;129:438.
67. Jeannet PY, Watts GD, Bird TD, Chance PF. Craniofacial and cutaneous findings expand the phenotype of hereditary neuralgic amyotrophy. Neurology. 2001;57:1963.
68. Foad SL, Mehlman CT, Ying J. The epidemiology of neonatal brachial plexus palsy in the United States. J Bone Joint Surg Am. 2008;90:1258.
69. van Dijk JG, Pondaag W, Malessy MJ. Obstetric lesions of the brachial plexus. Muscle Nerve. 2001;24:1451.
70. Wilbourn AJ. Plexopathies. Neurol Clin. 2007;25:139.
71. Kawabata H, Masada K, Tsuyuguchi Y, Kawai H, Ono K, Tada R. Early microsurgical reconstruction in birth palsy. Clin Orthop Relat Res. 1987;215:233–42.
72. Walters PM. Comparison of the natural history, the outcome of microsurgical repair, and the outcome of operative reconstruction in brachial plexus birth palsy. J Bone Joint Surg Am. 1999;81:649–59.
73. Capek L, Clarke HM, Curtis CG. Neuroma-in-continuity resection: early outcome in obstetrical brachial plexus palsy. Plast Reconstr Surg. 1998;102:1555–62.
74. Hazama A, Kinouchi K, Kitamura S, Fukumitsu K. Brachial plexus birth injuries: anaesthesia for surgical nerve reconstruction and preoperative myelography and computed tomographic myelography. Paediatr Anaesth. 1999;9:403–7.
75. Herod J, Denyer J, Goldman A, Howard R. Epidermolysis bullosa in children: pathophysiology, anaesthesia and pain management. Paediatr Anaesth. 2002;12:388–97.
76. James I, Wark H. Airway management during anesthesia in patients with epidermolysis bullosa dystrophica. Anesthesiology. 1982;56:323–6.
77. Milne JK, Rosales B. Anaesthesia for correction of oesophageal stricture in a patient with recessive epidermolysis bullosa dystrophica: case report. Can Anaesth Soc J. 1980;27(2):169–71.
78. Kelly RE, Koff HD, Rothaus KO, Carter DM, Artusio JF. Brachial plexus anesthesia in eight patients with recessive dystrophic epidermolysis bullosa. Anesth Analg. 1987;66:1318–20.
79. Holt M, Oram S. Familial heart disease with skeletal malformations. Br Heart J. 1960;22:236–42.
80. Basson CT, Cowley GS, Solomon SD, Weissman B, Poznanski AK, Traill TA, et al. The clinical and genetic spectrum of the Holt–Oram syndrome (heart–hand syndrome). N Engl J Med. 1994;331:885–91.
81. Sletten LJ, Pierpont ME. Variation in severity of cardiac disease in Holt-Oram syndrome. Am J Med Genet. 1996;65:128–32.
82. Newbury-Ecob RA, Leanage R, Raeburn JA, Young ID. Holt-Oram syndrome: a clinical genetic study. J Med Genet. 1996;33:300–7.
83. Bissonnette B, Luginbuehl I, Marciniak B, Dalens B. Syndromes: rapid recognition and perioperative Implications. New York: McGraw Hill; 2006.
84. Bruneau BG, Logan M, Davis N, Levi T, Tabin CJ, Seidman JG, et al. Chamber-specific cardiac expression of Tbx5 and heart defects in Holt-Oram syndrome. Dev Biol. 1999;211:100–8.
85. Poznanski AK, Gall Jr JC, Stern AM. Skeletal manifestations of the Holt–Oram syndrome. Radiology. 1970;94:45–53.
86. James MA, McCarroll Jr HR, Manske PR. Characteristics of patients with hypoplastic thumbs. J Hand Surg Am. 1996;21A:104–13.
87. Smith AT, Sack Jr GH, Taylor GJ. Holt–Oram syndrome. J Pediatr. 1979;95(4):538–43.
88. Huang T. Current advances in Holt-Oram syndrome. Curr Opin Pediatr. 2002;14(6):691–5.
89. Kevin P, David Jr CS. Disorders of sternum and the thoracic wall. 6th ed. Philadelphia: WB Saunders; 1995.
90. Poland A. Deficiency of the pectoral muscles. Guy's Hosp Rep. 1841;6:191.
91. Bing R. Uber angeborene Muskeldefekte. Arch Path Anat Physiol Klin Med. 1902;170:175.
92. Clarkson P. Poland's syndactyly. Guy's Hosp Rep. 1962;111:335–46.
93. Pearl M, Chow TF, Friedman E. Poland's syndrome. Radiology. 1971;101(3):619–23.
94. Bainbridge LC, Wright AR, Kanthan R. Computed tomography in the preoperative assessment of Poland's syndrome. Br J Plast Surg. 1991;44(8):604–7.
95. Mace JW, Kaplan KM, Schanberger JE, Gotlin RW. Poland's syndrome: report of seven cases and review of the literature. Clin Pediatr. 1972;11(2):98–102.
96. Martin LW, Helmsworth JA. The management of congenital deformities on the sternum. JAMA. 1962;179:82–4.
97. Duncan P. Neuromuscular diseases. In: Katz J, Steward DJ, editors. Anesthesia and uncommon pediatric diseases. 2nd ed. Philadelphia: WB Saunders Co.; 1993.
98. Khatavkar SS, Jagtap SR. Anaesthetic management for cataract surgery in VACTERL syndrome case report. Indian J Anaesth. 2009;53(1):94–7.
99. Maschke SD, Seitz W, Lawton J. Radial longitudinal deficiency. J Am Acad Orthop Surg. 2007;15(1):41–52.
100. Mariano ER, Chu LF, Albanese CT, Ramamoorthy C. Successful thoracoscopic repair of esophageal atresia with tracheoesophageal fistula in a newborn with single ventricle physiology. Anesth Analg. 2005;101:1000–2.

Physical Medicine and Rehabilitation Management of Children with Congenital Anomalies of the Upper Extremity

4

Scott E. Benjamin

Physical medicine and rehabilitation, otherwise known as physiatry, is the medical specialty most specifically interested in increasing functional independence. The goal of treatment is to assist the patient with adapting to and overcoming physical or cognitive impairments that limit function, to the extent actually possible. The physiatrist as a member of a multidisciplinary team is a key provider working toward these goals.

Physiatry works with physical therapists, occupational therapists, prothetist/orthotists, surgeons (orthopedic, plastic, neuro), families, case management, social work, psychology, speech and language pathologists, assistive technology, etc. to get people as functionally independent as possible. In the context of upper limb deformities, the physiatrist most closely works with the surgeons involved in any reconstruction, the occupational therapists, and the prosthetists, and, of course, the children and families. Intervention needs appropriate timing of medical, rehabilitation, and educational services.

Habilitation of the child with upper limb deformity must take into account multiple factors, such as the type of deformity—longitudinal, transverse, proximal, or distal. Consideration is taken of systemic or other deformities in certain syndromes. The team must consider the patients' goals, the families' goals and preconceptions, the practicality of the particular intervention, and the potential of the individual patient.

In the realm of prosthetics, as microchip computer technology and biomedical engineering continue to develop at a significant pace, the possibility for more advanced successful rehabilitation interventions with sophisticated equipment continues to grow. However, this must be weighed against the cost and insurance coverage for such technology. While there might be more technically advanced equipment available, the medical provider must question whether this truly provides a higher level of independence and ability, and whether the patient's insurance policy will cover this more expensive option. In the field of orthotics and prosthetics, insurance authorization for durable medical equipment is becoming more and more difficult to obtain. Health care professionals need to be able to document medical necessity of their care, and the specifics of this documentation are very important. On multiple occasions, this writer has had to re-document and argue for what would seem to be an obvious medical need.

Also, there needs to be an awareness of the fact that just because there is an available intervention that the intervention may not lead to an actual improvement in function and may simply be rejected by the patient or family.

In the case of the pediatric patient in particular, parental "buy in" to the treatment plan is imperative. Significant education, counseling, and emotional support may be needed. Dealing with a child with a chronic medical condition, physical impairment, or deformity can cause significant stress in the family, feelings of self-blame, shame, and helplessness for the parents; shame, frustration, and embarrassment for the child.

Rehabilitation psychology, child psychology, and parental counseling are all important concepts to remember when dealing with the upper limb deformity population.

Thus, many players and considerations are all important in the management of the upper limb deficient patient. Depending on the specific institution, the physiatrist may be the team leader responsible for coordinating care and educating the patient and family. Other providers, including therapists, surgeons, teachers, counselors, prosthetists all work together to provide care.

S.E. Benjamin, M.D. (✉)
Department of Orthopaedics and Rehabilitation, University of Vermont College of Medicine, Fletcher Allen Health Care, 790 College Parkway, Colchester, VT 05446, USA

Department of Pediatrics, University of Vermont College of Medicine, Fletcher Allen Health Care, 790 College Parkway, Colchester, VT 05446, USA
e-mail: Scott.benjamin@vtmednet.org

D.R. Laub Jr. (ed.), *Congenital Anomalies of the Upper Extremity: Etiology and Management*,
DOI 10.1007/978-1-4899-7504-1_4, © Springer Science+Business Media New York 2015

Exam of the Upper Limb Deficient Child

Standard pediatric history is obtained, including pregnancy, birth, and developmental history. Cause for limb deficiency, surgical history, concomitant medical history, e.g., vision, hearing, learning disabilities; cognitive abilities, hobbies, interests are all important considerations. Social history is obtained in regard to family support, living situation, family expectations, preconceptions, etc. One should discuss the family's reaction to acceptance of limb loss, and try to get a sense of the child's innate ability to adapt and accept.

General and focused exam of the child with limb deficiency is performed, noting length, passive range of motion, active movement and strength; sensation, proprioception, scarring, and tissue redundancy. Functional use of the limb in its current condition should be carefully assessed. Coordination, motor planning, tolerance to examination, ability to follow directions, and behavior are all-important aspects, as well.

Common Upper Limb Deficiencies and Management Considerations

Upper limb deficiency incidence is about 4.1–16 per 10,000, according to National Center for Health Statistics. Most of the time these are considered spontaneous events without a hereditary component, and the cause is usually unknown. However, first-trimester drug exposures, amniotic band, and some syndromes are known associations. There are five syndromes associated with upper limb deficiencies, particularly absence of the radius. These include TAR syndrome (Thrombocytopenia with Absence of the Radius), Fanconi's syndrome (anemia and leucopenia with absence of radius), Holt-Oram syndrome (atrial septal defects and/tetrology of Fallot), Baller Gerold syndrome (craniosynostosis) and VACTERL syndrome (vertebral, anal, cardiac, tracheoesophogeal atresia, renal, and limb defects (see Chap. 7).

The literature indicates that most children and types of upper extremity deficiencies are fitted for prosthesis at some point, but Kuyper et al. found that this did not necessarily lead to better functional outcome and suggested that some types of upper extremity deficiencies will ultimately lead to prosthetic rejection [1]. Thus, again, understanding the practical realities of prosthetic prescription is as important as the availability of such technology. For example, patients with linear defects tend not to receive prosthetics.

Prosthetic prescription is thought to be most appropriately introduced earlier rather than later to aid in acceptance. Parental and sibling response to the prosthetic management is important in early acceptance. First introduction of a prosthetic is around the time of independent sitting. The first prosthesis is passive, used mostly as an introduction and for aid in positional challenges while in the sitting position. Then subsequently active prostheses are introduced.

Of patients with various upper limb deficiencies, some are more likely to have successful functional outcomes with prosthetics, and others more function with surgical interventions without prosthetics, discussed elsewhere in this book.

A major part of management of the patient with upper limb deficiency is simply deciding on the appropriateness of prosthetic management. Some institutions, such as the De Hoostraat Rehabilitation Center in the Netherlands, have a restrained prescription policy. This is based on the experience of Kuyper et al., who show poor outcome with prostheses for more proximal deficiencies [1].

Transverse radial deficiency is a relatively common major deficiency, and tends to be the most successfully managed with prostheses. Upper third of the forearm is the most common level of transradial deficiency. Humeral shortening and some residual digits or nubbins are frequently present, but surgical intervention is rare. The radius in these patients can be unstable and sublux with elbow extension. Prosthetic fitting in the child with shorter transradial deficiencies is a little more challenging due to less socket surface area for fitting. The child with longer transradial deficiencies has better socket fitting and stronger lever arm.

Digital deficiencies are not uncommon, but rarely occur without other deformities. Surgical interventions are common to remove additional digits. In the case of amniotic band syndrome, other amputations may be present. Other syndromes, such as Moebius, have other anomalies in addition to the digits (i.e., cranial nerve deficiencies). Hypoplastic chest may occur with hand anomalies in the case of Poland syndrome. Prosthetic intervention with hand deficiencies, particularly unilateral, is generally not as helpful in increasing function and ultimately may be rejected. The older and adult patient may choose to eventually have a cosmetic prosthesis. Individual digit deficits come with surgical options and are discussed elsewhere. If the thumb is missing, this obviously creates a more serious deficit, best managed with surgery, such as pollicization.

Partial hand and wrist transverse deficiency are not uncommon. Distal nubbins are not usually a problem and are left alone. There is frequently shortening of the radius and ulna as well. Generally these children can be quite functional without intervention of surgery or prosthetics. They can use the distal residual limb to steady objects, drape over the forearm, or hold objects against the body.

Elbow disarticulation presents another problem in regard to prosthetic fitting. Because of the need for a prosthetic elbow, in the case of the true disarticulation the center of rotation of the elbow joint will be distal to the contralateral intact side due to lack of room to place a component and maintain symmetrical humeral length. The true elbow disarticulation has a distal growth plate. This does pose the consideration of at some point performing an epiphysiodesis (growth plate screw fixation) to allow for symmetrical elbow location.

Humeral deficiencies are frequently short and are at risk for diaphyseal overgrowth. Multiple surgeries are not uncommon. The result is frequently a short, fairly nonfunctional residual limb.

The child with shoulder deficiency is the most difficult situation to provide meaningful prosthetic function of a limb. The prosthetic fitting and management are extremely demanding technically, and the limb provided is cumbersome, heavy, and not particularly useful. Only if the patient and family desire it strongly should prosthetic fitting be offered. These children will figure out ways to hold items with the residual limb or using other body parts. If there is a portion of humerus, the axilla can be used to steady objects. Children will use their knees or mouth or chin to chest to hold objects for manipulation with the uninvolved side. In the case of bilateral deficiencies, feet may be used functionally to grasp and manipulate. Many body-powered prosthetics require active shoulder excursion. This is difficult to obtain in the case of the intrascapulo-thoracic deficiency, where there is only unilateral scapular motion. Prosthetic use may be quite limited in this situation and rejection is not uncommon.

The case of the bilateral upper limb deficient patient is yet another complicated case. There can be great variability in the types of deformities. Thus, there really is no specific protocol for management in these cases. No timetable for prosthetic fitting is suggested. As in any of the other types of deficiencies, prostheses are merely tools. If they are useful to the individual, they will be accepted and used. If not, they will be rejected [2]. As opposed to the patient with unilateral limb deficiency, a patient with bilateral prosthetics is without tactile sensation. Thus, if one limb has a longer deficiency, consideration of unilateral prosthesis would allow the child some tactile interaction with the environment not present in the prosthetic limb. Keeping the prostheses simple and as light as possible is important, as are comfort and some proprioceptive feedback.

Prosthetic Management

Functional Measures

Both body-powered and myoelectric prostheses are available, depending on the amputee. Body-powered terminal devices can be quite versatile, myoelectric, useful, and more cosmetic. With smaller computer components, myoelectric prosthetic options have indeed improved in weight and function. But whether or not that leads to improved acceptance and actual meaningful increases in functional independence is a different story. Thus, valid outcome measures for pediatric prosthetic users are helpful in the decision process. Furthermore, as reimbursement for expensive durable medical equipment is becoming more and more limited, having valid and "real" measures of endpoint improvements will be important. Literature review of functional measures indicates that there have been a number of measures developed over the last few decades but few in regular use. It matters little if one can measure prosthetic capability if the child still ends up rejecting the prosthesis [2–4].

The most well known and seemingly best-validated measure at this time is the PUFI (Prosthetic Upper Extremity Functional Index). This measures ease of task performance in bimanual activities, extent to which the child uses the prosthesis, ease of performance both with and without the prosthesis, and perceived usefulness. Gauthier et al. [3] and Wright et al. measured validity of the PUFI and found it "achieved acceptable discriminant, construct, and criterion validity," and describe prosthetic skill across age groups and different activities [2, 4].

Prosthetic Prescription

In the child with a transradial deficiency, first fitting is usually when the child begins to sit. A simple passive prosthesis is introduced to allow symmetrical two hand activities. This can also aid in postural responses in the sitting position. A closed hand (crawling hand) will assist with leading to more symmetrical crawling. Other goals for early fitting at this age include improved long-term wearing habits and prosthetic acceptance.

After the child's next major developmental milestone, walking, at around 11–13 months, it is appropriate to introduce a simple release-and-grasp terminal device or hand. It is best to only attempt a simple control mechanism at this age to maximize the chance for success. A single-electrode myoelectric hand is good simple option. By this age, the child should have adequate attention span for learning and understanding the grasp/release function. An occupational therapist can help facilitate this process. A child's individual tolerance to hands-on therapy and physical handling may limit the success of this, however.

As the child develops and develops more sophisticated ability to control a terminal device, develops particular interests and self-oriented goals, the physiatrist should make a decision about whether a different type of terminal device should be offered. Options include hooks of various shapes, mitts and hands, and custom task-specific devices for sports, and work. The preference of the family frequently is for a device that looks most like a normal hand. However, the cosmetic prosthesis may not be the most functional device. Hooks do, unfortunately, look just like hooks. However, they

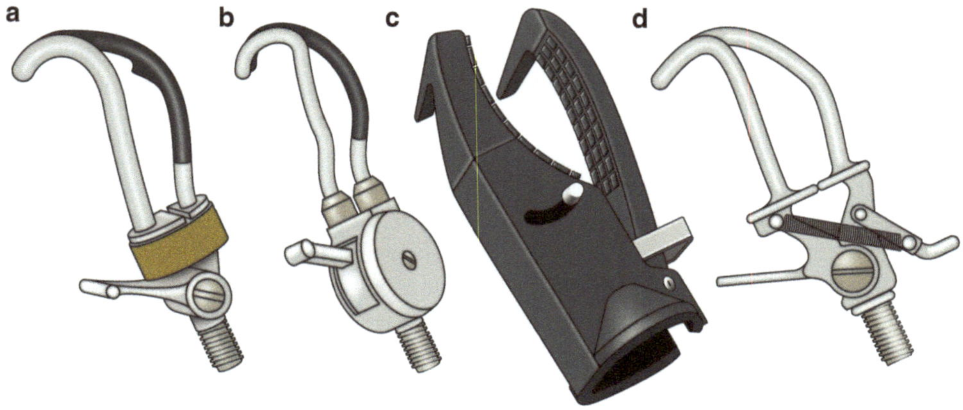

Fig. 4.1 (**a–d**) Prosthetic terminal devices: although not cosmetic, hook-type terminal grasping devices are functional and sturdy

can be quite versatile and durable. Usually cosmetic hand prostheses are provided as the first terminal device in order to maximize acceptance. As the child ages, he or she will make individual choices. See Fig. 4.1.

Transradial Deficiency

The child with a transradial deficiency will do best with a prosthesis with a socket that is self-suspending with or without a silicon sleeve. It generally will be supracondylar, going just above the elbow, using the condylar width to suspend the socket. The device can be body powered or myoelectric. A single-electrode myoelectric hand opening mechanism is relatively easy to use. The younger child may not have the strength, shoulder excursion, or cognitive development to work a body-powered device.

By the time the child starts school, they should be able to activate most types of devices. At this point, the device that is most functionally appropriate for the child should be chosen. Cosmetic considerations, while important, should not outweigh having the most useful device. Working with an experienced and open-minded prosthetist familiar with all types and brands of devices is helpful for the most thorough decision-making. A child may decide to switch the type of prosthesis depending on specific interests and activities.

Transhumeral Deficiency

A child with a transhumeral deficiency will be fitted with prosthesis even later in development. Because of elbow involvement, the transhumeral prosthesis is often too cumbersome for the infant to handle during the earlier motor developmental milestones such as rolling and crawling. A curved prosthesis with a passive hand and without an elbow hinge is a better choice for the first device. Similarly to the child with a transradial deficiency, at around the development of walking, a terminal activated device may be offered. The myoelectric hand offers good cosmesis, ease of function as the first terminal device. However, the transhumeral deficiency has the key difference of requiring a prosthetic elbow hinge, which poses a significant additional management challenge. The first elbow will be simple friction with limited range of motion to allow positioning of the terminal device, but blocking extensive flexion while weight bearing. Electric elbow components are also available and continue to evolve technologically. A harness or silicon sleeve suspends the device.

Components in More Detail

Common hook terminal devices remain the most cost-effective on practical tools in most cases. Technological advances in prosthetic design are one of the more exciting and "cutting edge" areas of rehabilitation management. However, the challenges of integrating newer technologies are cost, insurance coverage, and practical implementation. More advanced designs require higher degree of discreet control, more training, and more experience. These technologies may be most appropriate for the much older child and adult. A very exciting area of prosthetic management includes activity-specific prosthetics, such as sport-specific and work-specific attachments. Private funding for these devices is usually required, as insurance will not cover these indications.

Body-powered versus electric elbows, shoulders may be considered in the older upper limb deficient patient. The reader is referred to rehabilitation texts for discussion of technical details of these options.

Body-powered components include a figure-8 shoulder harness control over the elbow and/or terminal device is gained with glenohumeral motion and shoulder protraction

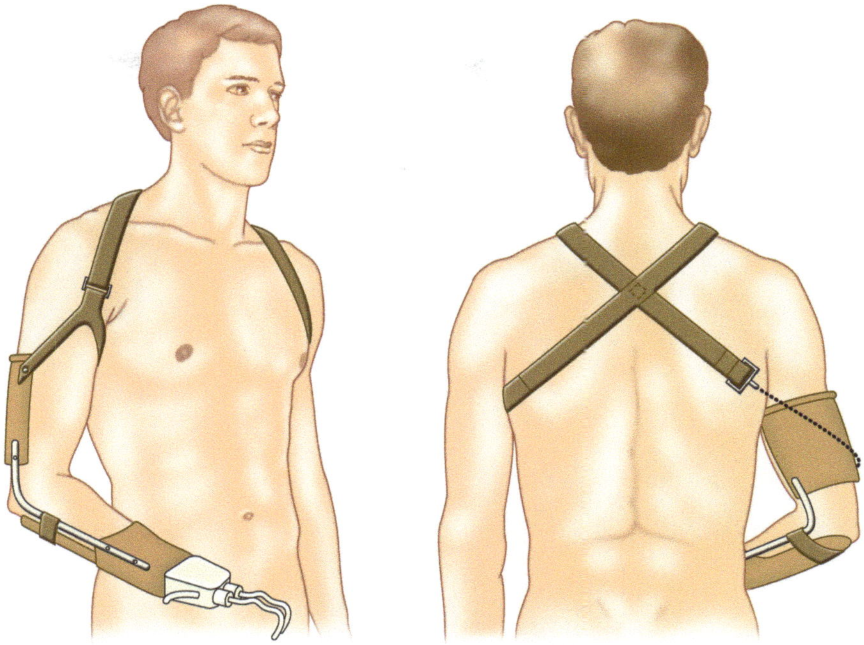

Fig. 4.2 Unilateral transradial prosthesis with figure-8 harness

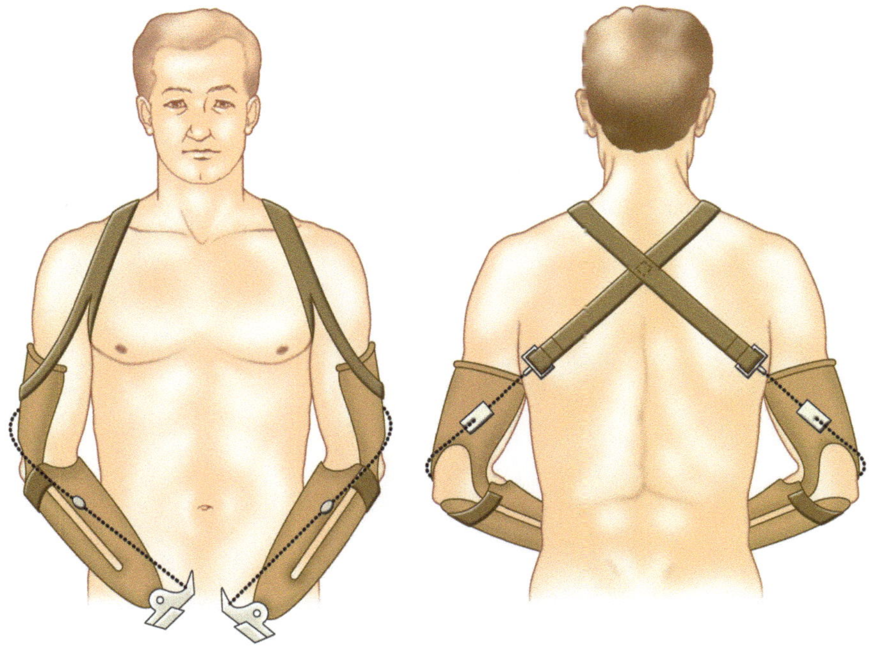

Fig. 4.3 Unilateral transradial prosthesis with gel pin suspension

and retraction. The elbow can be moved and then locked with one set of motions and then the terminal device activated with another. See Figs. 4.2 and 4.3.

With bilateral upper extremity deficiencies, there is no specific timetable of introduction of prosthesis. Introduction needs to be very specific and hand tailored to the individual based on developmental level and functional goals. Obviously bilateral upper limb deficiency patients are quite impaired and prosthetic fitting can be very useful if lightweight and simple to use. See Fig. 4.4.

There is of course growing fields of more sophisticated prosthetic devises as computer technology advances (more robotic-type prosthetic hands, etc.). These are very interesting and exciting areas of development, but these devices are heavy and quite expensive. However, they also may be the future of prosthetic management as well. Like most electronic development, the cost of these will hopefully decrease quite a bit as time goes on. Figures 4.5, 4.6, and 4.7 present a few examples of currently available "robotic" hands with myoelectric control from Touch Bionics.

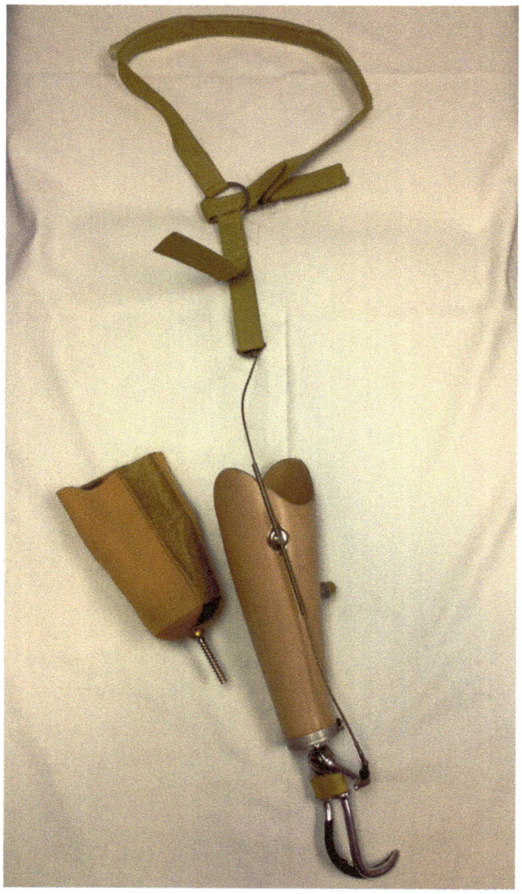

Fig. 4.4 Bilateral transradial prosthesis, body-powered

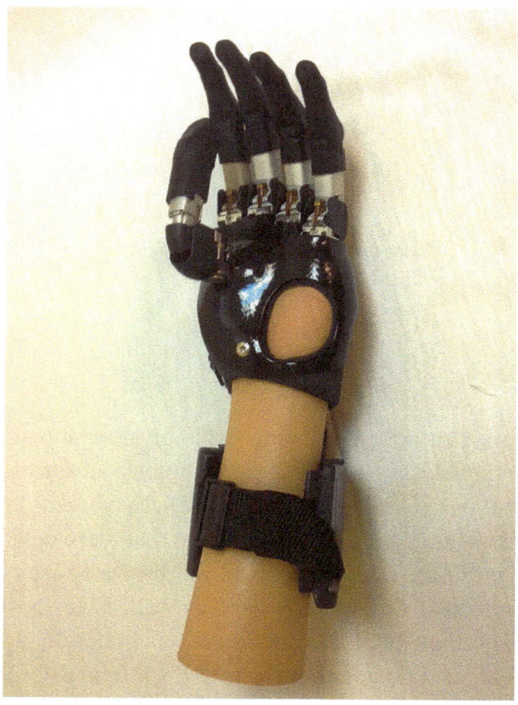

Fig. 4.5 iLimb Digits for use in partial hand amputations

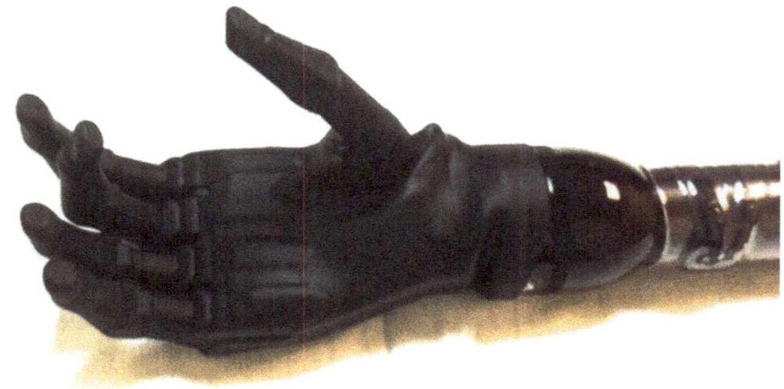

Fig. 4.6 iLimb Ultra for transradial amputees

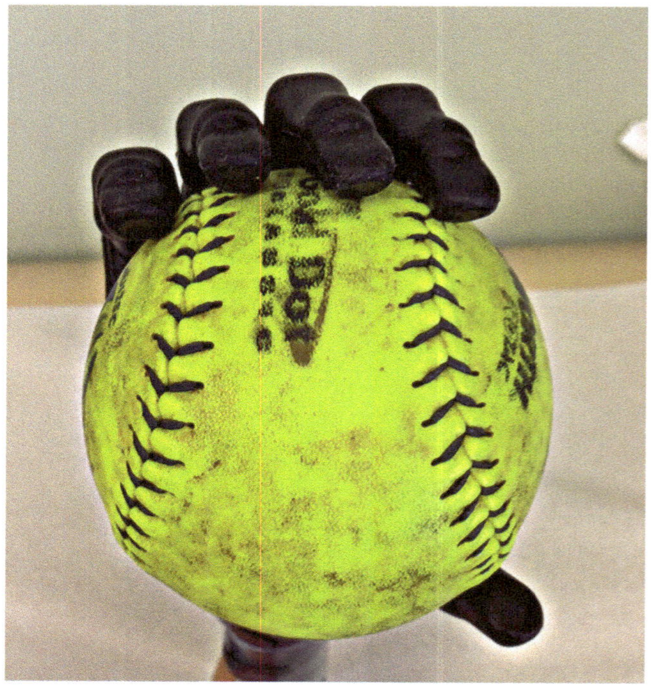

Fig. 4.7 iLimb Ultra holding softball

Psychosocial Adjustment

A child with a physical difference has significant potential challenges. Body image, shame, and embarrassment can lead to social isolation or even failure. Children bring their own unique coping strategies into play in this regard. Families' support systems, emotional reactions, and handling of the medical situation are also very important. Parents may have their own guilt and shame to deal with. The child will certainly perceive and react to the parent's emotions.

Acceptance and use of prostheses are related to the parent's reaction and support of prosthetic appearance. Of equal importance, or perhaps more importance, is the support of peers as the child ages. Having accepting and supporting peers once the child is school age will make a huge difference in the overall emotional health and social success of the child with upper limb deficiency. Hermansson et al. look at adjustment in Swedish children with a myoelectric prosthesis [4]. Children who had a myoelectric hand showed social competence, but tended to be more withdrawn, girls more so, and social activities were lower in older children. Prosthetic users tended to have less delinquency than nonusers. Varni et al. found that strain and depression of children with limb deficiencies was mediated by perceived social support. Analysis showed "evidence of the potentially powerful effects of the social environment of the school setting, with perceived classmate social support the only significant predictor variable across depressive symptomatology, trait anxiety and general self esteem" [5]. This does sound fairly accurate based on what I think is generally understood in regard to the power of peer acceptance and indicates how important it will be to work with the child, school, and classroom on these issues. One suggestion of this author would be to invite a prosthetist into the classroom with the most advanced and exciting prosthetic technology to share with the class. This would offer the opportunity for education and interest in advancing technologies that may lead to more interest and acceptance of the student with limb deficiency.

Summary

Rehabilitation management of the child with congenital upper limb deficiency presents an uncommon issue in the pediatric rehabilitation population outside of specialty centers that have clinics that draw from the surrounding region. This author at a regional university-affiliated hospital will refer to a larger urban center if the frequency of these patients and thus experience are higher in these centers. However, it is always important to have a good knowledge base in the outlying and even rural areas so that appropriateness of referral and local follow-up are possible for families. A team approach involving various physicians, therapists, counselors, prosthetists, and medical venders is an important part of the management of these patients and families. The ultimate goal, of course, is the maximal independent function, highest quality of life, and best possible psychosocial success.

References

1. Kuyper MA, Breedijk M, Mulders AHM, Post MWM, Prevo AJH. Prosthetic management of children in the Netherlands with upper limb deficiencies. Prosthet Orthot Int. 2001;25:228–34.
2. Lambregts SAM, Doornbosch F, Roebroeck ME, Rol M, Arendzen JH, Pexch-Batenburg JMFB, et al., editors. Functional outcome of adolescents and young adults with congenital upper limb reduction deficiency. Proceedings of the 2005 MyoElectric Controls/Powered Prosthetic Symposium. 2005 Aug 17–19 Fredericton, NB, Canada.
3. Wright V, Hubbard S, Naumann S, Jutai J. Evaluation of the validity of the prosthetic upper extremity functional index for children. Arch Phys Med Rehabil. 2003;84:518–27.
4. Hermansson L, Eliasson AC, Engstrom I. Psychosocial adjustment in Swedish children with upper-limb reduction deficiency and a myoelectric prosthetic hand. Acta Paediatr. 2005;94(4):479–88.
5. Varni J, Setoguchi Y, Rappaport LR, Talbot D. Psychological adjustment and perceived social support in children with congenital/acquired limb deficiencies. J Behav Med. 1992;15(1):31–44.

Suggested Reading

Gaebler-Spira D, Lipschutz R. Pediatric limb deficiencies. In: Alexander M, Matthews D, editors. Pediatric rehabilitation principles and practice. 4th ed. New York: Demos Medical; 2010. p. 339–47.

Gaebler-Spira D, Uellendahl J. Pediatric limb deficiencies. In: Molnar G, Alexander M, editors. Pediatric rehabilitation. 3rd ed. Philadelphia: Hanley and Belfus; 1999. p. 331–9.

Hubbard S. Pediatric upper limb outcome measures. J Prosthet Orthot. 2009;21(48):64–8.

Kelly BM, Davis AJ, Justice D, Miller QL, Nelson VS. Comprehensive care for the child with upper extremity limb deficiency. J Pediatr Rehabil Med. 2009;2:195–208.

Sener F, Yigiter K, Bayar K, Erbahceci F. Effectiveness of prosthetic rehabilitation of children with limb deficiencies present at birth. Prosthet Orthot Int. 1999;23:130–4.

Therapy Management of Children with Congenital Anomalies of the Upper Extremity

5

Ginny Gibson

This chapter will first introduce evaluation tools appropriate for children with congenital anomalies of the upper extremity (CAUE). Second general rehabilitation interventions will be described. Third attention will be given to interventions for children with selected CAUE who are often served by occupational or physical therapists.

Evaluation

Reviews, reports, and investigations have identified activities of daily living (ADL) and instrumental activities of daily living (IADL) that are problematic for children with CAUE including styling hair, squeezing toothpaste, completing toilet hygiene, tying shoelaces, closing and opening dressing fasteners, tucking shirts into pants at the waistline, donning socks, cutting and peeling food, and opening containers [1–4]. Educationally related activities that may prove difficult for children with CAUE include writing with a pen or pencil, using a keyboard, carrying books, cutting with scissors, managing a lunch tray, and full participation in playground activities and physical education [4, 5]. Outside of school, children with CAUE have reported difficulty with ball sports, dancing, martial arts, snow or ice sports, water sports, gymnastics, cycling, and playing with construction toys [5]. The evaluation of children with CAUE should consider impairment, activity performance, and activity participation, as there may or may not be a relationship between the three constructs [4, 6, 7].

Four studies have examined the relationship between impairment and body structure with activity performance or participation for children with radial longitudinal deficiency (RLD). Kotwal et al. [6] retrospectively compared children with RLD who underwent centralization or radialization to those who did not. Although the main purpose of the study was to discern if patients benefitted from surgical correction of wrist deformity, the researchers found strong correlations between Prosthetic Upper Extremity Functional Index (PUFI) scores and three measures of body function; including wrist range of motion (ROM) (r=0.65–0.81), long finger ROM (r=0.93–0.97), and grip strength (r=0.90–0.97). Buffart et al. [7] examined relationships between hand function impairment and activity performance. Grip and pinch strength, as well as AROM, were measured for the assisting hand. For children with unilateral involvement the affected hand was measured, and for those with bilateral involvement the more affected hand was measured. All children completed the Assisting Hand Assessment (AHA) and their parents completed the Ease of Performance Scale on the PUFI. Grip strength significantly correlated with activity performance for the AHA (rp=0.69, p=0.002) and PUFI (rp=0.52, p=0.003). Pinch strength significantly correlated with activity performance for the AHA (rp=0.77, p=0.001) only. AROM of the wrist and second digit significantly correlated with activity performance for the AHA (rp=0.59, p=0.006 and rp=0.87, p=0.001) and PUFI (rp=0.71, p=0.001 and rp=0.59, p=0.006, respectively) Ekblom et al. [8] found a relationship between outcomes on the AHA and total ROM of digits (p=0.042), and self-experienced time of performance on the Children's Hand-use Experience Questionnaire (CHEQ) and total active motion of the wrist (p=0.043). There was no relationship between the degree of radial deviation and outcomes of the Box and Block Test, AHA, or CHEQ. The aforementioned studies included children.

Holtslag et al. [4] investigated the functional implications of RLD for 17 adults who previously underwent surgical or conservative treatment. Measurements included grip and pinch strength, ROM, and hand function during standardized ADL using the Sequential Occupational Dexterity Assessment (SODA). Participation in activity was quantified using the

G. Gibson, O.T.D., O.T.R./L., C.H.T. (✉)
Pediatric Rehabilitation, UCSF Benioff Children's Hospital Oakland, 747 52nd Street, Oakland, CA 94609, USA

Department of Occupational Therapy, Samuel Merritt University, 450 30th Street, Oakland, CA 94609, USA
e-mail: ggibson@samuelmerritt.edu

D.R. Laub Jr. (ed.), *Congenital Anomalies of the Upper Extremity: Etiology and Management*, DOI 10.1007/978-1-4899-7504-1_5, © Springer Science+Business Media New York 2015

Table 5.1 Impairment-based measurement tools or techniques

Impairment	Measurement	Impairment	Measurement
Movement restriction	Goniometer Inclinometer	Impaired sensation/nerve injury	Monofilaments
	Wire tracing		Two-point discrimination
	Tape measure		Stereognosis
	Pollexograph		Moberg pickup test
			Ten test
			Ninhydrin sweat test
Weakness	Dynamometer	Prehension	Box and blocks
	Quantified muscle testing (QMT)		Nine hole peg test
	Manual muscle testing (MMT)		Functional dexterity test
Edema	Volumetry		Test of in-hand manipulation
	Tape measure		
Pain	Visual analog scale		
	Wong-Baker faces		
	Face, legs, activity, cry, consolability scale		

Table 5.2 Impairment ratings

		Normative data				
Impairment	Tool	First author and date	Citation	Measure	*N*	Age (years)
Movement restriction	Goniometer	Soucie (2011)	[9]	Shoulder, elbow, and forearm PROM	200	2–19
	Goniometer	Barad (2013)	[10]	Elbow PROM	1,361	1–16
	Pollexograph	de Kraker (2009)	[11]	Thumb abduction	100	4–12
	Distance measurement					
Weakness	Grippit	Häger-Ross (2002)	[12]	Grip strength	530	4–16
	Jamar dynamometer	Bowman (1984)	[13]	Grip strength	153	6–9
	Jamar dynamometer	Fullwood (1986)	[14]	Grip strength	214	5–12
	Jamar dynamometer	De Smet (2001)	[15]	Grip strength	487	5–15
	Jamar dynamometer	Holm (2008)	[16]	Grip strength	376	7–12
	Jamar dynamometer	Ploegmakers (2013)	[17]	Grip strength	2,241	4–15
	Jamar dynamometer	Mathiowetz (1986)	[18]	Grip strength	571	6–19
	B & L pinch gauge			Pinch strength		
	Preston pinch gauge	Lee-Valkov (2003)	[19]	Pinch strength	17	3–5
	Jamar dynamometer			Grip strength		
	Preston pinch gauge	Ager (1984)	[20]	Pinch strength	474	2–13
	Jamar dynamometer			Grip strength		
	B & L pinch gauge	Surrey et al. (2001)	[21]	Pinch strength	414	5–12
	Preston pinch gauge	De Smet (2006)	[22]	Pinch strength	262	5–12
Impaired sensation	Two-point discrimination	Cope (1992)	[23]	Discriminative touch	112	2–13
Prehension	Box and block test of manual dexterity	Mathiowetz (1985)	[24]	Manual dexterity	471	6–19
	Functional dexterity test	Gogola (2013)	[25]	Manual dexterity	175	3–17
	Nine hole Peg test	Smith (2000)	[26]	Manual dexterity	826	5–10
		Poole (2005)	[27]	Manual dexterity	409	4–19
	Purdue Pegboard	Wilson (1982)	[28]	Manual dexterity	206	2.6–5.1

Normative studies in typically developing children

Impact on Participation and Autonomy (IPA) questionnaire. Researchers found a positive correlation ($r=0.56$, $p=0.02$) between digital ROM and SODA outcomes, but no other relationship between body function and hand function or participation. Table 5.1 includes tests and measures of impairment, likely to be used when providing habilitative and rehabilitative services to children with CAUE, while Table 5.2 includes tests for which normative information is available.

Table 5.3 Performance-based assessment

Assessment tool	Target populations	Target age (years)	Studies describing psychometrics		
			Validity	Reliability	Responsiveness
ABILHAND-Kids	Children with cerebral palsy	6–15	[33]	[33, 35]	–
AHA	Children with typical function in one hand only	1.6–12.8	[36]	[33, 37, 38]	[37]
CHEQ	Children with typical function in one hand only	6–18	[39]	–	–
PedsQL	Children with acute or chronic illness	2–18	[40]	[40]	[41]
PEDI	Children with physical disability	6 months–7.5	[42–44]	[45]	–
PODCI	Children with orthopedic conditions	0–18	[46, 47]	[46]	[48, 49]
PUFI	Children who use an upper extremity prosthesis	3–18	[33, 50]	[33, 51]	–
UBET	Children with transverse reduction deficiency	2–21	[33]	[33, 52]	–

AHA Assisting Hand Assessment, *CHEQ* Children's Hand-use Experience Questionnaire, *PedsQL* Pediatric Quality of Life Inventory, *PEDI* Pediatric Evaluation of Disability Inventory, *PODCI* Pediatric Outcomes Data Collection Instrument, *PUFI* Prosthetic Upper Extremity Functional Index, *UBET* Unilateral Below Elbow Test

Skerik et al. [29] described a standardized process of assessment for all children with CAUE including analysis of available patterns of pinch and grip, observation of preferred patterns of usage, and measurement of ROM, pinch strength, and hand size. To measure outcomes following index finger pollicization, Percival et al. [30] developed a battery of seven tests for which a maximum score is 22. Included in this battery is a measure or observation of tip pinch and pulp pinch strength; opposition of the thumb to the middle, ring and small finger; grasping of two balls of different size, active movement of the thumb at three joints; two-point discrimination; and cosmesis (length and position of the thumb). Scores are characterized as excellent (>20) good (16–19), fair (12–15), or poor (<12). Ho and Clarke [31] conducted a systematic review of studies published between 1966 and 2003 aimed at evaluating outcomes following pollicization of the index finger or centralization for radial longitudinal deficiently. Of the ten studies reviewed, six attempted to measure ADL or functional use of the hand, but only one did so using a standardized instrument.

Since Ho and Clarke's review [31], other outcome studies have been published in which standardized assessment tools were employed. Buffart et al. [32] set out to identify appropriate assessment tools for use with children with transverse or longitudinal reduction deficiency using as criteria inclusion of bimanual tasks, measures of quality of movement, and appealing tasks. These researchers recommended the AHA, Unilateral Below Elbow Test (UBET), ABILHAND-Kids, and PUFI. In a follow-up study [33] the AHA, UBET, ABILHAND-Kids, and PUFI were administered to 20 children with RLD, aged 4–12 years. The AHA and PUFI were deemed most valid for children with RLD, due to the relationships found with type of RLD ($r=-0.82$ and -0.64, respectively), functional hand grips ($r=0.58$ and 0.46, respectively), and the therapist's global assessment of hand function ($r=0.85$ and 0.63, respectively). Kaplan and Jones [34] used the Pediatric Outcomes Data Collection Instrument (PODCI) to determine outcomes following microsurgical toe transfers for thumb reconstruction. Table 5.3 presents performance-based assessments specifically designed for children with CAUE, children with normal use of one hand only, or children with disability but no specific diagnostic population.

Assessments that attempt to measure satisfaction with or perceptions of activity performance and participation should include the child with CAUE, but in some cases the caregiver may need to serve as proxy. Researchers have studied the extent to which parents and children agree on satisfaction with or perception of activity performance and participation. Netscher et al. [53] examined ability to participate in activities following index finger pollicization. In addition to measuring impairment level and ability to participate in simulated tasks reflecting participation in a larger activity, researchers administered a non-validated novel questionnaire to nine children and their parents to determine perceptions of appearance, social participation, and performance skills. The mean score for children was 22, with 12 being the best score and 60 the worst. Although parents tended to assess their children's skills as slightly better than the children did of themselves, there was no statistically significant difference between parents' and children's scores, suggesting that parents may serve well as proxy. Ardon et al. [54] found similar results when parents and their children with CAUE separately completed the Pediatric Quality of Life Inventory (PedsQL). No statistically significant differences were observed for total score and the five domains (physical health, emotional functions, social functioning, school functioning, psychosocial health). The researchers noted analysis of individual scores showed children and parents tended to disagree and the variables that influenced disagreement included number of affected digits and bilateral involvement [54]. Similarly, in a large multi-center study significant differences were found between parents and their children with congenital below elbow deficiency (CBED) for upper extremity physical function ($p<0.001$), pain/comfort ($p<0.05$), and social functioning ($p<0.001$) using the PODCI and PedsQL [55]. In summary, use of a parent as proxy should be limited; effort to elicit children's participation is desirable.

Interventions to Address Impairments

Current estimates of the rate of congenital upper limb differences include 1 in 506 live births [56], 5.25 in 10,000 live births [57], and 21.5 per 10,000 live births [58]. In two reports of the incidence of all congenital limb reductions, 75–81 % involved the upper extremities [59, 60]. Within these estimates, not all children with CAUE will require surgical intervention and subsequent rehabilitation. When indicated, rehabilitation efforts may initially emphasize interventions to address impairment with simultaneous or subsequent attention to participation in activity. The studies presented in the following sections are not specific to children.

Edema

Edema management is often addressed via rest, ice, compression, and elevation. Postoperative dressings and casting provide rest and compression yet preclude icing. Chronic edema that persists after removal of postoperative immobilization may be treated with gentle compression. Younger children may not be amenable to elevation and the efficacy of elevation following hand surgery is unclear. In two prospective and randomized comparison trials, no statistically significant differences were noted in those who the limb and those who did not for adults undergoing Dupuytren's release [61] or carpal tunnel decompression [62]. Gentle compression may be achieved with self-adhering wrap [63]; however, only one case report of an adult with burn injury could be located to support its use [64].

Scar

In addition to being cosmetically unappealing, postoperative scar may lead to motion restriction, pain, and puritis. These impairments may in turn reduce function and participation in activities. Intervention should first concentrate on prevention of hypertrophic scars, but when hypertrophic scars are present, efforts should be made to reduce the extent of the existing scar. Scars from surgical incisions may respond well to treatment including massage, pressure, topical application of a gel product, and reduction of tension on scar.

Massage

Shin and Bordeaux [65] conducted a systematic review of studies investigating the effectiveness of scar massage regimes for scars due to burn and trauma, and included four randomized controlled studies, three prospective controlled studies, one prospective study, and two case reports. Across ten reports, the total number of subjects was 220 with 144 receiving scar massage. The standardized outcome measures included the Observer Scar Assessment Scale and the Vancouver Scar Scale (VSS), as well as subjective assessments of scar thickness, perfusion, color, pain, and itching. For patients who had surgical scars and received massage, 90 % improved. Foo and Tristani-Firouzi [66] recommend that postsurgical scar massage commence during the proliferative phase, 2–3 times per day, for 3–5 min, for 3–4 months.

Pressure

Pressure application may be applied using self-adherent wraps, neoprene splints, tubular elastic, and custom fit pressure garments. Pressure inhibits fibroblastic activity [66], via ischemia and hypoxia resulting in degeneration of fibroblasts and slowed synthesis of collagen [67]. Despite a long history of inclusion of pressure in the treatment of scar, definitive evidence regarding its efficacy is lacking.

In a meta-analysis of six published randomized controlled trials and one unpublished trial examining the benefit of pressure therapy for burn scar, researchers found no difference between scars treated with pressure therapy and controls [68]. More recently, a randomized controlled study of treatment of burn scar demonstrated significant improvement on the VSS using pressure therapy alone ($p<0.001$), but also found significant improvement with combined pressure therapy and application of silicone gel sheeting ($p=0.001$), and combined pressure therapy and silicone spray ($p<0.001$). Patients with two similar scars from split-thickness grafts were randomized into either a silicone gel sheeting group or silicone spray group, but all used pressure therapy. Differences between the groups were not significant [69]. Widgerow [83] suggests pressure garments are more appropriate for widespread scar seen in burn injury; however, in maintenance of tape or silicone gel sheeting on the hand of a young child can be challenging. Use of a pressure garment may discourage self-removal of treatment modalities held in place by the garment, including the garment itself. In a laboratory study of fibroblastic activity under pressure, researchers showed pressure application may be applied at higher levels over shorter periods of time or at lower levels for longer periods of time to reduce fibroblastic proliferation [66].

If using self-adherent wrap, care in wrapping and maintained supervision are indicated to avoid a tourniquet-like effect due to lifting, slippage, and rolling [72]. Use of neoprene patches or orthoses for at least 8 h per day was retrospectively studied in a small population of children and young adults with burn scar ($n=8$ participants, 12 scars). Duration of treatment ranged from 1 to 11 months. Scars were evaluated pre and post treatment and differences for mean VSS was significantly lower after treatment ($p=0.0001$). This study is useful to therapists working with children because neoprene splints are often used long term across several diagnostic groups for limb positioning and so could also serve to manage scar [73].

Silicone

Silicone gel may serve to prevent hypertrophic scars and improve characteristics of existing hypertrophic scar. In a narrative review of eight RCTs and an analysis of 27 trials, the International Advisory Panel on Scar Management concluded that use of silicone gel sheeting is "safe and effective"; however, the panel distinguished adhesive silicone gel sheeting from other adhesive gels, liquid silicone, and non-adhesive silicone gel sheeting [74]. O'Brien and Pandit [75] conducted a meta-analysis to determine the effectiveness of silicone dressings to prevent hypertrophic or keloid scarring in people with newly healed wounds and to treat established keloid or hypertrophic scars. The study included randomized or quasi-randomized controlled trials, and controlled clinical trials comparing silicone dressings to other nonsurgical treatment, no treatment or placebo. Included trials compared adhesive silicone dressings with control; non-silicone dressings; silicone gel plates with added vitamin E; laser therapy; triamcinolone acetonide injection, and nonadhesive silicone dressings. Scar quality was determined by blood flow, color change, hyperpigmentation, thickness, and shape. Studies that set out to determine effectiveness of silicone to treat existing scars measured change in scar size and did so using a ruler, taking an impression, or via ultrasound. Across 15 studies, 615 people between 2 and 81 years-of-age were included. Compared with no treatment silicone reduced the incidence of hypertrophic scar (RR 0.46, 95 % CI 0.21–0.98). For established keloid and hypertrophic scar SD significantly reduced scar thickness (RR −1.99, 95 % CI −2.13 to −1.85) and improved color (RR 3.05, 95 % CI 1.57–5.96). Silicone dressings produced superior results compared to controls in two trials, no difference was found in two trials, and the control group fared better in one trial. This study included clinical trials of varied rigor and most were subject to bias thus there is weak evidence for use of silicone dressing to prevent or improve scars. An update to this review was published in 2013; five new studies were included but the same conclusion was offered [76].

The proposed mechanism of action of silicone gel is thought to be hydration and occlusion [77], though non-silicone gels may be equally effective as silicone. In a prospective, randomized study patients ($n=24$) with existing hypertrophic or keloid scars ($n=41$) present for longer than 3 months, including incisional scars, were randomly assigned to one of three groups: treatment with silicone gel ($n=16$ scars), treatment with non-silicone gel ($n=14$ scars), or control ($n=11$ scars). Treatment was applied 24 h per day for 4.5 months. No statistically significant differences were found between SD and NSD groups for color, size, induration, and symptoms, although significant differences were noted when SD and NSD were compared to controls for color, size, induration, and scar pliability [78].

Tape

Tension on scar is believed to stimulate collagen production due to mechanosensitive fibroblasts [71, 79, 80]. Tape applied to scars may reduce tension and prove effective in preventing hypertrophic scar [81, 82]. Porous tape should be applied longitudinal to and directly over the scar to adequately provide support and reduce tension [83]. When scars cross joints, use of an orthosis may help to reduce tension on scar.

Motion Restriction

Clinicians utilize AROM, active assisted ROM, passive range of motion (PROM), joint mobilization and orthoses to achieve greater range of movement. Michlovitz et al. [84] conducted a systematic review of interventions to promote joint motion in the upper extremity. The review included 26 studies that examined interventions in adults, but excluded children and congenital hand differences. In their summary, the researchers noted moderate evidence for the use of orthoses or casts and passive exercise to increase ROM after joint trauma or immobilization. Following this study, Glasgow et al. [85] published a narrative review to develop a set of recommendations for mobilizing the stiff hand. After a review of 29 studies of varying levels, these authors recommended active and active assisted exercise during all stages of tissue healing, passive exercise during the proliferative and remodeling phases, and joint mobilization during the remodeling phase. Orthoses for management of stiffness via mobilization were recommended during the proliferative and remodeling phases.

When the purpose of an orthosis is to increase motion, orthosis prescription must consider tissue compliance and the length of time the restriction has been present. Therapists must decide on orthosis type (including no orthosis), wear time (hours per day and duration), and the magnitude of force to apply. Flowers [86] offered a hierarchy for decision-making when treating stiff joints using a modified Week's test [87]. After pre-conditioning, those whose PROM measures change by 20° may not need a splint; by 15° may require a static splint with no overpressure; by 10° may require a dynamic splint; and by 5° or less may required a static progressive splint with overpressure. This decision-making process may prove useful with older children; but may not be feasible with infants and toddlers due to required exposure to thermotherapy.

Consensus on wear time of an orthosis to resolve motion restrictions is lacking, although many studies provide guidance. Flowers and LaStayo [88] executed a study to determine if duration of orthosis use impacted outcomes for stiff joints. Patients ($n=15$) with 20 PIP flexion contractures between 15° and 60° were randomly assigned to continuous casting for 6 days then 3 days or 3 days then 6 days. There was a statistically significant difference ($p<0.005$) in gains made with 6 days of wear achieving a mean increase of 5.3° and 3 days of wear achieving 3°. Glascow et al. [89] prospectively investigated optimal hours of daily orthoses wear in 43 subjects with joint restrictions in the hand following trauma. Subjects with similar levels of stiffness—as determined via torque range of motion (TROM)—were randomly allocated to a <6 h or 6–12 h per day group. There was a statistically significant difference between the groups, with better TROM observed in the 6- to 12-h group. It is not clear if increasing time more than 12 h provides greater benefit. In a follow-up randomized study of 22 patients with PIP joint flexion contractures, no significant differences were found for PROM, AROM, or TROM between 6–12 h of wear and 12–16 h of orthosis wear after 8 weeks of treatment [90].

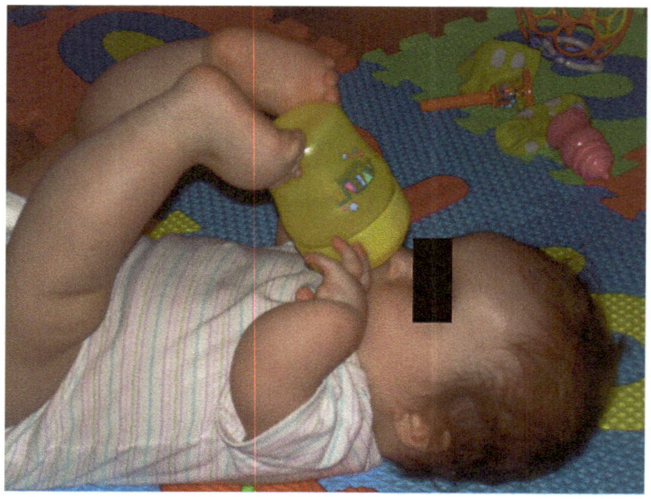

Fig. 5.1 This child with thrompocytopenia absent radii has self-identified strategies for participation in activities

Interventions to Address Activity Performance and Participation

Assuming a child with CAUE is otherwise typically developing, interventions to improve activity performance or participation may occur immediately following surgery or intermittently—when the child encounters specific problems with activity performance or participation. Following surgery, impairment-based may be emphasized concurrently with interventions to promote activity performance and participation via activity modification or introduction to assistive devices [4]. In a qualitative study investigating perceptions of children 8–20 years of age with unilateral CBED, participants described their own activity performance and participation and generally reported no limitations. Further, these children reported similar levels of participation as peers without CBED. The researchers suggested, for children in this study, perceptions of activity participation might have been limited to actual chosen activities rather than potential chosen activities (activities that may have been chosen if participants had two hands) [5]. In a descriptive study of eight people with ulnar longitudinal deficiency (ULD), age 3–41, adult patients reported no difficulty with self-dressing, washing, toileting, eating, closing and opening dressing fasteners, managing the telephone, typing, or opening containers with screw on caps and parents of children with ULD reported no difficulty with bimanual self-care, play, or school related activity [91].

Health professionals should recognize there are multiple strategies to manage limitations in activity performance and participation that may be acceptable to the child with CAUE including using other body parts (Fig. 5.1), activity modification, choosing varying levels of participation, receiving assistance from another, using assistive devices, and prosthetic wear [5]. In the study by de Jong et al. [5] health professionals were less apt to recognize as many strategies as did children and their parents, and identified assistive devices and prosthetics more frequently as potential solutions for success in activity performance and increased participation.

Diagnosis-Specific Intervention

Camptodactyly

Range of Motion Exercise

While orthotic management and surgery are intervention options for camptodactyly [92], ROM exercises may prove beneficial especially for children with an infantile onset of deformity. Rhee et al. [93] retrospectively evaluated the effectiveness of passive stretching to correct flexion deformities in children younger than 3 years with camptodactyly. Records of children with simple camptodactyly who had not received surgery or intervention with an orthosis were included, but those with flexion contractures of less than 10° were excluded. Parents were taught a PROM technique, to be implemented at home, requiring the PIP joint be extended with the wrist and metacarpophalangeal (MCP) joint in extension. Instructions were to complete gentle PROM, while the child was sleeping, 20 or more times per day with a hold time of 5 min. Exercise frequency was reduced to five or ten times per day when near full extension was achieved. Duration of intervention was individualized and poorly defined. The intervention could be realistically applied; however, the burden of applying PROM only when children are sleeping could compromise adherences rates. Pre- and post-intervention measurements, recorded by the same physician, were compared. Across groups, 13 males and 9 females with a mean age of 12 months (range 3–36 months) were included in the study. Digits were further classified into mild deformity (<30°, $n=12$ digits), moderate deformity (30–60°, $n=36$), and severe deformity (>60°, $n=13$) as per goniometric measures. Groups were expected to be different with regard to extent of deformity but no analysis was performed to assure they were similar for age, sex, and dominance. Final PROM for PIP extension was compared to initial measures. Mean change in PROM were as follows: −20° to −1° for the mild group, −39° to −12° for the moderate group, and −75° to −28° for the severe group. Differences from pretest to posttest were significant for all groups: mild ($p<0.001$), moderate ($p<0.001$), and severe ($p<0.001$). Mean time from start to end of intervention (either correction or cessation of change) for the mild group was 5 months, moderate group was 10 months, and severe group 13 months. Researchers found a relationship between degree of flexion contracture at the start of intervention and final measure. No relationship was found between initial flexion contracture, handedness, digit involvement, and number of digits or hands involved. Differences between pretest and posttest AROM values were statistically significant. No statistical analysis was performed to determine clinical significance, however all but two children (in the moderate group) improved and gains were maintained during a prolonged follow-up period (mean of 26 months, range of 12–47 months). The researchers concluded children under three who have camptodactyly should be treated with PROM only and orthoses are not necessary; however, this statement is unfounded since no comparison was made between PROM and use of an orthosis. The researchers recognized the weaknesses of the study including use of retrospective design and absence of a control group. The outcomes cannot be applied to all children with camptodactyly since only children under the age of three with simple syndactyly were studied, and children with syndromic or adolescent onset camptodactyly were not included [93].

Orthotics

In a descriptive case series, Hori et al. [94] evaluated the effectiveness of dynamic splinting on increasing digital extension in 24 (34 fingers) children with camptodactyly. A Capener type coil spring was applied initially for 24 h per day and then only 8 h per day during a maintenance period. Duration of treatment was individualized and not described. Measurement technique was unclear in 10 patients but an explicit statement regarding measurement was provided for 14 patients (21 fingers). The researchers noted "almost full correction" [94, p. 1062] in 14 patients (20 fingers). Eight patients (nine fingers) improved, three fingers were not improved, and two patients (two fingers) worsened. Of the 14 patients (21 fingers) measured, mean flexion contracture before and after intervention was 40° and 10°, respectively. Reoccurrence was noted in one patient. This study lacked a control group, randomization, and blinding. No statistical analysis was undertaken thus limiting generalizations to the larger population. Significant bias is likely since for some patients, AROM may have been determined by visual observation alone.

Miura et al. [95] also examined the effectiveness of dynamic splinting on increasing digital extension but did so prospectively and included a larger sample than Hori et al. [94]. The study included children ($n=142$) with non-traumatic flexion deformities. Of these, 62 had small finger involvement, 16 had small finger plus one or more other finger involvement, 41 had other finger involvement (not small finger), and 23 had syndromic camptodactyly. A dynamic orthosis (Capener type coil spring) was applied to children with contracture of the small finger only for 24 h per day, although only 12 h per day for children under 7 years of age. During a maintenance period wear time was reduced. Outcomes were dichotomized into *failed to respond* or *responded* to treatment. Of 142 patients, only five failed to respond to treatment. Reoccurrence was observed in two patients. From this study alone no definitive statements can be made regarding treatment of children with camptodactyly using orthoses; however, given the number of patients who made gains low-level evidence if offered [95]. Figure 5.2 depicts a serial static orthosis used to correct improve joint motion in camptodactyly.

Orthotics and PROM

Benson et al. [96] retrospectively evaluated the effectiveness of orthoses and PROM to conservatively treat camptodactyly across three subtypes involving the PIP joint. In this case series, in which only descriptive analysis was performed,

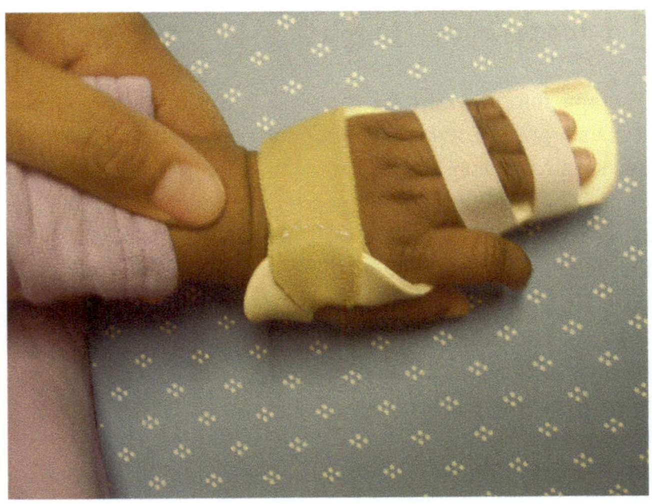

Fig. 5.2 Orthosis for camptodactyly involving multiple digits

researchers treated contracted digits of 18 patients (50 PIP joints) to promote PIP extension. Wear time for the orthosis ranged from 15–18 h per day for infants and 10–12 h per days for older children who were not inclined to sleep during the daytime. Parents performed PROM daily prior to application of the orthosis, although duration of treatment was individualized and poorly defined. Using goniometry, the same rater measured PROM before and after the intervention period. For analysis, children were assigned to one of three groups, including: (1) infantile camptodactyly between the age of 0.3–2.3 years ($n = 13$ patients, 24 digits); (2) adolescent camptodactyly between the age of 14.5–17.0 years ($n = 4$ patients, 5 digits); and (3) syndromic camptodactyly between the ages of 0.1–13.4 years ($n = 5$ patients, 30 digits). Full passive extension was achieved in 18 of 24 PIP joints for children with infantile camptodactyly. The group mean at start and end of treatment was −22.9° and end −4.3°, respectively. For children with adolescent onset of camptodactyly, only one (1 PIP joint) underwent a full program of orthosis wear and achieved full extension. Two others (2 PIP joints) elected surgery and worsened. The fourth patient (2 PIP joints) abandoned orthosis wear after 1 month and worsened. The group mean at start and end of treatment was −29.0° and −32.0°, respectively. In the syndromic group, four patients (24 PIP joints) were treated with an orthosis and demonstrated a group mean at the start and end of treatment of −23.0° and −1.0°, respectively. Two patients elected surgery and gained motion; one achieved full extension in two of two PIP joints and the other achieved and average of 41° of improvement across four digits. This study suggests conservative management with an orthosis may be prudent prior to electing surgery and perhaps more so with patients who present with infantile camptodactyly; however, in the absence of a control group, randomization, blinding, long-term follow-up, and inferential statistical analysis the outcomes are inconclusive [96].

Hypoplasia of the Thumb

Therapy interventions for children with thumb hypoplasia will vary greatly depending upon the severity of involvement and surgical management. This section will include interventions for children undergoing surgical procedures for Grade IIIA hypoplasia including web deepening, stabilization of the MCP joint and tendon transfers, and those for Grade IIIB, IV, and V including pollicization or free toe transfer.

Range of Motion Exercise

First Web Space Deepening, MCP Stabilization, Opponensplasty

At 6 weeks following abductor digiti minimi opponensplasty, supervised AROM and light activity is commenced [97, 98], with emphasis on opposition and palmer abduction, and PROM may commence 8 weeks following surgery [98] as well as resistive pinching [97]. Budding taping of the index finger to the middle finger may help to promote opposition of the index to the thumb by restricting lateral prehension between the index and middle finger.

Pollicization or Free Toe Transfer

For pollicization and free toe transfer, Egerszegi [99] recommends initiation of AROM at 3–4 weeks and PROM 1–2 weeks later; however, Goldfarb et al. [98] suggest PROM not begin until 8 weeks following surgery. Buddy taping of the middle finger to the ring finger may encourage opposition of the pollicized index finger to the middle finger by restricting lateral prehension between the middle and ring fingers.

Orthotics

First Web Space Deepening, MCP Stabilization, Opponensplasty

Following abductor digiti minimi opponensplasty, the hand and wrist should be completely immobilized for 4–6 weeks, after which an orthosis is fabricated to maintain a wide, open web space in opposition and palmer abduction [97, 98]. de Roode et al. [97] specifically recommend a neoprene orthosis. Regardless of type, the orthosis should be worn continuously until the eighth postoperative week [97, 98], and removed only for washing, and supervised activity and exercise. Goldfarb et al. [98] recommend discontinuing all orthoses 12 weeks following surgery, whereas de Roode et al. [97] recommend weaning of the splint to night-time wear only but do not indicate when or if night-time splinting should be discontinued. Goldfarb et al. [98] recommend similar immobilization regardless of opponensplasty technique; however, Kozin and Ezaki [100] recommend a long arm thumb spica cast with the elbow 90° flexion for only 2–3 weeks after flexor digitorum superficialis opponensplasty. These authors did not indicate need for a thermoplastic splint following cast removal.

Pollicization or Free Toe Transfer

Regarding pollicization, Egerszegi [99] recommends continuous immobilization for 3–4 weeks with a thermoplastic orthosis replacing the postsurgical splint and worn continuously for an additional week followed by an additional 6 weeks of orthotic use at night and during vigorous activity. In the case of free toe transfer, a similar program of orthosis wear is indicated except evidence of bony union signifies discontinuance of fulltime wear of an orthosis and transition to night-time wear. Goldfarb et al. [98] recommend an orthosis that places the thumb in opposition and palmar abduction.

Scar Management

Scar management may be initiated as early as 3–4 weeks with scar massage. A pressure garment with silicone sewn into the garment may prove useful for young children; whereas, gel and elastomer could be held in place with self-adherent elastic wrap for older children.

Radial Longitudinal Deficiency

Range of Motion Exercise

Children with RLD may have limitations in elbow motion in addition to wrist deformity [1, 101]. Brooks [2] recommends active and passive elbow ROM for 5–10 min, five times per day. In a series of 27 children with RLD and restriction in elbow flexion, Lamb [1] observed an increase in active elbow flexion for 20 children when an orthosis was applied to the wrist. Restricting wrist motion may facilitate greater elbow motion by preventing a functional pattern of wrist radial deviation to bring the hand toward the trunk and face. Initially, PROM alone may be indicated to preserve tissue length when the wrist can easily be brought into a neutral position. Bednar et al. [102] recommend passive ulnar deviation for 5–10 min, 4–5 times per day. If not passively correctable to neutral, the addition of orthotic management should be considered. Damore et al. [103] recommend passive ROM only until 3 months of age at which time a night-time only orthosis is introduced.

Following centralization procedures, Goldfarb et al. [98] recommend digital ROM begin immediately, and supervised light active use of the hand out of the orthosis by 6 weeks. Further wrist ROM (excluding passive radial deviation) may begin 6 months following surgery.

Orthotics

Conservative management of RLD includes use of casts or orthoses to preserve (Fig. 5.3) or increase tissue length and increase function [1, 104, 105]. The required duration of orthosis wear to achieve or approximate passive correction will depend upon the degree of deformity and the load required to bring the wrist toward neutral; however, this may need to be balanced by time out of the orthosis for play exploration and maintenance of skin integrity. Use of an orthosis may continue until skeletal maturity [2]. Fuller [105] recommends the orthosis be applied radially but cover 80 % of both the volar and dorsal forearm.

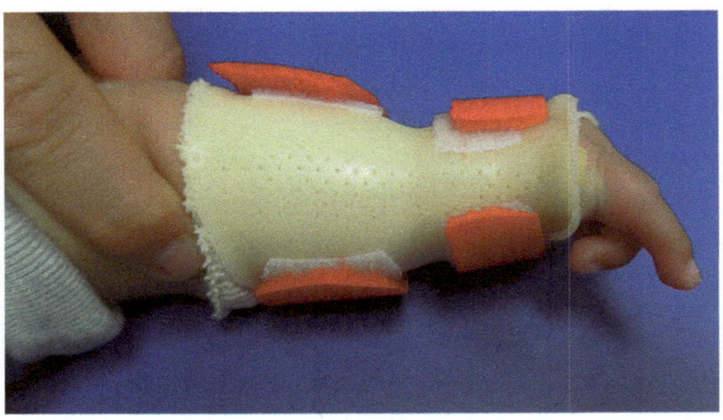

Fig. 5.3 Orthosis for RLD with thumb aplasia

Children with RLD who undergo centralization of the ulna or other soft tissue procedures will require prolonged use of an orthosis pre- and postoperatively [102, 106, 107]. Many authors recommend commencing with orthosis use or serial casting soon after birth and continuing until surgery [102–104, 106]. Kotwal et al. [6] proposed aggressive preoperative use of an orthosis minimizes the amount of tissue disruption and subsequent fibrosis that would otherwise contribute to further deforming forces on the wrist. Following centralization, radialization, or other soft tissue procedure to better align the wrist, fulltime orthosis wear followed by night-time only wear may be indicated. Following centralization and 6–8 weeks of pinning and postoperative splinting, Damore et al. [103] employs fulltime orthosis use followed by weaning toward night-time wear until skeletal maturity. Goldfarb et al. [98] recommend discontinuing use of the orthosis during the day by 6 months but continuing night-time wear until skeletal maturity. For both centralization and radialization, and after 8–12 weeks of internal fixation and splinting, Kotwal et al. [6] introduced fulltime use of an orthosis for 1 year followed by intermittent daytime use for an additional 1–2 years. No mention was made of night-time use during this latter period [6].

Kennedy [108] reported outcomes after applying orthoses to correct excessive radial deviation and minimize soft tissue reconstruction during corrective surgery, or to maintain or improve correction postoperatively. In this case series, children with RLD using an orthosis were treated preoperatively ($n=5$) or postoperatively ($n=4$). In the preoperative group, there were four males and one female with ages ranging from 3 weeks to 5 years. In the postoperative group, there were three males and one female with ages ranging from 2 years to 9 years. Each child received a custom fabricated neoprene orthosis with thermoplastic reinforcement to centrally align the hand to the carpus. Children wore the orthosis fulltime in all environments typical for the child. Duration of treatment for the preoperative group ranged from 3 weeks to 6 months to achieve correction, whereas duration of treatment for the postoperative group ranged from 6 weeks to 2 years to achieve correction. Wrist alignment was the desired outcome but the measurement technique was not described. For the preoperative group, all children obtained a neutral wrist with four children achieving 90° and one 45° of improvement. For the postoperative group mean correction of residual deformity in three children was 30°. Correction was maintained in the fourth child. The author reported subjective observations of improved activity participation with the orthosis including use of cutlery and tying shoelaces. This study lacked a control group, randomization, blinding, use of objective repeatable measures, and statistical analysis, but thoroughly describes a splint and provides descriptive outcomes for a small group of children with RLD [108].

Assistive Technology

Holtslag et al. [4] examined participation levels among adults with mild and severe RLD using the Participation and Autonomy questionnaire (IPA). No significant differences were noted between the groups, and both groups exhibited good levels of participation (median IPA score) 2.4 (a score of zero is very good and a score of four is poor). Some participants in this study indicated a need for activity modification or assistive device to perform fastening of buttons, squeezing a tube of toothpaste, carrying heavy objects, and cutting food. In a series of 117 patients with RLD, Lamb [1] noted no functional impairment for children with unilateral RLD, but for those with bilateral impairment fastening buttons, cutting meat, combing hair, and putting on socks proved difficult. Buffart et al. [7] also identified specific activities found to be difficult for children with RLD including fastening buttons, spreading jam, donning gloves, and cutting firm textured foods. These are important activities to practice with children and, perhaps, introduce assistive devices.

Syndactyly

Complications following syndactyly release include web creep, rotational and angular deformities, and limitations in AROM [109–113] for which ROM, application of an orthosis, and scar management may be indicated [113].

Range of Motion Exercise

Fuller [105] recommends parents be taught PROM. Extension deficits (flexion contractures) can be managed using an orthosis, while limitations in active flexion might be better managed with combined PROM and AROM during the day.

Orthotics

Goldfarb et al. [113] noted patterns of deformity following syndactyly release, for children with complex syndactyly not related to a syndrome or other CAUE, including a trend for the released digit to rotate away from and deviate toward the previously adjoined digit. After the postoperative dressings and splint have been discontinued, a thermoplastic splint may be indicated to maintain the MCP joint(s) in abduction, to correct an extension deficit, or to align the digits along the horizontal and frontal planes. Fuller [105] recommended a static forearm based orthosis with elevation of the material between adjacent digits and individual finger straps, whereas Moran and Tomhave [114] recommend a hand-based orthosis with individual finger straps.

Scar Management

Scar management options may be narrowed since children with syndactyly often undergo release during the infant or toddler years, and so choice of modality must include products that are less likely to pose a choking hazard. For this reason, a pressure garment with silicone sewn into the garment may prove useful for young children; whereas, gel or elastomer (Fig. 5.4) could be held in place with self-adherent elastic wrap for older children.

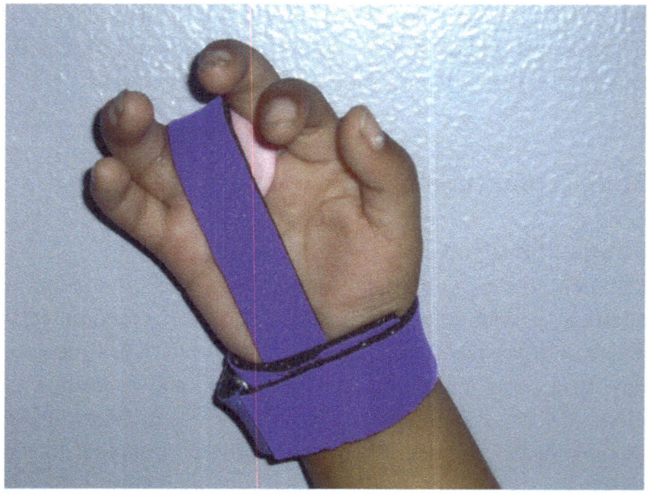

Fig. 5.4 Scar pad for web creep following syndactyly release

Trigger Thumb

Baek and Lee [115] conducted a prospective observational study of 71 trigger thumbs in 53 children whose mean age when diagnosed was 2 years with a mean flexion contracture of 26°. These children were followed for 49 months. Forty-five of 71 thumbs (63 %) spontaneous resolved. For this reason, children with trigger thumb are often observed or offered conservative treatment, including ROM and application of an orthosis.

Range of Motion Exercise

Two groups of researchers [116, 117] favor PROM over use of an orthosis for conservative treatment of trigger thumb. In a prospective, case series, Wantabe et al. [116] described 58 thumbs in 46 children treated with daily passive extension exercises only. Thumbs were identified as: Stage 0: No trigger or flexion posture; Stage 1: Locking, active movement with triggering; Stage 2: Locking, passive movement with triggering;, or Stage 3: Locked. A satisfactory result was noted in 96 % of cases at follow-up (mean 44 months), while complete recovery was noted in 27 % of thumbs at follow-up (mean 62 months). A cure rate of 80 % was reported for Stage 2 thumbs at follow-up (mean 56 months) and 25 % for Stage 3 thumbs at follow-up (mean 68 months). The cure rate for initial Stage 2 thumbs was significantly higher than for initial Stage 3 thumbs ($p<0.05$) [116].

In a similar prospective, consecutive case series, Jung et al. [117] examined treatment with PROM only in children ($n=30$), thumbs ($n=35$). PROM was applied 10–20 times per day. Digits were categorized as: Grade OA, extension beyond 0° without triggering; Grade OB, extension to 0° without triggering; Grade 1 active extension with triggering; Grade 2 passive extension with triggering; and Grade 3, locked. Pretest results found thumbs were identified as: Grade 1, 6 thumbs (17 %); Grade 2, 25 thumbs (71 %); and Grade 3, 3 thumbs (25 %). Posttest results found thumbs were identified as: Grade OA, 7 thumbs (20 %); Grade OB, 25 thumbs (21 %); Grade I, 5 thumbs (14 %); Grade II, 2 thumbs (6 %); No change = 1 thumb. The researchers found children with bilateral trigger thumb and children with a Grade III thumb were more likely to have an unfavorable outcome. Passive ROM seems useful for Grades 1 and 2, but may not be useful for Grade 3 trigger thumb. Additionally, PROM may be useful to correct deformity but triggering may persist [117]. These studies provide limited to moderate support for use of PROM to reduce triggering and improve motion for children with trigger thumb.

Orthotics

Two studies have described the effectiveness of orthoses to treat trigger thumb with varying outcomes [118, 119]. Koh et al. [118] conducted a retrospective, non-randomized, controlled study by reviewing medical records of children with locked interphalangeal (IP) joint. Parents self-selected whether to have their child wear an orthosis ($n=26$) or undergo observation alone ($n=38$). Children receiving a custom made, coil orthosis to hold the IP joint in extension while preventing hyperextension of the MCP joint wore the orthosis at night. Duration of treatment or observation was individualized until either resolution was achieved or surgery was indicated. The targeted outcome was full AROM of the thumb IP joint without snapping but no measurement technique was described. Of patients treated with an orthosis, 92 % experienced complete resolution within 22 months, whereas 60 % in the observation group had complete resolution in 59 months. After an additional 11 months, 97 % of patients in the observation group experienced resolution of snapping. All patients in both groups experienced complete resolution, but four (two from each group) required surgery due to continued snapping. Those receiving an orthosis had significantly higher rates of resolution ($p<0.05$) and shorter resolution time ($p<0.01$) compared to observation alone. This study suggests patients with locked trigger thumbs who wear a coil orthosis may have faster rates of resolution compared to those receiving no treatment [118]. Using a similar design, Lee et al. [119] compared treatment with an orthosis to observation alone for management of trigger thumb. In this non-randomized, non-blinded, and case controlled study, parents of children self-selected to receive an orthosis ($n=31$ thumbs) or be observed ($n=31$ thumbs). An orthosis that maintained the MCP joint and IP joint in extension was custom fabricated from thermoplastic for patients in the orthosis group, and was to be worn all day for 6–12 weeks in the child's usual environments. The orthosis was worn at night only once active extension was achieved. Mean duration of treatment was 11.7 weeks ± 6.6 weeks. The outcome classification was cured (full AROM), improved (full AROM with snapping less than once per week), or non-improved (persistent flexion deformity or surgery was requested). Regarding AROM, no measurement technique was described. In the group that received an orthosis, 12 were cured, 10 were improved, and nine were non-improved. In the observation alone group four were cured, three were improved, and 24 were unimproved. The difference between the groups was statistically significant ($p<0.05$). Response rates were 71 % for the orthosis group and 23 % for the observation alone group [119]. These studies provide limited support for use of an orthosis to manage trigger thumb when conservative treatment is desired.

References

1. Lamb DW. Radial club hand. J Bone Joint Surg. 1977;59A:1–13.
2. Brooks C. Rehabilitation of radial club hand. Tech Hand Up Extrem Surg. 1998;2(1):78–85.
3. Lake A. Hand therapy for children with congenital hand differences. Tech Hand Up Extrem Surg. 2010;14(2):78–84.
4. Holtslag I, van Wijk I, Hartog H, van der Molen AM, van der Sluis C. Long-term functional outcome of patients with longitudinal radial deficiency: cross-sectional evaluation of function, activity and participation. Disabil Rehabil. 2013;35(16):1401–7.
5. de Jong IG, Reinders-Messelink HA, Tates K, Janssen WG, Poelma MJ, van Wijk I, van der Sluis CK. Activity and participation of children and adolescents with unilateral congenital below elbow deficiency: an online focus group study. J Rehabil Med. 2012;44(10):885–92.
6. Kotwal PP, Varshney MK, Soral A. Comparison of surgical treatment and nonoperative management for radial longitudinal deficiency. J Hand Surg Eur Vol. 2012;37(2):161–9.
7. Buffart LM, Roebroeck ME, Janssen WG, Hoekstra A, Selles RW, Hovius SE, Stam HJ. Hand function and activity performance of children with longitudinal radial deficiency. J Bone Joint Surg Am. 2008;90(11):2408–15.
8. Ekblom AG, Dahlin LB, Rosberg HE, Wiig M, Werner M, Arner M. Hand function in children with radial longitudinal deficiency. BMC Musculoskelet Disord. 2013;14:116.
9. Soucie JM, Wang C, Forsyth A, Funk S, Denny M, Roach KE, Boone D. Range of motion measurements: reference values and a database for comparison. Haemophilia. 2011;17(3):500–7.
10. Barad JH, Kim RS, Ebramzadeh E, Silva M. Range of motion of the healthy pediatric elbow: cross-sectional study of a large population. J Pediatr Orthop B. 2013;22(2):117–22.
11. de Kraker MD, Selles RW, Molenaar TM, Schreuders TA, Hovius SE, Stam HJ. Palmar abduction measurements: reliability and introduction of normative data in healthy children. J Hand Surg Am. 2009;34A:1704–8.
12. Häger-Ross C, Rösblad B. Norms for grip strength in children aged 4–16. Acta Paediatr. 2002;91(6):617–25.

13. Bowman OJ, Katz B. Hand strength and prone extension in right-dominant, 6 to 9 year olds. Am J Occup Ther. 1984;38(6):367–76.
14. Fullwood D. Australian norms for hand and finger strength of boys and girls aged 5–12 years. Aust Occup Ther J. 1986;33:26–37.
15. De Smet L, Vercamment A. Grip strength in children. J Pediatr Orthop. 2001;10(4):352–4.
16. Holm I, Fredriksen P, Fosdahl M, Vøllestad N. A normative sample of isotonic and isokinetic muscle strength measurements in children 7 to 12 years of age. Acta Paediatr. 2008;97(5):602–7.
17. Ploegmakers JJ, Hepping AM, Geertzen JH, Bulstra SK, Stevens M. Grip strength is strongly associated with height, weight and gender in childhood: a cross sectional study of 2241 children and adolescents providing reference values. J Physiother. 2013;59(4):255–61.
18. Mathiowetz V, Wiemer DM, Federman SM. Grip and pinch strength: norms for 6- to 19-year-olds. Am J Occup Ther. 1986; 40(10):705–11.
19. Lee-Valkov PM, Aaron DH, Eladoumikdachi F, Thornby J, Netscher DT. Measuring normal hand dexterity values in normal 3-, 4-, and 5-year-old children and their relationship with grip and pinch strength. J Hand Ther. 2003;16(1):22–8.
20. Ager CL, Olivett BL, Johnson CL. Grasp and pinch strength in children 5 to 12 years old. Am J Occup Ther. 1984;38(2): 107–13.
21. Surrey LR, Hodson J, Robinson E, Schmidt S, Schulhof J, Stoll L, Wilson-Diekhoff N. Pinch strength norms for 5-to 12-year-olds. Phys Occup Ther Pediatr. 2001;21(1):37–49.
22. De Smet L, Decramer A. Key pinch force in children. J Pediatr Orthop B. 2006;15(6):426–7.
23. Cope EB, Antony JH. Normal values for the two-point discrimination test. Pediatr Neurol. 1992;8(4):251–4.
24. Mathiowetz V, Federman SM, Wiemer DM. Box and blocks test of manual dexterity: norms for 6–19 year olds. Can J Occup Ther. 1985;52(5):241–5.
25. Gogola GR, Velleman PF, Xu S, Morse AM, Lacy B, Aaron D. Hand dexterity in children: administration and normative values of the functional dexterity test. J Hand Surg Am. 2013;38(12):2426–31.
26. Smith YA, Hong E, Presson C. Normative and validation studies of the Nine-hole Peg Test with children. Percept Mot Skills. 2000;90(3 Pt 1):823–43.
27. Poole JL, Burtner PA, Torres TA, McMullen CK, Markham A, Marcum ML, et al. Measuring dexterity in children using the Nine-hole Peg Test. J Hand Ther. 2005;18(3):348–51.
28. Wilson BC, Iacoviello JM, Wilson JJ, Risucci D. Purdue Pegboard performance of normal preschool children. J Clin Neuropsychol. 1982;4(1):19–26.
29. Skerik SK, Weiss MW, Flatt AE. Functional evaluation of congenital hand anomalies. Am J Occup Ther. 1971;25(2):98–104.
30. Percival NJ, Sykes PJ, Chandraprakasam T. A method of assessment of pollicisation. J Hand Surg Br. 1991;16(2):141–3.
31. Ho ES, Clarke HM. Upper extremity function in children with congenital hand anomalies. J Hand Ther. 2005;18(3):352–64.
32. Buffart LM, Roebroeck ME, Pesch-Batenburg JM, Janssen WG, Stam HJ. Assessment of arm/hand functioning in children with a congenital transverse or longitudinal reduction deficiency of the upper limb. Disabil Rehabil. 2006;28(2):85–95.
33. Buffart LM, Roebroeck ME, Janssen WG, Hoekstra A, Hovius SE, Stam HJ. Comparison of instruments to assess hand function in children with radius deficiencies. J Hand Surg Am. 2007;32(4):531–40.
34. Kaplan JD, Jones NF. Outcome measures of microsurgical toe transfers for reconstruction of congenital and traumatic hand anomalies. J Pediatr Orthop. 2014;34:362–8.
35. Arnould C, Penta M, Renders A, Thonnard JL. ABILHAND-Kids: a measure of manual ability in children with cerebral palsy. Neurology. 2004;63(6):1045–52.
36. Krumlinde-Sundholm L, Holmefur M, Kottorp A, Eliasson AC. The Assisting Hand Assessment: current evidence of validity, reliability, and responsiveness to change. Dev Med Child Neurol. 2007;49(4):259–64.
37. Holmefur M, Krumlinde-Sundholm L, Eliasson AC. Interrater and intrarater reliability of the Assisting Hand Assessment. Am J Occup Ther. 2007;61(1):79–84.
38. Holmefur M, Aarts P, Hoare B, Krumlinde-Sundholm L. Test-retest and alternate forms reliability of the assisting hand assessment. J Rehabil Med. 2009;41(11):886–91.
39. Skold A, Hermansson LN, Krumlinde-Sundholm L, Eliasson AC. Development and evidence of validity for the Children's Hand-use Experience Questionnaire (CHEQ). Dev Med Child Neurol. 2011;53(5):436–42.
40. Varni JW, Seid M, Kurtin PS. PedsQL 4.0: reliability and validity of the Pediatric Quality of Life Inventory version 4.0 generic core scales in healthy and patient populations. Med Care. 2001;39(8): 800–12.
41. Schlenz AM, Schatz J, McClellan CB, Roberts CW. Responsiveness of the PedsQL to pain-related changes in health-related quality of life in pediatric sickle cell disease. J Pediatr Psychol. 2012;37(7):798–807.
42. Haley SM, Coster WJ, Faas RM. A content validity study of the Pediatric Evaluation of Disability Inventory. Pediatr Phys Ther. 1991;3:177–84.
43. Feldman AB, Haley SM, Coryell J. Concurrent and construct validity of the Pediatric Evaluation of Disability Inventory. Phys Ther. 1990;70(10):602–10.
44. Wright FV, Boschen KA. The Pediatric Evaluation of Disability Inventory (PEDI): validation of a new functional assessment outcome instrument. Can J Rehabil. 1993;7:41–2.
45. Nichols DS, Case-Smith J. Reliability and validity of the Pediatric Evaluation of Disability Inventory. Pediatr Phys Ther. 1996;8: 15–24.
46. Daltroy LH, Liang MH, Fossel AH, Goldberg MJ. The POSNA pediatric musculoskeletal functional health questionnaire: report on reliability, validity and sensitivity to change. J Pediatr Orthop. 1998;18(5):561–71.
47. Pencharz J, Young NL, Owen JL, Wright JG. Comparison of three outcomes instruments in children. J Pediatr Orthop. 2001;21(4): 425–32.
48. Amor CJ, Spaeth MC, Chafey DH, Gogola GR. Use of the Pediatric Outcomes Data Collection Instrument to evaluate functional outcomes in arthrogryposis. J Pediatr Orthop. 2011;31(3):293–6.
49. Haynes R, Sullivan E. The Paediatric Orthopaedic Society of North America paediatric orthopaedic functional health questionnaire: an analysis of normal. J Pediatr Orthop. 2001;21(5):619–21.
50. Wright FV, Hubbard S, Naumann S, Jutai J. Evaluation of the validity of the prosthetic upper extremity functional index for children. Arch Phys Med Rehabil. 2003;84(4):518–27.
51. Wright FV, Hubbard S, Jutai J, Naumann S. The Prosthetic Upper Extremity Functional Index: development and reliability testing of a new functional status questionnaire for children who use upper extremity prostheses. J Hand Ther. 2001;14(2):91–104.
52. Bagley AM, Molitor F, Wagner LV, Tomhave W, James MA. The unilateral below elbow test: a function test for children with unilateral congenital below elbow deficiency. Dev Med Child Neurol. 2006;48(7):569–75.
53. Netscher DT, Aliu O, Sandvall BK, Staines KG, Hamilton KL, Salazar-Reyes H, Thornby J. Functional outcomes of children with index pollicizations for thumb deficiency. J Hand Surg Am. 2013;38(2):250–7.
54. Ardon MS, Selles RW, Roebroeck ME, Hovius SE, Stam HJ, Janssen WG. Poor agreement on health-related quality of life between children with congenital hand differences and their parents. Arch Phys Med Rehabil. 2012;93(4):641–6.

55. Sheffler LC, Hanley C, Bagley A, Molitor F, James MA. Comparison of self-reports and parent proxy-reports of function and quality of life of children with below-the-elbow deficiency. J Bone Joint Surg Am. 2009;91(12):2852–9.
56. Giele H, Giele C, Bower C, Allison M. The incidence and epidemiology of congenital upper limb anomalies: a total population study. J Hand Surg Am. 2001;26(4):628–34.
57. Koskimies E, Lindfors N, Gissler M, Peltonen J, Nietosvaara Y. Congenital upper limb deficiencies and associated malformations in Finland: a population-based study. J Hand Surg Am. 2011;36(6):1058–65.
58. Ekblom AG, Laurell T, Arner M. Epidemiology of congenital upper limb anomalies in 562 children born in 1997 to 2007: a total population study from Stockholm, Sweden. J Hand Surg Am. 2010;35(11):1742–54.
59. Froster-Iskenius UG, Baird PA. Limb reduction defects in over one million consecutive live births. Teratology. 1998;39(2):127–35.
60. Evans JA, Vitez M, Czeizel A. Congenital abnormalities associated with limb deficiency defects: a population study based on cases from the Hungarian Congenital Malformation Registry (1975-1984). Am J Med Genet. 1994;49(1):52–66.
61. Baker RP, Field J, Gozzard C, Wyatt MC, Robertson Y. Does postoperative hand elevation reduce swelling? A randomized study. J Hand Surg Eur Vol. 2010;35(3):192–4.
62. Fagan DJ, Evans A, Ghandour A, Prabhkaran P, Clay NR. A controlled clinical trial of postoperative hand elevation at home following day case surgery. J Hand Surg Br. 2004;29:458–60.
63. Enos L, Lane R, MacDougal BA. Brief or new: the use of self-adherent wrap in hand rehabilitation. Am J Occup Ther. 1984;38(4):265–6.
64. Lowell M, Pirc P, Ward RS, et al. Effect of 3 M Coban self-adherent wraps on edema and function of the burned hand: a case study. J Burn Care Rehabil. 2003;24:253–8.
65. Shin TM, Bordeaux JS. The role of massage in scar management: a literature review. Dermatol Surg. 2012;38(3):414–23.
66. Foo CW, Tristani-Firouzi P. Topical modalities for treatment and prevention of postsurgical hypertrophic scars. Facial Plast Surg Clin North Am. 2011;19(3):551–7.
67. Chang LW, Deng WP, Yeong EK, Wu CY, Yeh SW. Pressure effects on the growth of human scar fibroblasts. J Burn Care Res. 2008;29(5):835–41.
68. Kischer CW, Shetlar MR, Shetlar CL. Alteration of hypertrophic scars induced by mechanical pressure. Arch Dermatol. 1975;111(1):60–4.
69. Anzarut A, Olson J, Singh P, Rowe BH, Tredget EE. The effectiveness of pressure garment therapy for the prevention of abnormal scarring after burn injury: a meta-analysis. J Plast Reconstr Aesthet Surg. 2009;62(1):77–84.
70. Steinstraesser L, Flak E, Witte B, Ring A, Tilkorn D, Hauser J, Langer S, Steinau HU, Al-Benna S. Pressure garment therapy alone and in combination with silicone for the prevention of hypertrophic scarring: randomized controlled trial with intraindividual comparison. Plast Reconstr Surg. 2011;128(4):306e–13.
71. Widgerow AD. Cellular/extracellular cross-talk in scar evolution and control. Wound Repair Regen. 2011;19:117–33.
72. Hart RG, Wolff TW, O'Neil WL. Preventing tourniquet effect when dressing finger wounds in children. Am J Emerg Med. 2004;22:594–5.
73. Yelvington M, Brown S, Castro MM, Nick TG. The use of neoprene as a scar management modality. Burns. 2013; pii:S0305-4179(12)00364-6.
74. Mustoe TA, Cooter RD, Gold MH, Hobbs FD, Ramelet AA, Shakespeare PG, Stella M, Téot L, Wood FM, Ziegler UE, International Advisory Panel on Scar Management. International clinical recommendations on scar management. Plast Reconstr Surg. 2002;110(2):560–71.
75. O'Brien L, Pandit A. Silicon gel sheeting for preventing and treating hypertrophic and keloid scars. Cochrane Database Syst Rev. 2006;1, CD003826.
76. O'Brien L, Jones DJ. Silicone gel sheeting for preventing and treating hypertrophic and keloid scars. Cochrane Database Syst Rev. 2013;9, CD003826.
77. Sawada Y, Sone K. Hydration and occlusion treatment for hypertrophic scars and keloids. Br J Plast Surg. 1992;45(8):599–603.
78. de Oliveira GV, Nunes TA, Magna LA, Cintra ML, Kitten GT, Zarpellon S, Raposo Do Amaral CM. Silicone versus nonsilicone gel dressings: a controlled trial. Dermatol Surg. 2001;27(8):721–6.
79. Rustad KC, Wong VW, Gurtner GC. The role of focal adhesion complexes in fibroblast mechanotransduction during scar formation. Differentiation. 2013;86(3):87–91.
80. Chiquet M, Gelman L, Lutz R, Maier S. From mechanotransduction to extracellular matrix gene expression in fibroblasts. Biochim Biophys Acta. 2009;1793:911–20.
81. Widgerow AD, Chait LA, Stals PJ, Stals R, Candy G. Multimodality scar management program. Aesthetic Plast Surg. 2009;33:533–43.
82. Atkinson JM, McKenna KT, Barnett AG, McGrath DJ, Rudd M. A randomized, controlled trial to determine the efficacy of paper tape in preventing hypertrophic scar formation in surgical incisions that traverse Langer's skin tension lines. Plast Reconstr Surg. 2005;116(6):1648–56.
83. Widgerow AD, Chait LA. Scar management practice and science: a comprehensive approach to controlling scar tissue and avoiding hypertrophic scarring. Adv Skin Wound Care. 2011;24(12):555–61.
84. Michlovitz SL, Harris BA, Watkins MP. Therapy interventions for improving joint range of motion: a systematic review. J Hand Ther. 2004;17(2):118–31.
85. Glasgow C, Tooth LR, Fleming J. Mobilizing the stiff hand: combining theory and evidence to improve clinical outcomes. J Hand Ther. 2010;23(4):392–400.
86. Flowers KR. A proposed decision hierarchy for splinting the stiff joint, with an emphasis on force application parameters. J Hand Ther. 2002;15(2):158–62.
87. Weeks PM, Wray RC. Management of acute hand injuries. 2nd ed. St. Louis: Mosby; 1978. p. 434–8.
88. Flowers KR, LaStayo PC. Effect of total end range time on improving passive range of motion. J Hand Ther. 1994;7(3):150–7.
89. Glasgow C, Wilton J, Tooth L. Optimal daily total end range time for contracture: resolution in hand splinting. J Hand Ther. 2003;16(3):207–18.
90. Glasgow C, Fleming J, Tooth LR, Peters S. Randomized controlled trial of daily total end range time (TERT) for capener splinting of the stiff proximal interphalangeal joint. Am J Occup Ther. 2012;66(2):243–8.
91. Blair WF, Shurr DG, Buckwalter JA. Functional status in ulnar deficiency. J Pediatr Orthop. 1983;3(1):37–40.
92. Ty J, James MA. Failure of differentiation: Part II (arthrogryposis, camptodactyly, clinodactyly, Madelung deformity, trigger finger, and trigger thumb). Hand Clin. 2009;25(2):195–214.
93. Rhee SH, Oh WS, Lee HJ, Roh YH, Lee JO, Baek GH. Effect of passive stretching on simple camptodactyly in children younger than three years of age. J Hand Surg Am. 2010;35(11):1768–73.
94. Hori M, Nakamura R, Inoue G, Imamura T, Horii E, Tanaka Y, Miura T. Nonoperative treatment of camptodactyly. J Hand Surg Am. 1987;12(6):1061–5.
95. Miura T, Nakamura R, Tamura Y. Long-standing extended dynamic splintage and release of an abnormal restraining structure in camptodactyly. J Hand Surg Br. 1992;17(6):665–72.
96. Benson LS, Waters PM, Kamil NI, Simmons BP, Upton 3rd J. Camptodactyly: classification and results of nonoperative treatment. J Pediatr Orthop. 1994;14(6):814–9.

97. de Roode CP, James MA, McCarroll HR. Abductor digit minimi opponensplasty: technique, modifications, and measurement of opposition. Tech Hand Up Extrem Surg. 2010;14(1):51–3.
98. Goldfarb CA, Calhoun VD, Daily L, Manske PR. Hand and upper extremity therapy: congenital, pediatric and adolescent: St Louis protocols. St. Louis: Shriners Hospital for Children; 2011.
99. Egerszegi EP. Reconstruction of congenital hand anomalies to provide stable pinch and/or grasp: case pictorial series. J Pediatr Rehabil Med. 2009;2(3):173–9.
100. Kozin SH, Ezaki M. Flexor digitorum superficialis opponensplasty with ulnar collateral ligament reconstruction for thumb deficiency. Tech Hand Up Extrem Surg. 2010;14(1):46–50.
101. Manske PR, Goldfarb CA. Congenital failure of formation of the upper limb. Hand Clin. 2009;25(2):157–70.
102. Bednar MS, James MA, Light TR. Congenital longitudinal deficiency. J Hand Surg Am. 2009;34(9):1739–47.
103. Damore E, Kozin SH, Thoder JJ, Porter S. The recurrence of deformity after surgical centralization for radial clubhand. J Hand Surg Am. 2000;25(4):745–51.
104. Banskota AK, Bijukachhe B, Rajbhandary T, Pradhan I, Singh A. Radial club hand deformity—the continuing challenges and controversies. Kathmandu Univ Med J (KUMJ). 2005;3(1):30–4.
105. Fuller M. Treatment of congenital differences of the upper extremity: therapists commentary. J Hand Ther. 1999;12(2):174–7.
106. Van Heest A. Wrist centralization using the dorsal rotation flap in radial longitudinal deficiency. Tech Hand Up Extrem Surg. 2010;14(2):94–9.
107. Wall LB, Ezaki M, Oishi SN. Management of congenital radial longitudinal deficiency: controversies and current concepts. Plast Reconstr Surg. 2013;132(1):122–8.
108. Kennedy SM. Neoprene wrist brace for correction of radial club hand in children. J Hand Ther. 1996;9(4):387–90.
109. Deunk J, Nicolai JP, Hamburg SM. Long-term results of syndactyly correction: full-thickness versus split-thickness skin grafts. J Hand Surg Br. 2003;28(2):125–30.
110. Lumenta DB, Kitzinger HB, Beck H, Frey M. Long-term outcomes of web creep, scar quality, and function after simple syndactyly surgical treatment. J Hand Surg Am. 2010;35(8):1323–9.
111. Vekris MD, Lykissas MG, Soucacos PN, Korompilias AV, Beris AE. Congenital syndactyly: outcome of surgical treatment in 131 webs. Tech Hand Up Extrem Surg. 2010;14(1):2–7.
112. Mallet C, Ilharreborde B, Jehanno P, Litzelmann E, Valenti P, Mazda K, Penneçot GF, Fitoussi F. Comparative study of 2 commissural dorsal flap techniques for the treatment of congenital syndactyly. J Pediatr Orthop. 2013;33(2):197–204.
113. Goldfarb CA, Steffen JA, Stutz CM. Complex syndactyly: aesthetic and objective outcomes. J Hand Surg Am. 2012;37(10):2068–73.
114. Moran SL, Tomhave W. Management of congenital hand anomalies. In: Skirven TM, Osterman AL, Fedorzyk JM, Amadio PC, editors. Rehabilitation of the hand and upper extremity. 6th ed. Philadelphia: Elsevier Mosby; 2011. p. 1631–50.
115. Baek GH, Lee HJ. The natural history of pediatric trigger thumb: a study with a minimum of five years follow-up. Clin Orthop Surg. 2011;3(2):157–9.
116. Wantabe H, Hamada Y, Toshima T, Nagasawa K. Conservative treatment for trigger thumb in children. Arch Orthop Trauma Surg. 2001;121(7):388–90.
117. Jung HJ, Lee JS, Song KS, Yang JJ. Conservative treatment of pediatric trigger thumb: follow-up for over 4 years. J Hand Surg Eur Vol. 2011;37E(3):220–4.
118. Koh S, Horii E, Hattori T, Hiroishi M, Otsula J. Pediatric trigger thumb with locked interphalangeal joint: can observation or splinting be a treatment option? J Pediatr Orthop. 2012;32(7):724–6.
119. Lee Z, Chang C, Yang W, Hung S, Shih C. Extension splint for trigger thumb in children. J Pediatr Orthop. 2006;26(6):785–7.

Psychological Considerations: Visible Distinctions and Congenital Anomalies of the Upper Extremities

6

Sondra Elice Solomon

> You came so nearly perfect from the hand of nature that this slightest possible defect, which we hesitate whether to term a defect or a beauty, shocks me as being the visible mark of earthly imperfection [1].

Introduction

In most cultures physical perfection is the standard by which a person's competence, intelligence, and humanity are assessed [2–5]. Visible attributes that challenge physical perfection are not well tolerated by normal-appearing others [3]. When a person possesses a visible attribute that does not conform to a narrowly defined metric of appearance acceptability, the bearer of that negatively valued visible attribute may be at risk for social exclusion, prejudice, discrimination, and stigma by perceived normal-appearing others [6–8]. Furthermore, when the visible attribute in question is determined by genetic or medical factors, psychological well-being may be affected [9].

Early consensus in the psychological literature suggested that individuals with visible atypical body or facial attributes would always be at a social disadvantage, since in addition to managing their own appearance-related thoughts, feelings, and behaviors, they had to manage the reactions of normal-appearing others towards their appearance [10]. Contemporary research acknowledges the complex interactions of individual, social, and cultural factors that shape the experiences and psychological well-being of individuals with atypical visible features [8, 11]. Facial appearance has been at the forefront of this research, and, at first blush, it is easy to understand why disruptions in facial appearance receive so much consideration. The face is a primary vehicle of human communication, and individuals make immediate judgments about others based on facial appearance. When facial integrity is disrupted social interaction is disrupted [7, 12]. However, hands and arms have salient cultural meaning as well. Hands and arms are essential for [1] interacting with and manipulating the physical world; [2] communicating with others; and [3] establishing and maintaining intimate physical contact with others. Like the face, hands and arms are difficult to conceal. Disruptions in the appearance of hands and arms have the potential to affect psychological well-being, yet there is limited research on the psychological functioning of individuals living with visible characteristics associated with congenital anomalies of the upper extremities (CAUE).

Definitions

In an effort to promote psychological well-being among individuals living with CAUE it might be useful to reevaluate the words we use to describe the population. The language we use to describe the people we treat has the potential to foster a strong therapeutic alliance as we work towards promoting long-term positive adjustment and psychological well-being for our patients. It is suggested that those who serve individuals living with CAUE employ the terminology offered in the following section. When possible and appropriate these terms will be used throughout this chapter.

Distinction

The term *distinction* will be used when referring to what the CAUE literature has characterized as aberrant, deformed, disfigured, defective, deficient, malformed, and abnormal attributes.

S.E. Solomon, Ph.D. (✉)
College of Arts and Sciences, Department of Psychological Sciences, University of Vermont, Dewey Hall, 346; 2 Colchester Avenue, Burlington, VT 05446, USA

College of Medicine, Department of Psychiatry, University of Vermont, Dewey Hall, 346; 2 Colchester Avenue, Burlington, VT 05446, USA
e-mail: Sondra.Solomon@uvm.edu

D.R. Laub Jr. (ed.), *Congenital Anomalies of the Upper Extremity: Etiology and Management*, DOI 10.1007/978-1-4899-7504-1_6,

The term *distinction* is relatively benign and can be substituted for the pejorative and negative labels that describe the visible characteristics of CAUE that affect appearance. It is recognized that some authors prefer the term *physical difference* [11, 13]; however, *distinction* is a relatively neutral word and is an appropriate descriptor for a visibly and culturally devalued attribute related to appearance.

Impairment and Disability

Most readers familiar with the genetics, rehabilitation, and disability literature will recognize the following definitions; however, it is useful to mention them again. *Impairment* is linked to a loss or a disruption of an anatomical structure or function and can be biologically determined or acquired via a disease process during a person's life, and *disability* is the consequence of the impairment and involves any restriction in the person's ability to perform an activity in the manner or within the range considered appropriate for individuals without the impairment [14–17]. The disability is the physical consequence of the impairment and is linked to how the impairment is manifested in the culture (i.e., the child with a congenital below the elbow anomaly has difficulty with motor function). The term *handicap* or *social handicap* should only be used when one considers how the person with the impairment is treated in the culture (i.e., the adult with a congenital below the elbow impairment is denied housing or employment due to processes that involve prejudice, exclusion, and discrimination).

Stigma and Stigmatization

Erving Goffman [18] began a discourse spanning 50 years, transforming the way we examine how human beings manage the minute and salient differences between us. These differences place most people in two camps based on various personal characteristics and attributes. People can join and or be excluded from the two camps based on where they happen to be at the time (cultural context) and which attributes are valued at the time (temporal salience). Also, it may be possible for a person to be a member of both camps at the same time. Undesirable attributes may be fixed and unquestionable (e.g., congenital disorders, facial distinctions, excessive weight, cognitive deficits, old age, ethnicity, disability, diagnoses of severe and/or chronic psychopathology, perceived to be engaged in non-normative behavior, etc.).

Goffman defined *stigma* as a spoiled identity or a deeply discrediting characteristic which may arise from physical deformities, blemishes of individual character that are interpreted to reflect weakness, unnatural passions, dishonesty; and one's lineage [18]. Possession of the devalued attribute or distinction places the affected individual at a social disadvantage. One early model to explain this disadvantaged social status suggests that stigma is a form of deviance that leads perceived normal-appearing others to judge individuals with the stigma as unworthy for participation in most social interchanges. They are viewed as incompetent, unpredictable, unreliable, or threatening [19]. This perception places the individual beyond the protection of a number of implicit norms that regulate social interaction. The disruptive impact of the distinction may be a function of how visible the distinction is to others, how much of the person's body is affected by the distinction, and how easily the distinction can be identified or seen by others [19, 20].

Researchers have been trying to understand and deconstruct the various processes contributing to devalued identities and subsequent spoiled interactions that devolve from possession of or contact with the undesirable attribute. Some have noted that it is difficult to identify a single defining feature of stigma and suggest that stigmatized people are believed to possess a feature, quality, or trait that portrays a social identity that is devalued in a particular social context [21]. In this view, stigma arises from one's membership in a group or category that is negatively valued in a specific situation (i.e., the adolescent with a below the elbow congenital anomaly is unable to participate in an activity in the same way that adolescents without the congenital anomaly).

Stigmatization may be conceptualized as a social process that seeks to reproduce inequality and exclusion [22–25]. There is an interaction between the environment and the individual with the distinction to recreate and perpetuate social and structural inequalities [25, 26]. Individuals with a devalued visible attribute may experience rejection, discrimination, and exclusion and these experiences have the potential to shape psychological, cognitive, and affective responses that affirm or impede healthy behaviors and psychological well-being [5].

Visible Distinctions and Stigma

An accepted definition of a *visible distinction* is that the attribute in question represents a departure from a culturally defined norm which is difficult to conceal from others and as a result the attribute has the potential to shape interpersonal interaction with perceived normal-appearing others [27]. The attribute is perceived by others to be atypical, non-normative, and noticeable and excludes those attributes that are consistent with a body dysmorphic presentation [11, 27]. A *visible distinction* can have a powerful influence on the affected individual. A *visible distinction* is a social disability, since in addition to influencing the thoughts, feelings, and behavior of the person with the visible distinction, it is also likely to shape the behavior of other people towards the affected individual [28, 29]. Research suggests that the extent to which a visible distinction results in social disability involves a complex interaction of social and individual factors [8, 11, 30]. We live in a culture that emphasizes physical perfection and individuals who possess visible attributes that are devalued occupy a special role in the culture and this role places them at a distinct advantage. The narrowly defined cultural appearance standard dictates who is accepted and who gets cast aside.

Stigma, Stigmatization, and Coping with Visible Distinctions

The stigmatized person is diminished in the eyes of the observer and may experience a variety of stressors. A stressor is an event in which environmental or internal demands tax or exceed the adaptive resources of the individual [31]. Stigma can increase demands on the affected individual because perceived normal individuals may hold stereotyped expectancies about what stigmatized people are like, harbor prejudiced attitudes towards stigmatized people, and behave in a discriminatory manner towards stigmatized people [32, 33]. Psychological responses such as anger, anxiety, hopelessness, resentment, and fear [3–5, 31, 34] may be experienced by the affected individual.

Visible distinctions are particularly stigmatizing because they remind the observer that the body is fragile, and depending on the etiology of the distinction may compel the observer to feel less compassion towards the individual with the distinction and to attribute more blame to them for having the distinction [35–37]. Children, adolescents, and adults living with CAUE frequently have visible attributes involving variations of limb formation, differentiation, duplication, overgrowth, and undergrowth; congenital constriction band syndrome; generalized skeletal irregularities; and comorbid facial irregularities [38]. Distinctions, such as those that can occur in CAUE, are particularly stigmatizing because the actual social identity—the attribute the individual possesses—does not meet society's normative expectations of the attribute the individual should possess [26]. Social identity is flawed and the affected individual is presumed unable to fulfill the basic requirements of social interaction. Physical perfection is the gold standard for social inclusion. Social exclusion and subsequent threats to psychological well-being may be inevitable if the devalued attribute is visible and involves the hands and arms.

Psychological Research on Visible Distinctions Associated with CAUE

Investigators have begun to explore how individuals adapt to a variety of stigmatizing attributes (e.g., diabetes, cancer, altered body appearance, HIV) [39–43]. An excellent review of the processes involved in managing visible distinctions acknowledged that successful outcomes are linked to (1) the individual's perception of the visible distinction; (2) their self-concept; (3) perceived and actual social support; (4) cultural contexts; (5) interpersonal encounters with others; (6) and the social skills they employ to manage difficult social encounters [11]. While this review was useful for a general understanding of psychological adjustment for those with visible distinctions (e.g., burns, dermatological disorders and cleft-palate) there was little to offer regarding those living with CAUE.

The broad spectrum of CAUE is rare but not entirely infrequent with a prevalence of 6.5–21.5 cases per 10,000 births [44]. They represent complex and variable pathologies with regard to the clinical severity of symptom presentation [45]. Some CAUE present in isolation and others present with associated systemic disorders and skeletal discrepancies [46]. Classification systems for the CAUE have been previously described [38, 46, 47]; however, the taxonomy endorsed by the International Federation of Societies for Surgery of the Hand is widely accepted [48, 49]. CAUE can be diagnosed in utero, at birth or during early childhood, and decisions regarding surgical intervention vary depending on the presentation of the specific genetic condition.

The Preferred Reporting Items for Systematic Reviews and Meta-analyses (PRIMSA) [50] criteria were followed in an attempt to identify studies on psychological sequelae for individual living with visible distinctions related to CAUE. Articles published as of August 2013 in English using literature searches of Pubmed, Web of Science, and Psych Info were sought. Searches of the literature were conducted using the terms: upper extremity congenital anomalies, limb deficiencies, and hand and arm, in conjunction with one or more of the following key terms: psychosocial, adjustment, coping, well-being, quality of life (QOL), and appearance. It was difficult to identify empirical studies published during the past decade in which psychological well-being, coping, and adjustment to CAUE appearance-related concerns were the primary outcome variables.

The preponderance of the research, energy, and attention on CAUE has focused on neonates, children, adolescents, and families. Most studies have been concerned with the timing of the surgery during childhood, surgical intervention, or postsurgical satisfaction [51–54]; and, longer-term functional outcomes [55–60]. There are few studies on adults living with CAUE [61–65].

Children and Adolescents Living with a CAUE

Some studies have demonstrated that living with a CAUE has an effect on the child's and adolescent's psychological well-being across several domains including self-esteem, internalizing behaviors (e.g., depression), and social interaction [66–70]. For example, one study of 66 children and adolescents living with a CAUE fitted with a myoelectric prosthetic hand reported that there were higher levels of withdrawn behavior for all children and adolescents living with a CAUE compared to a normative sample, and, that females living with a CAUE reported lower social interaction competence: when compared to their male counterparts [66]. This finding is not surprising given the prevailing negative cultural attitudes towards visible physical distinctions which are particularly salient for females.

Recently, participation in day-to-day activities and QOL has received attention in the literature on successful outcomes for children and adolescents living with a CAUE. Participation and QOL can be viewed as proxy measures for psychological well-being. Participation is the extent to which an individual is involved in various life situations and may include, but not be limited, to the cultural context or attitudes of community members; family interest in recreation; and the affected individual's personal characteristics (e.g., gender and social competence) [71]. QOL refers to an individual's perceptions of their position in life within cultural and value systems in which they live and in relation to their goals and expectations. QOL, which has been used in lieu of psychological symptomology, can comprise physical, psychological, spiritual, environmental, and interpersonal domains [72].

Depending on the severity of the disorder, it may be presumed that children and adolescents with CAUE may be at risk for limited participation in social activities and report poor QOL and psychological well-being, yet the literature reports inconsistent findings. A recent narrative review of 15 cross-sectional studies of children and adolescents with congenital limb deficiencies noted that the literature lacks sufficient information to support or refute this presumption and further acknowledged that while full participation and enhanced QOL are considered the main goals in pediatric rehabilitation the literature provides limited empirical data on how children and adolescents with CAUE participate and how they view their QOL [71]. These authors also note that while some of the studies in their review used sound psychometric measures, most studies used small sample sizes, and employed descriptive, exploratory and cross-sectional research designs [71]. They also reported that direct comparison between the studies was difficult due to the wide age range in the study samples (2–20 years) the lack of knowledge regarding the heterogeneity of CAUE [71]. A 2012 qualitative study [73] of 42 children and adolescents between the ages of 8 and 20 years of age with unilateral congenital below the elbow deficiencies (UCBED) found the majority of respondents did not report limitations in self-care, school, or recreational activities. While older respondents reported difficulties with novel social encounters, they were attributed to restrictions placed on them by their school or work environment and not to appearance-related concerns [73].

The experience of living with a visible distinction associated with a CAUE during adolescence has not been thoroughly examined. Research on the social psychology of facial appearance has documented that conditions that threaten appearance may place the adolescent at risk for psychosocial and interpersonal challenges [74]. Studies examining the significance of visible distinctions on psychological well-being have emphasized a number of psychosocial challenges, including those related to social interaction [42], and the potential impact of negative self-perceptions on the development of the self-concept [75], and the ability to initiate and maintain romantic relationships [74]. A recent study acknowledged that poor psychological adjustment, specifically internalizing behaviors (e.g., depression) and poor health-related QOL were predicted by the adolescent's reports of perceived stigmatization (e.g., absence of friendly behavior, staring, hostile behavior) [76]. Yet another study reported positive adjustments to visible facial distinctions [77] and noted that protective factors (e.g., positive self-schemas, strong family ties and external social supports) could counteract appearance-related distress. While it is encouraging to report these findings, it is distressing that the question of whether an adolescent living with a CAUE is more or less likely to experience psychological distress during this developmental period remains unanswered. Perhaps CAUE-related visible distinctions may also result in similar outcomes.

Adults Living with a CAUE

There are few studies on adults living with CAUE or on aging with CAUE. Case studies and reports on physical function are common [61–64]. One study commissioned by the Thalidomide Trust [61] reviewed the current health status and psychosocial sequelae of adults living with the consequences of Thalidomide in the United Kingdom. Of the 400 adults living with Thalidomide-related difficulties in the UK merely 12 men and 16 women participated in this study. The authors acknowledged these participants were married or had partners, many were employed reported good QOL and did not define themselves as disabled [61]. While these findings are encouraging it is difficult to determine if other adults would offer similar reports given the study's small and biased sample size. Furthermore, this study did not examine the appearance-related concerns related to living with a visible distinction.

Parental Coping and the Child with CAUE

Parental coping and adjustment to the birth of a child with a CAUE is an emotional family event [78]. Parental adjustment to the distinction, and associated medical, financial, social, and emotional demands may place enormous stressors on the family system [79, 80]. Parents face multiple challenges involving the management of grief-related emotions, finding an appropriate way to communicate with their children, and, making appropriate medical decisions [73]. Immediate- and longer-term factors contributing to the level of family distress may include but not necessarily be limited to (1) the extent and severity of the impairment and visibility of the distinction; (2) preexisting parental coping strategies; (3) the family's economic and psychological resources; (4) prevailing cultural attitudes towards the appearance of the child; and, (5) the developmental age of the child [81, 82].

Visible distinctions associated with CAUE may sometimes bias or otherwise impede a parent or caregiver's ability to effectively bond with their child [83, 84]. A successful transition through the first year of life characterized by bonding and parental affection and consistency in care are necessary conditions for the development of a child's sense of separate and valued self, and for the development of positive self-esteem [85, 86]. Researchers exploring family adjustment to the presence of a child with a visible distinction noted parents have reported heightened distress levels and that Parental psychological well-being prior to the birth of a child with a CAUE may be related to their child's long-term adjustment and psychological well-being [87]; however, it should be noted that findings are not consistent across studies due to inconsistencies in methodological approaches, small sample sizes, and scant longitudinal data. Such an approach may permit the development of integrated interventions within a biosocial medical model to improve functioning within this population.

Directions for Future Research

The research on the psychosocial sequelae of individuals living with visible distinctions associated with CAUE is limited and findings are inconsistent. CAUE research energy and attention has centered on children, adolescents, and families. Data on the transition between adolescence to the early adult years are not evident. Data on adults coping with visible distinctions associated with CAUE are modest and few investigators have made coping with CAUE in across the lifespan a priority. For adults living with a CAUE case studies or the personal narrative within the context of overcoming adversity prevails. Perhaps there is a presumption that the adult with a CAUE would have few, if any, appearance-related concerns because child and adolescent issues have been resolved and the adult should have "gotten over it by now." Published studies are hindered by the lack of psychometrically validated measures and methodological approaches that were descriptive or qualitative. It is also noted that sufficient funding to support basic, clinical/translational research and, clinical intervention trials is limited. While there is a need for high-quality research in this area we should not be discouraged. The open landscape offers an opportunity to develop a research agenda with an eye towards intervention.

We know from the extensive literature on psychological difficulties associated with facial appearance that the most common problems affected individuals encounter relate to negative self-perceptions, anticipatory anxiety regarding negative evaluations by others, and difficulties with social interactions [27]. Also, in contrast to early research examining the difficulties that individuals with visible facial distinctions encounter, investigators are devoting attention to the factors associated with adaptive coping strategies that affected individuals employ to manage a frequently hostile and unpredictable social landscape. The extensive literature on coping with stigmatizing attributes (e.g., obesity, HIV/AIDS) [25, 43, 88, 89] may provide some direction as well.

Coping has been defined as cognitive, emotional, and behavioral strategies that individuals employ to manage a variety of stressful experiences [31]. One coping model proposes two key responses: engagement and disengagement coping [90, 91]. Engagement coping can best be described by behaviors that engage with the stressful situation and/or by responses that help the individual to adapt to the stressful situation [43]. For example, the individual with a below the elbow anomaly may be confronted by persistent and unwelcome inquiries about his or her appearance. In response to these questions the affected individual may have at-the-ready a repertoire of responses to offer the curious observer. Disengagement coping involves responses that distance the individual from the stressor and includes avoidance, denial, and/or wishful thinking [43]. In this instance, the affected individual may avoid social encounters or engage in ruminative thoughts about his/her visible distinction.

Prior research also has demonstrated that the stigma associated with HIV poses various psychological challenges to people living with HIV, and that the consequences of stigma-related stressors on psychological well-being depend on the ability of affected individuals to employ engagement coping strategies [43, 92]. The stigma associated with CAUE appearance-related stigma may similarly pose psychological challenges to individuals living with visible distinctions associated with these anomalies yet little is known about these processes. It may be useful to employ stress and coping models to inform future research.

Researchers might examine the relationship between reports of appearance-related stigma; coping strategies used to manage the stigmatizing events, and associated psychological outcomes (e.g., depression, anxiety, anxiety sensitivity, resilience). What is the role of severity and visibility of the visible distinction? Are severity and visibility predictors of psychological difficulty? Are there risk or protective factors that may enhance positive outcomes? Are women, older adults, members of under-represented groups (e.g., African Americans, Latino/s, economically disadvantaged) at greater risk? What is the role of, social support, family and cultural context in the management of CAUE appearance-related stigma?

Investigators should use normative groups of similarly aged individuals without a CAUE or compare findings to the reports of a first-degree relative (e.g., same gendered non-affected sibling). Reliable and valid instruments to measure coping, perceptions of appearance-related stigma, and psychological outcomes must be used. Longitudinal studies would also be beneficial.

These factors should be considered in future research protocols. Findings from this preliminary wave of research may inform appropriate interventions.

Some Closing Comments and a Personal Story: It's Not About Me

The opportunity to write about the psychosocial aspects of living with a visible distinction associated with CAUE brought to mind my experience as a clinical psychologist, researcher, professor, and woman of color who lives with a genetic disorder and comorbid visible distinctions. Neurofibromatosis 1 (NF1), von Reckinghausen's disorder, or peripheral NF is one of several autosomal dominant neuro-cutaneous disorders caused by mutations of the gene on chromosome 17 (17q11.2) responsible for cell division [93]. Prevalence of NF1 is approximately 1 in 3,500 live births, and the disorder is highly random or variable regarding the clinical severity of symptom presentation [94, 95].

Clinical expressions of NF1 include café-au-lait spots, hamartomas (Lisch nodules), neurofibromas (Schwann cell tumors of four types: focal or diffuse cutaneous; subcutaneous; spinal; and, nodular or diffuse plexiform); optic gliomas; freckling in the axillary or inguinal regions; and distinctive bone lesions [93]. Common complications in individuals with NF1 are cognitive and learning disabilities [96]. While general intellectual functioning may be intact, identifiable and explicit cognitive deficits have been acknowledged among some affected individuals (e.g., perception, attention, executive functioning, language functions, learning disabilities, and visuo-spatial deficits) [97]. Surgical interventions to ameliorate or manage tumor growth have been reported in the literature. For example, surgical excision of plexiform neurofibromas of the face is complex and may require several medical interventions to debulk tumor growth; however, the cosmetic result is sometimes disappointing [98–100]. Also, individuals with NF1 are followed by various medical and mental health specialists (e.g., neurologists, neurosurgeons, ophthalmologists, orthopedic surgeons, reconstructive surgeons, genetic counselors, special educators, social workers, physical therapists, psychiatrists, neuropsychologists, psychologists, social workers) to manage symptoms, problems, or multiple impediments.

While most NF 1 tumors are benign, some individuals experience psychological distress as a result of the distinctive appearance associated with multiple visible tumors. Why mention NF 1 in a chapter devoted to CAUE? Individuals living with CAUE and NF1 may share some appearance-related concerns due to the visible distinctions associated with each disorder. I thought it would be useful to provide readers of this chapter with a first-hand account of what it is like to live with a visible distinction with an eye towards enriching clinical practice and research.

During my second year of doctoral training at the University of Vermont I was enrolled in a seminar in Community Clinical Psychology. On the first day of class we were asked to answer the following question: What is important to know about you? While not a fan of the "ice-breaker exercise" when it was my turn I complied and told my story. I said that I grew up in a housing project in New York City, in the north east Bronx. When I was a young girl, New York City housing projects were transitional housing for the upwardly mobile working class of the late 1950s, early 1960s. The Bronx River Housing Project was a diverse community of Europeans, African Americans, Latinos, South Americans, Pacific East Islanders, and Asians. Of course, we did not call ourselves by those names back then (we were Negro, Jew, Oriental, Irish, Italian, Greek, French, German, etc.). One day my father and mother announced to my sister and me that he had bought a home and we were going to move from the northeast Bronx to Riverdale. Riverdale was and remains an upscale residential community in the northwest Bronx. We were one of the first families of color to move to the area. To this day I do not know how my father was able to gather the financial resources to purchase a home for his family. At the time he worked for City of New York and earned $75.00–$100.00 a week. I told the class that my father inspired me and continues to inspire me. He never said these words to me explicitly, but the implicit message that my father's behavior modeled for me was that as long as you are alive you can do, shape, or change anything. As long as you have a goal, a dream, and a neuron firing in your skull you can achieve a vision. Your life condition does not matter. Your economic status, appearance privilege, weight, or age does not matter. As long as you can move and think you can shape a plan and implement that plan. I told the class that was the reason I decided to return to graduate school to become a psychologist when I was 41 years old. I told the class that the most important thing to know about me was that I was resilient.

Later that evening, a friend and fellow student called me. He said that he was baffled by the story I told in class, asked why I told that story, and wondered why I didn't talk about my NF. While I told the students in that seminar a story about me, what they wanted to hear was a story about my appearance. When people meet me they want to know: "What are those things on your skin?" "Why do you look like that?" "What is wrong with you?"

Individuals with visible distinctions must answer these questions every day. Parents have to answer these questions for their children. These questions are part of the stressors that individuals with visible distinctions encounter. More often than not individuals with visible distinctions have to make it easier for others to engage in social interactions with them. The burden of initiating and maintaining the social encounter is on the shoulders of the individual with the visible distinction. Perceived normal-appearing others ask questions that reduce their anxiety or personal curiosity. The bearer of a visible distinction is frequently in the spotlight, on display and under public scrutiny.

When asked about my visible distinction I must be ready to provide an answer. Children *always* receive my full attention and compassion because children are curious, and it is good practice to let them know that individuals who do not look like them should not be feared or avoided. The reader should know that I have encountered well-meaning individuals who said, "Sondra, I can't imagine how you do it." Others have said, "I can't imagine what I would do if I looked like you." As I listen to the familiar refrain I imagine they are waiting for me to share some special magical life skill I possess to manage my visible distinction related to NF 1. I used to engage in lengthy conversation with people. I noticed that when they were sufficiently satisfied with my answer they would walk away. Now, when I am asked that question I respond with a smile and say, "Yes, I imagine you can't." This response is my attempt to ally with the person who is confused and anxious about my appearance. This response shifts the burden away from me and directs it towards the person who was compelled to break the social contract. The question is not about me at all but is about the anxiety, fragility, and vulnerability experienced by normal-appearing others when they encounter children, adolescents, and adults who do not look like them. This response is part of a number of engagement coping strategies that I employ to deflect the slings and arrows of outrageous fortune that are part and parcel of living in a culture that demands perfection.

References

1. Hawthorne N. The birthmark. Mosses from an Old Manse. New York: Wiley and Putnam; 1846.
2. Sheridan J, Scior K. Attitudes towards people with intellectual disabilities: a comparison of young people from British South Asian and White British backgrounds. Res Dev Disabil. 2013;34(4):1240–7. PubMed PMID: WOS:000316532700016. English.
3. Kurzban R, Leary MR. Evolutionary origins of stigmatization: the functions of social exclusion. Psychol Bull. 2001;127(2):187–208. PubMed PMID: ISI:000170928000001.
4. MacDonald G, Leary MR. Why does social exclusion hurt? The relationship between social and physical pain. Psychol Bull. 2005;131(2):202–23. PubMed PMID: ISI:000227423200004.
5. Richman LS, Leary MR. Reactions to discrimination, stigmatization, ostracism, and other forms of interpersonal rejection: a multimotive model. Psychol Rev. 2009;116(2):365–83. PubMed PMID: ISI:000264913000004.
6. Harcourt D, Rumsey N, Paraskeva N. Appearance and body image. Psychologist. 2011;24(12):895–6. PubMed PMID: WOS:000297614100025. English.
7. Rumsey N. The psychology of appearance: why health psychologists should do looks. Psychol Health. 2008;23:16. PubMed PMID: WOS:000260047300010. English.
8. Rumsey N, Clarke A, White P, Wyn-Williams M, Garlick W. Altered body image: appearance-related concerns of people with visible disfigurement. J Adv Nurs. 2004;48(5):443–53. PubMed PMID: WOS:000225369600003. English.
9. Ablon J. The nature of stigma and medical conditions. Epilepsy Behav. 2002;3(6):S2–9. PubMed PMID: WOS:000184307700002. English.
10. Macgregor FC. After plastic surgery: adaptation and adjustment. New York: Praeger; 1979.
11. Thompson A, Kent G. Adjusting to disfigurement: processes involved in dealing with being visibly different. Clin Psychol Rev. 2001;21(5):663–82. PubMed PMID: WOS:000169442100001. English.
12. Wallace M, Harcourt D, Rumsey N. Experiences of healthcare provision in adolescents with an altered appearance. Psychol Health. 2008;23:270. PubMed PMID: WOS:000260047300633. English.
13. Egan K, Harcourt D, Rumsey N. Appearance RC. A qualitative study of the experiences of people who identify themselves as having adjusted positively to a visible difference. J Health Psychol. 2011;16(5):739–49. PubMed PMID: WOS:000291676700005. English.
14. Scheer J, Groce N. Impairment as a human constant—cross-cultural and historical perspectives on variation. J Soc Issues. 1988;44(1):23–37. PubMed PMID: WOS:A1988N062700003. English.
15. Susman J. Disability, stigma and deviance. Soc Sci Med. 1994;38(1):15–22. PubMed PMID: WOS:A1994MK27000003. English.
16. Zola IK. Self, identity and the naming question—reflections on the language of disability. Soc Sci Med. 1993;36(2):167–73. PubMed PMID: WOS:A1993KE81500009. English.
17. Van Brakel WH, Anderson AM, Mutatkar RK, Bakirtzief Z, Nicholls PG, Raju MS, et al. The participation scale: measuring a key concept in public health. Disabil Rehabil. 2006;28(4):193–203. PubMed PMID: WOS:000235427800002. English.
18. Goffman E. Stigma: notes on the management of spoiled identity. Englewood Cliffs, NJ: Prentice-Hall, Inc.; 1963. 147 p.
19. Elliott GC, Ziegler HL, Altman BM, Scott DR. Understanding stigma—dimensions of deviance and coping. Deviant Behav. 1982;3(3):275–300. PubMed PMID: WOS:A1982NV59700005. English.
20. Stafford MC, Scott RR. Stigma, deviance and social control. In: AInlay SC, Becker GB, Coleman SC, editors. The dilemma of difference: a multidisciplinary view of stigma. New York: Plenum Press; 1986. p. 77–90.
21. Crocker J, Major B, Steele C. Social stigma. In: Gilbert D, Fiske ST, Lindzey G, editors. Handbook of social psychology. 4th ed. Boston, MA: McGraw Hill; 1998.
22. Castro A, Farmer P. Understanding and addressing AIDS-related stigma: from anthropological theory to clinical practice in Haiti. Am J Public Health. 2005;95(1):53–9.
23. Link BG, Phelan JC. Conceptualizing stigma. Annu Rev Sociol. 2001;27:363–85.
24. Malcolm A, Aggleton P, Bronfman M, Galvao J, Mane P, Verrall J. HIV-related stigmatization and discrimination: its forms and contexts. Crit Public Health. 1998;8(4):347–70.

25. Parker R, Aggleton P. HIV and AIDS-related stigma and discrimination: a conceptual framework and implications for action. Soc Sci Med. 2003;57(1):13–24.
26. Mill JE, Edwards N, Jackson RC, MacLean L, Chaw-Kant J. Stigmatization as a social control mechanism for persons living with HIV and AIDS. Qual Health Res. 2010;20(11):1469–83. PubMed PMID: WOS:000283250900005. English.
27. Rumsey N, Harcourt D. The psychology of appearance. New York, NY: Open University Press; 2005. 237 p.
28. Macgregor FC. Social, psychological and cultural dimensions of cosmetic and reconstructive plastic-surgery. Aesthetic Plast Surg. 1989;13(1):1–8. PubMed PMID: WOS:A1989T620100001. English.
29. Macgregor FC. Patient dissatisfaction with results of technically satisfactory surgery. Aesthetic Plast Surg. 1981;5(1):27–32. PubMed PMID: WOS:A1981LM55500003. English.
30. Harcourt D, Rumsey N. Psychology and visible difference. Psychologist. 2008;21(6):486–9. PubMed PMID: WOS:000256831200018. English.
31. Folkman S, Lazarus RS, Dunkelschetter C, Delongis A, Gruen RJ. Dynamics of a stressful encounter: cognitive appraisal, coping and encounter outcomes. J Pers Soc Psychol. 1986;50(5):992–1003. PubMed PMID: WOS:A1986C306700013. English.
32. Crocker J, Major B. Social stigma and self-esteem: the self-protective properties of stigma. Psychol Rev. 1989;96(4):608–30. PubMed PMID: ISI:A1989AU66600004.
33. Miller CT, Kaiser CR. A theoretical perspective on coping with stigma. J Soc Issues. 2001;57(1):73–92. PubMed PMID: ISI:000168242500005.
34. Folkman S, Greer S. Promoting psychological well-being in the face of serious illness: when theory, research and practice inform each other. Psychooncology. 2000;9(1):11–9. PubMed PMID: ISI:000085499100002.
35. Ben-Naim S, Aviv G, Hirschberger G. Strained interaction: evidence that interpersonal contact moderates the death-disability rejection link. Rehabil Psychol. 2008;53(4):464–70. PubMed PMID: WOS:000261518900005. English.
36. Hirschberger G. Terror management and attributions of blame to innocent victims: reconciling compassionate and defensive responses. J Pers Soc Psychol. 2006;91(5):832–44. PubMed PMID: WOS:000241548100003. English.
37. Hirschberger G, Florian V, Mikulincer M. Fear and compassion: a terror management analysis of emotional reactions to physical disability. Rehabil Psychol. 2005;50(3):246–57. PubMed PMID: WOS:000231741200009. English.
38. Kozin SH. Upper-extremity congenital anomalies. J Bone Joint Surg Am. 2003;85A(8):1564–76. PubMed PMID: WOS:000184552100021. English.
39. Schabert J, Browne JL, Mosely K, Speight J. Social stigma in diabetes a framework to understand a growing problem for an increasing epidemic. Patient. 2013;6(1):1–10. PubMed PMID: WOS:000315586900001. English.
40. Sterba KR, Zapka J, Gore EI, Ford ME, Ford DW, Thomas M, et al. Exploring dimensions of coping in advanced colorectal cancer: implications for patient-centered care. J Psychosoc Oncol. 2013;31(5):517–39. PubMed PMID: WOS:000324001300003. English.
41. Rumsey N. Body image and congenital conditions with visible differences. In: Cash TF, Pruzinsky T, editors. Body image: a handbook of theory, research, and clinical practice. London: The Guilford Press; 2002.
42. Rumsey N, Clarke A, White P, Wyn-Williams M, Garlick W. Altered body image: appearance-related concerns of people with visible disfigurement. J Adv Nurs. 2004;48(5):443–53. PubMed PMID: MEDLINE:15533082. English.
43. Varni SE, Miller CT, McCuin T, Solomon S. Disengagement and engagement coping with HIV/AIDS stigma and psychological well-being of people with HIV/AIDS. J Soc Clin Psychol. 2012;31(2):123–50. PubMed PMID: WOS:000300333400002. English.
44. Giele H, Giele C, Bower C, Allison M. The incidence and epidemiology of congenital upper limb anomalies: a total population study. J Hand Surg. 2001;26(4):628–34.
45. Ardon MS, Janssen WG, Hovius SE, Stam HJ, Selles RW. Low impact of congenital hand differences on health-related quality of life. Arch Phys Med Rehabil. 2012;93(2):351–7. PubMed PMID: WOS:000300338900026. English.
46. Aucourt J, Budzik JF, Manouvrier-Hanu S, Mezel A, Cotten A, Boutry N. Congenital malformations of the hand and forearm in children: what radiologists should know. Semin Musculoskelet Radiol. 2012;16(2):146–58. PubMed PMID: WOS:000304677600009. English.
47. Linder JA, Pincus DJ, Panthaki Z, Thaller SR. Congenital anomalies of the hand: an overview. J Craniofac Surg. 2009; 20(4):999–1004. PubMed PMID: WOS:000268400400008. English.
48. Manske PR, Oberg KC. Classification and developmental biology of congenital anomalies of the hand and upper extremity. J Bone Joint Surg Am. 2009;91A:3–18. PubMed PMID: WOS:000267673900002. English.
49. Oberg KC, Feenstra JM, Manske PR, Tonkin MA. Developmental biology and classification of congenital anomalies of the hand and upper extremity. J Hand Surg Am. 2010;35A(12):2066–76. PubMed PMID: WOS:000285371300024. English.
50. Moher D, Liberati A, Tetzlaff J, Altman DG, Grp P. Preferred reporting items for systematic reviews and meta-analyses: the PRISMA statement. J Clin Epidemiol. 2009;62(10):1006–12. PubMed PMID: WOS:000270250500003. English.
51. Bellew M, Haworth J, Kay SP. Toe to hand transfer in children: ten year follow up of psychological aspects. J Plast Reconstr Aesthet Surg. 2011;64(6):766–75. PubMed PMID: WOS:000290562600020. English.
52. Vasluian E, de Jong IGM, Janssen WGM, Poelma MJ, van Wijk I, Reinders-Messelink HA, et al. Opinions of youngsters with congenital below-elbow deficiency, and those of their parents and professionals concerning prosthetic use and rehabilitation treatment. PLoS One. 2013;8(6):e67101. PubMed PMID: WOS:000321738400104. English.
53. Staines KG, Majzoub R, Thornby J, Netscher DT. Functional outcome for children with thumb aplasia undergoing pollicization. Plast Reconstr Surg. 2005;116(5):1314–23. PubMed PMID: WOS:000232421100017. English.
54. Hardwicke J, Khan MAA, Richards H, Warner RM, Lester R. Macrodactyly—options and outcomes. J Hand Surg Eur. 2013;38E(3):297–303. PubMed PMID: WOS:000317916800011. English.
55. Hadders-Algra M, Reinders-Messelink HA, Huizing K, van den Berg R, van der Sluis CK, Maathuis CGB. Use and functioning of the affected limb in children with unilateral congenital below-elbow deficiency during infancy and preschool age: a longitudinal observational multiple case study. Early Hum Dev. 2013;89(1): 49–54. PubMed PMID: WOS:000314073900010. English.
56. Ekblom AG, Dahlin LB, Rosberg HE, Wiig M, Werner M, Arner M. Hand function in children with radial longitudinal deficiency. BMC Musculoskelet Disord. 2013;14:116. PubMed PMID: WOS:000318296200001. English.
57. Korkmaz M, Erbahceci F, Ulger O, Topuz S. Evaluation of functionality in acquired and congenital upper extremity child amputees. Acta Orthop Traumatol Turc. 2012;46(4):262–8. PubMed PMID: WOS:000309801300007. English.

58. Nemec SF, Kasprian G, Brugger PC, Bettelheim D, Amann G, Nemec U, et al. Abnormalities of the upper extremities on fetal magnetic resonance imaging. Ultrasound Obstet Gynecol. 2011;38(5):559–67. PubMed PMID: WOS:000297512300014. English.
59. Oberg KC, Harris TE, Wongworawat MD, Wood VE. Combined congenital radial and ulnar longitudinal deficiencies: report of 2 cases. J Hand Surg Am. 2009;34A(7):1298–302. PubMed PMID: WOS:000269414600019. English.
60. Huizing K, Reinders-Messelink H, Maathuis C, Hadders-Algra M, van der Sluis CK. Age at first prosthetic fitting and later functional outcome in children and young adults with unilateral congenital below-elbow deficiency: a cross-sectional study. Prosthet Orthot Int. 2010;34(2):166–74. PubMed PMID: WOS:000283117200005. English.
61. Bent N, Tennant A, Neumann V, Chamberlain MA. Living with thalidomide: health status and quality of life at 40 years. Prosthet Orthot Int. 2007;31(2):147–56. PubMed PMID: WOS:000248726400004. English.
62. Holtslag I, van Wijk I, Hartog H, van der Molen AM, van der Sluis C. Long-term functional outcome of patients with longitudinal radial deficiency: cross-sectional evaluation of function, activity and participation. Disabil Rehabil. 2013;35(16):1401–7. PubMed PMID: WOS:000321465200011. English.
63. Goh ESY, Li CM, Horsburgh S, Kasai Y, Kolomietz E, Morel CF. The Roberts syndrome/SC phocomelia spectrum—a case report of an adult with review of the literature. Am J Med Genet A. 2010;152A(2):472–8. PubMed PMID: WOS:000274508300034. English.
64. Cetik O, Uslu M, Cirpar M, Eksioglu F. Experience with the surgical treatment of radial polydactyly in adults. Ann Plast Surg. 2005;55(4):363–6. PubMed PMID: WOS:000232282800006. English.
65. Eskandari MM, Oztuna V, Demirkan F. Late psychosocial effects of congenital hand anomaly. Hand Surg. 2004;9(2):257–9.
66. Hermansson L, Eliasson AC, Engstrom I. Psychosocial adjustment in Swedish children with upper-limb reduction deficiency and a myoelectric prosthetic hand. Acta Paediatr. 2005;94(4):479–88. PubMed PMID: WOS:000228451400018. English.
67. Varni JW, Rubenfeld LA, Talbot D, Setoguchi Y. Determinants of self-esteem in children with congenital acquired limb deficiencies. J Dev Behav Pediatr. 1989;10(1):13–6. PubMed PMID: WOS:A1989T156700003. English.
68. Varni JW, Setoguchi Y. Screening for behavioral and emotional problems in children and adolescents with congenital or acquired limb deficiencies. Am J Dis Child. 1992;146(1):103–7. PubMed PMID: WOS:A1992GY44600027. English.
69. Varni JW, Setoguchi Y. Effects of parental adjustment on the adaptation of children with congenital or acquired limb deficiencies. J Dev Behav Pediatr. 1993;14(1):13–20. PubMed PMID: WOS:A1993KK64300003. English.
70. Varni JW, Setoguchi Y. Perceived physical appearance and adjustment of adolescents with congenital/acquired limb deficiencies: a path-analytic model. J Clin Child Psychol. 1996;25(2):201–8. PubMed PMID: WOS:A1996UN35700009. English.
71. Michielsen A, Van Wijk I, Ketelaar M. Participation and quality of life in children and adolescents with congenital limb deficiencies: a narrative review. Prosthet Orthot Int. 2010;34(4):351–61. PubMed PMID: WOS:000284360400001. English.
72. Cohen JS, Biesecker BB. Quality of life in rare genetic conditions: a systematic review of the literature. Am J Med Genet A. 2010;152A(5):1136–56. PubMed PMID: WOS:000277739800008. English.
73. de Jong IGM, Reinders-Messelink HA, Janssen WGM, Poelma MJ, van Wijk I, van der Sluis CK. Mixed feelings of children and adolescents with unilateral congenital below elbow deficiency: an online focus group study. PLoS One. 2012;7(6):e37099. PubMed PMID: WOS:000305336800003. English.
74. Griffiths C, Williamson H, Rumsey N. The romantic experiences of adolescents with a visible difference: exploring concerns, protective factors and support needs. J Health Psychol. 2012;17(7):1053–64. PubMed PMID: WOS:000309354700015. English.
75. Gussy M, Kilpatrick N. The self-concept of adolescents with cleft lip and palate: a pilot study using a multidimensional/hierarchical measurement instrument. Int J Paediatr Dent. 2006;16(5):335–41. PubMed PMID: WOS:000239876500004. English.
76. Masnari O, Schiestl C, Rossler J, Gutlein SK, Neuhaus K, Weibel L, et al. Stigmatization predicts psychological adjustment and quality of life in children and adolescents with a facial difference. J Pediatr Psychol. 2013;38(2):162–72. PubMed PMID: WOS:000315417800007. English.
77. Feragen KB, Kvalem IL, Rumsey N, Borge AIH. Adolescents with and without a facial difference: the role of friendships and social acceptance in perceptions of appearance and emotional resilience. Body Image. 2010;7(4):271–9. PubMed PMID: WOS:000284348500002. English.
78. Bradbury ET, Kay SPJ, Hewison J. The psychological impact of microvascular free toe transfer for children and their parents. J Hand Surg Br Eur. 1994;19B(6):689–95. PubMed PMID: WOS:A1994QJ56000003. English.
79. Fonseca A, Nazare B, Canavarro MC. Parental psychological distress and quality of life after a prenatal or postnatal diagnosis of congenital anomaly: a controlled comparison study with parents of healthy infants. Disabil Health J. 2012;5(2):67–74. PubMed PMID: WOS:000301868700002. English.
80. Fonseca A, Nazare B, Canavarro MC. Clinical determinants of parents' emotional reactions to the disclosure of a diagnosis of congenital anomaly. J Obstet Gynecol Neonatal Nurs. 2013;42(2):178–90. PubMed PMID: WOS:000316279500009. English.
81. Warfield ME, Krauss MW, Hauser-Cram P, Upshur CC, Shonkoff JP. Adaptation during early childhood among mothers of children with disabilities. J Dev Behav Pediatr. 1999;20(1):9–16. PubMed PMID: WOS:000078764900002. English.
82. Hauser-Cram P, Warfield ME, Shonkoff JP, Krauss IV MW. Results: predictors of functioning and change in children's development and parent well-being. Monogr Soc Res Child Dev. 2001;66(3):54–78.
83. Wallander JL, Varni JW, Babani L, Banis HT, Wilcox KT. Family resources as resistance factors for psychological maladjustment in chronically ill and handicapped-children. J Pediatr Psychol. 1989;14(2):157–73. PubMed PMID: WOS:A1989AC65200002. English.
84. Wallander JL, Varni JW. Effects of pediatric chronic physical disorders on child and family adjustment. J Child Psychol Psychiatry. 1998;39(1):29–46. PubMed PMID WOS:000072047800003. English.
85. Beuf AH. Children coping with impaired appearance: social and psychological influences. Gen Hosp Psychiatry. 1990;6:294–301.
86. Hillbeuf A, Porter JDR. Children coping with impaired appearance—social and psychologic influences. Gen Hosp Psychiatry. 1984;6(4):294–301. PubMed PMID: WOS:A1984TM50000009. English.
87. Wiegner S, Donders J. Predictors of parental distress after congenital disabilities. J Dev Behav Pediatr. 2000;21(4):271–7. PubMed PMID: WOS:0000889[illegible]3700003. English.
88. Puhl RM, Brownell KD. Confronting and coping with weight stigma: an investigation of overweight and obese adults. Obesity. 2006;14(10):1802–15. PubMed PMID: WOS:000249605900017. English.
89. Myers A, Rosen JC. Obesity stigmatization and coping: relation to mental health symptoms, body image, and self-esteem. Int J Obes. 1999;23(3):221–30. PubMed PMID: WOS:000078796900001. English.

90. Compas BE, Connor-Smith JK, Saltzman H, Thomsen AH, Wadsworth ME. Coping with stress during childhood and adolescence: problems, progress, and potential in theory and research. Psychol Bull. 2001;127(1):87–127. PubMed PMID: ISI:000166843700005.
91. Connor-Smith JK, Compas BE, Wadsworth ME, Thomsen AH, Saltzman H. Responses to stress in adolescence: measurement of coping and involuntary stress responses. J Consult Clin Psychol. 2000;68(6):976–92.
92. Varni SE, Miller CT, Solomon SE. Sexual behavior as a function of stigma and coping with stigma among people with HIV/AIDS in rural New England. AIDS Behav. 2012;16(8):2330–9. PubMed PMID: WOS:000310316200024. English.
93. Evans D, Howard E, Giblin C, Clancy T, Spencer H, Huson S, et al. Birth incidence and prevalence of tumor-prone syndromes: estimates from a UK family genetic register service. Am J Med Genet A. 2010;152(2):327–32.
94. Lu-Emerson C, Plotkin S. The neurofibromatoses. Part 2: NF2 and schwannomatosis. Rev Neurol Dis. 2008;6(3):E81–6.
95. Lu-Emerson C, Plotkin S. The neurofibromatoses. Part 1: NF1. Rev Neurol Dis. 2009;6(2):E47.
96. Hyman SL, Shores A, North KN. The nature and frequency of cognitive deficits in children with neurofibromatosis type 1. Neurology. 2005;65(7):1037–44.
97. Van Es S, North K, McHugh K, De Silva M. MRI findings in children with neurofibromatosis type 1: a prospective study. Pediatr Radiol. 1996;26(7):478–87.
98. Chaudhry IA, Morales J, Shamsi FA, Al-Rashed W, Elzaridi E, Arat YO, et al. Orbitofacial neurofibromatosis: clinical characteristics and treatment outcome. Eye. 2012;26(4):583–92. PubMed PMID: WOS:000302938500015. English.
99. Lantieri L, Meningaud JP, Grimbert P, Bellivier F, Lefaucheur JP, Ortonne N, et al. Repair of the lower and middle parts of the face by composite tissue allotransplantation in a patient with massive plexiform neurofibroma: a 1-year follow-up study. Lancet. 2008;372(9639):639–45. PubMed PMID: WOS:000258622200027. English.
100. Miyawaki T, Billings B, Har-Shai Y, Agbenorku P, Kokuba E, Moreira-Gonzalez A, et al. Multicenter study of wound healing in neurofibromatosis and neurofibroma. J Craniofac Surg. 2007;18(5):1008–11. PubMed PMID: WOS:000249894600004. English.

Part II

Failure of Formation/Differentiation

Radial Longitudinal Deficiency: Radius Hypoplasia

7

Chris Stutz and Scott Oishi

Introduction

Radial longitudinal deficiency (RLD) comprises a spectrum of clinical manifestations involving phenotypic changes of the upper extremity that range from underdevelopment to complete absence of the radial sided structures. The majority of cases of RLD are sporadic in occurrence, but the deformity can be passed genetically as well. Treatment for this condition varies depending on the clinical presentation of the patient as well as any associated anomalies that may exist. This chapter will attempt to explain the background and etiology of RLD, outline the conditions that have been associated with the deformity, review the classification of the various phenotypic presentations, and review current treatment patterns and their associated outcomes.

Background

The first documented case of RLD, then termed "radial club hand" was reported by Petit in 1733 when he described the findings in an infant autopsy. The term "radial club hand" has been largely supplanted in the modern literature with the term "radial longitudinal deficiency." In 1894, Sayre published the first case of RLD treated with centralization to address the radial deviation deformity associated with the condition by outlining the steps of centralizing the carpus on the end of the distal ulna. Since the time of these early publications, there have been significant advances in the understanding of the diagnosis, the deformity, and its associated conditions. Despite these advances, there remains little consensus in opinion regarding the best operative or non-operative treatment of the radial deformity in children with RLD.

C. Stutz, M.D.
Department of Orthopaedics, Monroe Carell Jr Children's Hospital, Vanderbilt University Medical Center, 4202 Doctors' Office Tower, 2200 Children's Way, Nashville, TN 37204, USA
e-mail: Chris.Stutz@Vanderbilt.edu

S. Oishi, M.D. (✉)
Hand Service, Texas Scottish Rite Hospital for Children, 2222 Welborn Street, Dallas, TX 75219, USA
e-mail: scottoishi@aol.com; scott.oishi@TSRH.org

Etiology

The theories regarding the embryologic basis for RLD continue to evolve, as the specific mechanisms of limb bud development are uncovered. In animal models, the progressive reduction of apical ectodermal ridge associated fibroblastic growth factors causes a progressive reduction in the size and volume of the developing limb bud. These alterations in cellular communication result in deformities that resemble those seen clinically in RLD [1, 2]. Mutagenic agents given to pregnant rats at various time points in gestation resulted in a substantial portion of littermates exhibiting manifestations consistent with RLD. The manifestations correlated with the time of administration and the dose of the mutagenic agent [3]. The prevalence of RLD has been reported as 1 in 55,000 live births [4], with a male to female ratio of 3:2 [5–8].

Associated Conditions

The association of RLD with certain medical conditions is well established. Historically, patients diagnosed with RLD were given a poor general prognosis, likely related to the associated morbidity of the related medical conditions [9]. Goldfarb et al. [10] reported on 164 patients with RLD, 67 % of which had associated medical or musculoskeletal abnormalities. The investigators reported the relative incidence of associated medical conditions was directly related to the severity of the RLD, with the most common related conditions being cardiac anomalies (20 %), thrombocytopenia-absent radius syndrome (15 %), VACTERL association (13 %), Holt-Oram syndrome (4 %), and Fanconi anemia (1 %).

D.R. Laub Jr. (ed.), *Congenital Anomalies of the Upper Extremity: Etiology and Management*, DOI 10.1007/978-1-4899-7504-1_7, © Springer Science+Business Media New York 2015

Hall et al. defined thrombocytopenia-absent radius as a syndrome in 1969 [11]. The inheritance pattern was thought to be autosomal recessive, but reports of parent-to-child transmission and multiple affected relatives in families suggest either heterogeneity or a different mode of inheritance [12–14]. Further genetic investigations have found a specific microdeletion of chromosome 1q21.1, which is necessary, but in itself insufficient to cause the thrombocytopenia-absent radius phenotype [15]. The cardinal findings of TAR syndrome are the absence of radii with the presence of hypoplastic thumbs and thrombocytopenia [16]. The presence of an aberrant muscle, termed the brachiocarpalis, was identified by Oishi and colleagues in the upper extremities of children with TAR syndrome contributing to the radial angulation deformity of the carpus [17]. Unique to this diagnosis is that even though the thrombocytopenia can initially be severe, it usually spontaneously resolves over time without the need for intervention.

VACTERL association is a nonrandom association of birth defects involving vertebral anomalies, anal atresia, cardiovascular anomalies, trachea-esophageal fistula, renal and/or radial anomalies, and limb defects. VACTERL association is likely related to multiple factors, but can be seen with chromosomal defects such as Trisomy 18 and is encountered more commonly in children of diabetic mothers [18]. There has been no specific genetic cause identified in VACTERL association to date. RLD patients must have at least three, including RLD, of the possible associations to be considered a VACTERL patient.

Holt-Oram syndrome is an autosomal dominant condition hallmarked by cardiac abnormalities and upper limb anomalies involving the radial ray. The genetic abnormality responsible for the syndrome has been identified as a missense mutation in the TBX5 gene [19]. The upper extremity involvement in Holt-Oram is variable. There is commonly hypoplasia of the radial elements with or without bizarre synostoses between the radius and ulna (Fig. 7.1).

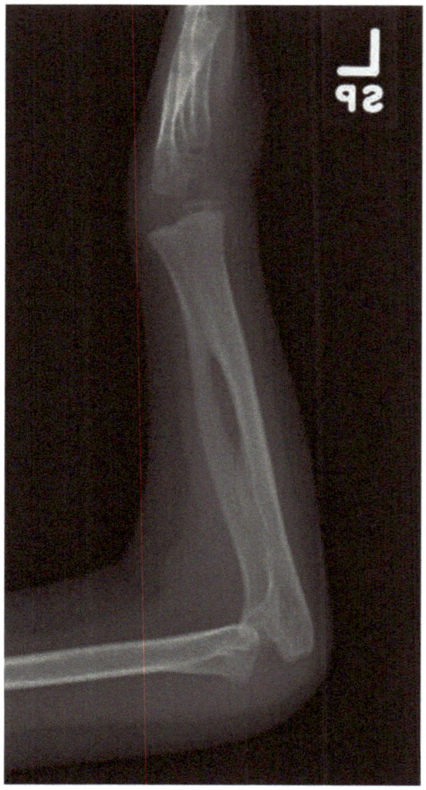

Fig. 7.1 Bizarre forearm synostosis in a patient with Holt-Oram syndrome

Fanconi anemia is the most common inherited cause of bone marrow failure [20]. The bone marrow failure most commonly occurs between the ages of 5 and 15. Phenotypic variations are common in presentation and include short stature, thumb and radius deformities, hyperpigmentation of skin, renal, cardiac, and genitourinary abnormalities [21]. The diagnosis can be made using a chromosome breakage analysis (diepoxybutane analysis). The test is expensive and its use as a routine screening tool in patients with apparent isolated RLD continues to be debated. However, the advent of successful pediatric bone marrow transplantation has led some authors to feel that diepoxybutane testing is important in every child with an RLD diagnosis.

Unique to many other conditions treated by the discipline of hand surgery, RLD often offers the hand surgeon the opportunity to be the first to make a diagnosis of other associated anomalies. This is related to the fact that the visible difference in upper extremity development often implores the parents and pediatrician to pursue evaluation for treatment of the affected limb. Hence, it is imperative that the hand surgeon be aware of these common associations and performs a complete evaluation of the child in all cases. This evaluation should include, at a minimum, a complete musculoskeletal and systemic evaluation, a complete blood count, echocardiogram, abdominal ultrasound, and subsequent evaluation for scoliosis.

Classification

The original classification of RLD was described by Bayne and Klug in 1987 [22]. They based the classification system on the radiographic appearance of the radius and divided the phenotype into four categories. Type I was defined as a short radius with delayed appearance of the distal radial epiphysis. Type II was defined as a "radius in miniature" with growth of both proximal and distal radial epiphyses affected. Type III denoted partial absence of the radius with no distal radial physis; Type IV was defined as complete absence of the radius.

The original classification of scheme of Bayne and Klug was modified by James et al. [23] in 1999 to include Types N and 0 with further delineation of what constituted Type I

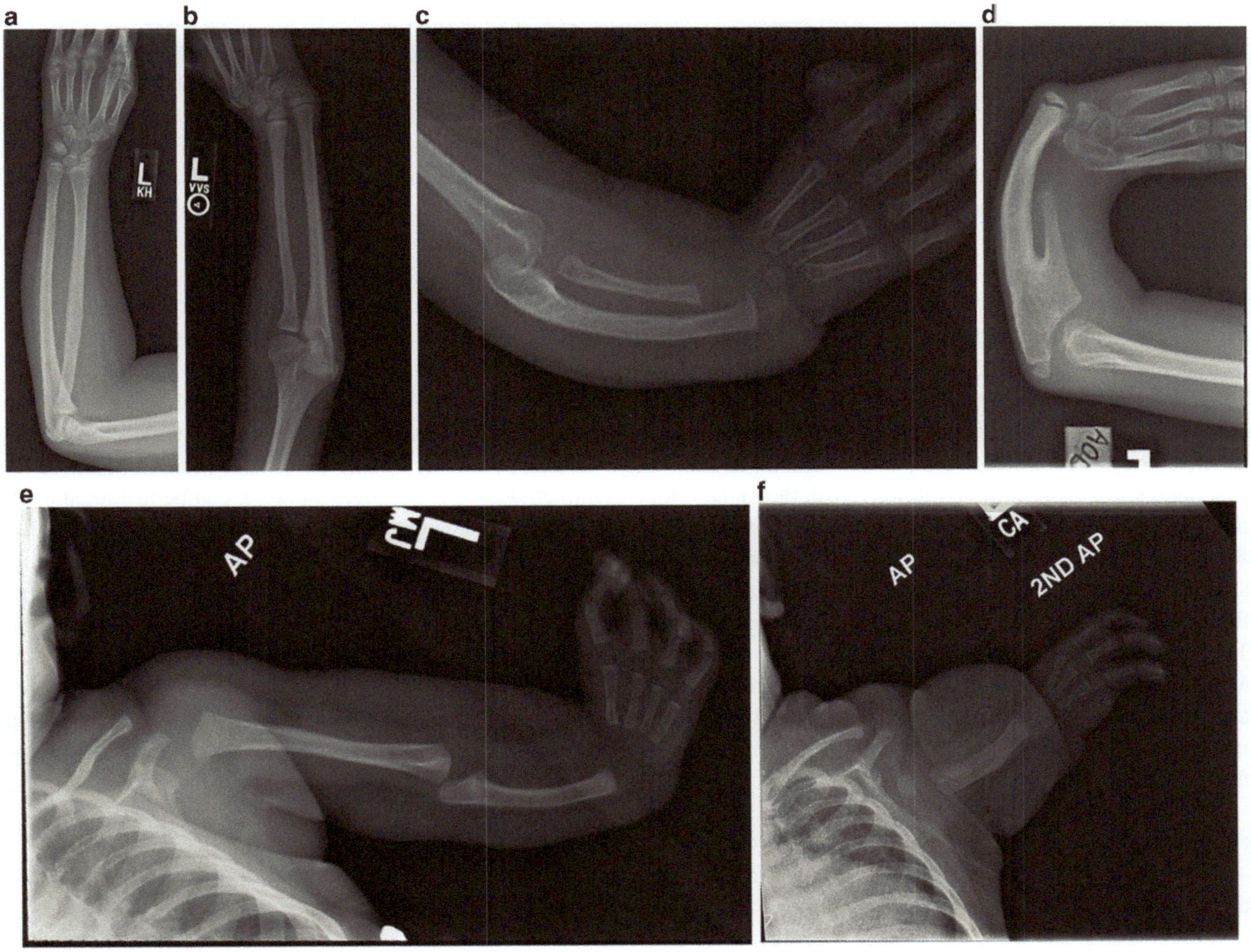

Fig. 7.2 (**a**) Type 0/N. (**b**) Type I. (**c**) Type II. (**d**) Type III. (**e**) Type IV. (**f**) Type V

RLD. The classification was further modified by Goldfarb et al. [24] in 2005 to include more severe proximal manifestations of RLD as Type V. The current state of RLD classification is as follows (Fig. 7.2):

Type N—The thumb is hypoplastic or absent in the presence of a normal carpus or radius. Radial angulation at the wrist is usually absent or minimal.

Type 0—The radius is of normal length with proximal and distal physes. The radial carpal bones are hypoplastic or absent. The degree of radial angulation of the wrist is variable. The angulatory deformity is owing to the abnormal carpal bones and the presence of tight soft tissue structures on the radial side of the wrist, including the wrist capsule and musculotendinous structures.

Type I—The radius is foreshortened by at least 2 mm compared to the distal ulna. The distal radial physis is present but its growth is slowed. The proximal radial physis is present and of normal morphology. Radio-ulnar synostosis or congenital radial head dislocation is variably present.

Type II—The radius is hypoplastic in its entirety with proximal and distal physes present—the so-called radius in miniature. This can be associated with notable ulnar bowing.

Type III—The distal portion of the radius is absent. There is no distal radial physis.

Type IV—The radius is absent in its entirety. This is the most common phenotypic presentation of RLD [22].

Type V—This represents a severe proximal form of RLD formerly considered phocomelia. Taking into account principles of developmental biology, the concept of a true intercalary defect has been challenged by recent authors [24, 25]. Extremities in this category have an abnormal glenoid, absence of the proximal portion of the humerus, articulation of the distal humerus with the ulna, and radial sided hand abnormalities.

Clinical Presentation

While the etiology of the condition hinges on the longitudinal dysplasia of the radius, the clinical presentation of patients with radial longitudinal dysplasia is diverse. Patients can often present with skeletal abnormalities that extend beyond the radial deficiency. These include shortening of the forearm and/or bowing of the ulna, absent or limited elbow flexion, and absence or hypoplasia of the scaphoid and other carpal bones. Thumb hypoplasia can be present and consist of hypoplasia of the thenar intrinsic and/or extrinsic musculature, hypoplasia of the skeletal elements with or without associated articular instability, rudimentary presence of the thumb ("pouce floutant"), or complete absence of the thumb. The fingers can exhibit limited flexion, with the radial digits more affected than the ulnar digits. In addition to the manifestations of RLD in the hand, the soft tissues on the radial side of the wrist and forearm are tight contributing to the radial angulation of the hand plate on the distal ulna. The extrinsic wrist extensors are often poorly developed, and the malformed radial soft tissues often form a fibrous tether to the radial side of the wrist. This combination results in the classic presentation of a radial deviated wrist held in a flexed posture.

The abnormalities have both aesthetic and functional consequences. In severe cases the appearance of the extremity can be unsightly secondary to the shortened forearm and the angled, flexed posture of the wrist and hand. On average, the forearm length is 54 % of normal, ranging from 37 to 67 % [26]. This limits the extremity's reach and can make two-handed activities with the normal, opposite extremity difficult. In patients with bilateral upper extremity involvement, the functional limitations can be more severe. James et al. [23] found the incidence of bilateral involvement to be 65 % in a study of 104 patients. If poorly functioning digits are present, this can further impede function. Unfortunately, when present, finger dysfunction is rarely amenable to surgical correction. This is in contradistinction to thumb limitations, where several options are available to improve function.

Non-operative Management

The non-operative care of a child with RLD often begins very early in life. Occupational therapy intervention is commonly instituted during the first few weeks of life, especially if the infant requires hospitalization for associated abnormalities. Those children whose health allows them to be discharged from hospital care in the first few days of life are often referred for outpatient therapy services very early on by their pediatricians.

Therapeutic intervention at this point includes stretching exercises aimed at lengthening the contracted tissues on the radial side of the wrist and improving the hand-forearm angle. Splinting is often used as an adjunct to stretching in an effort to maintain the wrist in the corrected position and provide static resistance to a resting position of radial deviation. Specific therapeutic protocols for treatment of RLD by non-operative means vary widely from surgeon to surgeon and therapist to therapist. There have been no published reports of therapeutic regimens proven to change the natural history of RLD, although its effectiveness in teaching children to use the affected limb in an efficient and useful manner has been seen clinically by many who care for these patients. Timing of intervention is also a topic of debate among those who treat these children. The authors feel that an early stretching regimen with nap and night splinting can be instituted early in life, but the parents should be encouraged to remove the splints for extended periods while the child is awake to allow him/her to interact appropriately with his/her surroundings and obtain the sensory interaction with the environment that is essential for proper development. Two-handed activities generally begin around the age of 3 months. At this time, splint wear during awake hours may become beneficial to place the hand in a less radially deviated position, functionally increasing the length of the affected extremity, and allowing for easier two-handed manipulation of objects.

Operative Management

There have been many procedures described for the management of the wrist and forearm deformity in RLD. Since the original description of centralization by Sayre in 1894, several authors have published similar techniques with slight variations to the original procedure [27–30]. In addition, newer techniques such as radialization, pre-centralization distraction, and microsurgical transfer of vascularized epiphyses have been introduced to treat the deformity [31–34]. No single procedure has proven superior to another. Hence there remains vast disparity in treatment recommendations between surgeons treating the condition. Recurrence of the radial angulation remains the Achilles heel for procedures aimed at correcting the deformity [35].

Reports centered on treatment of Types 0, N, I, and II RLD are sparse.

Type 0

Despite the relative frequency of Type 0 RLD reported by James et al. [23], a small number of these patients require surgical intervention. In 2004, Mo and Manske [36] reported on six wrists in five children treated with surgical correction.

They recommended surgical intervention for radial deviation deformity greater than 20°. In their subset of patients, the preoperative hand-forearm angle ranged from 35° to 70° with all wrists lacking active extension to neutral. The authors describe a dorsal approach to the wrist with exposure of the extensor carpi radialis tendon or tendons. The tendon is released from its distal insertion. Following release, the dorsal–radial wrist capsule, as well as the volar wrist capsule, is released allowing passive correction of the wrist to neutral position. The extensor carpi ulnaris tendon is released, leaving a distal stump for tenoraphy with the radial wrist extensors, effectively removing the radial deviation force and realigning it to gain neutral wrist extension. The proximal stump of the extensor carpi ulnaris tendon is sewn into the dorsal wrist capsule overlying the third metacarpal to further augment active wrist extension. Optionally, a pin can be placed across the carpus into the distal ulna to maintain the wrist in its corrected position. The patient is then casted in neutral to slight wrist extension for 6–8 weeks. The cast and pin, if present, are removed and the patient is allowed to begin active range-of-motion exercises. At rest the patient is splinted in the corrected position for an extended duration.

Mo and Manske [36] reported favorable outcomes using the above surgical technique. They reported an average improvement of radial deviation at rest from 58° to 12°, with active wrist extension improving an average of 53° and passive wrist extension improving and average of 28°. The average length of follow-up was 19 months (range, 2–38 months).

Types I and II

There have been few published reports on the treatment of Types I and II radial longitudinal deficiencies. Often, children with these types of RLD do not require surgical intervention. When necessary, the most common form of treatment is radial lengthening with release of the tight radial soft tissues and tendon transfer to support the realigned position. Lengthening of the radius is most commonly done by way of osteotomy and lengthening through an external fixator [37–40]. Others have reported on lengthening of the radius acutely, with gains of up to 1.6 cm [41]. Many authors have described techniques of lengthening through an external fixator with slight variations. Depending on surgeon preference, the lengthening can be performed with a single plane fixator [38] or by using a ring-type fixator [40]. When performing acute radius lengthening, Waters et al. [41] described a technique of using a temporary external fixator intraoperatively for distraction of the radius after performing a Z-cut osteotomy, followed by plate fixation of the bone in its new lengthened position.

Matsuno et al. [38] reported on two patients with Type II RLD who underwent radial lengthening with an external fixator. The outcomes demonstrated recurrence of the deformity following fixator removal with and increase the hand-forearm angle at final follow-up.

Types III and IV

The treatment of Types III and IV RLD is classically described as centralization of the carpus on the distal end of the ulna. Since Sayre first described the original procedure of centralization in 1894, multiple authors have published their experience using this technique, as well as several modifications to the procedure aimed at decreasing the recurrence of the radial angulation deformity. In addition, many others have suggested alternative procedures to accomplish the task of neutralizing the carpus on the end of the forearm. These procedures include radialization of the carpus, transfer of vascularized epiphyses to support the radial side of the carpus, and ulnocarpal fusion [31, 34, 42, 43].

Centralization

The centralization procedure is based on four surgical steps: (1) initial stretching of soft tissues ± pre-centralization distraction, (2) surgical alignment of the carpus on the ulna, (3) balancing of the deforming forces, and (4) maintenance of the corrected position.

Historically, stretching of the radial tissues was accomplished by serial cast application prior to surgical centralization, often carried out within the first several months of life. This technique fails to adequately distract the tight radial soft tissues or translate the carpus distally over the end of the ulna; instead it simply aligns the carpus alongside the distal ulna. In addition, the early application of casts precludes the use of the extremity by the child during the formative time of "learning" single and two-handed object manipulation. As a result, the use of external fixation to accomplish soft tissue distraction has been advocated in recent years by some surgeons. The application of uniplanar [44], biplanar [32, 45], and ring [33, 46, 47] external fixators have been described. The use of external fixation allows for the correction of the radial deviation deformity through distraction of the radial soft tissues and correction of the volar subluxation of the carpus in relation to the distal ulna. Distraction of the deformity is begun 3–5 days following the application of the fixator. The distraction is carried out at a rate of 0.5–1 mm per day until the desired position of the carpus is accomplished. The extremity is then maintained in the fixator for a period of 3 to 4 weeks prior to surgical stabilization of the carpus in its centralized position to allow the soft tissues to equilibrate.

Originally, the centralization procedure was performed through a longitudinal dorsal incision. Since that time, there have been multiple incisional techniques described to accomplish surgical centralization of the carpus [27, 28, 48].

The pre-centralization distraction of the soft tissues allows for ease in accomplishing surgical centralization while often obviating the need for transposition flaps for soft tissue coverage. Regardless of the incision used, the hypoplastic extensor tendons are carefully identified and retracted. The tight dorsal, radial, and volar wrist capsule and soft tissues are released to allow for a tension-free placement of the carpus onto the distal ulna aligned on the axis of the third metacarpal. Buck-Gramcko described "radialization" of the carpus in which he aligned the carpus on the axis of the second metacarpal in an effort to decrease the tendency towards recurrence of the deformity [31]. With the use of preoperative distraction, the need for "notching" [49] of the carpus to decrease soft tissue tension is usually unnecessary. The importance of obtaining a tension-free centralization has been reinforced by Sestero and Van Heest [50], who demonstrated that ulna in non-centralized radial longitudinal deficient extremities attained 64 % of normal length while the ulnar length in centralized extremities was 58 % of normal compared to 48 % of normal when notching of the carpus was performed. They postulated that the decrease in longitudinal growth capacity of the ulna was secondary to increased pressure applied to the distal ulnar physis by the centralized carpus. Once an appropriate centralized position is obtained, carpus is pinned to the ulna with longitudinal Kirschner wires (K-wires) taking care to avoid the distal ulnar physis. The pins are cut beneath the skin and often remain in place for up to 6 months postoperatively to maintain the corrected position. Soft tissue rebalancing procedures are then performed to redirect the forces across the centralized carpus. The extensor carpi ulnaris tendon is advanced to improve the ulnar and dorsal vector of pull to the wrist and hand [22, 30, 31]. If present, the radial wrist extensors are transferred ulnarly to alleviate the deforming force caused by their function. The digital extensors are translated in an ulnar direction using a sling of extensor retinaculum to align them along the longitudinal axis of the ulna, hence eliminating another deforming force.

Epiphyseal Transfer

The concept of supporting the hand and carpus by transferring bony elements to the radial side of the wrist to augment the support provided by the distal ulna was introduced in 1928 by Albee [51] and attempted by several subsequent authors [6, 8, 29]. Unfortunately, these early attempts were hindered by the limited growth potential possessed by the transferred nonvascularized tissue. With the advent and refinement of microsurgical techniques, the concept of vascularized epiphyseal transfer with retained growth potential [52–54] rejuvenated the interest in supporting the radial side of the carpus using a structural graft. In 1998, Vilkki [34] reported on the use of the second metatarsophalangeal joint to support the radial side of the carpus.

In contrast to the centralization procedure, the epiphyseal transfer is generally performed at an age of 4–5 years. Prior to embarking on the microsurgical portion of the reconstruction, the child often undergoes a soft tissue release with detethering of the radial side of the carpus with concomitant volar bilobed flap, transposing the excess ulnar sided soft tissue to the deficient radial side [55]. This early intervention (done at approximately 12–18 months of age) has the advantage of maintaining wrist motion while minimizing risk to the distal ulnar physis. Following release and soft tissue transfer, a protocol of stretching and splinting is maintained through the early childhood years in an effort to preserve the increase in motion.

At an age of 5–6 years, the child is evaluated for the possibility of microsurgical epiphyseal transfer. Often the child and his family decline additional surgery because very few functional limitations exist and cosmesis would be the primary indication for surgery. That said, if further surgical reconstruction is warranted, the microsurgical epiphyseal transfer is preceded by soft tissue distraction using an external fixator as described earlier in the chapter. The frame is applied and the carpus is slowly distracted (0.5–1 mm per day) until the desired anatomic position of the hand is accomplished over the distal ulnar. This can take 6–8 weeks to accomplish. The second toe metatarsophalangeal joint is harvested from the ipsilateral limb maintaining two arterial sources—first and second dorsal metatarsal artery and second and third plantar metatarsal artery [56]. Flexor and extensor tendons are preserved and sutured to the remaining proximal phalanx. The dorsal cutaneous nerves are also preserved to the dorsal skin paddle. The middle and distal phalanges of the toe are excised. Exquisite care must be taken to preserve the vessels to the epiphysis of the proximal phalanx and metatarsal during harvest.

The metatarsophalangeal joint is transferred to the wrist through a dorsal ± volar incision. The metatarsal is anchored to the ulna using K-wires, which are cut and bent beneath the skin. The proximal phalanx is anchored to the base of the second metacarpal, or against the scaphoid if present, in a position of 15–20° of flexion to increase stability. The preserved tendons of the toe are then sutured to the radial flexor and extensor tendons or muscle bellies to confer additional stability. After securing the bony construct, the metatarsophalangeal joint is revascularized.

Oftentimes the radial artery is absent in limbs affected by RLD; hence, the arterial supply for the epiphyseal transfer is provided by a persistent median artery or the ulnar artery. If present, the median artery or radial artery is anastomosed to the dominant vessel of the metatarsophalangeal joint in end-to-end fashion. In those cases where the median and radial artery is absent, the dominant vessel of the metatarsophalangeal joint is anastomosed to the ulnar artery in end-to-side fashion. Following acquisition of arterial inflow, the venous drainage is accomplished by anastomosis of dorsal veins.

The distraction device and K-wires are removed after radiographs have confirmed bony consolidation, usually 6–8 weeks. The arm is then casted for an additional month to protect the maturing transfer.

Ulnocarpal Arthrodesis

Ulnocarpal arthrodesis [43], or epiphyseal ulnocarpal arthrodesis [42] for the skeletally immature, is the procedure that most effectively stabilizes the wrist and improves the appearance of the radial angulation deformity. Despite the improvement in appearance, some have questioned the benefit of arthrodesis citing the maintenance of wrist motion as a substantial benefit in the function of the radial deficient limb [7]. Hence, the procedure is often thought of as a salvage procedure for severe, recurrent deformity. Rayan reported on two cases of recurrent deformity in skeletally mature patients who underwent ulnocarpal arthrodesis with improvement in both appearance and function [43]. Pike et al. [42] reported on 12 post-centralization wrists treated with ulnocarpal epiphyseal arthrodesis for recurrent radial angulation >45° and/or inability to extend the wrist beyond 25°. Post-operatively, the wrists were stable at an average of 20° radial angulation and 11° of flexion. All reported improvement in appearance and function post-operatively. A trial of ulnocarpal pinning can be considered for patients/parents who have concern regarding postoperative function prior to performing definitive arthrodesis procedure.

Distraction-Lengthening of the Ulna

In order to address the functional limitation of impaired "reach" of the affected extremity, authors have reported lengthening of the ulna using a ring or uniplanar external fixator in several small series ranging from 4 to 9 patients [39, 57–59]. The distraction time ranged from 11 to 15 weeks, followed by a 23–32-week consolidation period. Average length gained in each extremity was 4.4–6 cm (46–54 % of total length). Complications of lengthening included callus fracture, delayed union, digital and wrist stiffness, pain, pin tract infection, and recurrence of radial angulation. There were no rigid outcomes reported documenting improvement in function of the lengthened extremity.

Outcomes/Complications

Regardless of the type of surgery utilized, the common denominator in the outcomes of the surgical management of RLD is the recurrence of the radial angulation deformity. Multiple studies have documented the recurrence of radial angulation deformity following centralization [26, 35, 60]. An average radial-forearm angle of 21–26° immediately after centralization has been noted in these studies, with an additional 9- to 38-degree increase in radial angulation occurring over time. The avoidance of recurrent deformity has not been alleviated by the use of pre-centralization distraction as shown by Dana et al. [61]. In 2008, Vilkki [62] presented the long-term study of 19 wrists treated with microsurgical epiphyseal transfer with an average of 11 years follow-up. The average hand-forearm angle was 28° of radial deviation with mean total active wrist motion of 83°. Of the nine wrists included in his original report [34], seven were noted to have increased radial angulation (mean of 12°) over a follow-up period of 15.2 years. Goldfarb et al. [26] reported significant functional limitations of the post-centralized hand, noting a 62 % increase in the Jebsen-Taylor timed activity tests compared to normal. Interestingly, the DASH scores showed only mild functional limitation. Buffart et al. [63] observed grip and pinch strength values of 36 % and 30 %, respectively, when compared to normal controls. Both of the previous studies represent post-centralization scores compared to normal controls. There are no comparisons to pre-centralization function, thus making it impossible to determine the effects of surgical deformity correction.

Complications of the surgical treatment of radial deficient limbs are both all inclusive and dependent of the surgical technique used. Recurrence of deformity is a complication that is ubiquitous despite the treatment modality. Pin tract infections, callus fracture, delayed union, and stiffness are common to all techniques utilizing external fixation. Damage to the distal ulnar physis, further impairing its ability to accomplish longitudinal growth, is the most feared complication of centralization. Hence, the concept of carpal notching has been largely supplanted by newer techniques of pre-distraction centralization, in an effort to diminish the forces exerted across the distal ulnar physis.

Future Directions

The best treatment of RLD and its multiple phenotypes remains a popular topic among surgeons commonly treating the condition. To date, treatment algorithms have encompassed the full circle of management strategies, from non-operative to operative care at various stages of life for various clinical presentations utilizing a vast array of surgical procedures. Certainly, the definitive "best" treatment has yet to be determined, and likely is not the same for every patient. Future comparisons of those treated for RLD with surgical intervention versus those treated by nonoperative means may shed the most meaningful light on what interventions benefit these children the most.

References

1. Mariani FV, Ahn CP, Martin GR. Genetic evidence that FGFs have an instructive role in limb proximal-distal patterning. Nature. 2008;453(7193):401–5. doi:10.1038/nature06876. Epub 2008/05/02. PubMed PMID: 18449196; PubMed Central PMCID: PMC2631409.
2. Sun X, Mariani FV, Martin GR. Functions of FGF signalling from the apical ectodermal ridge in limb development. Nature. 2002; 418(6897):501–8. doi:10.1038/nature00902. Epub 2002/08/02. PubMed PMID: 12152071.
3. Kato H, Ogino T, Minami A, Ohshio I. Experimental study of radial ray deficiency. J Hand Surg Br. 1990;15(4):470–6. Epub 1990/11/01. PubMed PMID: 2269841.
4. Lourie GM, Lins RE. Radial longitudinal deficiency. A review and update. Hand Clin. 1998;14(1):85–99. Epub 1998/04/04. PubMed PMID: 9526159.
5. Flatt A. Radial clubhand. The care of congential hand anomalies. 2nd ed. St. Louis: Quality Medical Publishing; 1993. p. 366–410.
6. Heikel HV. Aplasia and hypoplasa of the radius: studies on 64 cases and on epiphyseal transplantation in rabbits with the imitated defect. Acta Orthop Scand. 1959;39:1–155. PubMed PMID: 14400621.
7. Lamb DW. Radial club hand. A continuing study of sixty-eight patients with one hundred and seventeen club hands. J Bone Joint Surg. 1977;59(1):1–13. PubMed PMID: 833156.
8. Riordan DC. Congenital absence of the radius. J Bone Joint Surg. 1955;37-A(6):1129–39; discussion, 39–40. PubMed PMID: 13271460.
9. Kelikian H. Radial ray defect. Congenital deformities of the hand and forearm. Philadelphia: WB Saunders Company; 1974. p. 780–824.
10. Goldfarb CA, Wall L, Manske PR. Radial longitudinal deficiency: the incidence of associated medical and musculoskeletal conditions. J Hand Surg. 2006;31(7):1176–82. PubMed PMID: 16945723.
11. Hall JG, Levin J, Kuhn JP, Ottenheimer EJ, van Berkum KA, McKusick VA. Thrombocytopenia with absent radius (TAR). Medicine. 1969;48(6):411–39. Epub 1969/11/01. PubMed PMID: 4951233.
12. Ward RE, Bixler D, Provisor AJ, Bader P. Parent to child transmission of the thrombocytopenia absent radius (TAR) syndrome. Am J Med Genet Suppl. 1986;2:207–14. Epub 1986/01/01. PubMed PMID: 3146292.
13. Schnur RE, Eunpu DL, Zackai EH. Thrombocytopenia with absent radius in a boy and his uncle. Am J Med Genet. 1987;28(1):117–23. doi:10.1002/ajmg.1320280117. Epub 1987/09/01. PubMed PMID: 3314504.
14. Edelberg SB, Cohn J, Brandt NJ. Congenital hypomegakaryocytic thrombocytopenia associated with bilateral absence of the radius—the TAR syndrome. Hum Hered. 1977;27(2):147–52. Epub 1977/01/01. PubMed PMID: 863461.
15. Klopocki E, Schulze H, Strauss G, Ott CE, Hall J, Trotier F, et al. Complex inheritance pattern resembling autosomal recessive inheritance involving a microdeletion in thrombocytopenia-absent radius syndrome. Am J Hum Genet. 2007;80(2):232–40. doi:10.1086/510919. Epub 2007/01/20. PubMed PMID: 17236129; PubMed Central PMCID: PMC1785342.
16. Toriello HV. Thrombocytopenia-absent radius syndrome. Semin Thromb Hemost. 2011;37(6):707–12. doi:10.1055/s-0031-1291381. Epub 2011/11/22. PubMed PMID: 22102274.
17. Oishi SN, Carter P, Bidwell T, Mills J, Ezaki M. Thrombocytopenia absent radius syndrome: presence of brachiocarpalis muscle and its importance. J Hand Surg. 2009;34(9):1696–9. PubMed PMID: 19773129.
18. Stevenson RE, Hunter AG. Considering the embryopathogenesis of VACTERL Association. Mol Syndromol. 2013;4(1–2):7–15. doi:10.1159/000346192. Epub 2013/05/09. PubMed PMID: 23653571; PubMed Central PMCID: PMC3638783.
19. Huang T. Current advances in Holt-Oram syndrome. Curr Opin Pediatr. 2002;14(6):691–5. Epub 2002/11/19. PubMed PMID: 12436037.
20. Shimamura A, Alter BP. Pathophysiology and management of inherited bone marrow failure syndromes. Blood Rev. 2010;24(3):101–22. doi:10.1016/j.blre.2010.03.002. Epub 2010/04/27. PubMed PMID: 20417588; PubMed Central PMCID: PMC3733544.
21. Soulier J. Fanconi anemia. Hematology Am Soc Hematol Educ Program. 2011;2011:492–7. doi:10.1182/asheducation-2011.1.492. Epub 2011/12/14. PubMed PMID: 22160080.
22. Bayne LG, Klug MS. Long-term review of the surgical treatment of radial deficiencies. J Hand Surg. 1987;12(2):169–79. PubMed PMID: 3559066.
23. James MA, McCarroll Jr HR, Manske PR. The spectrum of radial longitudinal deficiency: a modified classification. J Hand Surg. 1999;24(6):1145–55. PubMed PMID: 10584934.
24. Goldfarb CA, Manske PR, Busa R, Mills J, Carter P, Ezaki M. Upper-extremity phocomelia reexamined: a longitudinal dysplasia. J Bone Joint Surg. 2005;87(12):2639–48. PubMed PMID: 16322613.
25. Tytherleigh-Strong G, Hooper G. The classification of phocomelia. J Hand Surg Br. 2003;28(3):215–7. PubMed PMID: 12809650.
26. Goldfarb CA, Klepps SJ, Dailey LA, Manske PR. Functional outcome after centralization for radius dysplasia. J Hand Surg. 2002;27(1):118–24. PubMed PMID: 11810625.
27. Evans DM, Gateley DR, Lewis JS. The use of a bilobed flap in the correction of radial club hand. J Hand Surg Br. 1995;20(3):333–7. PubMed PMID: 7561408.
28. Manske PR, McCarroll Jr HR, Swanson K. Centralization of the radial club hand: an ulnar surgical approach. J Hand Surg. 1981;6(5):423–33. PubMed PMID: 7276473.
29. Starr D. Congenital absence of the radius. A method of surgical correction. J Bone Joint Surg. 1945;27A:572–7.
30. Watson HK, Beebe RD, Cruz NI. A centralization procedure for radial clubhand. J Hand Surg. 1984;9(4):541–7. PubMed PMID: 6747239.
31. Buck-Gramcko D. Radialization as a new treatment for radial club hand. J Hand Surg. 1985;10(6 Pt 2):964–8. PubMed PMID: 4078287.
32. Kanojia RK, Sharma N, Kapoor SK. Preliminary soft tissue distraction using external fixator in radial club hand. J Hand Surg Eur Vol. 2008;33(5):622–7. PubMed PMID: 18977832.
33. Sabharwal S, Finuoli AL, Ghobadi F. Pre-centralization soft tissue distraction for Bayne type IV congenital radial deficiency in children. J Pediatr Orthop. 2005;25(3):377–81. PubMed PMID: 15832159.
34. Vilkki SK. Distraction and microvascular epiphysis transfer for radial club hand. J Hand Surg Br. 1998;23(4):445–52. PubMed PMID: 9726542.
35. Damore E, Kozin SH, Thoder JJ, Porter S. The recurrence of deformity after surgical centralization for radial clubhand. J Hand Surg. 2000;25(4):745–51. PubMed PMID: 10913218.
36. Mo JH, Manske PR. Surgical treatment of type 0 radial longitudinal deficiency. J Hand Surg. 2004;29(6):1002–9. doi:10.1016/j.jhsa.2004.06.010. Epub 2004/12/04. PubMed PMID: 15576208.
37. Cheng JC. Distraction lengthening of the forearm. J Hand Surg Br. 1991;16(4):441–5. Epub 1991/11/01. PubMed PMID: 1779163.
38. Matsuno T, Ishida O, Sunagawa T, Suzuki O, Ikuta Y, Ochi M. Radius lengthening for the treatment of Bayne and Klug type II and type III radial longitudinal deficiency. J Hand Surg. 2006;31(5):822–9. PubMed PMID: 16713850.
39. Raimondo RA, Skaggs DL, Rosenwasser MP, Dick HM. Lengthening of pediatric forearm deformities using the Ilizarov technique: functional and cosmetic results. J Hand Surg. 1999;24(2):331–8. PubMed PMID: 10194019.

40. Villa A, Paley D, Catagni MA, Bell D, Cattaneo R. Lengthening of the forearm by the Ilizarov technique. Clin Orthop Relat Res. 1990;250:125–37. Epub 1990/01/01. PubMed PMID: 2293920.
41. Waters PM, Van Heest AE, Emans J. Acute forearm lengthenings. J Pediatr Orthop. 1997;17(4):444–9. Epub 1997/07/01. PubMed PMID: 9364380.
42. Pike JM, Manske PR, Steffen JA, Goldfarb CA. Ulnocarpal epiphyseal arthrodesis for recurrent deformity after centralization for radial longitudinal deficiency. J Hand Surg. 2010;35(11):1755–61. doi:10.1016/j.jhsa.2010.07.022. Epub 2010/10/12. PubMed PMID: 20932693.
43. Rayan GM. Ulnocarpal arthrodesis for recurrent radial clubhand deformity in adolescents. J Hand Surg. 1992;17(1):24–7. PubMed PMID: 1538107.
44. Taghinia AH, Al-Sheikh AA, Upton J. Preoperative soft-tissue distraction for radial longitudinal deficiency: an analysis of indications and outcomes. Plast Reconstr Surg. 2007;120(5):1305–12; discussion 13–4. PubMed PMID: 17898604.
45. Thatte MR, Mehta R. Treatment of radial dysplasia by a combination of distraction, radialisation and a bilobed flap—the results at 5-year follow-up. J Hand Surg Eur Vol. 2008;33(5):616–21. PubMed PMID: 18694912.
46. Goldfarb CA, Murtha YM, Gordon JE, Manske PR. Soft-tissue distraction with a ring external fixator before centralization for radial longitudinal deficiency. J Hand Surg. 2006;31(6):952–9. PubMed PMID: 16843155.
47. Thirkannad SM, Burgess RC. A technique for using the Ilizarov fixator for primary centralization in radial clubhand. Tech Hand Up Extrem Surg. 2008;12(2):71–8. PubMed PMID: 18528232.
48. VanHeest A, Grierson Y. Dorsal rotation flap for centralization in radial longitudinal deficiency. J Hand Surg. 2007;32(6):871–5. PubMed PMID: 17606069.
49. Lidge R. Congenital radial deficient club hand. J Bone Joint Surg. 1969;69A:1041–2.
50. Sestero AM, Van Heest A, Agel J. Ulnar growth patterns in radial longitudinal deficiency. J Hand Surg. 2006;31(6):960–7. PubMed PMID: 16843156.
51. Albee FH. Formation of radius congenitally absent: condition seven years after implantation of bone graft. Ann Surg. 1928;87(1):105–10. PubMed PMID: 17865806.
52. Bowen CV, Ethridge CP, O'Brien BM, Frykman GK, Gumley GJ. Experimental microvascular growth plate transfers. Part I—Investigation of vascularity. J Bone Joint Surg Br. 1988;70(2): 305–10.
53. Bowen CV, O'Brien BM, Gumley GJ. Experimental microvascular growth plate transfers. Part 2—Investigation of feasibility. J Bone Joint Surg Br. 1988;70(2):311–4.
54. Donski PK, O'Brien BM. Free microvascular epiphyseal transplantation: an experimental study in dogs. Br J Plast Surg. 1980;33(2):169–78. PubMed PMID: 7388206.
55. Wall LB, Ezaki M, Oishi SN. Management of congenital radial longitudinal deficiency: controversies and current concepts. Plast Reconstr Surg. 2013;132(1):122–8. doi:10.1097/PRS.0b013e318290fca5. Epub 2013/06/29. PubMed PMID: 23806915.
56. de Jong JP, Moran SL, Vilkki SK. Changing paradigms in the treatment of radial club hand: microvascular joint transfer for correction of radial deviation and preservation of long-term growth. Clin Orthop Surg. 2012;4(1):36–44. doi:10.4055/cios.2012.4.1.36. Epub 2012/03/02. PubMed PMID: 22379554; PubMed Central PMCID: PMC3288493.
57. Horii E, Nakamura R, Nakao E, Kato H, Yajima H. Distraction lengthening of the forearm for congenital and developmental problems. J Hand Surg Br. 2000;25(1):15–21. PubMed PMID: 10763716.
58. Peterson BM, McCarroll Jr HR, James MA. Distraction lengthening of the ulna in children with radial longitudinal deficiency. J Hand Surg. 2007;32(9):1402–7. PubMed PMID: 17996775.
59. Pickford MA, Scheker LR. Distraction lengthening of the ulna in radial club hand using the Ilizarov technique. J Hand Surg Br. 1998;23(2):186–91. PubMed PMID: 9607657.
60. Geck MJ, Dorey F, Lawrence JF, Johnson MK. Congenital radius deficiency: radiographic outcome and survivorship analysis. J Hand Surg. 1999;24(6):1132–44. PubMed PMID: 10584933.
61. Dana C, Auregan JC, Salon A, Guero S, Glorion C, Pannier S. Recurrence of radial bowing after soft tissue distraction and subsequent radialization for radial longitudinal deficiency. J Hand Surg. 2012;37(10):2082–7. doi:10.1016/j.jhsa.2012.07.018. Epub 2012/10/02. PubMed PMID: 23021174.
62. Vilkki SK. Vascularized metatarsophalangeal joint transfer for radial hypoplasia. Semin Plast Surg. 2008;22(3):195–212. doi:10.1055/s-2008-1081403. Epub 2008/08/01. PubMed PMID: 20567714; PubMed Central PMCID: PMC2884879.
63. Buffart LM, Roebroeck ME, Janssen WG, Hoekstra A, Selles RW, Hovius SE, et al. Hand function and activity performance of children with longitudinal radial deficiency. J Bone Joint Surg. 2008;90(11):2408–15. PubMed PMID: 18978409.

Radial Longitudinal Deficiency: Thumb Hypoplasia

8

Michael A. Tonkin

Introduction

Thumb hypoplasia (underdevelopment) accompanies many congenital conditions, including thumb duplication, transverse deficiencies and symbrachydactyly, brachydactyly, cleft hand complex and ulnar longitudinal deficiency, congenital constriction ring syndrome and other miscellaneous conditions such as the thumbs of Apert and Rubinstein–Taybi syndromes. Each condition represents its own specific challenges, but the principles remain the same. An optimal thumb demands appropriate size and shape, stability and mobility. No matter what the cause, surgery is directed towards the addition or removal of tissue, correction of deformity, stabilisation of unstable joints and/or the creation of joint mobility. At times there is a conflict between stability and mobility. Although generalisations are not necessarily applicable to all individual cases, the achievement of optimal mobility at the carpometacarpal (CMC) joint is perhaps the major determinant of effective thumb mobility, with less importance placed on the metacarpophalangeal (MCP) and interphalangeal (IP) joints. In principle, mobility may be sacrificed for stability at these levels.

Classical thumb hypoplasia, as part of a radial longitudinal deficiency, is a specific entity. It may accompany varying degrees of forearm radial hypoplasia or absence, or may occur alone. In the former instance this has been classified in the Swanson/International Federation of Societies for Surgery of the Hand (IFSSH) system within Group I: "Failure of Formation", but in the latter instance has been variably placed within this group and within Group V: "Undergrowth" [1, 2]. In the more recently proposed OMT system, it is classified as a "Failure of Axis Formation/Differentiation—affecting the radial-ulnar axis of the entire upper limb" or the "radial-ulnar axis of the hand plate" when the thumb alone is affected [3, 4]. This latter circumstance is uncommon, as a close clinical and radiological examination will nearly always reveal some proximal hypoplasia, even if subtle.

Thumb hypoplasia is often bilateral, although mild grades may be overlooked. Associations, syndromic and non-syndromic, are not uncommon (Table 8.1) [5]. Assessment of cardiac, gastrointestinal, renal, vertebral and other musculoskeletal anomalies, and investigation of possible blood disorders, such as those associated with thrombocytopenic absent radius (TAR) and Fanconi's anaemia are routine and have generally been performed by the referring paediatrician. Genetic counselling may be warranted.

Classification

Müller, in 1937, introduced the concept of a teratogenic sequence resulting in increasing severity of thumb hypoplasia [6]. He didn't specify the precise anomalies associated with a particular grade of severity, although many subsequent reviews have attributed four grades of hypoplasia to his name. In 1967, Blauth refined Müller's concept, defining five grades of thumb hypoplasia (Fig. 8.1) [7, 8]. A number of modifications to this classification have been suggested. That of Manske is most commonly quoted in the literature, but does involve significant changes to the definitions of Blauth [9, 10]. Blauth viewed the hypoplastic thumb according to grades of severity, with increasing bone and joint hypoplasia accompanied by increasing soft tissue hypoplasia. He distinguished Grade 2 from Grade 3 according to the presence or absence of a CMC joint, retaining the thumb in the former case but advising reconstruction of an alternative CMC joint in the latter. Manske moved this distinction into a sub-classification of Grade 3, in which Grade 3A has a CMC joint and Grade 3B does not. Buck-Gramcko added a 3C in which only the distal one-third of the metacarpal remained (Fig. 8.2) [11]. The Manske classification distinguishes

M.A. Tonkin, M.B.B.S., M.D., F.R.A.C.S., F.R.C.S. (Ed Orth) (✉)
Department of Hand Surgery and Peripheral Nerve Surgery,
Royal North Shore Hospital, The Children's Hospital at Westmead,
University of Sydney, Sydney, NSW 2065, Australia
e-mail: mtonkin@med.usyd.edu.au

D.R. Laub Jr. (ed.), *Congenital Anomalies of the Upper Extremity: Etiology and Management*,
DOI 10.1007/978-1-4899-7504-1_8, © Springer Science+Business Media New York 2015

between Grades 2 and 3A by the absence or presence of extrinsic musculotendinous anomalies. Such a subclassification suggests that extrinsic anomalies develop with more severe grades of hypoplasia but are not present in less severe grades (Grades 1 and 2), and that these occur after the insult to intrinsic musculotendinous units. In my experience, if surgical reconstructions of thumb intrinsics, MCP joint instability and first web hypoplasia are indicated, there are always some extrinsic anomalies. These may or may not deserve reconstruction. It is of interest that neither the classification of Blauth nor Manske considered the stability or mobility of the CMC joint in those grades in which the proximal metacarpal is present (Blauth Grade 2, Manske Grades 2 and 3A). Manske specifically equated the presence of the proximal metacarpal with a stable CMC joint and proximal metacarpal absence with an unstable joint. Buck-Gramcko defined the 3A thumb as having an unstable CMC joint and described significant extrinsic anomalies within Grade 2.

I favour Müller's concept of increasing hypoplasia of all thumb elements, of soft tissues, bones and joints, occurring concurrently, and Blauth's distinction between Grades 2 and 3 according to the presence or absence of the proximal metacarpal. In its original form, the Blauth classification also provides logical guidelines for treatment by grade. In the main, Grade 2 thumbs are reconstructed; Grade 3 thumbs are removed and the index finger is pollicised. Manske and Buck-Gramcko moved these alternative treatment recommendations to within Grade 3, distinguishing between 3A and 3B.

Some who are classification "splitters" may choose to subclassify Grade 2 according to which components of the thumb would be improved by surgical reconstruction and the techniques whereby this is achieved. Smith advised a Grade 2A or 2B on the basis of uniaxial or global MCP joint instability [12, 13]. This could be extended to specify differences in other aspects of Grade 2 hypoplasias. The classification "lumpers" may prefer to designate the classification of Grade 2 to all such thumbs, regardless of the reconstructive techniques utilised. However, as Buck-Gramcko states "the assessment of results is difficult, especially because the outcome depends on the preoperative condition in the severity of the deformity" [11]. It is clear that the surgical reconstruction of a thumb with uniaxial MCP joint instability, intrinsic hypoplasia and a mildly hypoplastic first web, when accompanied by minor extrinsic anomalies not requiring reconstruction, is

Table 8.1 Associations of thumb hypoplasia, aplasia and triphalangism[a]

Frequent in:
Aase S.
Baller-Gerold S.
Congenital microgastria-limb reduction complex
Deletion 13q S.
Fanconi pancytopenia S.
Holt-Oram S.
Levy-Hollister S.
Nager S.
Oculo-auriculo-verterbral spectrum
Radial aplasia-thrombocytopenia S.
Roberts-SC phocomelia
Rothmund-Thomson S.
Townes-Brocks S.
VATERR Association
Yunis-Varon S.
Occasional in:
De Lange S.
Foetal aminopterin/methotrexate S.
Foetal valproate S.
Fibrodysplasia ossificans progressiva S.
Fraser S.
Fryns S.
Hypomelanosis of Ito
Lenz microphthalmia S.
Miller S.
Monozygotic (MZ) twinning and structural defects—general
MURCS Association
Popliteal pterygium S.
Trisomy 18S.

[a]Adapted from [5]

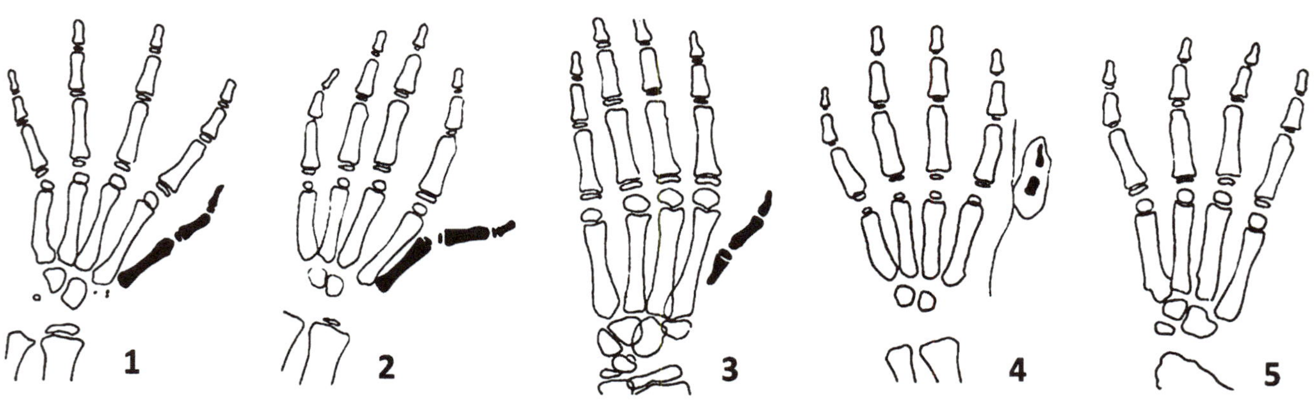

Fig. 8.1 Blauth grades of thumb hypoplasia 1–5. Published with kind permission of Michael A. Tonkin ©2014.

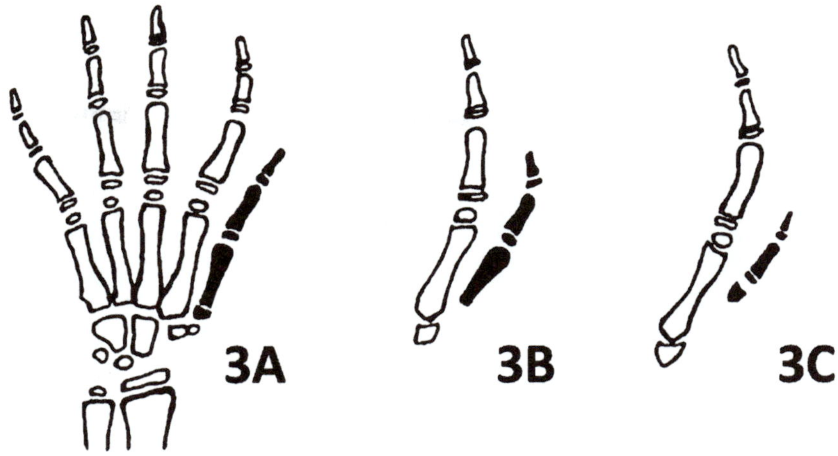

Fig. 8.2 Classification of thumb hypoplasia as modified by Manske (Grades 3A and 3B) and Buck-Gramcko (Grade 3C). Published with kind permission of Michael A. Tonkin ©2014. All rights reserved

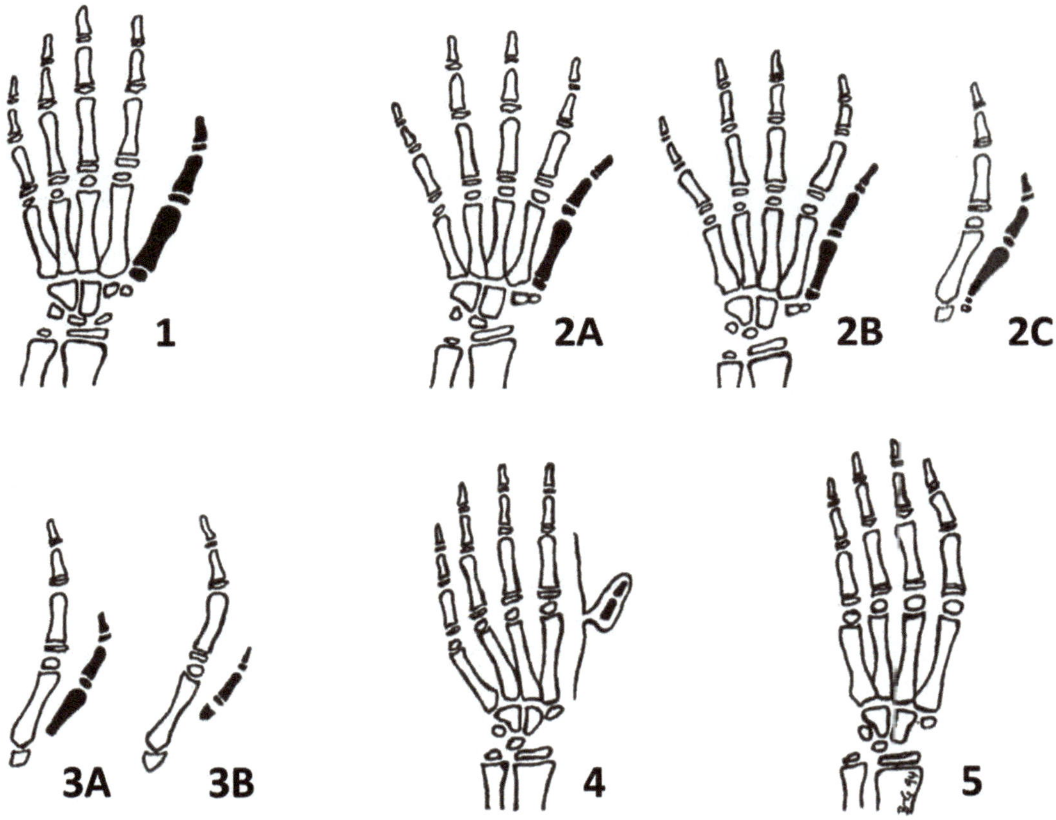

Fig. 8.3 Proposed modified Blauth classification. Published with kind permission of Michael A. Tonkin ©2014. All rights reserved

quite different from the reconstruction of a thumb with global MCP joint instability, severe hypoplasia of the first web and intrinsic absence, in association with a pollex abductus anomaly and/or hypoplasia or aplasia of the extrinsic flexors and extensors and/or abnormal alignment and insertion of these.

The following classification is offered as one maintaining the integrity of Blauth's skeletal classification and the teratological sequence of increasing severity of hypoplasia proposed by Müller, Blauth and others (Fig. 8.3). The subdivisions within grades do not create separate categories for each anatomical anomaly and its treatment, but allow the results of surgical reconstructions to be compared for "similar" thumbs:

Grade 1: The thumb is small, there is some hypoplasia of the thenar musculature and there may be mild extrinsic anomalies. However, the joints are stable and mobile. No surgery is indicated.

Grade 2: Thumb hypoplasia is more severe and would benefit from reconstruction. The CMC joint is present. Intrinsic and extrinsic anomalies are more significant and

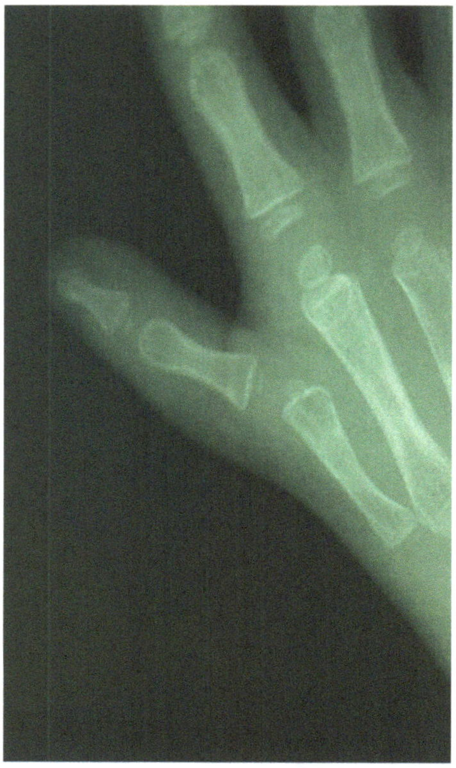

Fig. 8.4 Blauth Grade 2 (A, B) thumb hypoplasia with proximal metacarpal flare. Published with kind permission of Michael A. Tonkin ©2014. All rights reserved

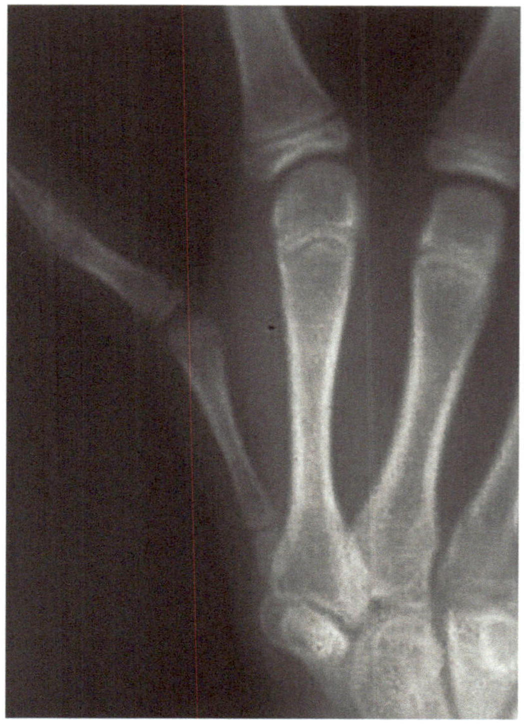

Fig. 8.5 Blauth Grade 2C thumb hypoplasia with an inadequate CMC joint. Published with kind permission of Michael A. Tonkin ©2014. All rights reserved

there is MCP joint instability and first web underdevelopment. An increasing severity of hypoplasia is recognised according to the clinical and radiological examinations:

2A: Mild. Hypoplasia of intrinsic muscles; uniaxial MCP joint instability; and adduction of the first metacarpal with first web deficiency. Management includes release of the first web, MCP joint ulnar collateral ligament (UCL) reconstruction and an opposition transfer as appropriate. Mild extrinsic anomalies do not demand attention.

2B: Moderate. The intrinsic hypoplasia and first web insufficiency are more severe. MCP joint instability is multiplanar, requiring reconstruction of soft tissues other than the UCL alone. Chondrodesis or formal fusion may be necessary in a minority. Extrinsic anomalies demand reconstruction for optimal thumb function and prevention of recurrence of deformity. CMC joint stability and mobility are adequate as indicated by radiological evidence of a proximal flare at the first metacarpal base (Fig. 8.4).

2C: Severe. Increasing hypoplasia of all structures, with severe global MCP joint instability ("elephant's trunk sign"), gross extrinsic hypoplasia, and an inadequate CMC joint—clinically unstable or immobile. These thumbs may also be identified by the radiological appearance of loss of the proximal metacarpal base flare, which tapers proximally (the "pencil sign") (Fig. 8.5). The thumb requires a more significant first web release and skin transposition, an opposition transfer and extrinsic reconstruction. A chondrodesis or fusion of the MCP joint, and reconstruction of the CMC joint through stabilisation or mobilisation creates a satisfactory albeit compromised thumb ray. Rarely, pollicisation may be considered to provide a superior result for the most severe of these Grade 2C hypoplasias.

Grade 3: Increasing hypoplasia of all structures. The CMC joint is absent (Fig. 8.6).

3A: Absence of the proximal metacarpal.

3B: Distal metacarpal remnant is the only remaining metacarpal component.

Grade 4: Metacarpal absence. The floating thumb with phalanges is connected by a skin bridge to the index finger ray.

Grade 5: Thumb absence.

Pollicisation remains the optimal surgical reconstruction for Grades 3, 4 and 5. However, such a decision for children with Grade 3 and 4 thumbs may be complicated by concerns about the creation of a four-digit hand. More recently, alternative methods of construction of a CMC joint, through transfer of vascularised and non-vascularised joints and/or bone, have shown some encouraging results and may be indicated when the need to retain five digits is paramount [14–17]. The precise reconstructive procedure may be tailored to the degree of hypoplasia and the amount of bone available within the thumb to be retained. The surgical techniques are easier to perform

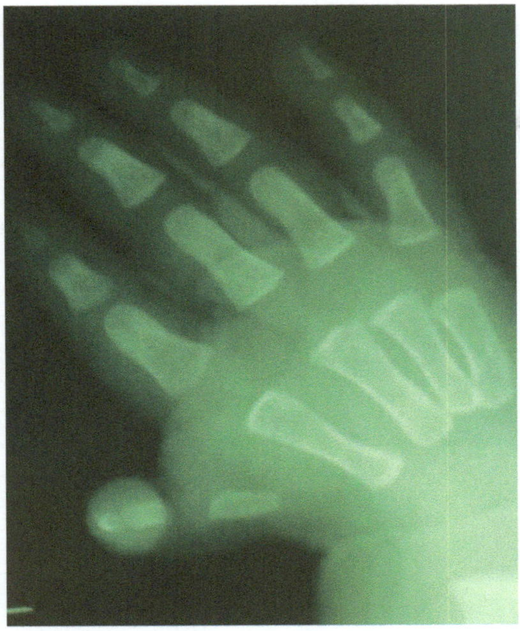

Fig. 8.6 Grade 3A—absent proximal metacarpal. Published with kind permission of Michael A. Tonkin ©2014. All rights reserved

and the results of such surgery are likely to be better for Grade 3A thumbs than for those of Grade 3B or 4. In Grade 5 hypoplasia, a vascularised toe transfer is perhaps the only feasible method of creating five digits.

Surgery

When the child is under anaesthesia, a further preoperative examination assists decision making. CMC joint stability and mobility, or the lack thereof, MCP joint instability and the passive range of IP joint motion can be confirmed at this time (Fig. 8.7a–c). Final decisions await the detail of anomalous anatomy revealed at surgical exploration.

Surgical Techniques

First Web Insufficiency

A four- or five-flap web-plasty are the most common techniques of first web deepening (Fig. 8.8a–d). Rotation and

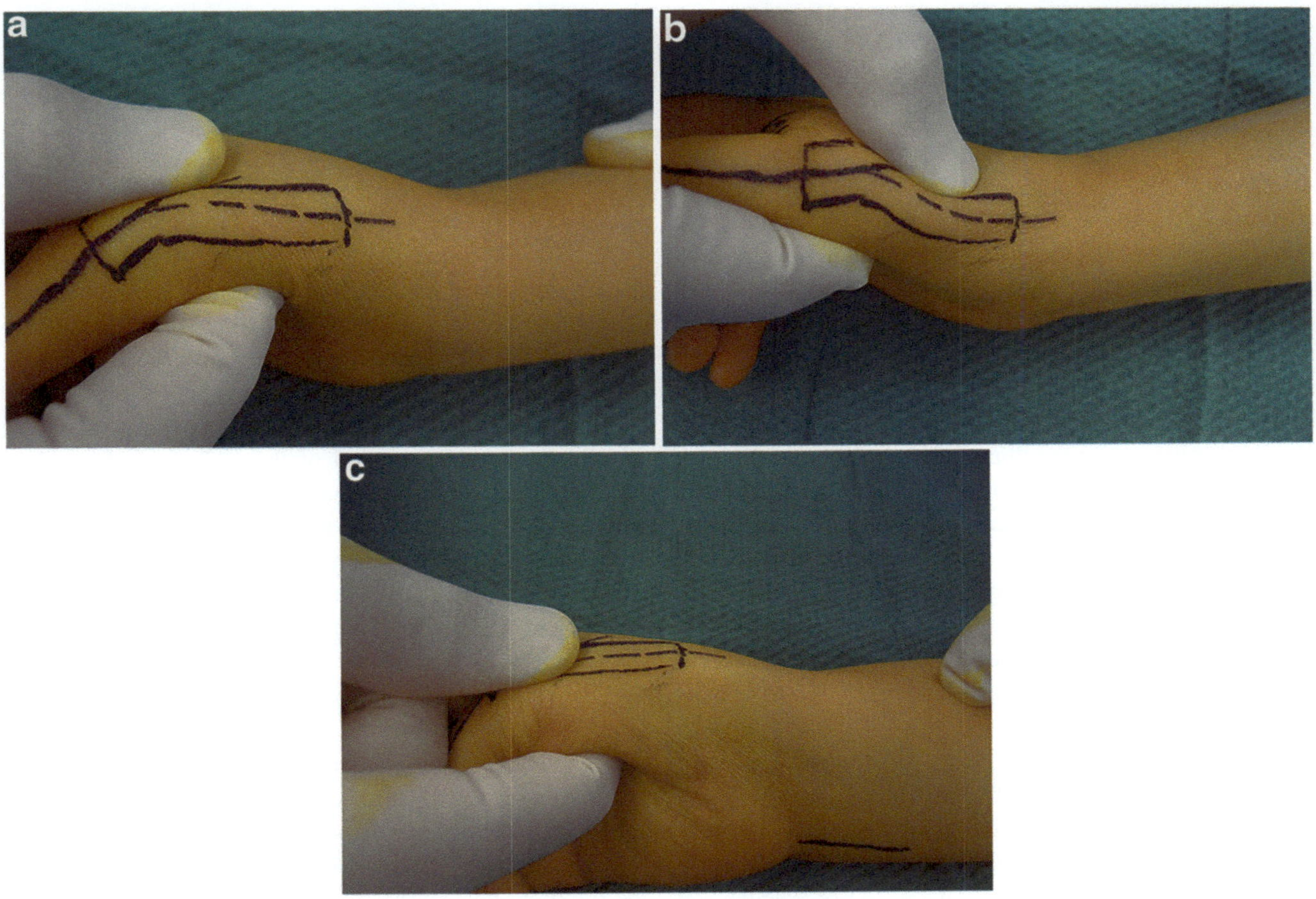

Fig. 8.7 (a–c) Assessment of CMC joint stability/motion at surgery. Published with kind permission of Michael A. Tonkin ©2014. All rights reserved

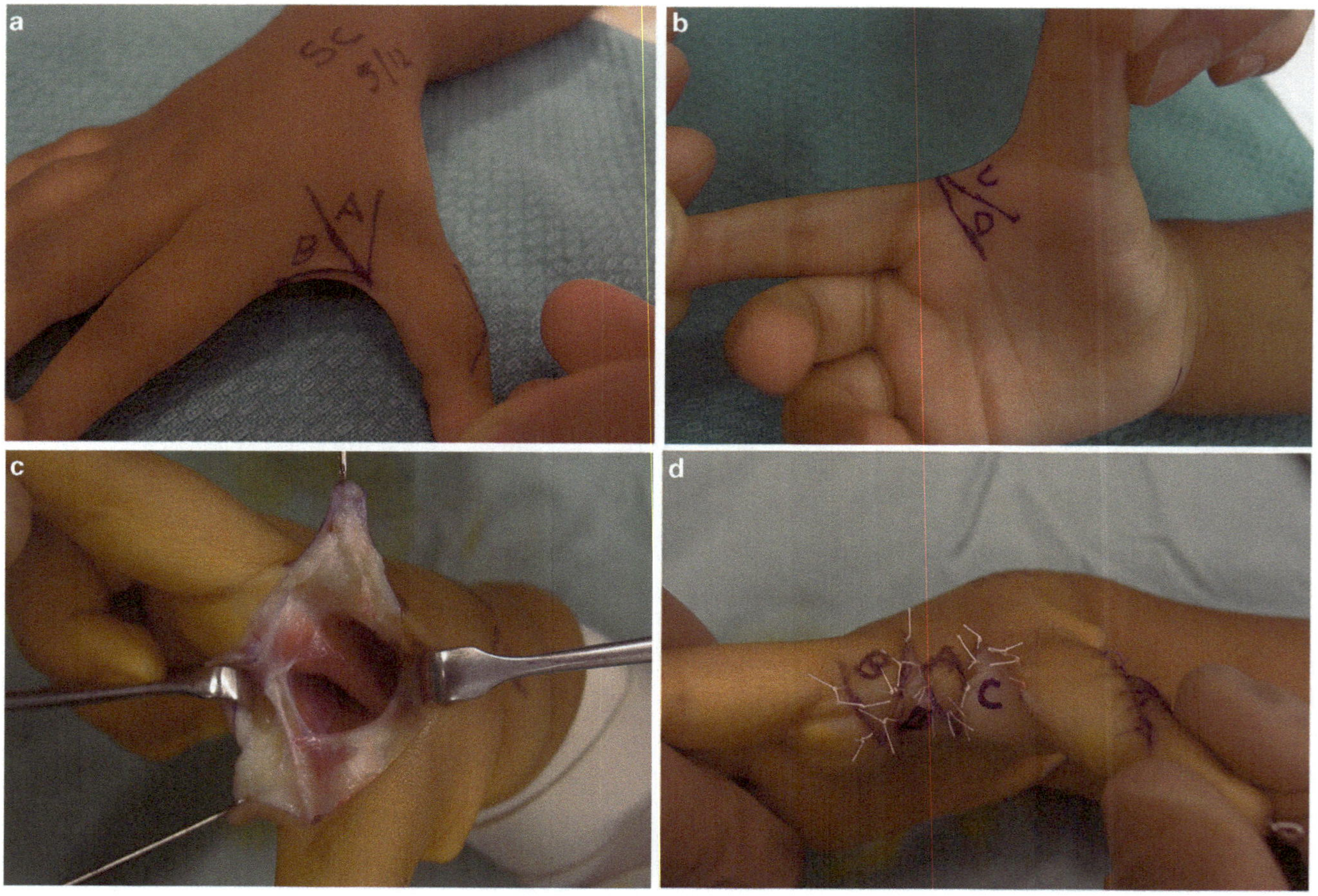

Fig. 8.8 (a–d) Four flap first web-plasty. Published with kind permission of Michael A. Tonkin ©2014. All rights reserved

advancement of tissue from the dorsum of the hand may be indicated for more severe first web deficiency. It is very uncommon to require tissue from distant sources, such as a pedicled posterior interosseous artery flap or radial forearm flap, or even a free tissue transfer. They may be considered if reconstruction in Grades 3, 4 and 5 is undertaken.

The adductor pollicis and first dorsal interosseous muscles, both supplied by the ulnar nerve, are intact but play a role in the adduction of the first metacarpal and first web insufficiency. The thumb is weak and too aggressive a release of these muscles may position the thumb better but weaken it further. The fascia over each muscle should be divided (see Fig. 8.8c). Some gentle recession of the first dorsal interosseous from the thumb metacarpal or of the transverse component of the adductor pollicis may be indicated, but tenotomies should be avoided.

Metacarpophalangeal Joint Instability

In determining the optimal stabilisation procedure, consideration must be given as to whether the instability is predominantly a loss of UCL integrity (Grade 2A) or whether the instability is global (Grade 2B), requiring a more sophisticated reconstruction or even a chondrodesis or fusion of the joint (Fig. 8.9).

There are two common methods of reconstruction of the UCL. One is to use available local tissue, imbricating capsule and ligamentous structures, such as they are, on the ulnar side of the joint. The other is to introduce tissue which is extrinsic to the joint to cater for the deficiencies of the local structures. The terminal part of a flexor digitorum superficialis (FDS) tendon used for an opposition transfer is a popular source.

Whichever reconstruction of the UCL is performed, it will fail if there is an abnormal abduction force crossing the MCP joint on its radial side, most commonly in association with a pollex abductus anomaly in which there is a flexor to extensor connection [18]. Attention must be directed to this if the joint forces are to be balanced and the UCL reconstruction protected.

My preference is to assess the calibre of the MCP joint ulnar soft tissues at the time of surgery. If they are satisfactory, I proceed to a double-breasting of these structures and protect the joint with a fine Kirschner-wire (K-wire). A strip of palmar plate can supplement this reconstruction. A 2- to 3-mm width may be mobilised, maintaining its insertion at the proximal phalanx base, transferring its proximal origin dorsally to the metacarpal head-neck junction. A similar technique may be applied for radial collateral ligament instability. If local tissue is adequate for collateral ligament

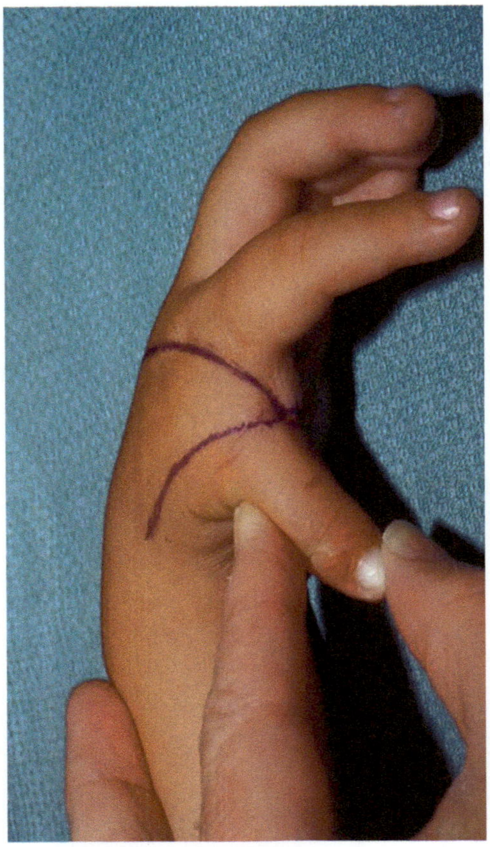

Fig. 8.9 Assessment of metacarpophalangeal (MCP) joint instability at surgery. Published with kind permission of Michael A. Tonkin ©2014. All rights reserved

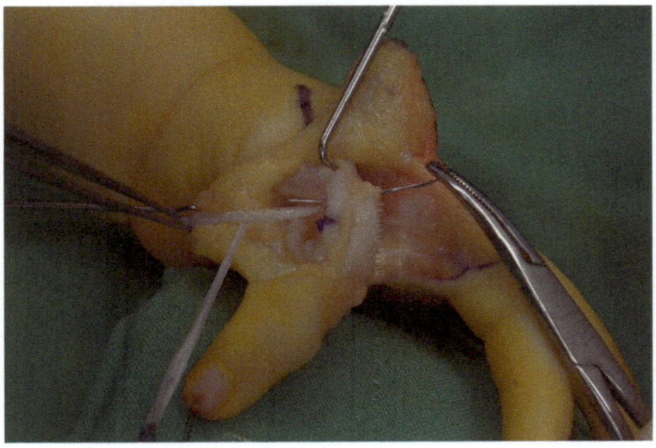

Fig. 8.10 Use of an FDS slip to create an MCP joint ulnar collateral ligament. Published with kind permission of Michael A. Tonkin ©2014. All rights reserved

reconstruction, the abductor digiti minimi (ADM) is used as an opposition transfer as described below. If the soft tissues are inadequate, then I will proceed to an FDS opposition transfer. One slip of the terminal part of the FDS is passed through a drill hole at the head-neck junction of the metacarpal, from radial to ulnar side, and is sutured to the base of the proximal phalanx and to soft tissues attached to this. Lister and subsequently Smith have advocated placing drill holes through the proximal phalanx, but I have tended to avoid this in the child because of the proximity of the growth plate and the small size of the bone.

One alternative for moderate global instability (Grade 2B) is to use two slips of FDS to reconstruct ulnar and radial collateral ligaments (Fig. 8.10). For MCP joint hyperextension instability, the whole of the palmar plate may be advanced proximally and fixed at the head-neck junction of the metacarpal, creating a check rein (Fig. 8.11a, b). I prefer this complex combination of soft tissue reconstructions to chondrodesis or fusion, unless the underdevelopment of articular surfaces is profound indeed. There is severe global instability. The "elephant's trunk sign" is indicative (Fig. 8.12a, b). The condyles of the head of the metacarpal are severely underdeveloped on the palmar aspects, with the shape of the metacarpal head, viewed end-on, triangular in appearance, curving palmarwards in the manner of an elephant's trunk. The base of the proximal phalanx is of small diameter and is planar with no concavity. A formal arthrodesis can be performed but this does shorten the thumb and is only possible if there is epiphyseal ossification. A chondrodesis, fixing the cartilaginous surfaces with one or two fine wires, will stabilise the joint, at least temporarily. This is necessary for the degree of underdevelopment present in Grade 2C thumbs.

Correction of MCP joint instability is vital to the protection of the underdeveloped CMC joint. Radial deviation at the MCP joint results in adduction of the metacarpal and basal subluxation at the CMC joint, a zig-zag deformity. If an MCP joint fusion or chondrodesis is necessary, this lengthens the lever arm, which places increased stress across the CMC joint. An unstable CMC joint may be further compromised. In this instance, one must consider the necessity of a soft tissue stabilisation at the CMC joint level, a relatively difficult reconstruction using free tendon graft in a figure-of-eight fashion. A soft tissue release for an immobile CMC joint is possible but care must be taken for fear of instability. Rarely, in circumstances of severe MCP joint instability and significant proximal hypoplasia, in spite of the presence of a CMC joint, alternative methods of CMC joint reconstruction such as pollicisation may be considered.

Opposition Transfers

The main alternatives are an ADM (Huber) transfer and an FDS transfer. There are proponents of both but there is no clear indication of the superiority of one over the other. The use of the ADM diminishes the power of abduction of the little finger but provides some thenar bulk. It is a better pronator of the thumb ray. The FDS transfer removes a flexor from the usually more mobile ulnar digits (ring finger), perhaps decreasing grip strength, and fails to provide any bulk to the thenar eminence. The FDS is superior in providing

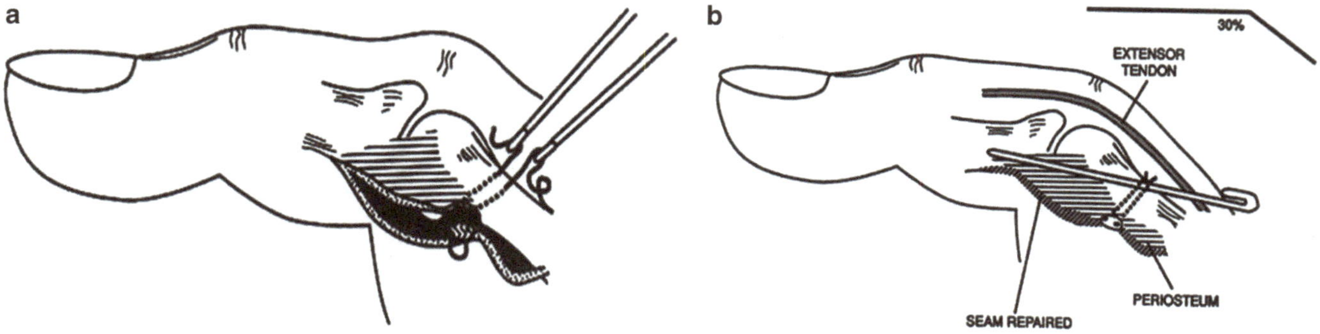

Fig. 8.11 (**a, b**) Advancement of the palmar plate proximally to prevent hyperextension instability of the MCP joint. Published with kind permission of Michael A. Tonkin ©2014. All rights reserved

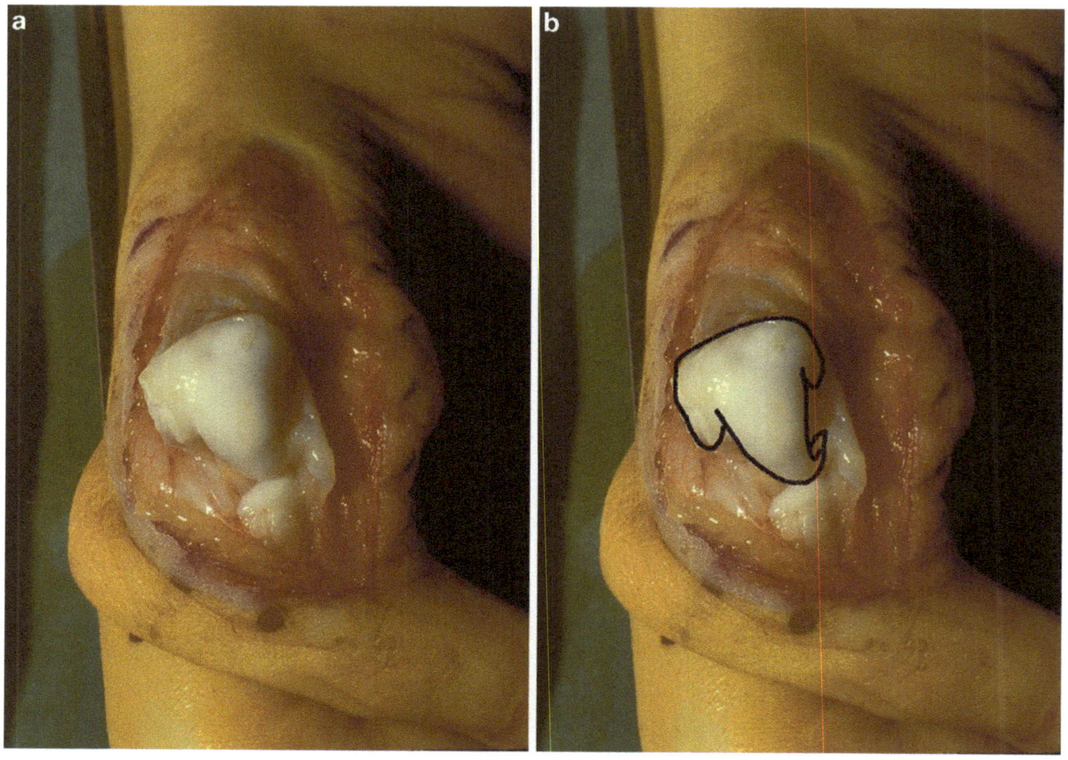

Fig. 8.12 (**a, b**) The "elephant's trunk" sign of global MCP joint instability. Published with kind permission of Michael A. Tonkin ©2014. All rights reserved

palmar abduction but pronates less effectively. When additional tissue is needed to stabilise the MCP joint, the FDS can provide this as described above.

Abductor Digiti Minimi Transfer

The incisions are shown in Fig. 8.13. The ulnar incision at the junction of glabrous and dorsal skin provides a very pleasing cosmetic result (Fig. 8.14). Proximally, the incision should curve around the wrist crease at the level of the pisiform so that the origin of the ADM may be mobilised, if necessary, for length. Distally, the insertion of the abductor should be incised from the base of the proximal phalanx but the tendon contribution to the extensor mechanism dorsally should also be harvested to provide adequate length (Fig. 8.15). This tissue is not of adequate quality to be extended to the ulnar side of the joint for ligament construction. I do not transfer the origin of the ADM to the flexor retinaculum as suggested by some for fear of interference with the neurovascular pedicle. Its origin may be mobilised fairly aggressively, maintaining some attachment to both the flexor carpi ulnaris (FCU) and the pisiform proximally. Tunnelling of the muscle is a little more difficult with the ulnar incision than with a para-hypothenar incision. It is necessary to make certain that no retinacular fibres of the aponeurosis impede

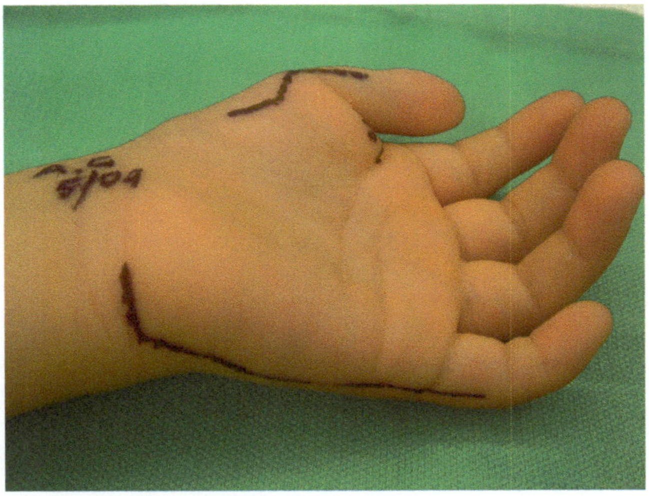

Fig. 8.13 Medial incision for abductor digiti minimi (ADM) transfer. Published with kind permission of Michael A. Tonkin ©2014. All rights reserved

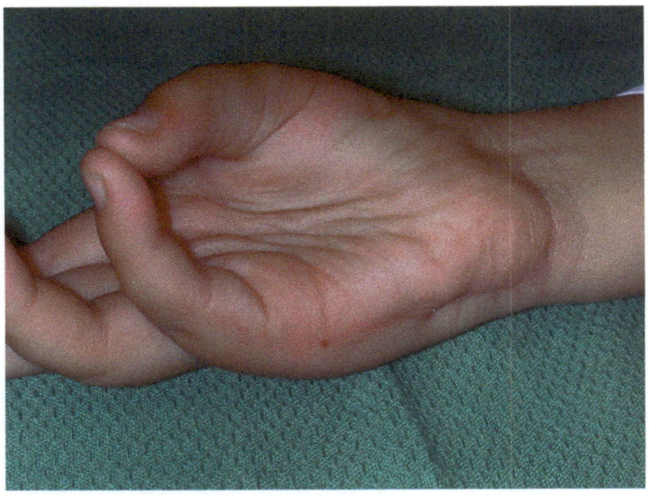

Fig. 8.14 Scar from medial incision following ADM transfer; note opposition and thenar bulk. Published with kind permission of Michael A. Tonkin ©2014. All rights reserved

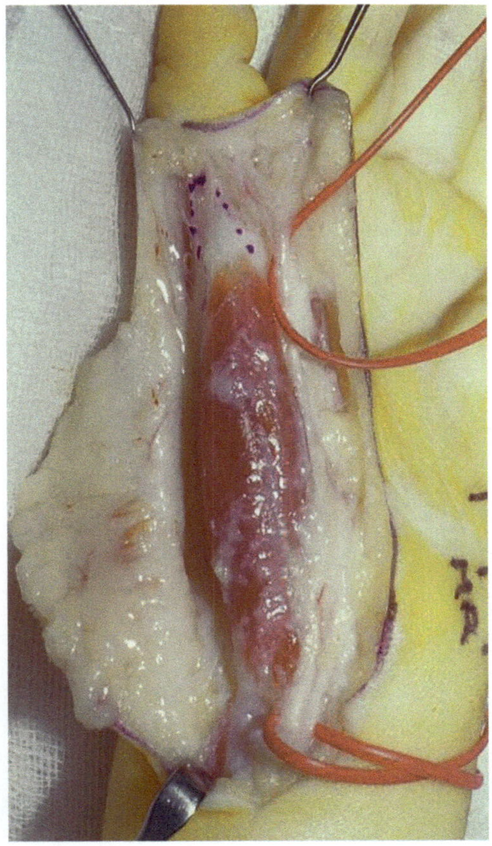

Fig. 8.15 Dissection for ADM transfer with distal extension to gain tendon length. Published with kind permission of Michael A. Tonkin ©2014. All rights reserved

its passage and that the neurovascular bundle is not kinked during its transfer. Insertion at the thumb is into the abductor pollicis brevis (APB) remnant if it is present. Otherwise it is better to attach the transfer to the head-neck junction of the metacarpal rather than to the proximal phalanx, as the latter insertion tends to create a radial deviating force which may challenge the UCL reconstruction.

Flexor Digitorum Superficialis Transfer

Incisions are shown in Fig. 8.16. The FDS transfer is sutured to the periosteum at the head-neck junction with one slip passed through the metacarpal to be used for UCL reconstruction (see Fig. 8.10). The FDS transfer demands reconstruction of a pulley to allow an optimal direction of pull so that pronation of the thumb ray is possible. This is achieved with a distally based slip of FCU (Fig. 8.17). It is possible to also prolong a radial slip to assist in reconstruction of the radial collateral ligament for global instability, sometimes in association with a proximal advancement of the palmar plate, as described previously. This aggressive soft tissue reconstruction at the MCP joint reduces the necessity to consider a primary MCP joint chondrodesis or a fusion, or at least allows delay of such a procedure until a later stage if failure of the soft tissue reconstruction demands a more permanent solution.

Extrinsic Tendon Reconstruction

Failure to correct a pollex abductus anomaly (flexor to extensor connection) will lead to a recurrence of MCP joint UCL instability, metacarpal adduction and possible CMC joint instability. Flexor pollicis longus (FPL) anomalies are common. Traction on the FPL at the level of the MCP joint will alert the surgeon to eccentric distal insertions and abnormal origins. In the former, deviation of the IP joint or lack of full flexion is evident. In the latter, there is minimal excursion of the musculotendinous unit with proximal traction. Any connection between the flexor and extensor mechanism must be divided (Fig. 8.18). In these instances the pulley system is

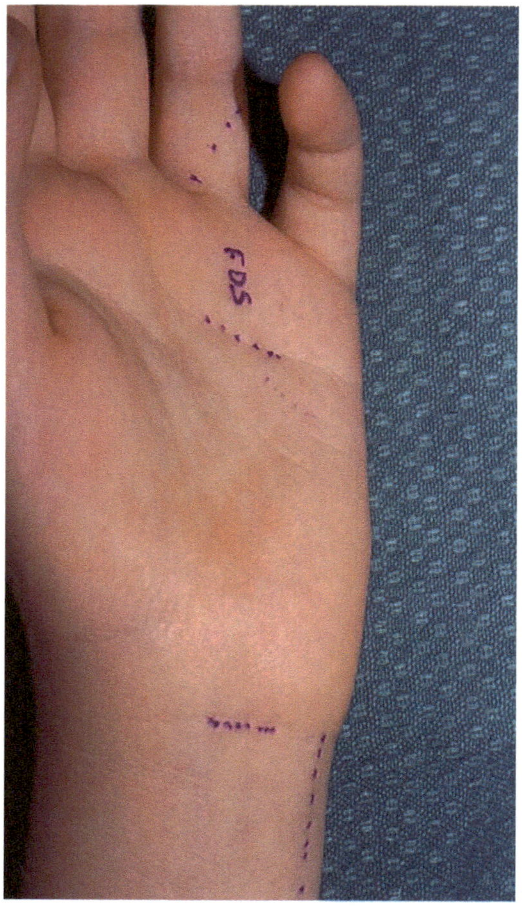

Fig. 8.16 Incisions for FDS transfer. Published with kind permission of Michael A. Tonkin ©2014. All rights reserved

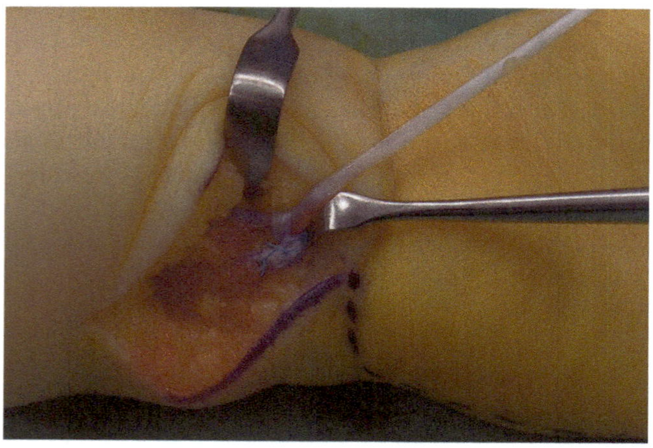

Fig. 8.17 FDS opposition transfer through an FCU pulley. Published with kind permission of Michael A. Tonkin ©2014. All rights reserved

often incompetent. This may be reconstructed at proximal phalangeal level with a strip of extensor retinaculum or a strip of local tendon (Fig. 8.19). Sometimes, particularly following release of a pollex abductus anomaly, the FPL tendon will continue to bowstring across the radial aspect of the MCP

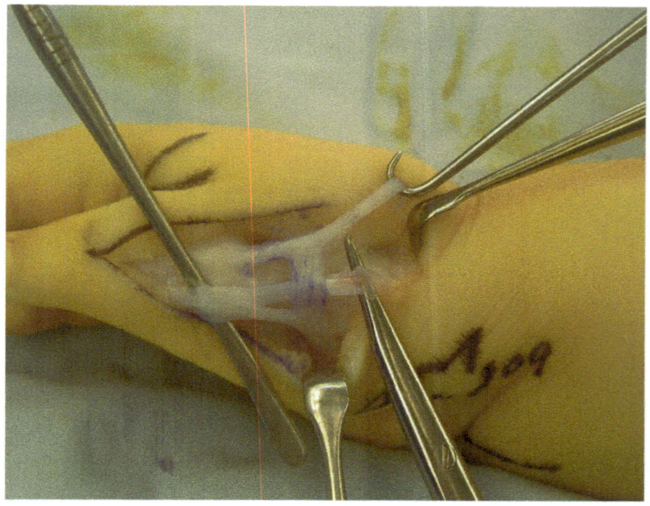

Fig. 8.18 Pollex abductus connection between extrinsic extensors and flexor. Published with kind permission of Michael A. Tonkin ©2014. All rights reserved

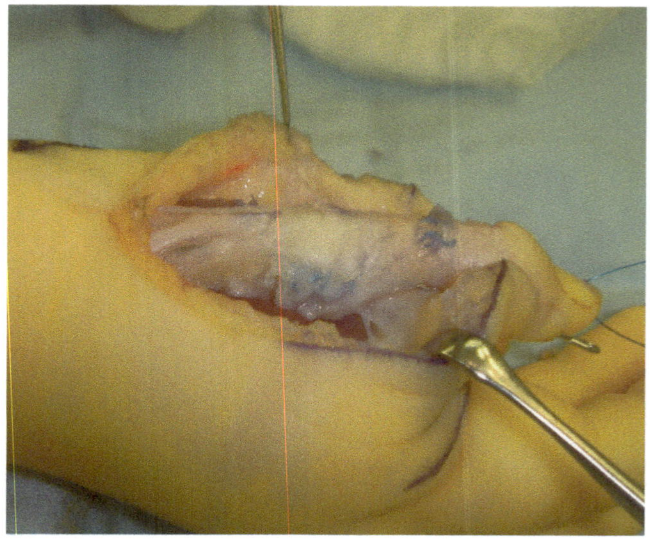

Fig. 8.19 Realignment of flexor pollicis longus and pulley reconstruction. Published with kind permission of Michael A. Tonkin ©2014. All rights reserved

joint, placing at risk the efficacy of both the UCL reconstruction and the opposition transfer, as the deviating force will tend to recreate the radial deviation deformity at the MCP joint. I believe that, just as in reconstruction for thumb duplications, axial malalignment of extrinsic tendons is one of the main causes of surgical failure. It is possible that axial realignment of FPL following the first web release and MCP joint stabilisation may well compromise gliding of the tendon and, if it is present passively, active IP joint flexion. This loss is less important than the presence of a deforming force post-operatively. The radial-most aspect of the tendinous insertion of flexor pollicis brevis (FPB), or perhaps the adductor pollicis, may be elevated from its insertion, allowing transposition

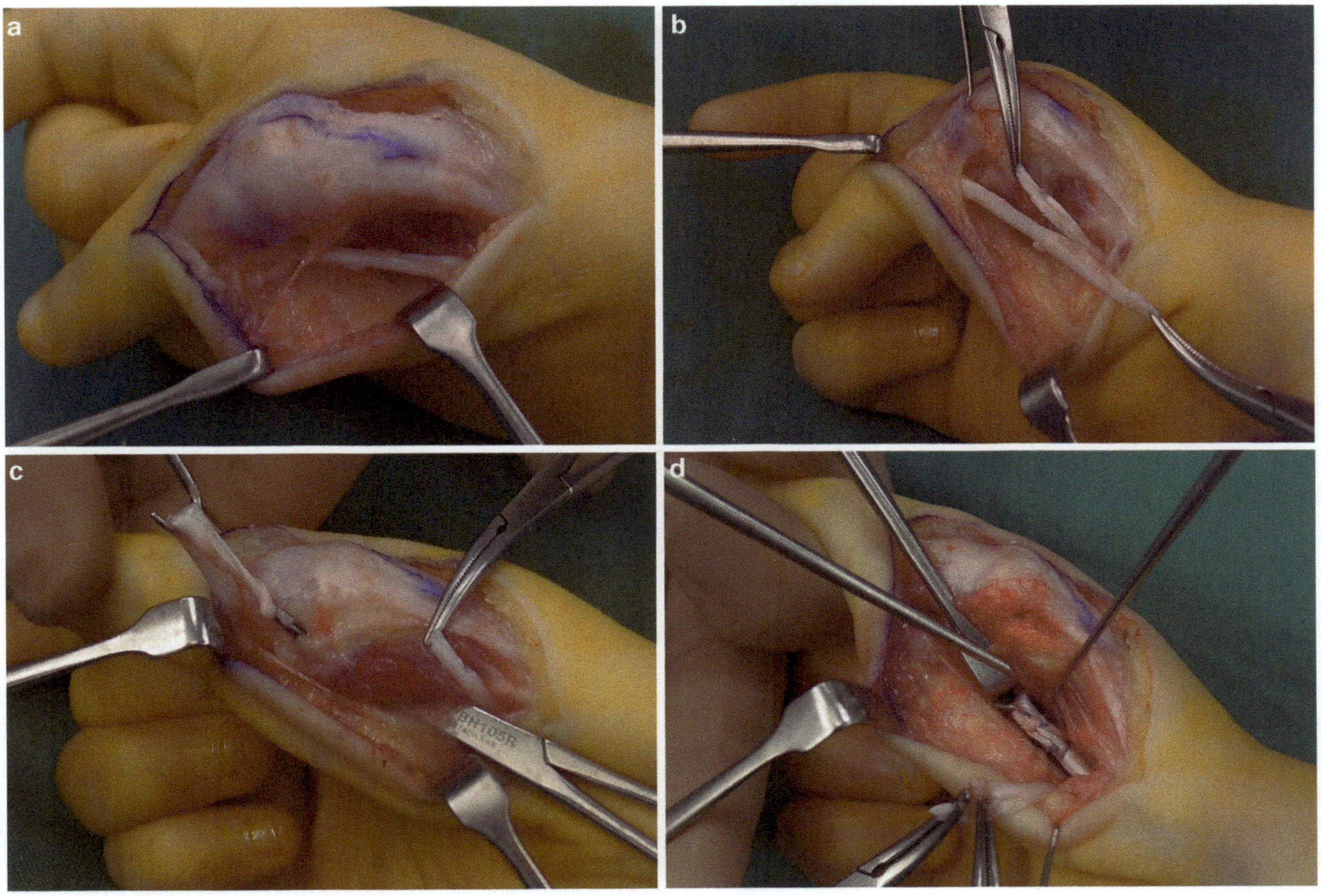

Fig. 8.20 (**a–d**) Z-division and realignment of FPL in the correct longitudinal axis. Published with kind permission of Michael A. Tonkin ©2014.

of FPL ulnarwards. The intrinsics, resutured distally, create a pulley and prevent subluxation of FPL radially. Rarely, I have divided the FPL in a Z fashion, either proximal to the wrist or distal to the carpal tunnel, to allow realignment and stabilisation in the longitudinal axis of the thumb. The tendon ends are sutured side to side (Fig. 8.20a–d).

If there is minimal passive IP joint motion, I do not proceed to sophisticated extrinsic flexor reconstruction. A superficialis transfer to a well-formed FPL tendon without an adequate proximal muscle belly is a possibility when there is a satisfactory passive range of motion. A staged flexor tendon reconstruction with preliminary insertion of a silastic rod, pulley reconstruction and subsequent superficialis transfer is rarely necessary but may be considered in certain circumstances. Eccentric extensor and flexor insertions should be centralised. An extensor indicis proprius (EIP) transfer may replace extensor pollicis longus (EPL) or extensor pollicis brevis (EPB) function, when occasionally indicated.

Pollicisation

I believe that pollicisation provides optimal thumb function and a very satisfactory appearance when the CMC joint is absent in Grades 3, 4 and 5 hypoplasia. Such a procedure may also be considered, uncommonly, in cases of Grade 2C hypoplasia in which, in spite of the presence of a proximal metacarpal, the global hypoplasia is so severe that reconstruction would provide an inferior thumb to that achieved by pollicisation (positive "elephant's trunk" and "pencil" signs). The necessity to retain five digits for social, racial or religious reasons must not be underestimated. In these instances, the alternative reconstructions outlined below are considered.

The technique of Buck-Gramcko is that followed by most surgeons [19]. A number of modifications have been offered, with alterations in placement of incisions and specific techniques of CMC joint and tendon reconstruction. However, the younger surgeon will find a reliable friend if he/she adheres to Buck-Gramcko's method.

Incisions

The surgery is performed under tourniquet. Some prefer not to utilise a Martin or Esmarch bandage to exsanguinate the limb, so that venous and arterial vasculature patterns are more obvious. My preference is to use a bandage to exsanguinate

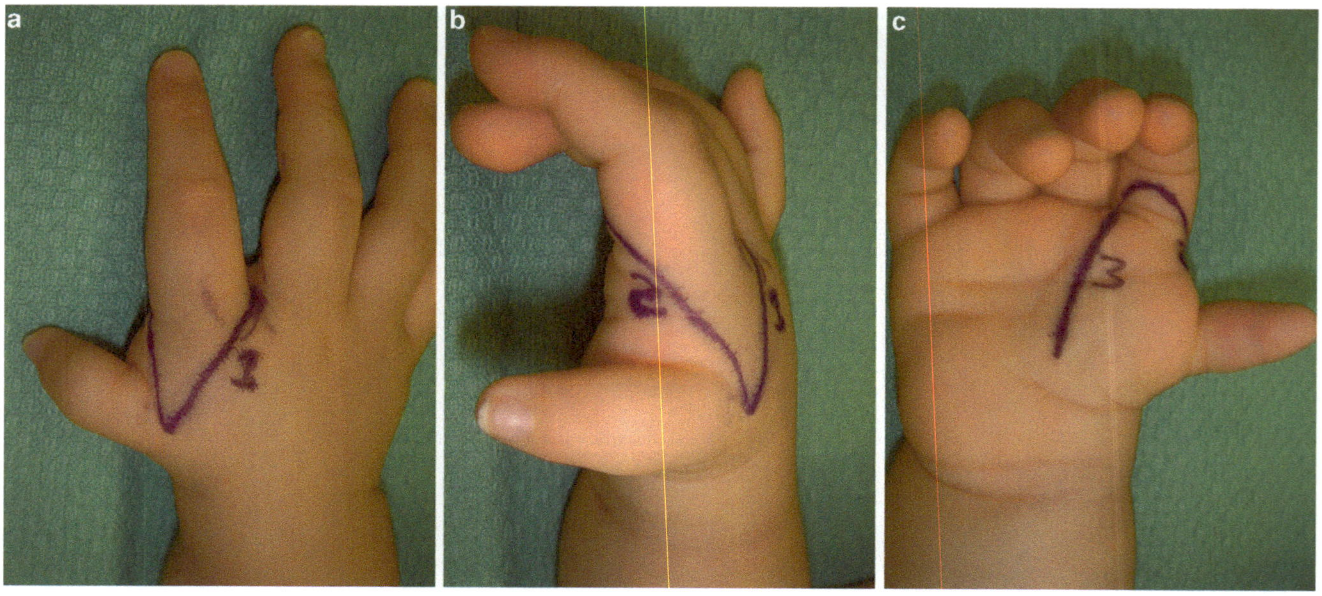

Fig. 8.21 (**a–c**) Z concept of pollicisation skin incision with the three limbs marked. Published with kind permission of Michael A. Tonkin ©2014. All rights reserved

the limb. Over a relatively short period of time, the vessels fill with blood allowing identification and I believe this to be preferable to the excessive bleeding which may occur as the tourniquet time progresses. The surgeon may move from palmar to dorsal dissection sites whilst this phenomenon evolves.

The concept of the incisions forming a modified z-plasty may be helpful (Fig. 8.21a–c). The first limb begins dorsally and distally at the index-middle web, and extends proximally and obliquely to the radial border of the hand proximal to the index finger MCP joint. The second limb extends from the proximal point of the first limb onto the palmar aspect of the proximal phalanx to meet the origin of the first limb in the index-middle web space. The third limb extends proximally from the palmar limb, in the line of the index-middle intermetacarpal space. These flaps are transposed when the index finger is rotated and recessed proximally. A number of subtleties of modification cater for specific demands. The palmar incision in the digit should be extended to just proximal to the proximal interphalangeal (PIP) joint when the index finger is well developed and mobile (see Fig. 8.21c). A longer thumb is preferable if there is significant index finger stiffness as greater length compensates for lack of mobility. In this instance the palmar incision is moved proximally towards the basal finger crease. A longitudinal incision extended distally from the dorsal limb incision to the PIP joint allows access to the extensor mechanism and its lateral bands for construction of thumb intrinsic mechanisms and the extrinsics, EPB and abductor pollicis longus (APL) (Fig. 8.22). The third palmar limb may be moved radially to incorporate excision of a Grade 3 or Grade 4 thumb (Fig. 8.23). Alternatively, the excision of such may be incorporated into the second, more radial limb (Figs. 8.22 and 8.24).

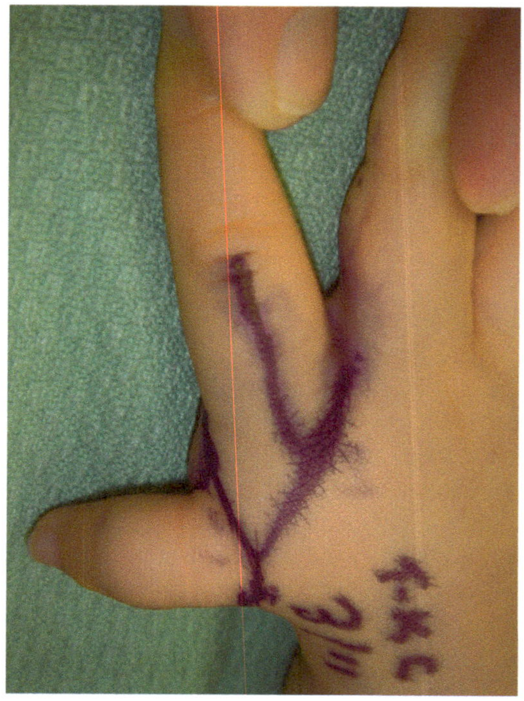

Fig. 8.22 Dorsal incision for intrinsic reconstruction. Published with kind permission of Michael A. Tonkin ©2014. All rights reserved

Palmar Dissection

I prefer to begin with the palmar dissection. The neurovascular bundle of the index-middle web is identified. A radial neurovascular bundle is usually present. However, the radial digital artery to the index finger may be very small, perhaps even absent, in Grade 5 hypoplasia which is accompanied by index finger hypoplasia. The neurovascular bundles on either side of the digit are mobilised using microsurgical

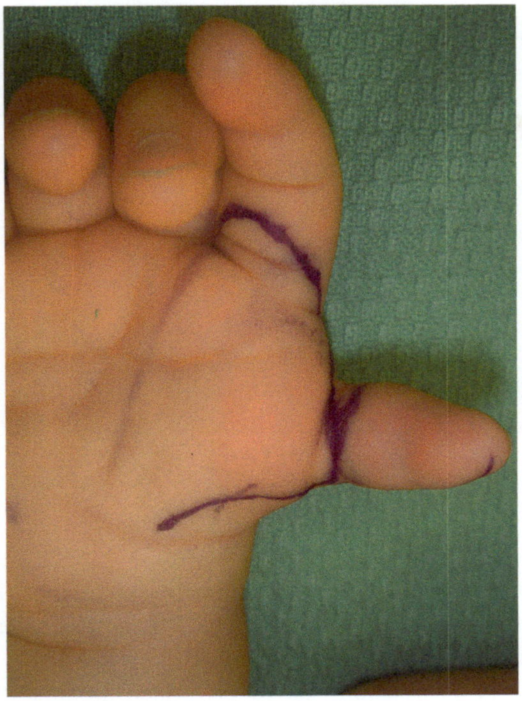

Fig. 8.23 Incorporation of Grade 3 thumb to be excised into third limb of pollicisation incisions. Published with kind permission of Michael A. Tonkin ©2014. All rights reserved

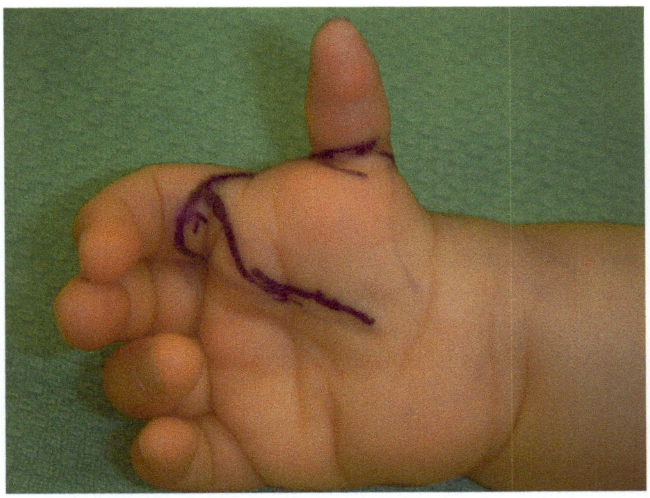

Fig. 8.24 Incorporation of Grade 3 thumb to be excised into second limb of pollicisation incisions. Published with kind permission of Michael A. Tonkin ©2014. All rights reserved

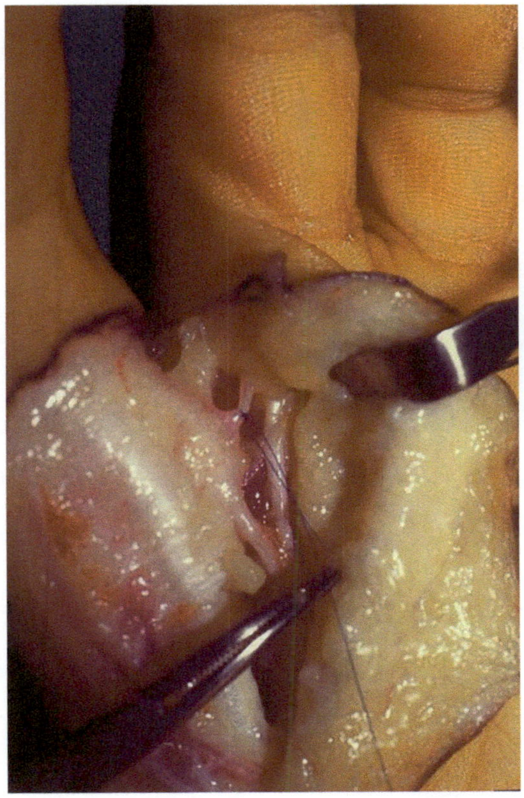

Fig. 8.25 The radial digital artery to the middle finger is tied off. Published with kind permission of Michael A. Tonkin ©2014. All rights reserved

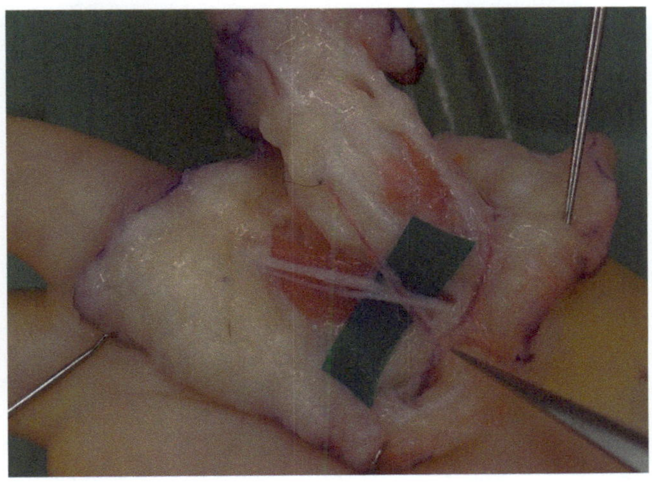

Fig. 8.26 Dissection of a neural ring to prevent common digital artery compromise. Published with kind permission of Michael A. Tonkin ©2014. All rights reserved

instruments and magnification. Inspection of the second common digital artery will determine the level of bifurcation into digital arteries to the adjacent sides of the index and middle fingers. The radial digital artery to the middle finger is tied off (Fig. 8.25). The neurovascular pedicle is dissected proximally. A neural ring is relatively common but can usually be attended to by intraneural dissection of the common digital nerve (Fig. 8.26). An awareness of the possibility of arterial compromise with proximal recession of the digit, either due to a neural ring or fascial structures, should prevent this complication.

Rarely, anomalies of the common digital artery demand an alteration in strategy. The vessel may arise from the deep palmar arch. In this instance the artery is short and may not allow proximal recession of the digit without compromising its arterial supply. It may be necessary to divide the deep

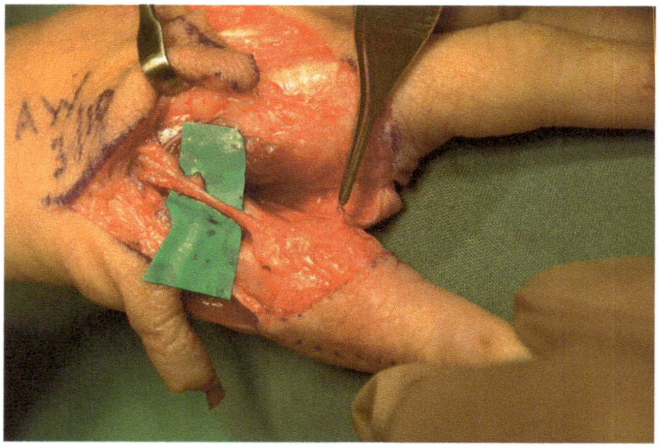

Fig. 8.27 Dorsal metacarpal artery connecting with palmar digital system. Published with kind permission of Michael A. Tonkin ©2014. All rights reserved

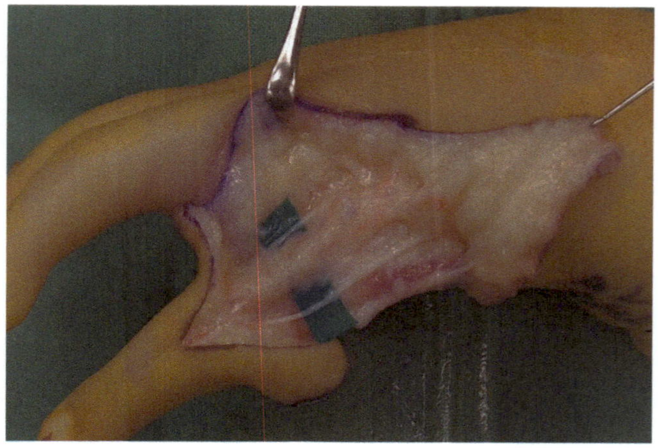

Fig. 8.29 Dorsal veins and nerves. Published with kind permission of Michael A. Tonkin ©2014. All rights reserved

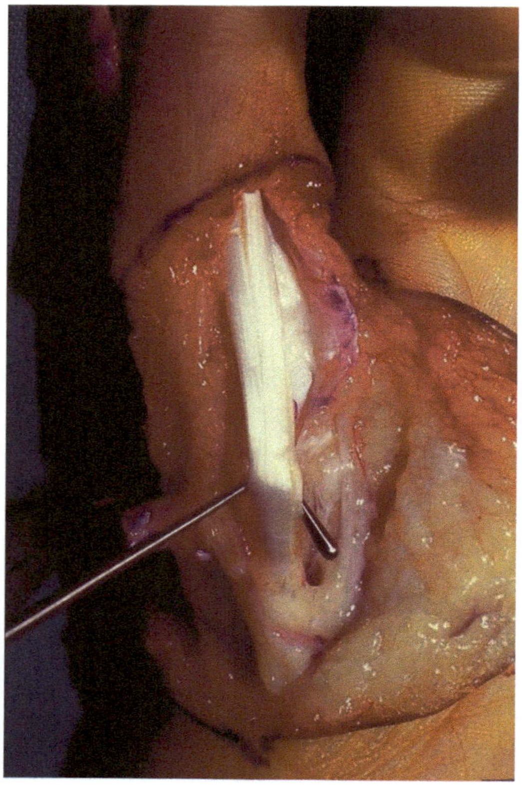

Fig. 8.28 Release of A1 and A2 pulleys. Published with kind permission of Michael A. Tonkin ©2014. All rights reserved

arch, following preliminary clamping and assessment of any compromise in vascularity to the hand, to gain length. In one instance, I have found absence of a palmar common digital artery but with a large dorsal metacarpal artery connecting to the palmar system at the head-neck junction (Fig. 8.27). Pollicisation was performed with the digit nourished by this vascular pedicle.

A1 and A2 pulleys are divided (Fig. 8.28). The A3, A4 and A5 pulleys become the thumb A1, oblique and A2 pulleys, respectively. Some routinely shorten the flexor digitorum profundus (FDP), but I have not found this necessary unless pollicisation is performed at greater than 5 years of age. A z-shortening can be performed proximal to the wrist to avoid increasing the possibility of adhesions within the dissected area of the palm.

The dissection of the intrinsic muscles, the first dorsal and first palmar interossei, begins on the palmar side, mobilising the musculotendinous units to the MCP joint level, but protecting the neural supply of each.

Dorsal Dissection

Thin dorsal flaps are elevated until the dorsal venous architecture is identified so that one or two veins, along with superficial dorsal nerves, can be mobilised separately from the flaps and the underlying digit (Fig. 8.29). This prevents kinking of vessels, compromising venous return, when the digit is recessed proximally.

The extensor mechanism is inspected to assess the presence or absence of EIP and the quality of extensor digitorum communis (EDC) (Fig. 8.30). Excursion is often poor when radial deficiency accompanies thumb hypoplasia. Subsequent dissection of the extrinsic extensors and the intrinsic contributions to the extensor mechanism are performed before division of the extensors and with the skeleton intact. This allows distal mobilisation of the extensor mechanism to the level of the PIP joint, separating the lateral band contributions to this level, but maintaining continuity with the first dorsal interosseous and the first palmar interosseous muscles on radial and ulnar sides, respectively (Fig. 8.31). Release of the intrinsic attachments to either side of the base of the proximal phalanx must respect the integrity of the capsule and ligaments of what will become the new CMC joint (Fig. 8.32a, b). Although some recommend ablation of the blood supply to the physis of the metacarpal, others prefer not to interfere with any contribution which may maintain

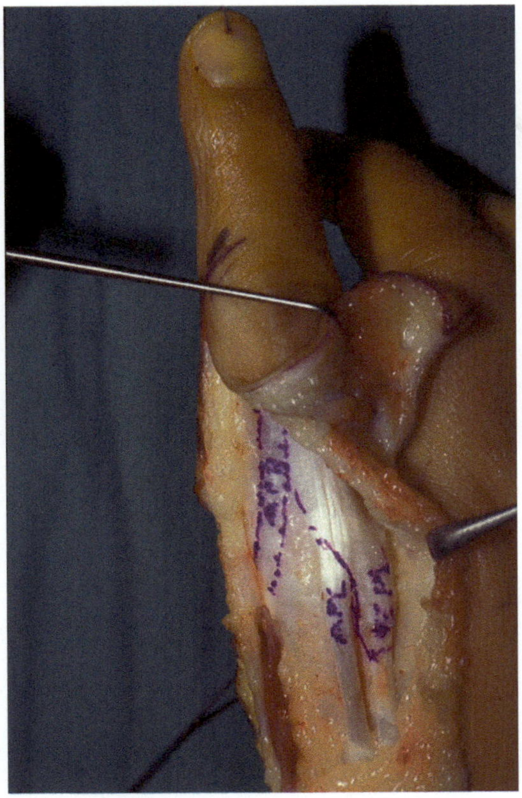

Fig. 8.30 Intrinsic and extrinsic tendons outlined prior to reconstruction. Published with kind permission of Michael A. Tonkin ©2014. All rights reserved

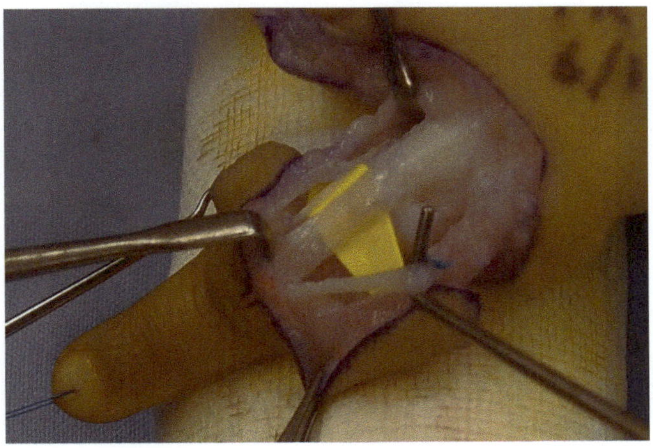

Fig. 8.31 Dissection of radial and ulnar lateral bands without division. Published with kind permission of Michael A. Tonkin ©2014. All rights reserved

the integrity of the physis of the proximal phalanx. Premature physeal closure and a short first metacarpal in the reconstructed thumb is a consequence of growth plate compromise of the index finger proximal phalanx.

At this point, the EIP and EDC may be divided at the level of the MCP joint. Any remaining attachments of the intrinsic musculature are then dissected in a sub-muscular extra-periosteal manner from the metacarpal diaphysis. Retractors are then placed around the head-neck junction of the metacarpal, protecting all other structures, particularly the palmar neurovascular bundles, whilst an osteotomy is performed at the head-neck junction of the metacarpal. In the young child, a Beaver blade or small osteotome is most satisfactory for the purpose. Some bone nibblers can be used to flower the metaphyseal perimeter of the head of the metacarpal by simply breaking bone fragments, which remain attached to the periosteum. This leaves bone with osteogenic potential to assist in bone union of the new trapezium to the metacarpal base (see below). The physis is removed using a fine curette and Beaver blade so that the new trapezium will not grow longitudinally. If ossification has occurred in the head of the metacarpal, it is easy to establish that the growth plate has been adequately removed. Care needs to be taken when ossification has not occurred, so that the articular surface of the metacarpal head is not breached.

CMC Joint Reconstruction

An integral part of the success of a pollicisation is the creation of a new CMC joint and there are a number of principles in reconstruction which are important:

- Optimal positioning of the new thumb ray in palmar abduction, radial abduction and appropriate rotation.
- Placement of the thumb ray in an anterior plane to that of the finger CMC joints.
- Hyperextension of the index finger MCP joint to prevent a hyperextension deformity of the new CMC joint.

It is difficult to satisfy all of the above parameters and obtain bony apposition between the index finger metacarpal head and base. Buck-Gramcko suggested retention of the metacarpal base to be necessary only in cases with relatively short phalanges. In these cases, the metacarpal head was fixed to the base using one or two K-wires. If the phalanges were of normal length, his initial description did not retain the metacarpal base and the metacarpal head was sutured to the joint capsule and carpal bones. Subsequently, most, including Buck-Gramcko, have preferred to retain the base. The plane of osteotomy incision of the metacarpal is varied, with both a transverse osteotomy at the metacarpal base and an oblique osteotomy in either coronal or sagittal planes being described. Some prefer K-wire fixation to promote head to base union as described by Buck-Gramcko [19–22]. Some eschew this [23]. Manske wrote of the importance of a fibrous union rather than a bony union between the retained base and head [24, 25], creating a pseudarthrosis at this articulation. He proposed that using sutures rather than K-wires for fixation permitted increased mobility of the new thumb.

A concern is one of possible instability of the new trapezium. However, the effect on functional outcomes according to the presence or absence of bone union between the metacarpal head (new trapezium) and the metacarpal base has not

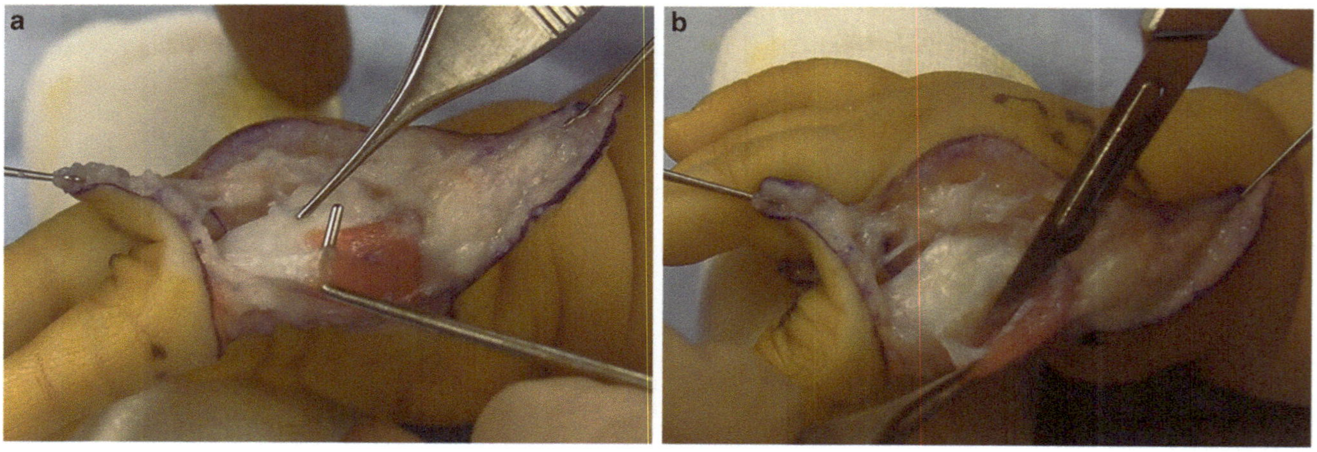

Fig. 8.32 (**a**, **b**) Dissection of first dorsal interosseous from capsule of MCP joint. Published with kind permission of Michael A. Tonkin ©2014.

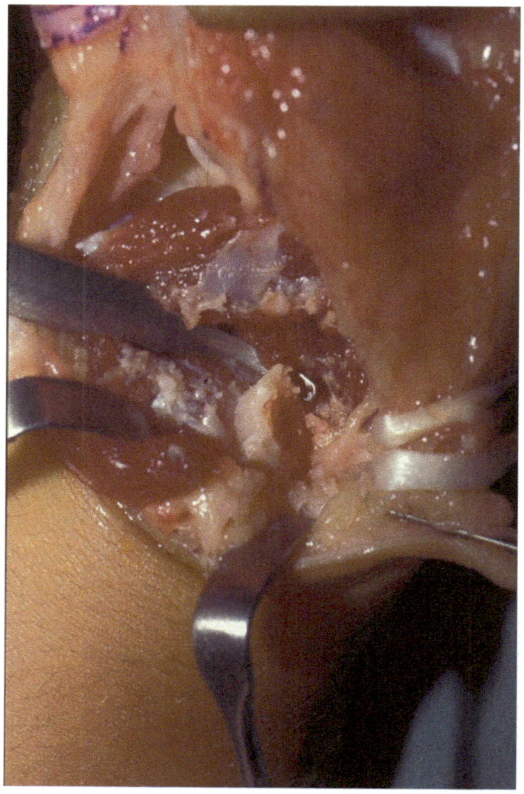

Fig. 8.33 Oblique osteotomy at base of index finger metacarpal. Published with kind permission of Michael A. Tonkin ©2014.

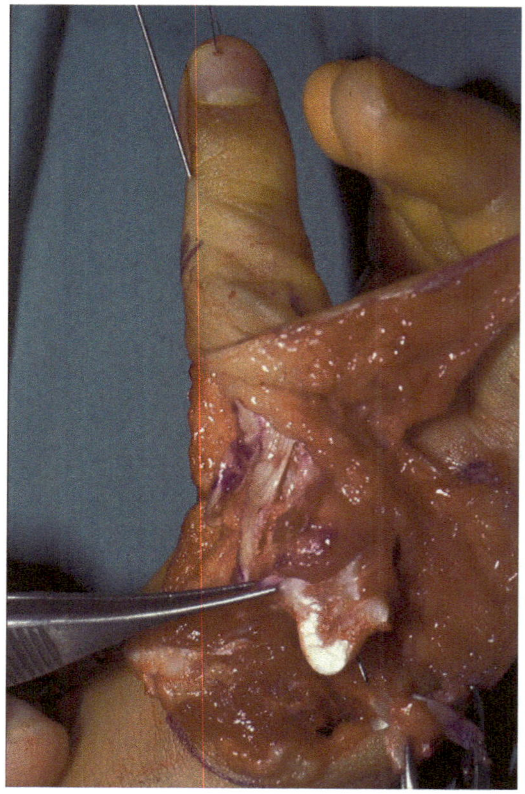

Fig. 8.34 K-wire placement through index finger with metacarpal head flexed. Published with kind permission of Michael A. Tonkin ©2014.

been determined. My preference is to aim for bone union whilst satisfying the above criteria of positioning.

An oblique osteotomy leaving the bone longer dorsoradially allows a satisfactory compromise in positioning the thumb optimally and maintaining some bone to bone contact (Fig. 8.33). A fine K-wire is placed antegrade through the flexed metacarpal head and phalanges of the index finger and then driven retrograde into the carpus with the thumb in the desired position, removing the wire at 5 weeks (Fig. 8.34). Before fixing the thumb to the carpus in this manner, two gauge 2-0 Ticron sutures are placed through the base of the metacarpal and into the metacarpal head, to be tightened following wire fixation of the thumb to the carpus. This method compromises the position of pronation, as 90° only is possible if one is to maintain an anterior lie of the new trapezium in relationship to the metacarpal base and some bone to bone apposition. Thirty degrees of radial abduction and 40° of palmar abduction is ideal. The less mobile digit may be fixed at lesser angles of radial and palmar abduction. Passive joint motion and the quality of the extrinsic and intrinsic motors play a role in this decision.

Tendon Reconstruction

The EIP, if present, is shortened and re-sutured to the central extensor mechanism to the PIP joint of the index finger. Most refer to this as a construction of EPL function. However, the insertion of the central slip into the middle phalangeal base of the index finger mimics EPB anatomy of the thumb, rather than EPL anatomy. The new tendon does simulate the adductor-retropulsion action of EPL. The tension of repair should be firm but less than full. Too tight a repair will result in retropulsion of the pollicised digit, particularly if a balance is not achieved following the reconstruction of APB. EDC helps stabilise the position of the new thumb metacarpal, moreso if its route and positioning are modified to better mimic the function of APL. It is attached to the periosteum at the dorso-radial aspect of the index proximal phalanx, avoiding the growth plate. If EIP is absent, EDC is used for EPB construction.

Although Buck-Gramcko advises dividing the lateral bands, shortening and resuturing them to create an APB and an adductor from the first dorsal interosseous and the first palmar interosseous, respectively, I tend to concertina these tendons without dividing them and suture them together under as firm a tension as is possible. It is necessary to mobilise both lateral bands to beyond the PIP joint of the index finger, particularly that from the first dorsal interosseous so that its ability to abduct and rotate is optimal. This also decreases a tendency of the lateral bands to hyperextend the new MCP joint of the thumb. A gauge 5-0 Ticron suture is used to secure the tendon reconstructions.

When thumb hypoplasia is accompanied by radial hypoplasia, there is often a camptodactyly of the index finger. My preference is to deal with any significant flexion deformity of the new thumb MCP joint at a second procedure, for fear of interfering with the viability of the pollicised digit.

The tourniquet is released to check the vascularity of the thumb. Flaps are then refashioned so that they may be sutured into position with a pleasing contour. The skin tension within the flaps will assist the musculotendinous reconstruction in maintaining the position of the thumb once the wire is removed (Fig. 8.35).

Reconstruction of Grades 3, 4 and 5 Thumb Hypoplasia

When pollicisation is unacceptable to parents and/or patient, reconstruction of Grades 3, 4 and 5 thumbs is possible [14–17]. A vascularised second toe metatarsophalangeal (MTP) joint may be transferred to the carpus or to the base of the shaft of the second metacarpal. The metatarsal head becomes the new trapezium and the proximal phalanx becomes the thumb metacarpal. Non-vascularised transfers are also utilised. An extrinsic extensor can be reconstructed using EIP from the index finger. A superficialis tendon can be transferred as a flexor and an opposition transfer is created in the manner described for Grade 2 hypoplasia.

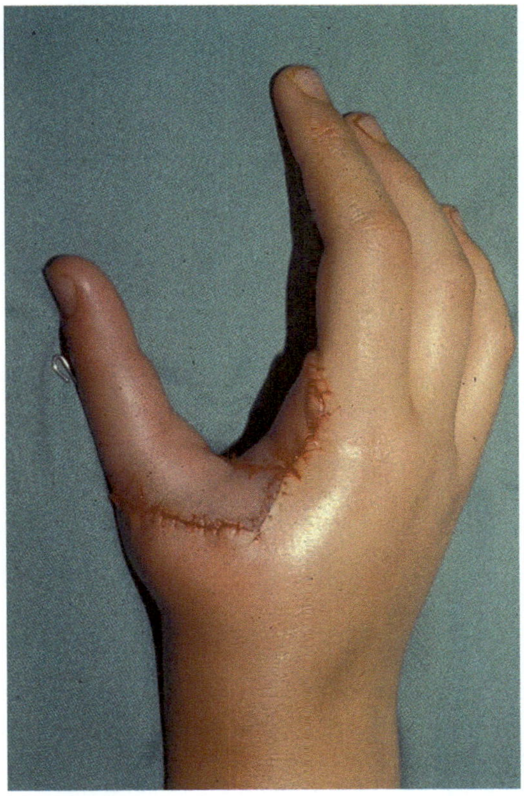

Fig. 8.35 Position of reconstructed thumb. Published with kind permission of Michael A. Tonkin ©2014. All rights reserved

An alternative is to transfer the distal two-thirds of the fourth metatarsal bone (non-vascularised), reversing this and using the metatarsal head as the new joint. The shaft is fixed distally to the remnant of the metacarpal or proximal phalanx of the Grade 3 or 4 thumb [26].

Flaps are necessary to recreate the first web in all such cases.

Multiple surgeries are often necessary to create a stable thumb with some mobility. The patient has five digits. The width of the hand is maintained, which assists grip. However, the problems are many: scarring is significant; the "new" thumb remains small and may require lengthening; joints are often unstable, requiring fusion subsequently; and mobility is poor.

Full toe transfers have been utilised by some for Grade 5 hypoplasia. However, the lack of normal proximal tissues and the lack of cortical representation, render the function of such transfers less than satisfactory. Skin transfer through pedicle or free flaps are necessary for first web construction.

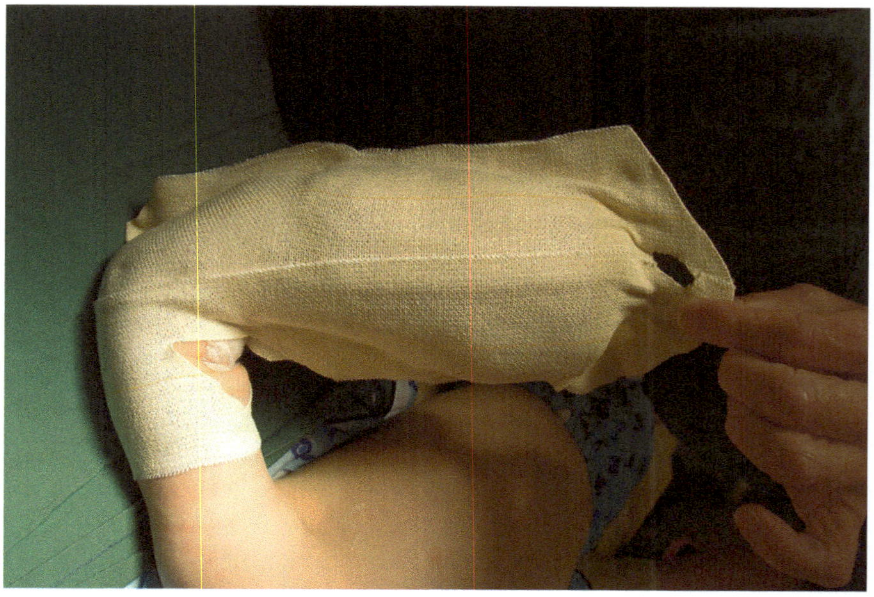

Fig. 8.36 Post-operative dressing. Published with kind permission of Michael A. Tonkin ©2014. All rights reserved

It is not my practice to apply these reconstructive procedures to young children. If pollicisation is refused, some of the above techniques may be indicated at a later age if the child is using the thumb. Carefully selected surgery may stabilise a joint or even provide a joint through an MTP transfer. An opposition tendon transfer may improve function. Such reconstructions should be limited to those who have not excluded the rudimentary thumb but use it for some activities. The results remain inferior to those obtained from a well-performed pollicisation. However, five digits are retained.

Post-operative Management

Following reconstructive surgery of Grade 2 thumbs and pollicisation procedures, I retain the forearm and hand in an inclusive plaster for 5 weeks. Occasionally the child escapes from the plaster, but the technique taught by Foucher is effective. Two U-slabs of plaster cover the hand and forearm to elbow. Three-inch Elastoplast tape is used as a stirrup around the elbow to prevent the plaster cast from slipping (Fig. 8.36).

Wires are removed in the clinic at 5 weeks. A soft dressing is used for 1 or 2 weeks with twice-daily bathing and massage of scars. A low-profile elastic splint, as practised by Manske and others, helps maintain opposition without interfering greatly with mobilisation (Fig. 8.37) [25]. A deviating force should not be applied beyond the MCP joint. Radial deviation may simulate opposition but is a false friend. Buddy strapping of the two radial fingers discourages side-to-side use of these for pinch and encourages use of the new thumb. The therapists may assist in retraining by introducing the child to games which utilise desired thumb activities. In the main, the child is his/her best therapist. FPL function usually returns from 3 months or thereabouts.

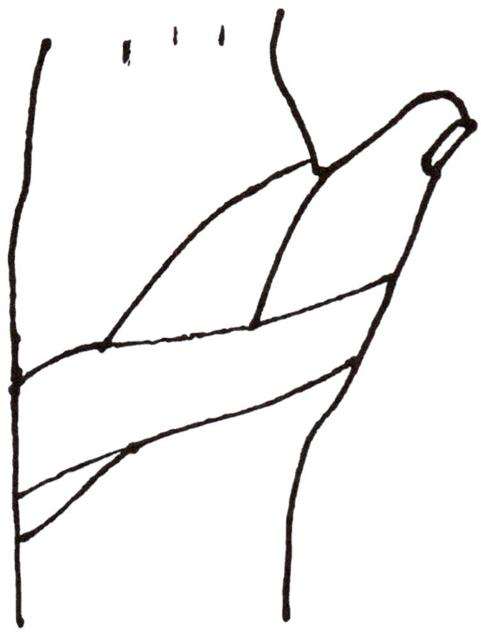

Fig. 8.37 Soft tissue splint. Published with kind permission of Michael A. Tonkin ©2014. All rights reserved

Results and Complications

Functional results following pollicisation are entirely dependent upon the preoperative status. Those with a significant radial longitudinal deficiency are severely disadvantaged. The wrist may be unstable, in spite of the best attempts to stabilise the carpus on the end of the ulna. Extrinsic musculotendinous units to the index finger, in particular, have poor excursion; joints tend to be stiff with camptodactyly of the index finger a common finding. The index finger is hypoplastic. As a consequence, the thumb function and appearance are compromised. Nevertheless, it is my experience and that of others that in nearly all instances the child will use the pollicised digit for certain activities. Side-to-side pinch utilising the more mobile ulnar digits may be preferred for smaller diameter objects. Strength and motion are significantly diminished in comparison to age-related normal values. These results contrast with those following pollicisation of a near-normal index finger in a limb with minimal, if any, discernible radial longitudinal deficiency.

Kozin [27] found a grip strength of 67 % of the opposite side and Clark [21] reported 43 % of the opposite side. My review of 42 pollicisations found results very similar to those of Manske [24]. Grip strength was reduced to 40 % of age-related normal values when the preoperative status of the limb and index finger was normal or near-normal, in comparison to Manske's 31 %. These values decreased alarmingly with significant radial longitudinal deficiency when the index finger was of poor quality, with values of 6 % and 15 % for my patients and those of Manske, respectively. Strength of pinch was similar in the two studies and with the same significant decrease in those with poor quality limbs and index fingers. In the latter instance, lateral pinch measured 9 % (Manske 14 %) of age-related normal values. This improved to 30 % (Manske 38 %) in those children not disadvantaged by the accompanying deficiencies. These trends are also apparent for measurements of total active motion of the digit, with an average of 26° of motion at the MCP joint when combining all patients undergoing pollicisation (Manske 42°) and 26° at the IP joint (Manske 25°). Radial abduction averaged 44°. Sixty percent of patients could oppose to the pulp of the little finger, 17 % to the ring finger and 23 % to the middle finger only, again with motion being significantly improved in those without concomitant deformities. The Jebsen timed test for functional tasks found an increased time as a percentage of published normal values, 200 % for those patients with concomitant deficiency and 130 % in those with good preoperative status. These figures were a little poorer than those of Manske.

The results in both studies were not significantly altered by the age of the patient at the time of the operation. In my group, 14 patients repeated the study 3 years apart. The strength measurements and time to completion of Jebsen tasks improved with age, but they remained the same relative to age-related normal values.

These results are consistent with those published by others [19–25, 27–34].

Percival introduced a scale to measure function incorporating strength, motion, ability to perform certain tasks, sensibility and appearance [28]. In his 30 pollicisations, 73 % were graded good or excellent, 17 % fair and 10 % poor. Vekris and others found similar results in 21 pollicisations, with 75 % excellent, 19 % good and 6 % poor [33].

Goldfarb, in conjunction with Manske and others, evaluated the objective features and aesthetic outcomes of 31 pollicised digits, comparing these with normal thumbs [35]. They found the average length of the pollicised digit relative to the long finger proximal phalanx to be 90 % compared to an age-matched normal average of 71 %. The girth of the pollicised digit relative to the long finger was 92 % compared to an age-matched normal average of 132 %. The nail width of the pollicised digit relative to the nail width of the long finger was 96 % compared with an age-matched normal thumb average of 104 %. The visual analogue scale for subjective aesthetic analysis of these pollicised digits averaged 7.3 for the caregiver, 6 for the therapist and 6.4 for the surgeon. They concluded that pollicised digits are longer, but have reduced girth and nail width compared with age-matched normal thumbs.

Intra-operative complications are associated with vascular compromise, arterial and/or venous; denervation of the dorsal and/or palmar interossei during mobilisation; and poor position of the digit—often in association with inadequate motors or inappropriate tension in musculotendinous reconstructions and skin suture. Failure to flex the MC head may create a radial abduction (hyperextension) deformity of the metacarpal. Partial flap necrosis is uncommon, but is reported. Secondary surgery is not uncommon with some reports of a high incidence of opposition transfers to better position and move the digit. Instability of both the new trapezium or the new CMC joint may follow a failure to adequately stabilise the MC head to the MC base or capsule, or from loss of structural integrity of the index finger MCP joint collateral ligaments during harvest (Figs. 8.38a, b and 8.39). Flexion contractures of the MCP joint may be secondary to excessive CMC joint radial abduction or to the preoperative status of the index finger.

In 96 pollicisations, I have stabilised a mobile trapezium in two cases, revised two webs which were too deep and v-shaped, performed one tendon transfer to increase radial abduction, one metacarpal osteotomy to better position the thumb, and three MCP joint fusions for flexion contractures.

Functional results of reconstruction of Grade 2 hypoplastic thumbs may be assessed utilising the same parameters as those used to assess the results of pollicisation. However, the disparate anomalies within this grade of thumb hypoplasia render comparisons difficult. As discussed under the subheading of Classification, different definitions of characteristics according to grade and, consequently, the alternative reconstructions which have been performed, do not allow comparison of like with like. Sub-classification along the lines that have been suggested in this chapter would assist in addressing this difficulty. Some have reported results according to Manske's classification but the comparison still

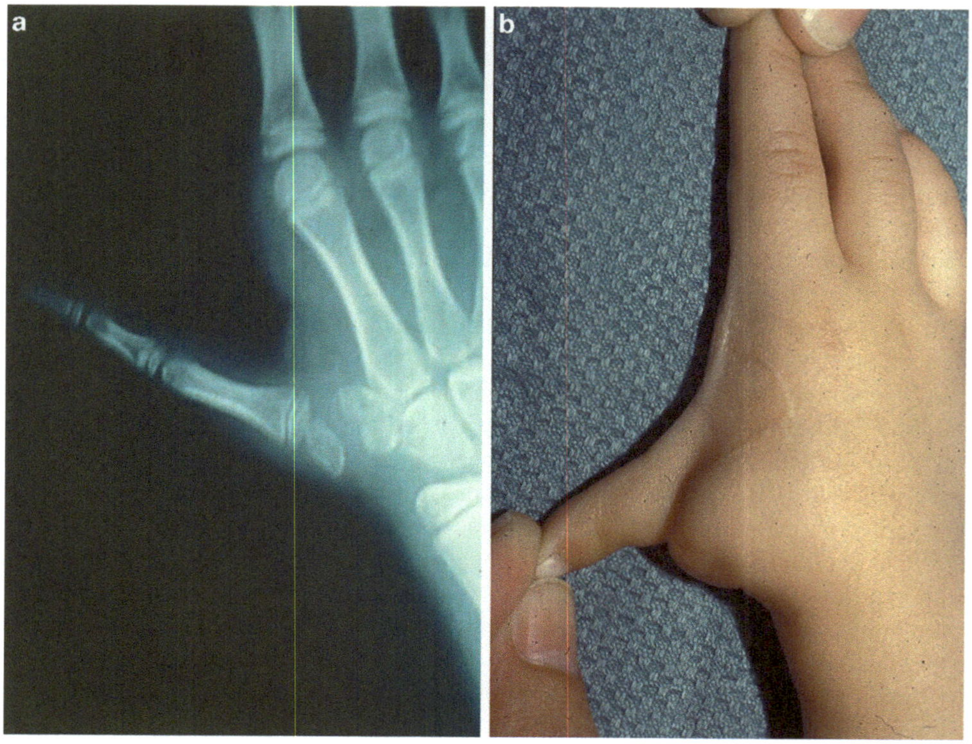

Fig. 8.38 (a, b) Instability of the new trapezium. Published with kind permission of Michael A. Tonkin ©2014. All rights reserved

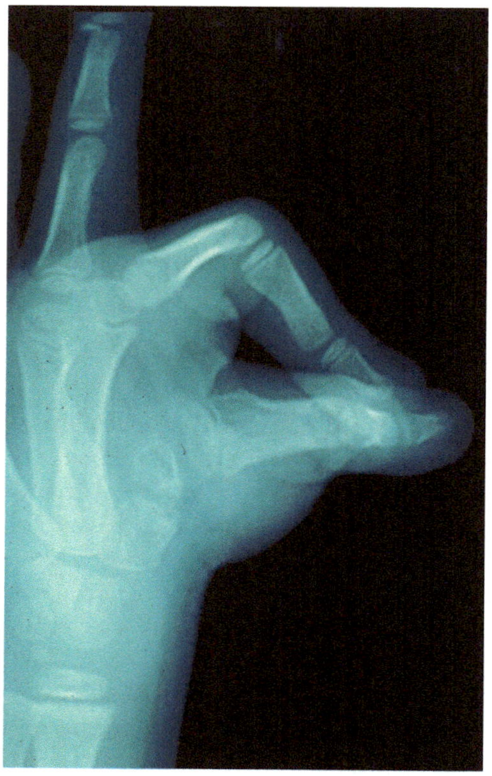

Fig. 8.39 Instability of the "new" CMC joint. Published with kind permission of Michael A. Tonkin ©2014. All rights reserved

remains less than perfect as some include correction of extrinsic anomalies within Grade 2 thumbs. Graham and Louis reported the results of reconstruction of 14 Manske Grade 3A thumbs with improved thumb IP joint motion of an average of 20°, but with two patients with mild MCP joint UCL instability [36]. Abdel-Ghani and Amro reported excellent stability of the thumb MCP joint in 71 % of patients. Opposition of the thumb to the little finger was excellent in eight of nine patients [37].

I have reviewed 22 patients with 21 opposition transfers, 15 first web plasties, 2 metacarpal osteotomies for realignment and 7 with attention to extrinsic anomalies. MCP joint stabilisation was performed by double breasting of the tissues present on the ulnar side of the joint in 15, reconstruction with an FDS slip in 3, and chondrodesis in 1. Assessment of active motion in comparison to the opposite unaffected thumb (when appropriate) found 34 % of IP joint motion, 60 % of MCP joint motion, 51 % of palmar abduction and 58 % of radial abduction. Kapandji's opposition assessment revealed a mean score of 6.6. Lateral pinch was 51 % of the opposite unaffected thumb, tripod pinch 59 % and power grip 82 % of the unaffected side. There was no significant difference in metacarpal lengths according to a thumb-index finger metacarpal length ratio between affected and opposite unaffected thumbs. The metacarpal width as a ratio of thumb to index was 78 % in affected thumbs and 84 % in opposite unaffected thumbs. Mild hypoplasia (Grade 1) of the opposite thumb does compromise the validity of these results. When compared with age-related normal values the difference may be greater. Mild instability at the IP joint was found in one. Moderate instability was present at the MCP joint level in seven. In three further patients, global instability was apparent at the time of assessment. These results suggest, as do the findings of others, that although MCP joint motion may be decreased, good mobility can be obtained at the CMC joint and retained at the IP joint if present preoperatively, and that stability and strength are improved. A Visual Analogue Scale assessment by parent and patient provided a mean score of 6.6 for function and a mean score for appearance of 7.

Complications of reconstructions of Grade 2 thumbs relate to continuing or recurrent MCP joint instability and poor function of the opposition transfer—denervation of ADM or adhesion formation impairing FDS gliding. Both problems tend to result in a recurrence of first metacarpal adduction and radial deviation at the MCP joint. Malalignment of extrinsic tendons plays a significant role in this deformation.

In my series, there was one patient with mild instability at the IP joint and ten with instability at the MCP joint. Four of the latter were considered to be severe enough to revise to arthrodesis, three with global MCP joint instability. One further patient underwent first web revision surgery.

It is generally considered that reconstruction of Grade 3 and 4 thumbs provides poorer results than those obtained by pollicisation. The first web space often remains deficient. Mobility is poor and strength is compromised in comparison to a pollicised index finger. However, some report encouraging results with microsurgical reconstruction, which is more likely to provide growth than those reconstructions relying on non-vascularised bone grafts. Foucher et al. reviewed five patients with vascularised transfer of the second MTP joint to reconstruct a CMC joint [15]. Mobility was poor; hypoplasia of the thumb was seen in all five patients, ranging from 59 to 85 % of the opposite thumb; flexion contractures were present in two patients; grip strength measurements averaged 33 % and pinch strength 13 % of measurements in the opposite hand. Shibata et al. found marginally better function and grip than in pollicised digits, but poorer pinch strength and total active motion [16]. Tu et al. also found poor motion with a mean total active range of 60°. In many cases, the patients do not use the thumb consistently for pinch [38]. However, five digits are retained.

In all, results of surgical treatment of the hypoplastic thumb are dependent on the state of the digit to be reconstructed or to be pollicised and the presence or absence of accompanying limb deformities. Valid assessments and comparisons of results await the development of a more sophisticated scoring scale along the lines of that proposed by Percival, one that incorporates the preoperative status of the digit to be reconstructed or pollicised. Attention to technical details brings beneficial outcomes for patients and is rewarding for surgeons.

References

1. Swanson AB. A classification for congenital malformations of the hand. N J Bull Acad Med. 1964;10:166–9.
2. Swanson AB. A classification for congenital limb malformations. J Hand Surg Am. 1976;1(1):8–22.
3. Oberg KC, Feenstra JM, Manske PR, Tonkin MA. Developmental biology and classification of congenital anomalies of the hand and upper extremity. J Hand Surg Am. 2010;35(12):2066–76.
4. Tonkin MA, Tolerton SK, Quick TJ, Harvey I, Lawson RD, Smith NC, et al. Classification of congenital anomalies of the hand and upper limb: development and assessment of a new system. J Hand Surg Am. 2013;38(9):1845–53. doi:10.1016/j.jhsa.2013.03.019.
5. Jones KL. Smith's recognizable patterns of human malformation. 6th ed. Philadelphia, PA: Elsevier Saunders; 2006. p. 908.
6. Müller W. Die angeborenen Fehlbildungen der menschlichen Hand. Leipzig: Thieme; 1937.
7. Blauth W. Der hypoplastische Daumen. Arch Orthop Unfallchir. 1967;62:225–46.
8. Blauth W, Schneider-Sickert F. Congenital deformities of the hand. An atlas of their surgical treatment. Translated by UH Weil. Berlin: Springer; 1981. p. 120–1.
9. Manske PR, McCarroll Jr HR. Reconstruction of the congenitally deficient thumb. Hand Clin. 1992;8(1):177–96.
10. Manske PR, McCarroll Jr HR, James M. Type III-A hypoplastic thumb. J Hand Surg Am. 1995;20(2):246–53.
11. Buck-Gramcko D. Congenital malformations of the hand and forearm. State of the Art Part III. European medical bibliography. Hand Surg. 1993;3(4):15–21.
12. Smith P. Lister's the hand. Diagnosis and indications. 4th ed. London: Churchill Livingstone; 2002. p. 505–512.
13. Smith P, Sivakumar B, Hall R, Fleming A. Blauth II thumb hypoplasia: a management algorithm for the unstable metacarpophalangeal joint. J Hand Surg Eur Vol. 2012;37(8):745–50.
14. Yamauchi Y, Fujimaki A, Yanagihara Y, Yoshizaki K. Reconstruction of floating thumb. Especially on the use of metatarsophalangeal joint grafting. Seikeigeka (Orthop Surg). 1979;30:1645–8.
15. Foucher G, Medina J, Navarro R. Microsurgical reconstruction of the hypoplastic thumb, type IIIB. J Reconstr Microsurg. 2001; 17(1):9–15.
16. Shibata M, Yoshizu T, Seki T, Goto M, Saito H, Tajima T. Reconstruction of a congenital hypoplastic thumb with use of a free vascularized metatarsophalangeal joint. J Bone Joint Surg Am. 1998;80(10):1469–76.
17. Matsuzaki H, Toishi S, Yoshizu T. A Blauth IIIB hypoplastic thumb reconstructed with a vascularized metatarso-phalangeal joint transfer: a case report with 28 years of follow up. Hand Surg. 2009;14(1):63–8.
18. Tupper JW. Pollex abductus due to congenital malposition of the flexor pollicis longus. J Bone Joint Surg Am. 1969;51(7):1285–90.
19. Buck-Gramcko D. Pollicization of the index finger. Method and results in aplasia and hypoplasia of the thumb. J Bone Joint Surg Am. 1971;53(8):1605–17.
20. Kozin SH. Pollicization: the concept, technical details, and outcome. Clin Orthop Surg. 2012;4(1):18–35.
21. Clark DI, Chell J, Davis TR. Pollicisation of the index finger. A 27-year follow-up study. J Bone Joint Surg Br. 1998;80(4):631–5.
22. Egloff DV, Verdan C. Pollicization of the index finger for reconstruction of the congenitally hypoplastic or absent thumb. J Hand Surg Am. 1983;8(6):839–48.
23. Taghinia AH, Upton J. Index finger pollicization. J Hand Surg Am. 2011;36(2):333–9.
24. Manske PR, Rotman MB, Dailey LA. Long-term functional results after pollicization for the congenitally deficient thumb. J Hand Surg Am. 1992;17(6):1064–72.
25. Manske PR. Index pollicization for thumb deficiency. Tech Hand Up Extrem Surg. 2010;14(1):22–32.
26. Chow CS, Ho PC, Tse WL, Hung LK. Reconstruction of hypoplastic thumb using hemi-longitudinal metatarsal transfer. J Hand Surg Eur Vol. 2012;37(8):738–44.
27. Kozin SH, Weiss AA, Webber JB, Betz RR, Clancy M, Steel HH. Index finger pollicization for congenital aplasia or hypoplasia of the thumb. J Hand Surg Am. 1992;17(5):880–4.

28. Percival NJ, Sykes PJ, Chandraprakasam T. A method of assessment of pollicisation. J Hand Surg Br. 1991;16(2):141–3.
29. Staines KG, Majzoub R, Thornby J, Netscher DT. Functional outcome for children with thumb aplasia undergoing pollicization. Plast Reconstr Surg. 2005;116(5):1314–23.
30. Netscher DT, Aliu O, Sandvall BK, Staines KG, Hamilton KL, Salazar-Reyes H, Thornby J. Functional outcomes of children with index pollicizations for thumb deficiency. J Hand Surg Am. 2013;38(2):250–7.
31. Ceulemans L, Degreef I, Debeer P, De Smet L. Outcome of index finger pollicisation for the congenital absent or severely hypoplastic thumb. Acta Orthop Belg. 2009;75(2):175–80.
32. Foucher G, Medina J, Lorea P, Pivato G, Szabó Z. Pollicization in congenital differences. Handchir Mikrochir Plast Chir. 2004;36(2–3):146–51.
33. Vekris MD, Beris AE, Lykissas MG, Soucacos PN. Index finger pollicization in the treatment of congenitally deficient thumb. Ann Plast Surg. 2011;66(2):137–42.
34. Sykes PJ, Chandraprakasam T, Percival NJ. Pollicisation of the index finger in congenital anomalies. A retrospective analysis. J Hand Surg Br. 1991;16(2):144–7.
35. Goldfarb CA, Deardorff V, Chia B, Meander A, Manske PR. Objective features and aesthetic outcome of pollicized digits compared with normal thumbs. J Hand Surg Am. 2007;32(7):1031–6.
36. Graham TJ, Louis DS. A comprehensive approach to surgical management of the type IIIA hypoplastic thumb. J Hand Surg Am. 1998;23(1):3–13.
37. Abdel-Ghani H, Amro S. Characteristics of patients with hypoplastic thumb: a prospective study of 51 patients with the results of surgical treatment. J Pediatr Orthop B. 2004;13(2):127–38.
38. Tu YK, Yeh WL, Sananpanich K, Ueng SW, Chou YC, Ma CH, Lee ZL. Microsurgical second toe-metatarsal bone transfer for reconstructing congenital radial deficiency with hypoplastic thumb. J Reconstr Microsurg. 2004;20(3):215–25.

Congenital Radioulnar Synostosis

9

Tarun Taneja and Manoj Ramachandran

Introduction

Congenital radioulnar synostosis is a rare congenital anomaly due to a failure of segmentation resulting in restricted forearm rotation. The forearm is fixed in a position ranging from neutral to severe pronation [1]. Sandifort originally described the condition in 1793 in *Museum Anatomicus* [2]. When the deformity is mild, a child can compensate using the ipsilateral shoulder and wrist and the deformity may hardly be noticed [1, 3]. A severe pronation deformity can cause disabilities and difficulty in performing ordinary everyday tasks such as eating, washing, turning a door knob, accepting objects in the palm and similar activities.

Embryology

Congenital radioulnar synostosis results from an anomaly of longitudinal segmentation. The upper limb bud arises at about 26 days of embryonic development. The segmentation begins distally. The proximal ends of the radius and ulna share a common perichondrium for some time and genetic or teratogenic factors can lead to disruption in the formation of the radioulnar joint. During the phase of intrauterine development, the forearm is anatomically placed in varying degrees of pronation [4]. A failure of segmentation leading to disruption in the formation of the proximal radioulnar joint will leave the forearm in its foetal position of pronation. This is consistent with the clinical picture seen in children, where the synostosis invariably results in a pronated position of the forearm [4].

T. Taneja, M.B.B.S., M.S., F.R.C.S. (Orth)
M. Ramachandran, B.Sc., M.B.B.S., F.R.C.S. (Orth) (✉)
Centre for Orthopaedics, The Royal London and Barts & The London Children's Hospitals, Whitechapel Road, Whitechapel, London E1 1BB, UK
e-mail: taruntaneja@hotmail.com; manoj.ramachandran@bartshealth.nhs.uk

Epidemiology and Natural History

The condition is usually sporadic, though positive family history has been identified in cases [1, 5, 6]. About 60–80 % of cases are bilateral. It is more common in males with a male: female ratio of 3:2. It can be associated with other conditions such as Apert syndrome, Klinefelter's syndrome, acropolysyndactyly (Carpenter syndrome), arthrogryposis, Holt-Oram syndrome, microcephaly and foetal alcohol syndrome [7–9].

There can be associated clinical anomalies affecting the cardiovascular, musculoskeletal, renal, gastrointestinal, and thoracic and central nervous systems. Musculoskeletal anomalies found include clubfeet, dislocated hips, syndactyly, polydactyly and Madelung deformity [10–12]. Cardiac anomalies include ventricular septal defect and tetralogy of Fallot. Associated thoracic abnormalities include hypoplasia of the pectoralis musculature and the first and second ribs. Central nervous system anomalies include hydrocephalus, microcephaly and encephalocoele.

Presentation and Clinical Features

These children will often present when a parent or teacher notes their functional deficit. Children with bilateral involvement and a more severe pronation deformity tend to present earlier. The age at presentation can vary between 2.5 and 5 years, and most children would have presented by school age.

The complaints often relate to difficulty in being able to accept objects in the palm and holding a small object such as a pencil. Dressing might be a problem, including being unable to manipulate buttons. Feeding might present problems due to the pronation deformity. Other problems include participating in certain sports that require skilled use of upper limbs and backhanded positioning when holding objects.

On physical examination, there is often a minimal flexion contracture at the elbow with a decreased carrying angle.

D.R. Laub Jr. (ed.), *Congenital Anomalies of the Upper Extremity: Etiology and Management*, DOI 10.1007/978-1-4899-7504-1_9, © Springer Science+Business Media New York 2015

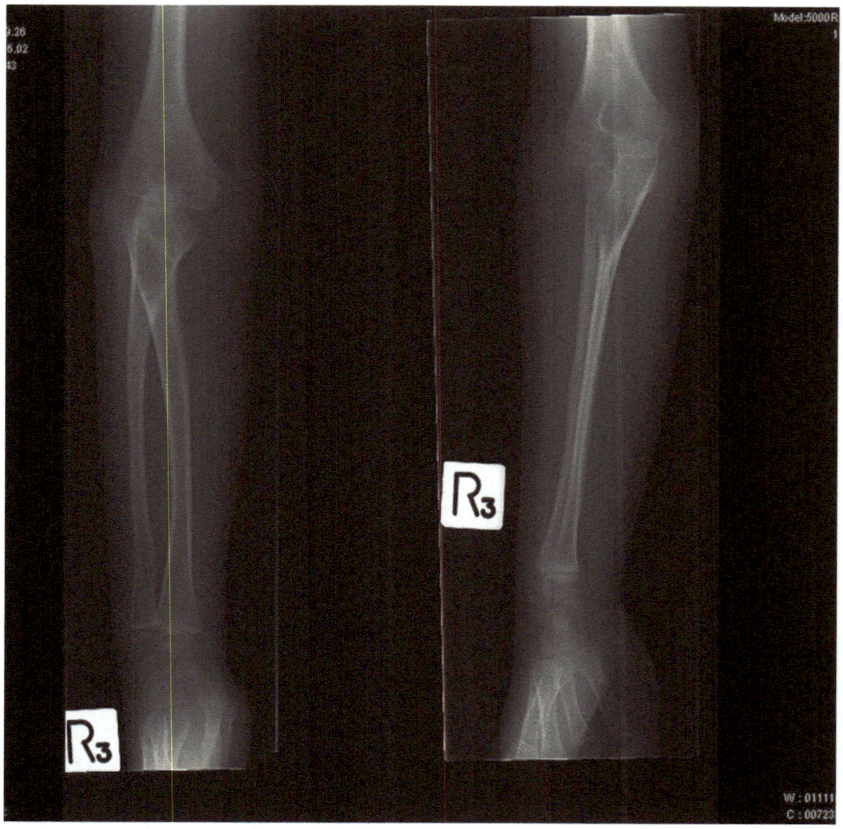

Fig. 9.1 Plain radiographs showing complete radioulnar synostosis

The forearm shortening is more obvious in unilateral cases. The forearm is fixed in varying degrees of pronation ranging from 15 to 150°. In Ramachandran et al.'s study, the mean pronation deformity was 68° [13]. In the study by Simmons et al. [12], 40 % of patients had a pronation deformity of more than 60°, 20 % had deformities ranging from 30 to 60°, while 40 % had a deformity of less than 30°. The loss of rotation is often compensated for to an extent by rotational hypermobility at the wrist [1, 3].

Imaging

There may be a wide anatomical spectrum of deformities ranging from simply a radial head deformity, synostosis of just the proximal forearm to complete synostosis for the forearm bones (Fig. 9.1) [11]. There may be shortening of the forearm, and there is usually an anterior bowing of the radius. Part of the synostosis may be cartilaginous and is best demonstrated on an MRI scan. Occasionally, a fibrous tether may become obvious on the MRI [10].

Classification

Wilkie, Tachdjan and Cleary and Omer have proposed various classification systems.

Wilkie [2] described two types of congenital synostosis, based on the proximal radioulnar junction. Type 1 is a complete synostosis, with the radius and ulna fused proximally for a variable distance. Type 2 is a partial synostosis involving the region just distal to the proximal radial epiphysis and is associated with radial head dislocation.

Classification according to *Tachdjian's criteria* [14]:

Type 1: The radial head may be fused to the ulna or may be completely absent (known as the "headless type")

Type 2: The radial head is malformed and often dislocated

Cleary and *Omer* [1] proposed a four-part radiological classification:

Type 1: Synostosis did not involve bone and was associated with an abnormal looking radial head

Type 2: A visible osseous synostosis was present, otherwise normal findings

Type 3: Osseous synostosis with hypoplastic and posteriorly dislocated radial head

Type 4: Short osseous synostosis with anteriorly dislocated radial head, which is usually mushroom shaped

Cleary and Omer Type 3 is the most common type reported in various studies. In Ramachandran et al.'s study [13], out of the six cases in their series, five forearms were classified as Cleary and Omer Type 3 (with a posteriorly dislocated radial head), while one was classified as Type 2. In the paper by Rubin et al. [15], all cases were classified as Cleary and Omer Type 3. Since there is not much functional difference between the different types and the appearances may change with time, the classifications may have not much role in deciding the management and are thus of limited clinical significance [13].

Management

Many children with forearm synostosis will not have much functional limitation and they can be treated conservatively. These children will often have mild pronation deformities less than 60°, unilateral disease and are able to compensate with radiocarpal and intercarpal wrist rotation. Often these children present to clinic when their parents or school teachers have noticed that they perform routine tasks differently from their peers.

Indication for Surgery

Most authors suggest a pronation deformity of 60° to be significant enough to merit operative intervention. In the paper by Ramachandran et al. [13] all of the patients had a mean pronation deformity of 68°. Simmons et al. [12] considered pronation of 60° as definite indication for osteotomy, while 15–60° was considered a relative indication depending on individual need of that patient. Ogino and Hikino [3] proposed that a pronation deformity of 60° created disability that needed surgery, whereas patients with a mean deformity of 20° did not complain of significant disability. These figures have varied in different studies, and some papers have considered ethnic and cultural factors that could influence decision-making.

Age at Surgery

Most children will present at school-going age. There is some variation in the literature about the age at surgery for these children. In the study by Ramachandran et al. [13], the mean age of the patients was 4.9 years (3.5–8.5 years). In the study by Rubin et al. [15], the average age at surgery was 11 years (range 9–13 years.). Hung [16] performed surgery at an average age of 6 years 3 months. There were a total of 34 patients and 52 forearms in this series. Eighteen patients (52.9 %) had bilateral deformities. They considered the ideal age for surgery to be between 3 and 6 years as it is easy to perform an osteotomy and there is significant potential for remodelling left at this age. Griffet et al. [17] considered an average age of 4–10 years as appropriate for surgery. In the study by Kanaya and Ibaraki [18] the average age was 8 years and 2 months (range 6 years 4 months to 11 years 10 months).

Operative Management

Various types of surgeries have been described. The two broad categories include either operative mobilization to restore forearm rotation or to perform an osteotomy to place the forearm in a position appropriate for day-to-day activities of the child.

Resection of the synostosis to restore forearm rotation has generally produced unsatisfactory results with subsequent loss of correction and vascular complications [18, 19]. Interposition of a free vascularized fascial flap between the separated bones has been attempted to reduce the risk of reformation of the synostosis [18, 20, 21]. Joint replacement using metallic swivel prostheses in the intramedullary canal of the radius between the supinator and pronator teres did not show good results [22].

The second group of procedures involves an osteotomy. Three types have been described to correct the deformity. The first is an osteotomy at the site of the synostosis followed by an acute correction. As the rotation here takes place over a narrow space, this may lead to excessive soft tissue tightness, loss of correction, vascular complications and neurological deficit including posterior interosseus nerve palsy [12, 23]. The second type is an osteotomy at a single site at the distal radius diaphysis [24]. The third type involves osteotomy of the diaphysis of both the radius and ulna [16, 25].

Other authors have used circular external fixators such as Illizarov to gradually correct the deformity [26]. Other techniques included osteotomies followed by derotation 10 days later [27, 28] and bone shortening by resection of bone from the synostosis [3].

Murase et al. [25] performed osteotomies in the distal third of the radius and proximal third of the ulna in patients with deformities more than 70° of pronation. They achieved good correction and only lost about 20° of correction in one case. Ramachandran et al. [13] performed a distal radius osteotomy achieving correction in all their cases (see operative technique below). Hung [16] performed a shortening by resection of 1.5 cm of bone. They measured the length of the synostosis mass in their cases and found the average length between 15 and 18 mm. Yammine et al. [29] recommended shortening the forearm by <2 cm.

Various authors have attempted separation of the synostosis with mixed results. Muira et al. [19] interposed the anconeus after synostosis separation but could not prevent recurrence with this technique. Most authors have used some sort of interposition graft after separation of the synostosis. Gill et al. [30] noted that free fat grafts worked well to prevent recurrence and performed better than Gelfoam in dogs. They also noted that pedicle fat graft was superior to free fat graft for this purpose. Langenskiold and Valle [31] demonstrated the viability of free fat grafts transplanted onto the dura up to 18 years later in four patients. Kanaya and Ibaraki [18] reported excellent results with the use of a free vascularized fascio-fat graft with no recurrence in their seven cases. They chose the lateral aspect of the ipsilateral arm as the donor site for their fascio-fat graft to ensure that surgery was confined to one limb only.

The Illizarov technique has been successfully used for this deformity. Rubin et al. [15] performed an osteotomy followed by gradual correction of deformity using the Illizarov frame achieving excellent results. They pointed out that correction should be achieved gradually as two of their patients did develop radial nerve neurapraxias when they attempted acute corrections. Bolano [26] also used the Illizarov frame but performed an immediate acute correction of 60° followed by a gradual derotation. Because of the complications encountered by Rubin et al. [15] using this technique of acute correction, they did not recommend it.

Operative Technique from Ramachandran et al. [13]

The patient is positioned supine and a well-padded tourniquet applied. An osteotomy is performed in the ulna at the mid shaft level through a subcutaneous posterior approach. A 1.8-mm Illizarov wire is passed retrogradely from the osteotomy to exit through the olecranon, and then antegradely across the osteotomy into the distal ulna. A second osteotomy is then performed in the radius at the distal diaphyseal-metaphyseal junction through a volar approach using an oscillating saw. The tourniquet is released and the forearm rotated to a position of 10° of supination. The deep fascia of the forearm is incised proximally and distally at the osteotomy sites to allow for expansion of the muscle bellies. The Illizarov wire is bent and left proud of the skin. An above-elbow plaster cast is applied with the elbow flexed to 90° and the forearm in the corrected position (Fig. 9.2). The patient is observed post-operatively for any evidence of compartment syndrome and neurovascular deficit.

The wire is removed 2 weeks post-operatively in theatre under general anaesthesia. The plaster is changed to a below-elbow cast. A plain radiograph is performed to confirm callus at the osteotomy sites and the patients are then allowed to mobilize the elbow. At a further 3 weeks, if the radiographs confirm bony union, the cast is removed. In case of delayed healing, the cast is retained till bony union is achieved.

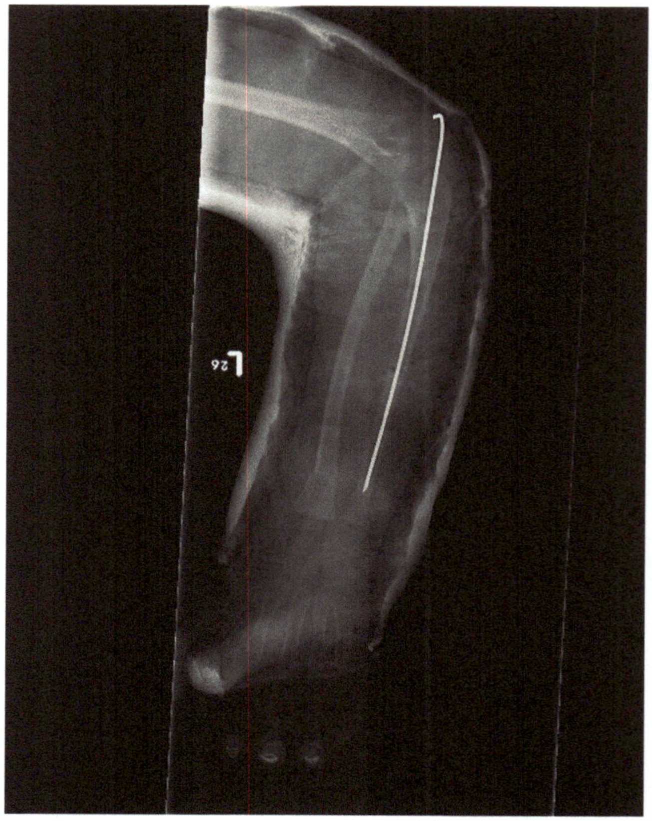

Fig. 9.2 Plain radiographs showing the ulna osteotomy fixed with a wire and a separate distal radial osteotomy

Green and Mital [4] proposed that one should be aiming for a position of 30–45° of pronation in the dominant forearm and 20–35° of supination in the non-dominant arm in bilateral cases. In unilateral cases they considered 10–20° of supination as the ideal position. Simmons et al. [12] proposed that the dominant arm be corrected to 10–20° of pronation and the non-dominant arm to neutral rotation in bilateral cases. In unilateral cases they considered 0–15° of pronation to be the ideal position. Rubin et al. [15] proposed that in right-handed patients with bilateral involvement, the left forearm be corrected to 15° (0–30°) of supination. They considered this to be a good functional position that would help in holding objects and for use in activities of daily living. Hung [16] considered 0–30° of pronation for the dominant arm and neutral for the non-dominant limb. Their best end position was 70–100° of pronation.

Post-operative Correction

In the study by Ramachandran et al. [13], all patients achieved a post-operative correction of 10° of supination.

Complications

The most significant complication of the corrective procedures is compartment syndrome. It is related to changes in the vascularity and volume of the forearm compartments with significant derotation osteotomies in the range of 60–90° [12]. Prophylactic fasciotomies or resection of a segment of the synostotic bone will reduce the incidence of this complication.

In children, high levels of anxiety and increasing analgesic requirements are the most diagnostic signs for compartment syndrome [32]. Green and Mital [4] reported one case of Volkmann's ischemic contracture out of a total of 13 cases. Simmons et al. [12] reported a single case of Volkmann's ischemia out of 33 cases.

Other complications include neurological deficit. To shorten the time spent in the Illizarov frame, Rubin et al. [15] performed a trial of partial immediate correction of deformity by 30° at the end of the operation in two patients. They noticed neurapraxia of the radial nerve in both patients in the recovery room. They returned the forearm to the original position in the recovery room under sedation. This led to complete neurological recovery. Ramachandran et al. [13] reported a delayed union in one case (bilateral staged forearm case). No loss of correction was noted in any case. There was one case of hematoma collection resulting in compartment syndrome requiring fasciotomy. No neurovascular complications were noted at follow up. One of their patients developed a pin tract infection.

Hung [16] reported slight loss of correction (15–20°) during cast immobilization in five forearms.

In Kanaya and Ibaraki's [18] series, the patients in whom a radial osteotomy was not performed developed a radial head dislocation. The arc of motion in this subgroup was less (40°) in comparison to the group in which a radial osteotomy was performed (83°).

With regard to separation of synostosis and interposition of fat or muscle, several authors have reported recurrence of the ankylosis. Muira et al. [19] reported recurrence in all of their series of eight patients after they had used the anconeus muscle as an interposition graft. Kanaya and Ibaraki [18] did not report any recurrence with their technique of using a free vascularized fascio-fat graft.

References

1. Cleary JE, Omer GE. Congenital proximal radioulnar synostosis: natural history and functional assessment. J Bone Joint Surg Am. 1985;67(4):539–45.
2. Wilkie DPD. Congenital radioulnar synostosis. Br J Surg. 1914;1:366–75.
3. Ogino T, Hikino K. Congenital radioulnar synostosis compensatory rotation around the wrist and rotation osteotomy. J Hand Surg Br. 1987;12:173–8.
4. Green WT, Mital MA. Congenital radioulnar synostosis: surgical treatment. J Bone Joint Surg Am. 1979;61(5):738–43.
5. Bergsma D. Birth defects compendium. 2nd ed. New York: Alan R Liss (The National Foundation, March of Dimes); 1979.
6. Henson HO, Anderson ON. Congenital radioulnar synostosis. Acta Orthop Scand. 1970;41:255.
7. Dawson HGW. A congenital deformity of the forearm and its operative treatment. Br Med J. 1912;2:833–5.
8. Jaffer Z, Nelson M, Beighton P. Bone fusion in the foetal alcohol syndrome. J Bone Joint Surg Br. 1981;63B(4):569–71.
9. Giuffre L, Corsello G, Giuffre M, Piccione M, Albanese A. New syndrome: autosomal dominant microcephaly and radioulnar synostosis. Am J Med Genet. 1994;51(3):266–9.
10. Waters PM, Simmons BP. Congenital abnormalities: elbow region. In: Peimer CA, editor. Surgery of the hand and upper extremity. New York: McGraw-Hill; 1996. p. 2049.
11. Mital MA. Congenital radioulnar synostosis and congenital dislocation of the radial head. Orthop Clin North Am. 1976;7:375.
12. Simmons BP, Southmayd WW, Riseborough EJ. Congenital radioulnar synostosis. J Hand Surg Am. 1983;8:829–38.
13. Ramachandran M, Lau K, Jones DHA. Rotational osteotomies for congenital radioulnar synostosis. J Bone Joint Surg. 2005;87-B:1406–10.
14. Herring JA, Tachdjian MO, editors. Tachdjian's paediatric orthopaedics. Philadelphia: WB Saunders; 1972.
15. Rubin G, Rozen N, Bor N. Gradual correction of congenital radioulnar synostosis by an osteotomy and Illizarov external fixation. J Hand Surg Am. 2013;38(3):447–52.
16. Hung NN. Derotation osteotomy of the proximal radius and the distal ulna for congenital radioulnar synostosis. J Child Orthop. 2008;2(6):481–9.
17. Griffet J, Berard J, Michel CR, Caton J. Les synostoses congenital radio-cubitales supeiurse. Int Orthop. 1986;10(4):265–9. Apropos de 43.
18. Kanaya F, Ibaraki K. Mobilization of a congenital proximal radioulnar synostosis with use of a free vascularized fascio-fat graft. J Bone Joint Surg Am. 1998;80(8):1186–92.
19. Muira T, Nakamura R, Suzuki M, Kanie J. Congenital radioulnar synostosis. J Hand Surg Am. 1984;9-B:153–5.
20. Funakoshi T, Kato H, Minami A, Suenaga N, Iwasaki N. The use of pedicled posterior interroseus fat graft for mobilisation of congenital radio ulnar synostosis : a case report. J Shoulder Elbow Surg. 2004;13:230–4.
21. Kawaguchi S, Kitamura M, Usui M. Proximal radioulnar synostosis treated with a free vascularized fascio fat graft—report of 2 cases. J Hand Surg. 2000;5(2):161–4.
22. Kelikian H. Congenital deformities of the hand and forearm. Philadelphia: WB Saunders; 1974.
23. Hankin FM, Smith PA, Kling TF, Louis DS. Ulnar nerve palsy following rotational osteotomy of congenital radioulnar synostosis. J Pediatr Orthop. 1987;7:103–6.
24. Fujimoto M, Kato H, Minami A. Rotational osteotomy at the diaphysis of the radius in the treatment of congenital radioulnar synostosis. J Pediatr Orthop. 2005;25(5):676–9.
25. Murase T, Tada K, Yoshida T, Morimoto H. Derotation osteotomy at the shafts of the radius and ulna for congenital radioulnar synostosis. J Hand Surg Am. 2003;28:133–7.
26. Bolano LE. Congenital radioulnar synostosis: treatment with the Illizarov method. J Hand Surg Am. 1994;19:977–8.
27. Manske PR, McCarroll Jr HR, Hale R. Biceps tendon rerouting and percutaneous osteoclasis in the treatment of supination deformity in obstetrical palsy. J Hand Surg Am. 1980;5:153–9.
28. Lin HH, Strecker WB, Manske PR, Schnoecker PL, Seyer DM. A surgical technique of radioulnar osteoclasis to correct severe forearm rotation deformities. J Pediatr Orthop. 1995;15:53–8.
29. Yammine K, Salon A, Poiliquen JC. Congenital radioulnar synostosis. Study of a series of 37 children and adolescents. Ann Hand Upper Limb Surg. 1998;17(4):300–8.
30. Gill GG, Sakovich L, Thompson E. Pedicle fat grafts for the prevention of scar formation after laminectomy. An experimental study in dogs. Spine. 1979;4:176–86.
31. Langenskiold A, Valle M. Epidurally placed free fat grafts visualized by CT scanning. 15–18 years after discectomy. Spine. 1985;10:97–8.
32. Kadiyala K, Waters P. Upper extremity compartment syndromes. Hand Clin. 1998;14:467.

Ulnar Longitudinal Deficiency

10

Hilton Phillip Gottschalk and Michael S. Bednar

Introduction

Ulnar longitudinal deficiency (ULD) is a rare condition that usually affects the entire upper limb, including the elbow, forearm, and hand. It has been reported to occur in 1:25,000 live births and ULD is most commonly unilateral [1, 2]. It is a sporadic, non-inherited condition, but can be associated with other musculoskeletal anomalies, such as proximal femoral focal deficiency, fibular and tibial deficiency, scoliosis, and finger differences [1, 2].

Embryology

To better understand the clinical appearance and variation in the spectrum of ULD, one must first review the development of the upper limb. Starting around days 26–52 after fertilization, the limb bud develops around three axes: proximal-distal, dorsal-ventral, and radial-ulnar [1, 3–5]. Each axis has its own signaling center:

1. Apical ectodermal ridge (AER) coordinates the proximal-distal outgrowth
2. Zone of polarizing activity (ZPA) controls radial-ulnar asymmetry
3. Progress zone (PZ) for dorsal-ventral differentiation [3, 6]

Integral to these specialized zones are several signaling molecules. They include fibroblast growth factors, sonic hedgehog, and bone morphogenic proteins. These molecules affect each other through feedback loops [3]. In regard to ULD, sonic hedgehog is responsible for development of ulnar-sided forearm structures as well as the four ulnar-sided digits [1]. The thumb abnormalities occasionally seen in ulnar dysplasia can be explained by the sonic hedgehog-fibroblast growth factor feedback loop [6].

H.P. Gottschalk, M.D. (✉)
Department of Pediatric Orthopaedics, Dell Children's Medical Center, 1301 Barbara Jordan Blvd. Ste 300, Austin, TX 78723, USA
e-mail: hpgottschalk@gmail.com

M.S. Bednar, M.D.
Department of Orthopedic Surgery and Rehabilitation, Loyola University Medical Center, 2160 South First Ave., Maywood, IL 60153, USA
e-mail: mbednar@lumc.edu

Classification and Clinical Picture

The spectrum of clinical presentation for ULD is quite variable. The entire upper limb is involved in the majority of cases with classification schemes focusing on the elbow/forearm abnormalities [7–11], hand [12], and more specifically the thumb and first web space [13].

The commonly used Bayne classification [7] describes the progression of deficiency noted at the elbow and forearm. Its original description had four types and was later modified by Havenhill et al. [8]. This modified classification of ULD is as follows:

1. Normal length ulna with ulnar-sided hand anomalies
2. Hypoplasia of the ulna (presence of distal and proximal ulnar epiphysis)
3. Partial aplasia of the ulna (absence of the distal or middle one third of the ulna)
4. Total aplasia of the ulna (complete absence of the ulna)
5. Complete absence of the ulna with radiohumeral synostosis (fusion of the radius to the humerus)

Goldfarb et al. [14] proposed a type V ulnar longitudinal dysplasia that would incorporate cases of severe radiohumeral synostosis with humeral bifurcation or a large medial epicondyle. Given the rarity of the disease along with the variable presentation, Buck-Gramcko [15] stated that the pathological findings in ulnar deficiency are so different in the involvement and distribution in the arm, it is impossible to divide them into a classification system. Although Bayne and others describe the elbow and forearm abnormalities, treatment has really been focused more on the hand and digits. As such, Cole and Manske [13] presented a classification

D.R. Laub Jr. (ed.), *Congenital Anomalies of the Upper Extremity: Etiology and Management*, DOI 10.1007/978-1-4899-7504-1_10, © Springer Science+Business Media New York 2015

system based upon the characteristics of the thumb and first web:

1. Normal first web space and thumb
2. Mild first web and thumb deficiency
3. Moderate to severe first web and thumb deficiency; potential loss of opposition; malrotation of the thumb into the plane of the other digits; thumb–index syndactyly; absent extrinsic tendon function
4. Absent thumb

The authors of this classification scheme opine that it is the complexity of the radial-sided problems that require the majority of surgical procedures, and as such this classification will focus the surgeon's attention on those deficiencies that are most important for the restoration of function. They concluded that ULD be classified by an elbow/forearm system and supplemented by the hand classification [13].

Associated Anomalies

Unlike radial longitudinal deficiency, patients with ULD rarely have heart or hematopoietic anomalies. However, these patients may have associated musculoskeletal anomalies such as proximal femoral focal deficiency, additional hip pathology (coxa vara), tibial or fibular ray deficiency, phocomelia, scoliosis, clubfeet, and spina bifida [1, 16].

Upper Arm and Shoulder

With regard to the proximal humerus and shoulder region, hypoplasia can occur. Despite the abnormality, most patients do not have restricted motion [15].

Elbow

There is quite a bit of variation with regard to clinical presentation. The elbow may be stable, unstable, or fused. The articular surfaces can range from normal to hypoplastic to severely deformed. Congenital dislocation of the radial head can be present and subsequent deformity to the distal end of the humerus present [15]. El Hassan et al. [17] reported that 12 % of ULD had a radiohumeral synostosis. In their series, the elbows were fixed in 20–90° of flexion, with no elbows in full extension [17]. Others have described the elbow fixed in full extension [11] or severe flexion and rotation of the elbow so that the hand is positioned behind the child and away from the opposite, uninvolved hand, the so-called hand on flank deformity [18].

Forearm

Buck-Gramcko [15] reported that the different types of ulna defect show no correlation to the severity of the involvement of other parts of the arm and can be combined with all variations of hand and elbow anomalies. The majority of patients with ULD will have a shorter forearm than normal (Fig. 10.1). Havenhill et al. [8] described a variation of patients with a normal forearm but deficiencies isolated to the ulnar side of the hand—Type 0. In ULD, ulnar hypoplasia is most common (60 %) with partial absence of the ulna reported 22.5 % and complete absence in 18 % of patients [15]. Some patients with ULD will have a fibrocartilaginous mass, possibly representing the anlage of the absent portion of the ulna [16]. This is commonly seen in Bayne Types II and IV and may be the cause for radial bowing and wrist deviation, although this point has been debated [16–22].

Wrist

Angulation of the wrist can occur, but is typically not as severe as seen in radial longitudinal deficiency. (Fig. 10.1c). El Hassan et al. [17] reported that the wrist was positioned in neutral in 71 % of patients, with the remaining wrists resting in 5–40° of ulnar deviation. Those patients with the wrist in neutral position had essentially normal wrist range of motion. However, when the wrist was in ulnar deviation, limitations were documented with regard to radial deviation, wrist flexion, and extension [17]. Controversy over the role of the ulnar anlage and the amount of wrist deviation exists [15–17]. Carpal bones can be absent in correlation with missing digital rays, and synostoses can occur in 30–40 % of cases [15].

Hand

Approximately 90 % of hands with ULD have missing digits and 30 % have syndactyly [1]. Multiple digital anomalies can be seen with the hand ranging from a full complement of digits to just one digit. Ectrodactyly has been well documented in patients with ULD [1, 13, 15, 17]. Many of the existing digits are usually not normal, with variations of hypoplasia, missing phalanges or metacarpals, and variations of syndactyly and synostoses between phalanges and metacarpals [15].

Seventy percent of patients with ULD have abnormalities related to the thumb [1]. El Hassan et al. [17] reported that 11 of 17 limbs with ULD had digital anomalies, with four of those limbs having absent thumbs. Swanson et al. [11] and Broudy and Smith [21] reported that 68 and 100 % of their

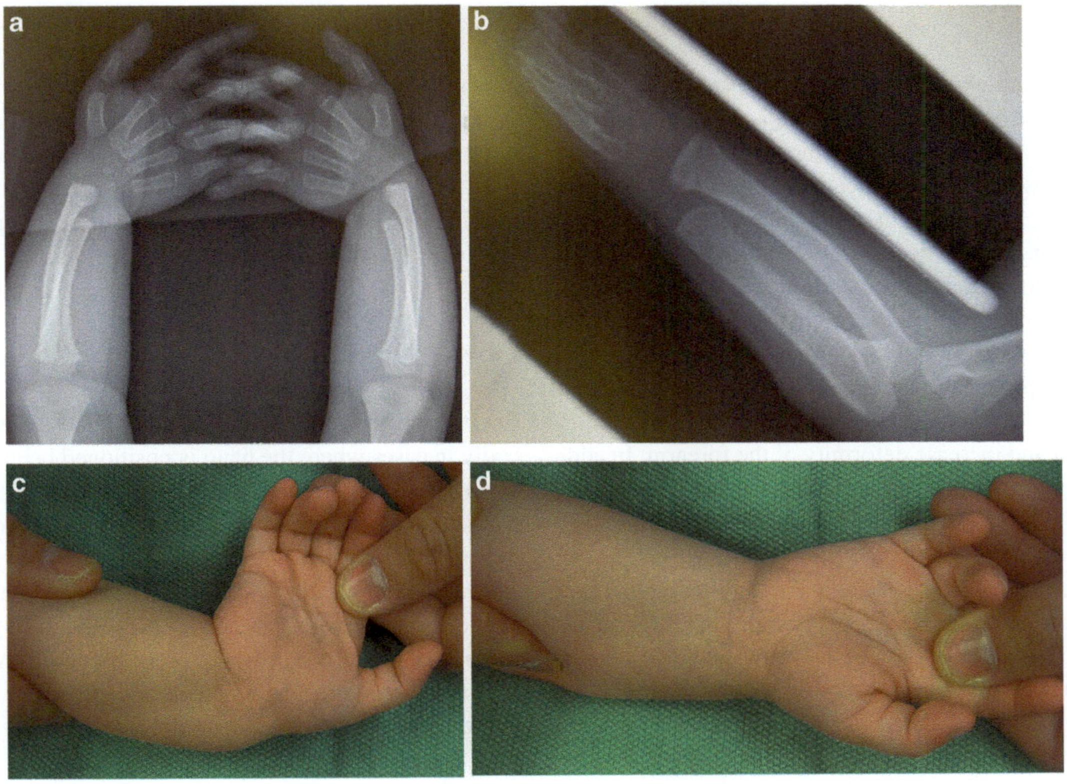

Fig. 10.1 (**a**) Anteroposterior and (**b**) lateral radiographs of a 2-year-old boy with bilateral ulnar longitudinal deficiency type II/A. (**c**) Clinical photograph showing excessive wrist ulnar deviation. (**d**) The wrist position rests in neutral

patients with ULD had radial-sided hand abnormalities, respectively. Cole and Manske [13] reported that 73 % of the 55 hands evaluated had an abnormal thumb or first web space. Their classification system describes the spectrum of thumb and first web space involvement from normal all the way to aplastic [13]. Evaluating the thumb and first web space deficiencies is important because surgical intervention to alter the radial-sided abnormalities in the hand may provide more substantial functional gains than operations elsewhere along the arm [1, 13, 15–17].

Treatment

Treatment of patients with ULD depends on the function of the limb. Non-operative intervention typically consists of early stretching and splinting starting at a young age. Depending on the function of the hand, surgical intervention may be warranted. Thus, the majority of surgical interventions in patients with ULD are performed on the hand, including syndactyly releases, deepening of the first web space, and first metacarpal rotational osteotomy [1, 13, 15, 16]. In special circumstances, other procedures including excision of the ulnar anlage, humeral rotational osteotomy, and creation of a one-bone forearm may be indicated.

Hand

Hand function can be improved with syndactyly releases, reconstruction of the thumb (opponensplasty, pollicization), and deepening of the first web space [1, 16, 23]. Ezaki and Carter [16] recommend delaying hand surgery until the second year of life. The reconstruction procedures of the hand are very important in improving the function of these children, and they recommend waiting for the hands to get larger to allow for a more precise surgery and thus better result [16].

First metacarpal rotational osteotomy is indicated in hands where the digits all lie in the same plane. The goal of rotation is to allow for prehension with the pulp of the digits. Rotation of other metacarpals and even phalanges to achieve this goal should be performed. Ezaki and Carter [16] report that there is a tendency for a slow loss of rotation after surgical intervention, and they recommend concomitant realignment of muscle power with tendon transfers to help prevent derotation.

Wrist

Controversy over excision of the ulnar anlage has been debated within the literature [11, 15–17, 21, 22]. However, there is some agreement as to which patient may benefit from early anlage excision. Indications for ulnar anlage excision [1, 15–17, 22] include the following:

1. Greater than 30° of fixed ulnar deviation
2. Clinically documented progression of ulnar deviation

It is recommended that excision of the ulnar anlage be performed at age 6 months. Proponents of early excision state it may improve both the function and appearance of the arm [1, 7, 22]. The anlage acts as a tether and will restrict radial growth and increase deformity of the forearm. In addition, the forearm will double in length by age 3 years, and resection of the anlage will provide the best possibility for unrestricted growth of the limb [16, 22].

To excise the ulnar anlage, either a longitudinal or lazy "S" incision is used over the ulnar border of the forearm and wrist. Usually the flexor carpi ulnaris is absent and the neurovascular bundle (if present) is directly under the skin and needs to be protected. Distally, it is crucial to dissect the anlage off of the carpus and radius completely. Following distal resection, the wrist should be passively corrected to a neutral position. Resection of the entire fibrous anlage proximally is not required, and usually resection of the distal third is adequate [16]. If excessive bowing of the radius is present, then an osteotomy can be performed at the same time. Postoperative course includes immobilization of the wrist in a neutral position for 6 weeks followed by stretching and splinting for at least 6 months, although some authors have recommended nighttime splinting with a short arm orthosis until skeletal maturity [23].

Forearm

The forearm in patients with ULD can be challenging to treat. Multiple procedures have been described: creation of a one-bone forearm [1, 15, 23, 24], radial osteotomies [18–20], and forearm lengthening [25, 26].

Several authors [1, 16, 27, 28] have advocated that the only indication for creating a one-bone forearm in patients with ULD is in the presence of forearm instability that is disabling. Thus, this procedure should rarely be done, knowing that any possible improvement in cosmetic appearance will be offset by the loss of function.

Radial osteotomies have been described [18–20] and may be performed at the same time of excision of the ulnar anlage if excessive bowing exists [16]. Although the forearm may be malrotated, most children do not require a forearm rotational osteotomy to improve their function [1].

Chen et al. [26] describe a case using an external fixator to gradually lengthen the ulna in a Bayne Type II. This patient also had a radial head dislocation. They reported an 81-mm lengthening over 7 months, with gradual reduction of the radial head. Elbow range of motion increased by 40° from 10° to 110° and preservation of preoperative forearm rotation was documented. This seems to be an option in this very specific subset of patients.

Elbow/Humerus

Rotational osteotomy about the elbow may be useful, especially in cases where the hand is positioned behind the child, as in the hand-on-flank deformity [1, 16–18, 23]. These patients typically have a radiohumeral synostosis with a hyperpronated forearm, bowing of the radius, and flexion and rotation of the elbow [17, 18]. The procedure can be performed at the level of the distal humerus through a lateral incision. Careful dissection is used to expose the humerus. Kirshner wires are placed distal and proximal to the proposed osteotomy site in a parallel fashion. The distal fragment is rotated so that hand is now positioned in front of the trunk. Care must be taken when performing the rotation, as serious damage to the vessels can occur. If needed, it is better to shorten the humerus as well. The osteotomy should be fixed with either transverse wires or plate and screws depending on the size of the patient. The arm can be protected in a long arm cast for 4–6 weeks.

References

1. Bauer AS, Bednar MS, James MA. Disruption of the radial/ulnar axis-congenital longitudinal deficiencies. J Hand Surg Am. 2013;38(11):2293–302.
2. Koskimies E, Lindfors N, Gissler M, Peltonen J, Nietosvaara Y. Congenital upper limb deficiencies and associated malformations in Finland: a population-based study. J Hand Surg Am. 2011; 36A:1058–65.
3. Oberg KC, Feenstra JM, Manske PR, Tonkin MA. Developmental biology and classification of congenital anomalies of the hand and upper extremity. J Hand Surg Am. 2010;35A:2066–76.
4. Tickle C, Summerbell D, Wolpert L. Positional signaling and specification of digits in chick limb morphogenesis. Nature. 1975; 254:199–202.
5. Tickle C. Experimental embryology as applied to the upper limb. J Hand Surg Am. 1987;12B:294–300.
6. Yang Y, Kozin SH. Cell signaling regulation of vertebrate limb growth and patterning. J Bone Joint Surg. 2009;91A Suppl 4:76–80.
7. Bayne LG. Ulnar club hand (ulnar deficiencies). In: Green DP, Hotchkiss RN, Pederson WC, editors. Operative Hand Surgery. 3rd ed. New York: Churchill Livingstone; 1993. p. 288–303.
8. Havenhill TG, Manske PR, Patel A, Goldfarb CA. Type 0 ulnar longitudinal deficiency. J Hand Surg Am. 2005;30A:1288–93.

9. Kummel W. Die missbildungen der extremitaeten durch defect, verwachsung und ueberzahl. Bibliotheca Medica (Casse). 1895;Heft 3:1–83.
10. Ogden JA, Watson HK, Bohne W. Ulnar dysmelia. J Bone Joint Surg. 1976;58A:467–75.
11. Swanson AB, Tada K, Yonenobu K. Ulnar ray deficiency: its various manifestations. J Hand Surg Am. 1984;9A:658–64.
12. Ogino T, Kato H. Clinical and experimental studies on ulnar ray deficiency. J Pediatr Orthop. 1983;3:37–40.
13. Cole RJ, Manske PR. Classification of ulnar deficiency according to the thumb and first web. J Hand Surg Am. 1997;22A:479–88.
14. Goldfarb CA, Manske PR, Busa R, Mills J, Carter P, Ezaki M. Upper-extremity phocomelia reexamined: a longitudinal dysplasia. J Bone Joint Surg. 2005;87A:2639–48.
15. Buck-Gramcko D. Congenital malformations of the hand and forearm. Chir Main. 2002;21:70–101.
16. Carter PR, Ezaki M, Oishi S, Herring JA. Disorders of the upper extremity. In: Herring JA, editor. Tachdjian's pediatric orthopaedics, vol. 4. 1st ed. Philadelphia: Saunders; 2008. p. 536–9.
17. El Hassan B, Biafora S, Light T. Clinical manifestations of type IV ulna longitudinal dysplasia. J Hand Surg Am. 2007;32A:1024–30.
18. Miller JK, Wenner SM, Kruger LM. Ulnar deficiency. J Hand Surg Am. 1986;11A:822–9.
19. Carroll RE, Bowers WH. Congenital deficiency of the ulna. J Hand Surg Am. 1977;2:169–74.
20. Straub LR. Congenital absence of the ulna. Am J Surg. 1965;109:300–5.
21. Broudy AS, Smith RJ. Deformities of the hand and wrist with ulnar deficiency. J Hand Surg Am. 1979;4A:304.
22. Flatt AE. The Care of congenital hand anomalies. St Louis: Quality Medical Publishers; 1994.
23. James MA, Bednar M. Deformities of the wrist and forearm. In: Green DP, Hotchkiss RN, Pederson WC, Wolfe SW, editors. Green's Operative Hand Surgery. 5th ed. New York: Churchill Livingstone; 2005. p. 1479–83.
24. Vitale CC. Reconstructive surgery for defects in the shaft of the ulna in children. J Bone Joint Surg. 1952;34A:804–10.
25. Smith AA, Greene TL. Preliminary soft tissue distraction in congenital forearm deficiency. J Hand Surg Am. 1995;20A:420–4.
26. Chen GX, Zhou ZA, Yang L. Ulnar lengthening using a half ring sulcated external fixator for ulnar longitudinal deficiency: a case report. Cell Biochem Biophys. 2013. doi:10.1007/s12013-013-9566-z.
27. Laurin CA, Farmer AW. Congenital absence of the ulna. Can J Surg. 1959;2:204–7.
28. Blair WF, Shurr DG, Buckwalter JA. Functional status in ulnar deficiency. J Pediatr Orthop. 1983;3:37–40.

11 Symbrachydactyly

William J. Dahl and Neil F. Jones

Definition

Symbrachydactyly is a congenital hand difference that can present with a variety of findings including brachydactyly, syndactyly, and hypoplasia of the hand. The condition is typically unilateral and may be associated with absence of the pectoralis major muscle in some cases. The fingers in symbrachydactyly are shortened and stiff with varying degrees of bone loss depending on the size of the middle phalanx [1].

Classification

Swanson [2] and the International Federation of Societies for Surgery of the Hand [3] classify symbrachydactyly as a deformity resulting from a failure of formation. Manske and Oberg in 2009 [4] modified this classification system based on increased knowledge about the molecular basis of congenital hand differences. Symbrachydactyly was placed in the transverse deficiency subset under the group I failure of axis formation and/or differentiation. In 2010, Oberg further modified the 2009 classification system creating the Oberg Manske Tonkin (OMT) classification system [5]. It placed symbrachydactyly under the malformations group and the subgroup of failure of axis formation/differentiation involving the entire upper limb. The OMT classification system was further modified in 2013 [6]. Symbrachydactyly continued to be grouped under the malformations group and the subgroup of failure of axis formation/differentiation involving the entire upper limb, but this subgroup was further subdivided into three divisions: proximal distal outgrowth, radial-ulnar axis, and dorsal-ventral axis. Symbrachydactyly was placed into the proximal distal outgrowth division.

Several classification systems have been proposed to better characterize the often-wide spectrum of involvement seen in symbrachydactyly patients. The original classification of symbrachydactyly was introduced by Pol in 1921 [7] and modified by Blauth and Gekeler in 1971, based on an analysis of 19 of their cases and 179 cases in the literature [8]. They divided symbrachydactyly into four types based mainly on morphological characteristics. The first category in their teratologic sequence is brachymesophalangia or short finger type I. The fingers in this group are often missing middle phalanges and display incomplete syndactyly. Functionally, fingers in this group tend to be stiff with limited flexion and unstable proximal interphalangeal joints. The second group in their classification system is the oligodactylic or "atypical cleft hand" type II, in which the hand is missing some or all of the central three fingers (Fig. 11.1) as well as partial loss of the small finger. The third or monodactylic group consists of hands missing all four fingers except the thumb (Fig. 11.2). The finger metacarpals may also be partially or completely absent. The most involved group in their teratologic sequence is the peromelic or adactylic group IV, in which the hand is missing all five digital rays, with only nubbins or nail remnants (Fig. 11.3).

Suguira refined the Blauth and Gekeler classification in 1976 [9]. He further subclassified the type one or short-fingered hands based on the number of phalanges in each digit. The least involved digits were the triphalangeal type. Diphalangeal and monophalangeal types have two phalanges and one phalanx respectively.

Ogino et al. analyzed 76 children with symbrachydactyly [10]. All were unilateral; 48 were classified as type I, 9 were type II, 8 were type III, and 11 were type IV. Ogino argued that type I symbrachydactyly is a mild form of an intercalary transverse deficiency, whereas types II through IV represent terminal transverse deficiencies.

W.J. Dahl, M.D.
Department of Orthopaedic Surgery, University of California, Irvine, 101 The City Drive South, Pavilion III, Orange, CA 92868, USA
e-mail: wjdahl@gmail.com

N.F. Jones, M.D., F.R.C.S. (✉)
Department of Orthopedic Surgery, University of California Irvine Medical Center and Shriners Hospital Los Angeles, 101, The City Drive South, Orange, CA 92868, USA
e-mail: nfjones@uci.edu

D.R. Laub Jr. (ed.), *Congenital Anomalies of the Upper Extremity: Etiology and Management*, DOI 10.1007/978-1-4899-7504-1_11, © Springer Science+Business Media New York 2015

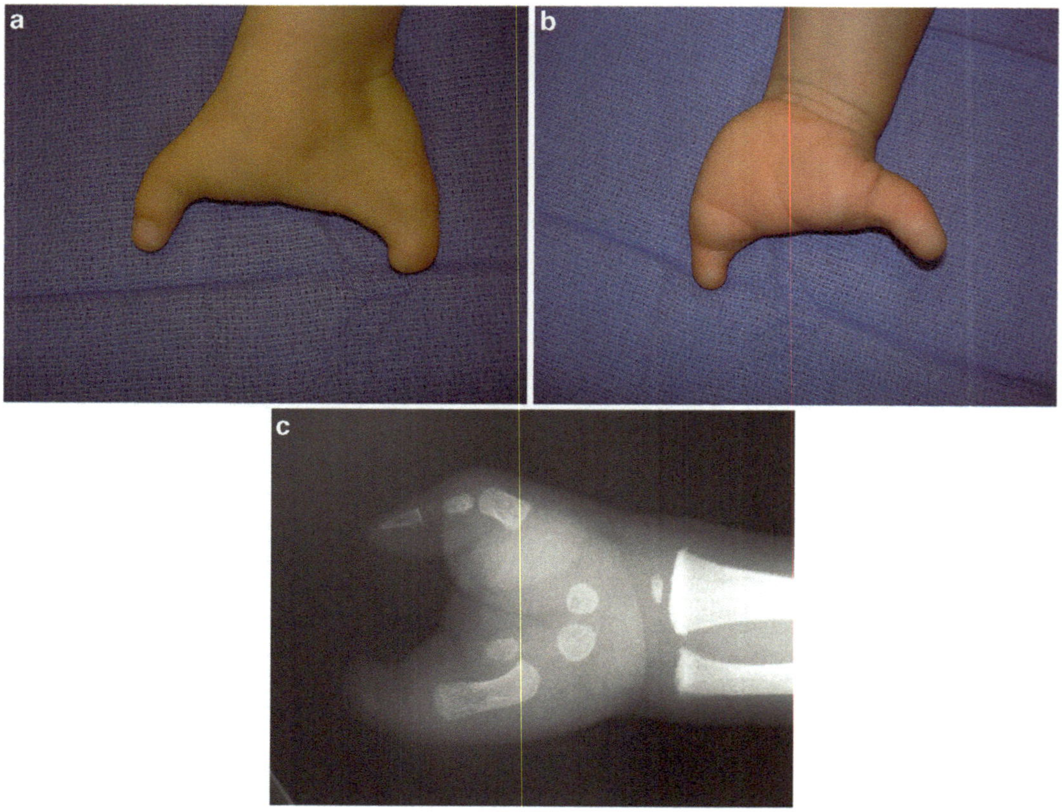

Fig. 11.1 (a–c) Dorsal and palmar photographs and radiograph of an "atypical" cleft hand, now classified as a central absence or oligodactylic type II symbrachydactyly, affecting the left hand of a 4-year-old boy. Published with kind permission of Neil F. Jones ©2014. All rights reserved

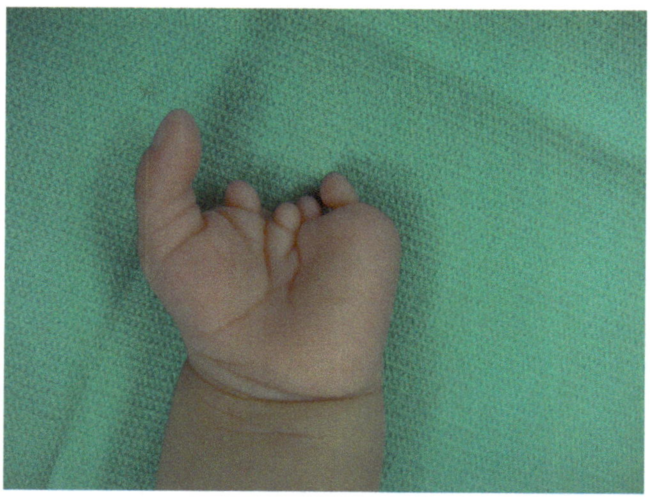

Fig. 11.2 Monodactylic type III symbrachydactyly of the left hand in a 2-year-old girl. The four fingers are represented by nubbins and this would be classified as a U4R1 hand. Published with kind permission of Neil F. Jones ©2014. All rights reserved

Yamauchi further divided the classification of symbrachydactyly into seven types [11]. In type 1 or triphalangia type, the hand has its full complement of bony structures although the middle phalanges are usually short. Type 2 or diphalangia type hands have one phalanx, usually the middle phalanx, missing. Type 3 or monophalangia type hands have a digit or digits containing only one phalanx. Type 4 or aphalangia type hands have a digit or digits that are missing all three phalanges. Type 5 or ametacarpia type hands have absence of the metacarpal and all three phalanges in one digit or several digits. Type 6 or acarpia hands have absence of all the digits and a partial or complete absence of the carpus. Type 7 or forearm amputation have absence of the distal part of the forearm.

All of the classification systems have inherent weaknesses. In particular, the IFSSH classification originally placed the two transverse abnormalities in two different categories, with transverse arrest being placed in category I failure of formation and symbrachydactyly under category V undergrowth. Swanson wrote in his original paper "failure of formation may be manifest as an almost transverse arrest of the entire hand with only rudimentary radial and ulnar digits present," yet showed a case of symbrachydactyly as an example. The Japanese Society for Surgery of the Hand considers symbrachydactyly to be synonymous with transverse failure of formation and therefore believes that symbrachydactyly be moved to category I of the IFSSH classification. Symbrachydactyly is now being seen as a distal manifestation of transverse deficiency, whereas transverse arrest is seen as a more proximal manifestation of transverse

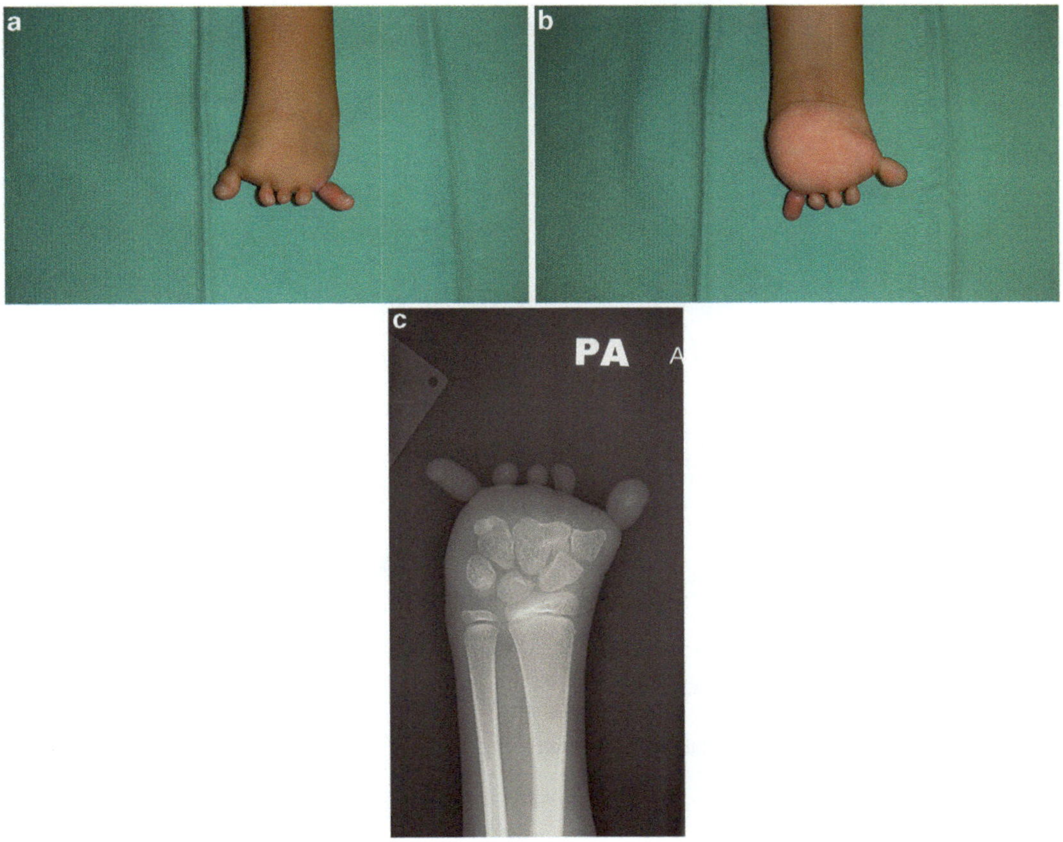

Fig. 11.3 (a–c) Dorsal and palmar photographs and radiograph of a 2-year-old girl with adactylic type IV symbrachydactyly of her left hand. All five digits are represented just by nubbins and are missing from the level of the carpometacarpal joints. This would be classified as an R5 hand. Published with kind permission of Neil F. Jones ©2014. All rights reserved

deficiency. However, this understanding combines symbrachydactyly in which the initial deficiency is hypoplasia of the middle phalanges with preservation of the distal elements, with transverse deficiency in which the distal elements are missing completely.

Jones and Kaplan [12] suggested a new documentation system for congenital absent digits based on their review of photographs and PA radiographs of 235 hands in 204 children born with absent digits. This documentation system does not attempt to imply any underlying embryological causation, but unlike most other classifications, it provides a simple description of either the morphological or radiographic appearance of a child's hand to facilitate communication between physicians. Three letters can describe each hand: R (radial), C (central), and U (ulnar) as well as five numbers. The first letter and number describe which rays are missing and the second and third letters and numbers describe the rays that are present. A normal hand is therefore described as R0. An absent thumb would be described as R1U4. The spectrum of radial deficiencies includes R2U3, R3U2, and R4U1 (Fig. 11.4). The spectrum of transverse deficiencies and ulnar deficiencies include U1R4, U2R3, U3R2, and U4R1 (Fig. 11.5). A hand with a thumb but absent fingers would be designated as U4R1. This is the most common phenotype and corresponds to the Blauth and Gekeler monodactylic type III form of symbrachydactyly (see Fig. 11.2). Typical cleft hand or central longitudinal deficiency as it is now known, would be designated as C1R2U2. Other central deficiencies (Fig. 11.6) include C1R1U3, C1R3U1, C2R1U2, C2R2U1, and C3R1U1 (the old "atypical" cleft hand, which corresponds to the Blauth and Gekeler oligodactylic type II form of symbrachydactyly). Complete absence of all five digits would be designated as R5, which corresponds to the Blauth and Gekeler peromelic type IV form of symbrachydactyly (see Fig. 11.3). The documentation system can be further refined by describing the level at which the rays are absent: w—radio carpal joint to carpometacarpal joint, m-distal to the carpometacarpal joint to just distal to the metacarpophalangeal joint, p—distal to the metacarpophalangeal joint out to the proximal third of the middle phalanx or the tip of the thumb, and d—distal to the proximal third of the middle phalanx to the tip of the finger.

The Jones and Kaplan system incorporates all the previous subclassification systems that have attempted to describe congenital absent digits in transverse deficiencies, central deficiencies, and symbrachydactyly and simplifies

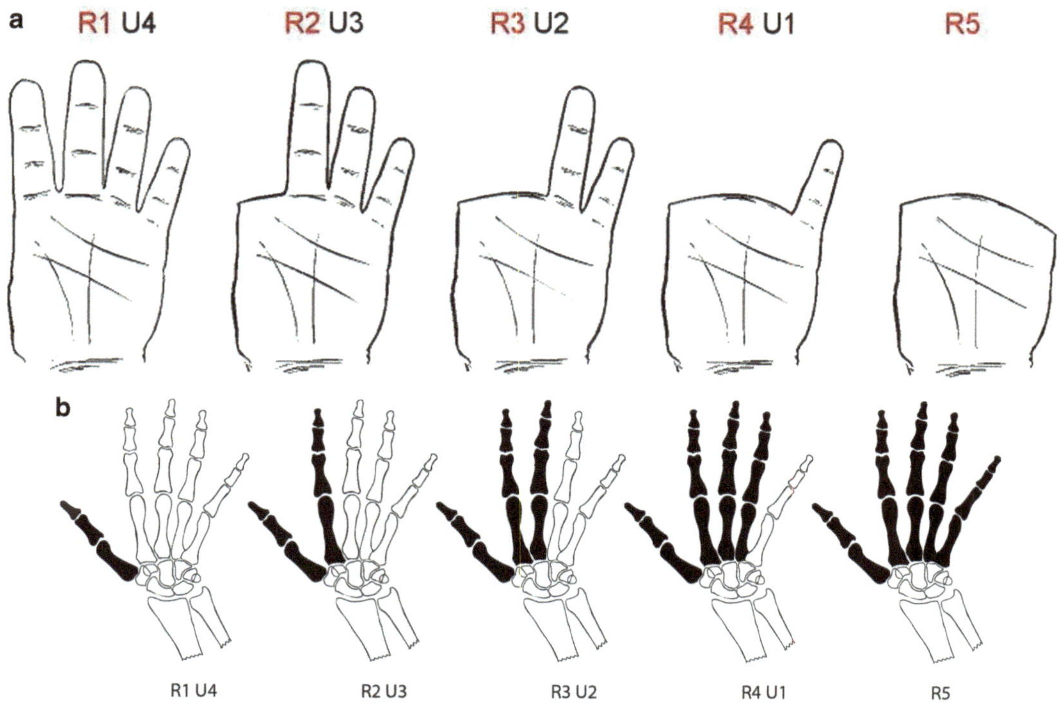

Fig. 11.4 (**a**, **b**) Schematic representation of congenital absent digits affecting the radial side of the hand. Published with kind permission of Neil F. Jones ©2014. All rights reserved

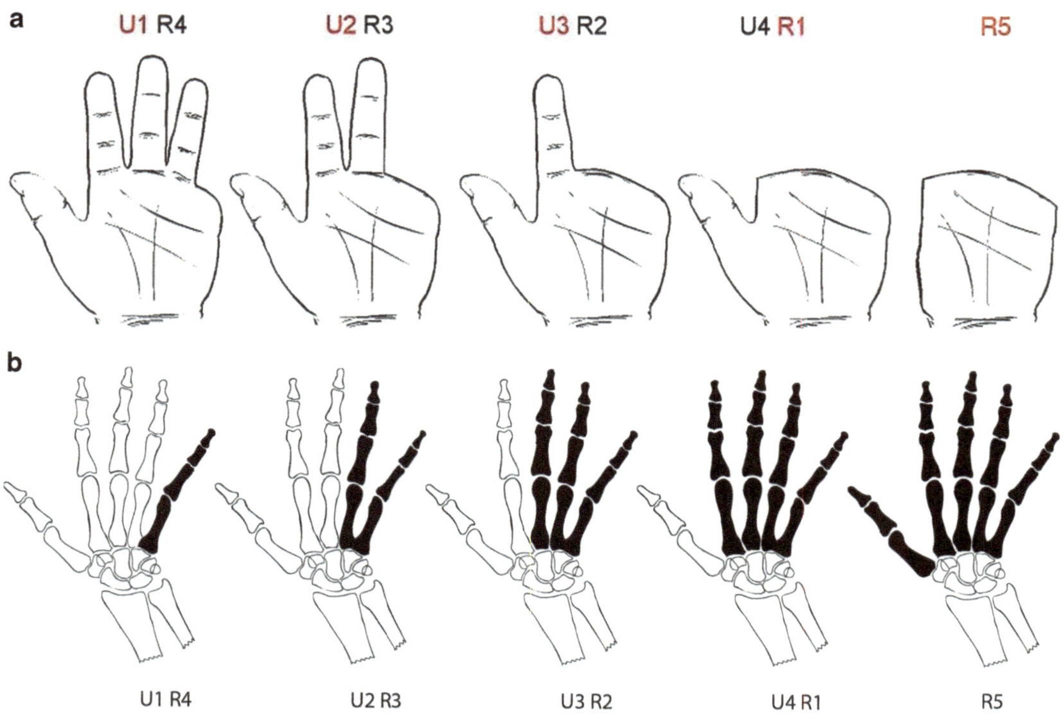

Fig. 11.5 (**a**, **b**) Schematic representation of congenital absent digits affecting the ulnar side of the hand. Published with kind permission of Neil F. Jones ©2014. All rights reserved

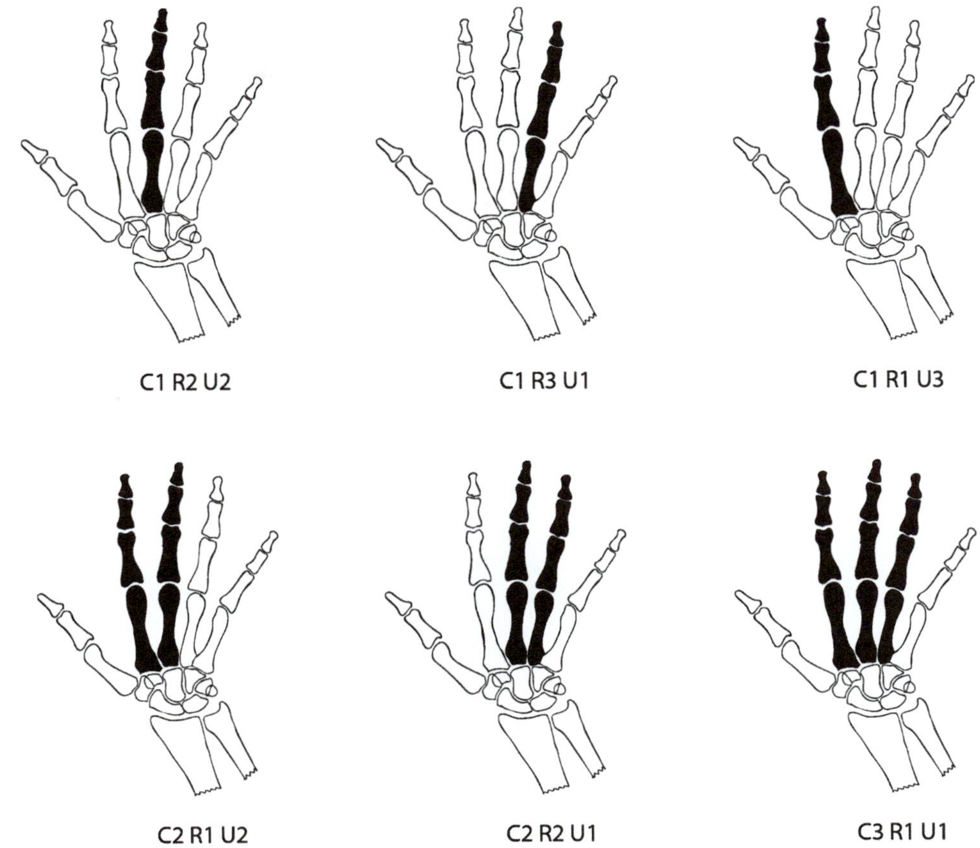

Fig. 11.6 Schematic representation of congenital absent digits affecting the central part of the hand. Published with kind permission of Neil F. Jones ©2014. All rights reserved

the documentation of these children's hands. Blauth and Gekeler [8] and Buck-Gramcko [13] postulated a "reduction theory" in symbrachydactyly which starts at the level of the middle phalanges producing hypoplasia of the middle phalanges ("brachymesophalangia") and then proceeds proximally, so that the distal phalanges or parts of the distal phalanges are always present as digital nubbins with rudimentary nails. With progression, there is absence of the proximal and middle phalanges of the central three fingers, the index, middle, and ring fingers, resulting in the oligodactylic type II "atypical cleft hand" form of symbrachydactyly, which corresponds to the C3R1U1 phenotype (see Fig. 11.1). Reduction progresses to involve the small finger resulting in the type III monodactylic form of symbrachydactyly, which corresponds to the U4R1 phenotype (see Fig. 11.2) and finally extends to the thumb resulting in the type IV peromelic or adactylic form of symbrachydactyly with absence of all digits, corresponding to the R5 phenotype (see Fig. 11.3). Therefore, symbrachydactyly is represented by the C3R1U1, U4R1, and R5 phenotypes.

Another issue is the reclassification of cleft hand within symbrachydactyly. The description "typical cleft hand" has now been replaced with the term "central longitudinal deficiency." But the old term "atypical" cleft hand (see Fig. 11.1) has now been reclassified as "symbrachydactyly central absence type" within category I transverse deficiency [14, 15]. However, reduction of rays proceeds ulnarly from the central three digits in the oligodactylic type II form of symbrachydactyly, leaving only a thumb and no fingers, resulting in the monodactylic type III form of symbrachydactyly and corresponding to a U4R1 phenotype (see Fig. 11.2); whereas in an "atypical" cleft hand, reduction proceeds radially leaving the ring and small fingers or only a single small finger on the ulnar side of the hand, resulting in a R3U2 or R4U1 phenotype (Fig. 11.7). In the authors' opinion, these are two completely different phenotypes that are being placed together in the same category!

Clinical Features

The hand affected by symbrachydactyly can present with a variety of findings. A common feature is short digits frequently involved in varying degrees of simple incomplete to complex complete syndactyly, or instead of fingers just "nubbins" [16]. Another feature associated with symbrachydactyly is skin invagination in the palm, thought to represent the attachments of forearm extrinsic muscle-tendon units [17]. The extensor tendons in symbrachydactyly are more normal and extend out over the hypoplastic metacarpals, but the flexor tendons often form a single amorphous tendon mass within the carpal tunnel [18].

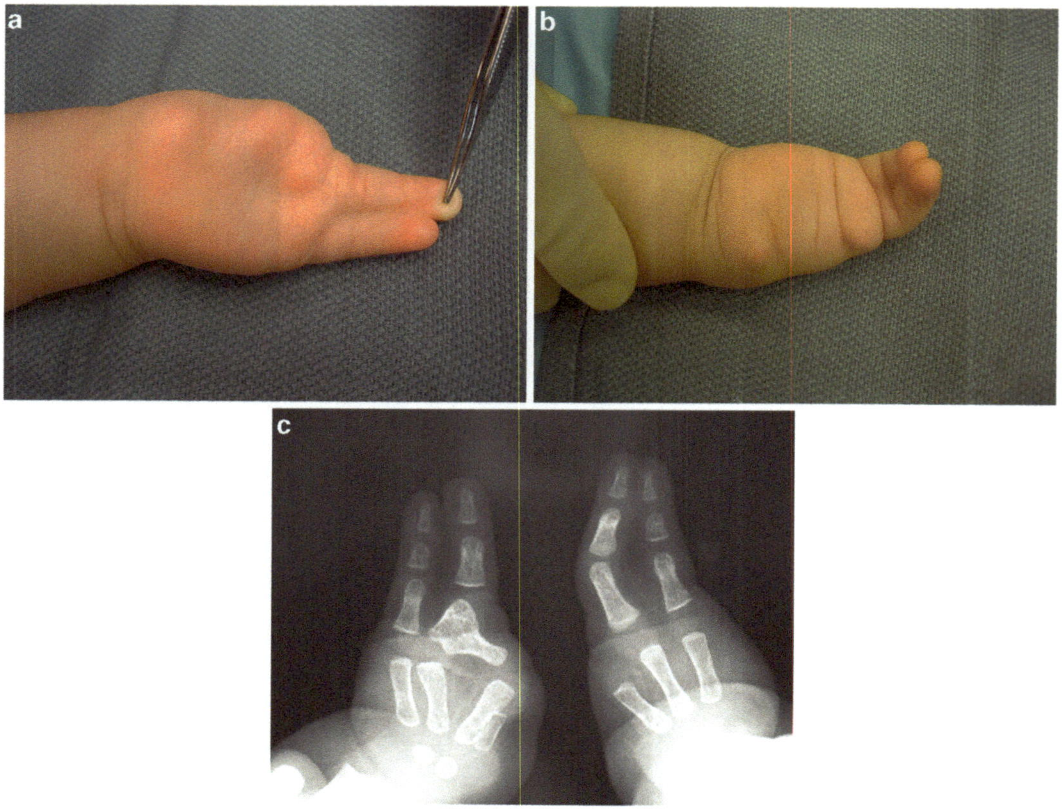

Fig. 11.7 (a–c) Two-year-old boy with bilateral cleft hands, missing the thumb, index, and middle fingers. The ring and small fingers are involved in a complete simple syndactyly. This would be classified as a R3U2 hand. Published with kind permission of Neil F. Jones ©2014. All rights reserved

Distinguishing symbrachydactyly from other conditions caused by other transverse failures of formation can be difficult. Kallemeier et al. [19] examined the relationship between transverse deficiency and symbrachydactyly in 271 children with a diagnosis of transverse deficiency at the level of the forearm; 207 of these children (93 %) had manifestations of symbrachydactyly—soft tissue "nubbins" or skin invagination at the distal aspect of their limbs. They concluded that symbrachydactyly and congenital transverse deficiency of the forearm represent two points on a single continuum, in that transverse deficiency at the level of the forearm represents a more proximal form of symbrachydactyly.

Miura and Suzuki [20] also highlighted these difficulties when they attempted to differentiate between typical cleft hand and the "atypical" cleft hand (central absence type) seen in symbrachydactyly. They examined the length of the metacarpals in normal hands, syndactyly, cleft hands, symbrachydactyly, and constriction band syndrome and found that hands with symbrachydactyly and failure of formation of parts had shortened metacarpals; whereas hands with syndactyly, constriction band syndrome, and typical cleft hand had normal length metacarpals.

Pediatricians and even some surgeons have difficulty differentiating transverse failure of formation, symbrachydactyly, and congenital constriction ring syndrome. A child's hand affected by a transverse failure of formation usually has shortened digits with smooth "amputation" stumps, without "nubbins" or evidence of constriction rings (Fig. 11.8). Radiographs may show tapering of the phalanges or shortened metacarpals. A child's hand affected by symbrachydactyly usually shows either a thumb and a small finger separated by "nubbins" or a wide cleft (see Fig. 11.1); or a thumb but missing all four fingers just represented by "nubbins" (see Fig. 11.2); or absence of all five digits represented just by "nubbins" (see Fig. 11.3). Radiographs will reveal shortened or absent metacarpals in the affected digits. Finally, a child's hand affected by congenital constriction ring syndrome will show a relatively smooth amputation of one or several fingers with evidence of constriction rings affecting other digits or more proximally the wrist or forearm (Fig. 11.9a); or amputation of several fingers with adhesion of the amputation stumps together distally (acrosyndactyly) with sinuses representing the web spaces more proximally (see Fig. 11.9b). Radiographs typically show normal bony architecture proximal to the constriction rings.

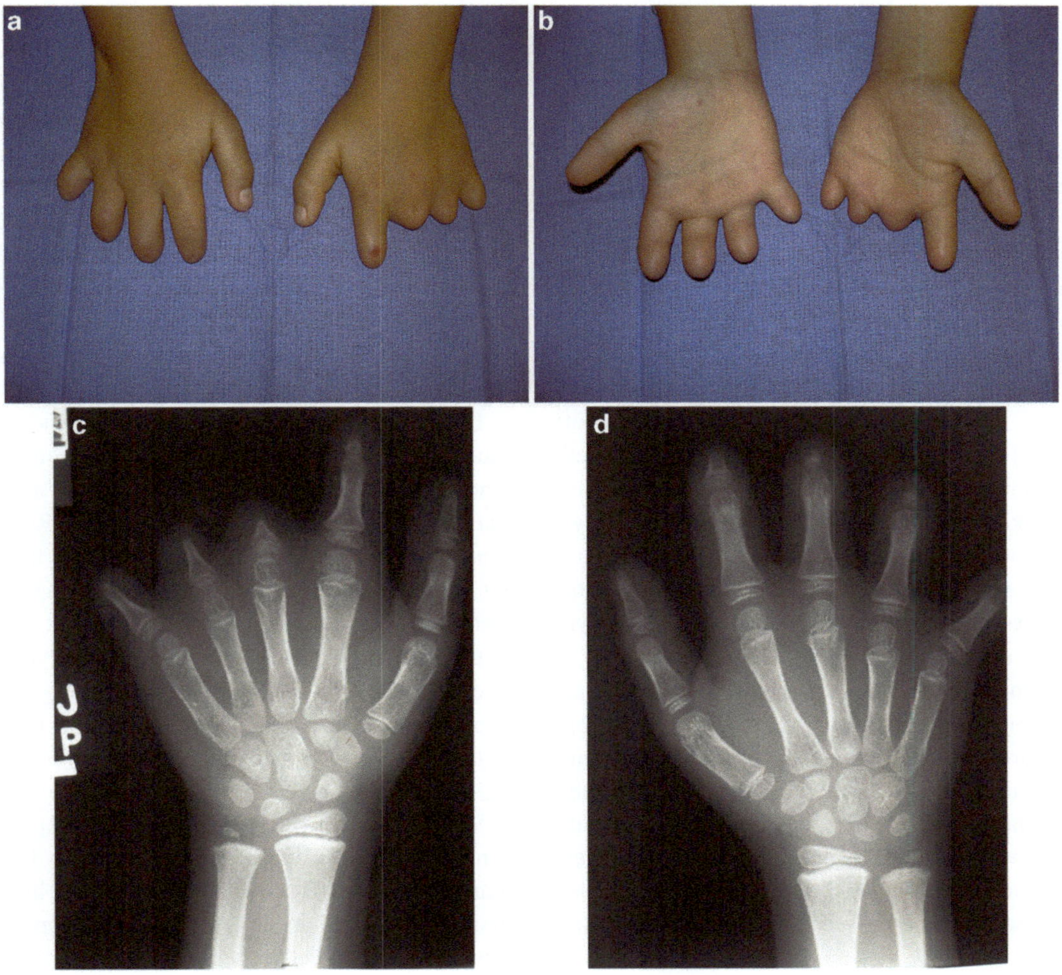

Fig. 11.8 Dorsal and palmar photographs (**a**, **b**) and radiographs (**c**, **d**) of a 6-year-old boy with a transverse failure of formation affecting both hands. In the right hand the failure of formation is at the level of the base of the middle phalanges. In the left hand the level of failure of formation is at the level of the proximal phalanges in the middle, ring and small fingers and at the base of the middle phalanx in the index finger. Published with kind permission of Neil F. Jones ©2014. All rights reserved

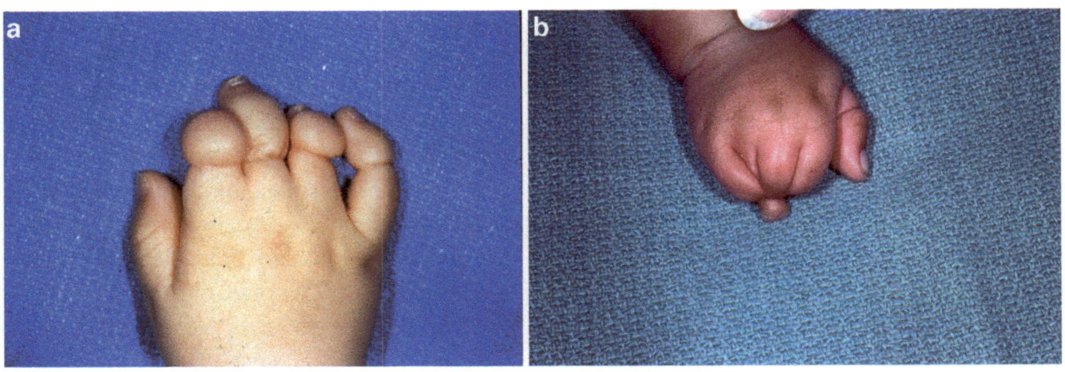

Fig. 11.9 Congenital constriction ring syndrome affecting the index, middle, ring and small fingers of the right hand (**a**). Acrosyndactyly of the right hand with amputation of the distal phalanges and coalescence of the terminal portions of the fingers together with sinuses represent the web spaces more proximally (**b**). Published with kind permission of Neil F. Jones ©2014. All rights reserved

Etiology

The exact cause of symbrachydactyly is not known. Mesenchymal stem cell defects in the hand plate are presumed to be the cause due to the hypoplastic nature of the hand in symbrachydactyly [21]. The likely mesodermal nature of the defect explains the persistence of ectodermal structure such as the finger pulp, nail fold, and nail even in severe presentations [22]. Bavnick and Weaver proposed that subclavian artery disruption at different points in embryological development could explain a variety of mesodermal anomalies seen in Poland's syndrome, Mobius syndrome, and Klippel-Feil syndrome [23]. There is no known hereditary pattern of inheritance described for symbrachydactyly.

There is no known animal model for symbrachydactyly. There are however, mice with functional null mutations in growth and differentiation factor 5 (Gdf5) that display shortened limb bones with a phenotype very similar to symbrachydactyly in humans. They are referred to as brachypodism mice [24]. The metacarpals, metatarsals, and proximal phalanges are significantly shortened, and the middle phalanges are often absent. Kanauchi et al. [24] examined the bony histology of the hypoplastic bones in these brachypodism mice. The hypoplastic bones showed an endochondral ossification pattern but lacked a growth plate and epiphysis. The authors speculated that a similar mechanism explains the hypoplastic bones seen in symbrachydactyly.

Surgical Treatment

Surgical options for reconstruction of children with transverse failure or symbrachydactyly include nonvascularized toe phalangeal bone grafting, distraction osteogenesis, and microsurgical toe-to-hand transfers.

Nonvascularized Toe Phalangeal Bone Grafts

The first treatment option advocated for the treatment of short digits in symbrachydactyly was the nonvascularized transfer of toe phalanges.

The first report of nonvascularized toe phalangeal transfer was by the German surgeon Wolff in 1910 [25] and 1911 [26]. He reported the transfer of the second toe proximal phalanx to the proximal phalanx of a finger that had been destroyed by a tuberculosis infection. Entin [27] first used this technique in 1959 in the treatment of severe transverse deficiency. The technique was reintroduced by Carroll and Green in 1975 [28]. They reported on 159 toe phalanges transferred in 79 patients. They found that no open physes continued to grow, but did not see evidence of resorption. Complications of this technique in their series included skin necrosis at the tip of the lengthened digit in four patients and a pin tract infection in one patient.

Goldberg and Watson [29] examined their experience with 20 patients and 36 digits treated with nonvascularized toe phalangeal transfer. In contrast to the findings of Carroll and Green [28], 90 % of the growth plates in children under the age of 18 months remained open at an average follow-up of almost 4 years. This rate dropped to 67 % in patients 18 months to 5 years old and to 50 % in patients over the age of 5 years. They reported growth rates 90 % of the contralateral non-transferred phalanges when growth plates remained open.

Buck-Gramcko [30] reported on his experience with 40 patients with symbrachydactyly and constriction band syndrome who underwent transfer of 63 nonvascularized phalangeal bone grafts. He reported 100 % "take" of the bone graft provided that the periosteum over the phalanx was not disrupted and the graft was not split. He found that the best timing for transfer of the phalanges was between 19 and 48 months. Attempts to recreate a functional joint led to variable results with a range of motion ranging from 0 to 90°. Complications in his series included skin necrosis in five patients and joint subluxation requiring reduction in two patients.

Radocha et al. [31] described their experience in the transfer of 73 phalanges with a minimum follow-up of 1 year. They found a 94 % rate of open physes in patients operated on before 1 year of age. The rate dropped to 71 % for those operated on between 1 and 2 years of age and dropped further to 48 % for those older than 2 years of age. Growth rates per age group were found to be 1 mm/year in the two younger age groups and 0.5 mm/year in the group over the age of two. The authors stressed the importance of extraperiosteal dissection during harvesting of the phalanx; ligament, and tendon repair in the recipient digit and a young age (under 12 months) as important factors in maintaining an open physis and therefore the potential for further growth.

Cavallo et al. [32] reported on the transfer of 64 phalanges in 22 children with aphalangia from symbrachydactyly and constriction band syndrome. They found a total digital elongation of 6 mm at an average of 5 years of follow-up. The average range of motion at the newly created joint was found to be 60°. The most common complication in their series was graft instability or malposition, seen in 17 % of the cases, more commonly in cases of atypical cleft hand.

Gohla et al. [33] reported on the transfer of 113 nonvascularized toe phalanges in 48 patients with diagnoses of symbrachydactyly and constriction band syndrome. The operative technique used was similar, and the patients were grouped as previously described by Buck-Gramcko [30]. Epiphyseal plate survival was highest in those patients treated before 18 months of age with an 87 % rate of open physes at follow-up examination. The rate of open physes dropped only to 86 % in patients aged 19 months to 4 years and to 64 % in patients over the age of 4 years. They also looked at rates of bone resorption and found a 45 % rate of resorption in patients over the age of 4 years compared to a rate of only 4 % in patients under 18 months old. Eighteen of the 48 patients developed a complication, including four cases with necrosis of the skin resulting in the loss of the phalangeal bone grafts. Six children had scarring significant enough to require secondary procedures such as Z-plasties or local flaps. Six other transfers were complicated by digital instability or graft displacement.

Donor Site Morbidity and Patient/Parental Satisfaction

The transfer of nonvascularized bone into a soft tissue envelope has been complicated by bone resorption, lack of bone growth, and donor site morbidity. Unglaub in 2006 [34] looked at outcomes of toe phalangeal transfers including growth, resorption, donor site morbidity, patient satisfaction, and parental satisfaction. He divided patients into similar groups as did Buck-Gramcko [30]: under 1.5 years old, 1.5–4 years old, and older than 4 years. Patients under 1.5 years showed good growth of the transferred phalanges with very few cases of resorption. Patients in the middle age group showed no growth in the transferred bone. Patients over 4 years of age had a 54 % rate of graft resorption. He found little morbidity attributable to the donor site. He felt that the functional gains of the procedure were mostly from increased length as little active motion was achieved in the transferred joints in his series. Seventy-five percent of the parents in this series were highly satisfied with the functional gains and "manual skillfulness" provided by the nonvascularized toe phalangeal bone graft procedure.

The issue of donor site morbidity was also addressed by Bourke and Kay [35] who noted that all the toes with phalanges harvested by the technique described by Buck-Gramcko [30] were shortened, floppy, and had a tendency to cross over other toes. They introduced a technique of placing a nonvascularized iliac crest bone graft in the donor toe with epiphysis present. This tubular bone graft was placed between the epiphysis at the base of the resected phalanx and a small cap of bone left from the harvested phalanx and pinned in place with a longitudinal Kirschner wire (K wire). They reported that their series of 11 patients had better preservation of toe length and stability.

Garagnani et al. [36] studied donor site morbidity clinically and radiographically in a series of 40 patients with hypoplastic digits. A total of 136 phalanges were harvested using supraperiosteal dissection as previously described, with repair of the extensor tendon after removal of the phalanx. The mean follow-up for the series was 122 months with a minimum follow-up of 36 months. The Oxford Ankle-Foot Questionnaire (OAFQ) is a validated questionnaire for children aged 5–16 years old that assesses subjective patient and parental satisfaction. Over 80 % of patients and families reported some degree of emotional problems related to their feet. Footwear related problems were noted by over 60 % of both patients and families. All of the patients interviewed reported a tendency to hide their feet. From a clinical perspective, shortening of the harvested toes was universal, and malrotation was seen in 76–100 % of the toes. Not surprisingly, clinical deformity increased when multiple phalanges were harvested from a single foot. Radiographic examination revealed hypoplasia of surrounding bony structures including the distal phalanx, middle phalanx, and metatarsal. One patient in their series even underwent amputation of bilateral overriding and unstable fourth toes with significant postoperative improvement in the appearance of the feet.

Indications and Patient Selection

Jones [37] described three specific indications for the transfer of nonvascularized toe phalanges. The first is stabilization of a floppy hypoplastic digit consisting of only a soft tissue envelope. The second is lengthening and stabilization of a digit that contains a remnant of the proximal phalanx. The third indication is stabilization of an intercalated defect between the distal phalanx and the metacarpal of a thumb. Based on the outcomes described earlier, the ideal patient for nonvascularized toe phalangeal transfers is a child under the age of 18 months with multiple short digits and a bony skeleton out to at least the level of the distal metacarpals with a sufficient soft tissue envelope [38].

Surgical Technique

Under tourniquet control, the hypoplastic digit is explored through a dorsal longitudinal incision. If a significant palmar soft tissue contracture is present, a volar approach could be chosen. Blunt dissection within the soft tissue is used to create a cavity for the donor bone. It is crucial to maintain a sufficient pad of soft tissue at the distal aspect of the digit to prevent necrosis caused by pressure from the donor bone. Typically, the flexor and extensor tendons are confluent over the hypoplastic metacarpal head. They are sharply divided to create independent flexor and extensor tendons and radial and ulnar collateral ligaments.

Typically the proximal phalanx from the third or fourth toe is used as a donor phalanx. The second toe can be used if a microsurgical second toe transfer is not planned for the future. A gently curved incision is used over the dorsum of the toe because a straight incision over the dorsum of the toe can result in an extension contracture of the toe. The extensor tendon is split longitudinally to expose the proximal phalanx. Previous experience [29–31] has shown that an extraperiosteal dissection of the proximal phalanx in a child under the age of 18 months provides the best chance for preventing resorption of the transferred bone. The collateral ligaments of the PIP joint are divided off the proximal phalanx while the collateral ligaments and volar plate of the metatarsophalangeal joint are harvested with the proximal phalanx.

The tourniquet on the leg is then released and hemostasis achieved. A variety of methods have been described to prevent shortening of the donor toe [30, 31, 35]. The simplest of these is suturing the extensor tendon to the flexor tendon. Iliac crest bone graft with its associated apophysis as described by Bourke and Kay [35] can be inserted to help maintain the length and stability of the toe. A 0.035-in K wire is then introduced retrograde through the toe into the metatarsal head and left in place for 4–5 weeks to hold the toe out to length.

The toe phalanx is transferred to the hand and the bone graft can be positioned in one of three basic constructs. In digits with a partial proximal phalanx, the graft can be placed distally in the "on top" position. In digits with an intercalary defect between a hypoplastic distal phalanx and metacarpal, the graft can be interposed between the two bones. Finally, the graft can potentially be used to simultaneously reconstruct the metacarpophalangeal joint and provide length to the floppy digit in children lacking all skeletal elements distal to the metacarpal head.

A 0.035-in or 0.028-in K wire is inserted through the phalanx. Nonabsorbable sutures are placed but not tied between the flexor tendon and the volar plate of the transferred phalanx as well as between the radial and ulnar capsule of the MCP joint and the radial and ulnar collateral ligaments of the transferred phalanx. The K wire is then advanced distally out through the distal soft tissues of the digit. The phalangeal bone graft is reduced into the soft tissue envelope of the digit and held in appropriate position relative to the metacarpal. The previously placed sutures are tied. The K wire is then advanced retrograde into the metacarpal. The extensor tendon and dorsal capsule of the MCP joint are repaired to the dorsal capsule of the donor phalanx. The hand is immobilized in a plaster splint and the K wire is left in place for 4–6 weeks postoperatively.

Because of only modest growth of nonvascularized toe phalangeal bone grafts; the problems of subluxation, instability, and resorption of the bone graft; and problems of the donor toe; we now rarely use this technique. Currently, we only use nonvascularized toe phalangeal transfer for elongating and stabilizing soft tissue finger stumps with bone out to the level of the metacarpal heads or just distal to the PIP joints and for intercalated bone grafting in a thumb missing the proximal phalanx (Figs. 11.10 and 11.11).

Limitations

The main limitations of the toe phalangeal transfer technique are the pre-existing soft tissue envelope of the hand and the limited growth potential of the transferred bone. The pre-existing soft tissue envelope of the hand dictates the amount of bone length that can be achieved with a single-stage operation. Attempting to over lengthen the soft tissue envelope acutely can result in the complications noted by Carroll and Green [28]. The growth potential of the transferred phalanx is quite limited. Even in the best-case scenario, a toe proximal phalanx lengthens the digit at an average of 5.8 mm [32] with the maximum lengthening seen with growth to be 18 mm [33].

Bone Distraction Osteogenesis

Bone distraction osteogenesis has also been used in the treatment of symbrachydactyly in an attempt to overcome the limitations of nonvascularized toe phalangeal transfers and to potentially avoid the need for additional bone grafting in some cases (Figs. 11.12 and 11.13).

Codivilla reported the first use of distraction osteogenesis in 1905 [39] with lengthening of the lower extremities in cases of congenital deficiencies. Matev reported the first use of distraction osteogenesis in the hand in 1970 [40] with lengthening of three patient's thumb amputations through a metacarpal osteotomy. Kessler [41] reported the use of bone distraction to treat 11 children with congenital aplasia or hypoplasia of the digits. Iliac crest bone grafting and internal fixation were required to achieve final stability. Wenner in 1986 [42] recommended the use of intramedullary K wires to prevent unwanted angulation during distraction osteogenesis.

Seitz and Froimson [43] described distraction of 12 digits for a variety of diagnoses including congenital differences. Nine of the 12 patients achieved complete consolidation of their regenerate without requiring secondary bone grafting. Complications included one pin tract infection and one premature cessation of growth. They advocated using a uniplanar fixator for lengthening the non-weight bearing upper extremity. In a further series published in 1995 [44], Seitz and Froimson reported 14 single-stage lengthenings using a half frame construct. Digital lengthening of 2–3.5 cm was achieved without the use of bone graft in 13 cases. They recommended a slow rate of lengthening (0.25 mm four times per day) to minimize the discomfort associated with the procedure.

Ogino et al. [45] reported their experience of lengthening 15 digits in patients with symbrachydactyly, brachydactyly, and congenital constriction band syndrome. They only lengthened in one symbrachydactyly patient in a total of six patients using distraction osteogenesis. Other methods used were single-stage lengthening with iliac crest or local bone graft and "on-the-top-plasty." They used a fixator as described by Matev and distracted the bone at a rate of 0.5–1 mm per day. After the fixator was in place for 13–34 days, they removed the fixator and used internal fixation and iliac crest bone graft to maintain the length gained with the fixator. The digits treated with distraction osteogenesis showed the

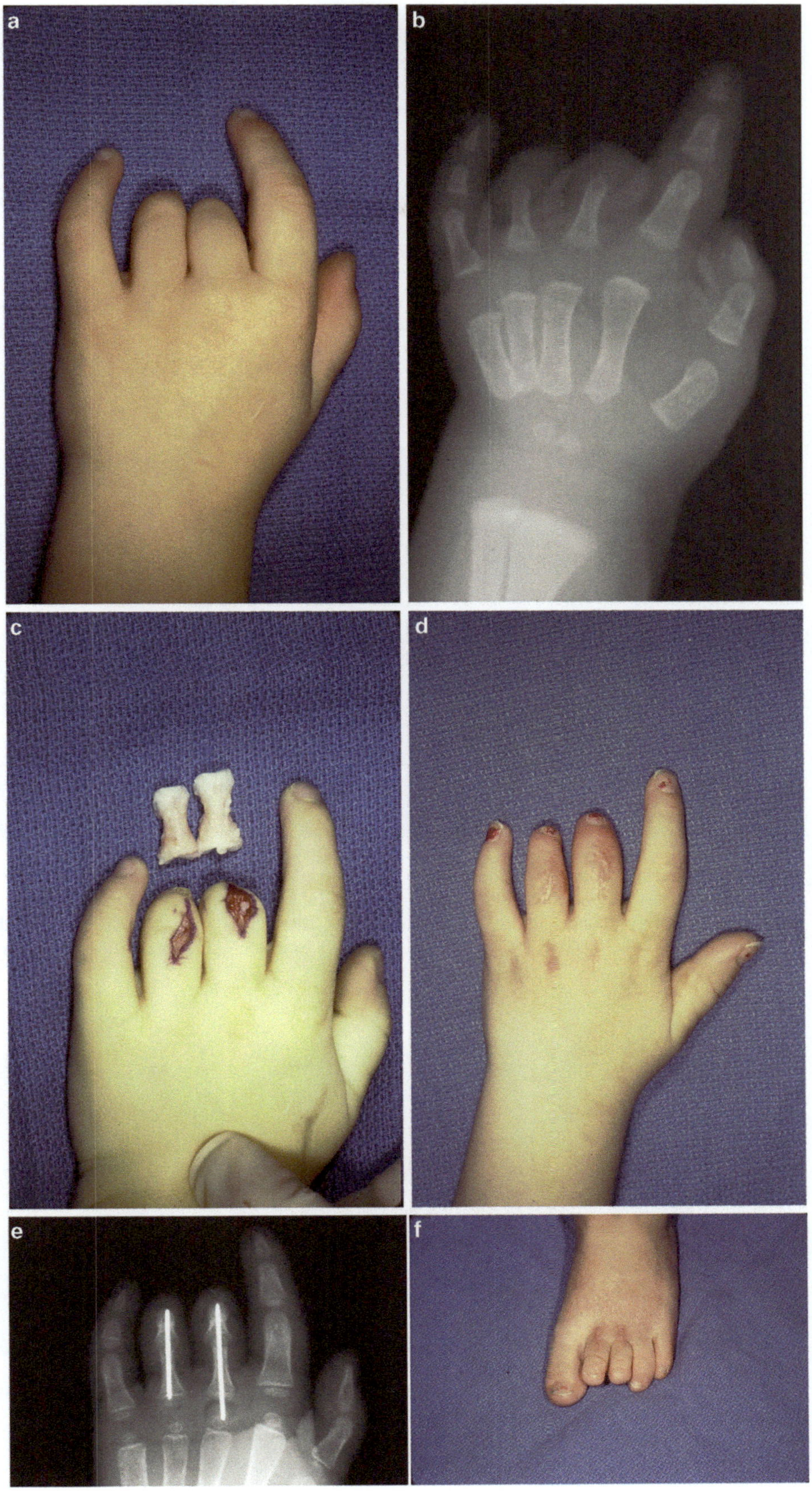

Fig. 11.10 Dorsal and palmar photographs and radiograph of a 4-year-old girl with a transverse failure of formation of her left middle and ring fingers at the level of the proximal phalanges (**a, b**). The soft tissue envelopes of these two fingers were stabilized and elongated using nonvascularized bone grafts from the proximal phalanges of the left second and third toes (**c**). Resultant lengthening of the left middle and ring fingers with the nonvascularized toe phalangeal bone grafts (**d, e**). The donor site in the left foot (**f**). Published with kind permission of Neil F. Jones

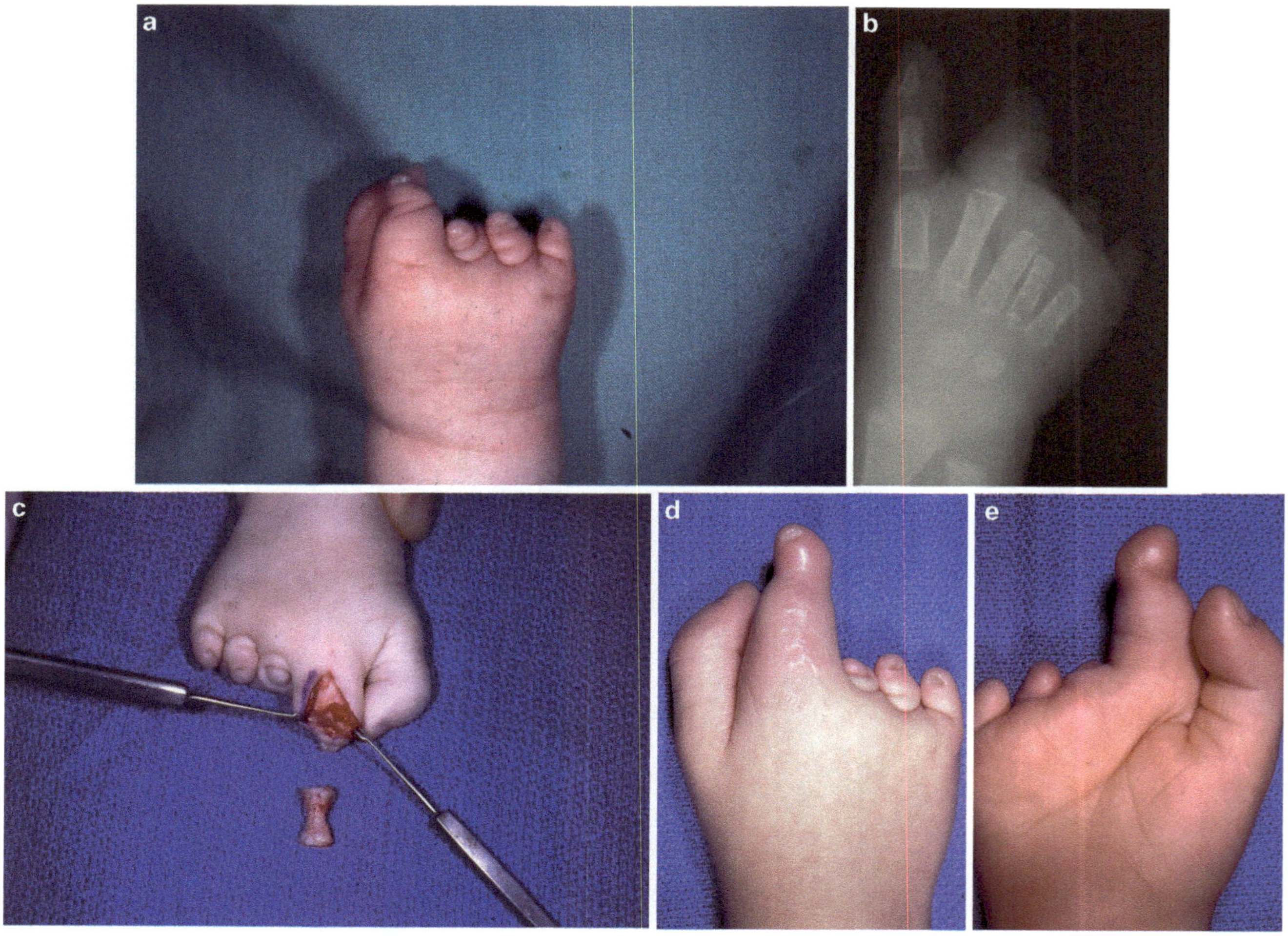

Fig. 11.11 One-year-old boy with monodactylic type III symbrachydactyly affecting his right hand, classified as a U4R1 hand (**a**, **b**). His parents initially refused a microsurgical toe-to-hand transfer. Therefore he underwent a nonvascularized toe phalangeal bone graft from the right third toe to elongate and stabilize the right index finger (**c**). The postoperative result after nonvascularized toe phalangeal bone grafting of the right index finger (**d**, **e**). Published with kind permission of Neil F. Jones ©2014.

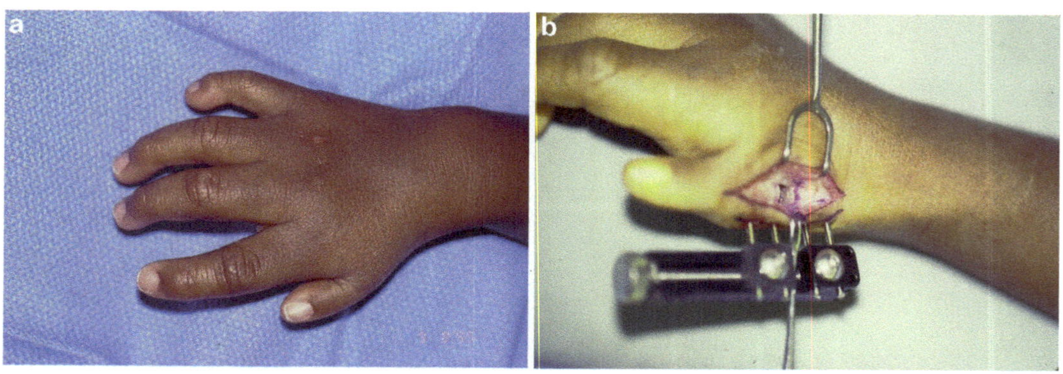

Fig. 11.12 (**a**, **b**) Three-year-old boy with a hypoplastic right thumb (Blauth stage IIIB). The parents refused pollicization of the index finger and therefore he is undergoing distraction lengthening of the thumb metacarpal. Published with kind permission of Neil F. Jones ©2014.

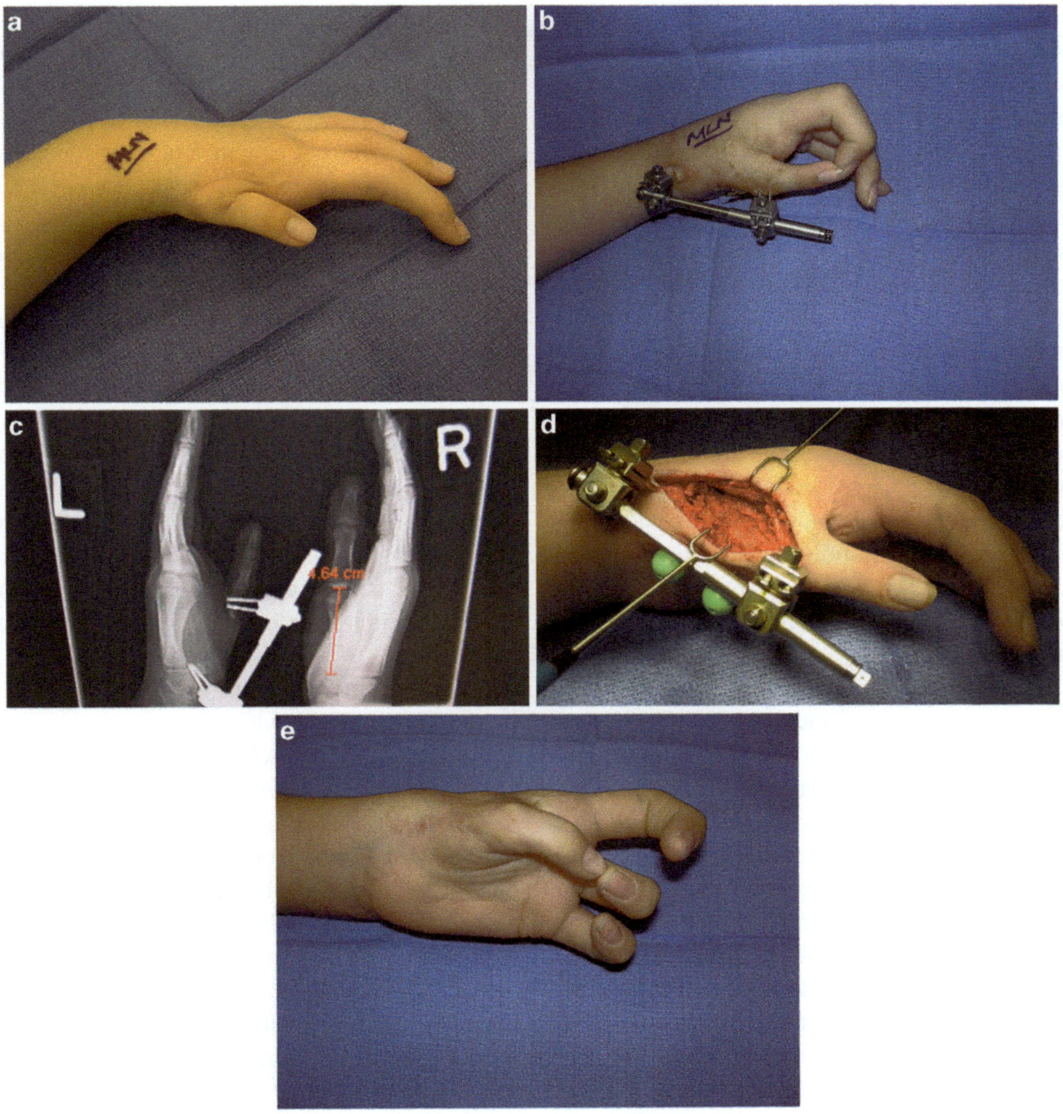

Fig. 11.13 Eight-year-old boy with an unsatisfactory result following pollicization of his left index finger with inadequate length to the new thumb (**a**). He underwent distraction lengthening of 27 mm of the "thumb metacarpal" (index finger proximal phalanx) (**b**, **c**). He subsequently underwent secondary corticocancellous bone grafting of the resultant defect (**d**) and after bony consolidation, he was able to oppose the tip of the thumb to the tips of the little and ring fingers (Kapandji stage 4) (**e**). Published with kind permission of Neil F. Jones ©2014. All rights reserved

greatest average increase in length of 17 mm with no cases of delayed union, whereas two cases of nonunion occurred with single-stage lengthening.

Pensler et al. [46] reported using distraction osteogenesis to treat 12 digits in children with Apert's syndrome. The average age at the time of operation was 4.7 years and the average duration of distraction was 31.1 days. The fixator was generally left in place for 2 days for every 1 mm of lengthening that was performed. The average lengthening was 23.6 mm. Seventeen percent of the digits (2 of 12) required intraoperative manipulation to correct angular deformities that had developed during the course of lengthening.

The first use of distraction osteogenesis specifically for the treatment of symbrachydactyly was reported by Hulsbergen-Kruger et al. [47] who treated three patients with symbrachydactyly with the goal of obtaining pinch grip in the affected hands. They first attempted to lengthen previously transferred proximal toe phalanges, but met with complications due to the tight soft tissue envelope and pin exposure. In their second case, an infection developed during lengthening of the thumb ray. Despite this complication, they were able to achieve 2.2 cm of lengthening. In their third case, a more stable fixator construct was designed and 2.6 cm of lengthening was achieved.

Dhalla et al. [48] compared two different techniques of distraction osteogenesis in a mixed patient population including 10 digits in children with some form of transverse arrest. They compared the use of two half pins on either side of the osteotomy site in 7 digits with a second group of 20 digits in which a single half pin was used on either side of the osteotomy (because the bone was too small to accommodate four half pins) and lengthened over a centrally placed K wire. The mean preoperative bone length in the dual half pin group was 30 mm compared to 18 mm in the single half pin group. The mean gain in length for the dual half pin group was 14 mm compared to 12 mm in the single half pin group. The rate of complications in the single half pin group was 75 % (15) compared to 43 % (3) in the dual half pin group. Only seven of the complications required reoperation. All of the infections were seen in the single half pin group. This study highlights the feasibility of successfully lengthening even very short bones, albeit with a high rate of complications. The authors recommended the use of prophylactic antibiotics in the single half pin fixator cases.

Miyawaki et al. [49] reported their experience with bone distraction osteogenesis of seven metacarpals in four hands with symbrachydactyly. They used a mini-fixator with a distraction rate of 1 mm per day. Lengthening occurred over a mean of 37.3 days and the fixator remained in place for a mean duration of 84 days. An intramedullary 1.0-mm K-wire was used to help maintain alignment. In three hands, a single fixator was used to lengthen the fourth and fifth metacarpals simultaneously. The mean increase in bone length was 22.3 mm. The only major complication was a fracture of a fifth metacarpal that occurred during distraction. No growth disturbances were observed in the lengthened bones at an average of 3.9 years of follow-up. A functional benefit of the procedure was that pinch strength improved in all of the treated hands.

Matsuno et al. [50] examined the bone growth that occurred after distraction osteogenesis in a variety of congenital hand diagnoses including symbrachydactyly. They found that earlier bone lengthening tended to result in greater bone growth after distraction and consolidation. Growth plates closed soon after lengthening in patients older than 10 years of age. In their series, seven metacarpals in three symbrachydactyly patients were lengthened at an average of 8 mm with a total time in the fixator of 104 days. These metacarpals grew at an average of 7.6 mm during the average follow-up period of 59 months. Complications in the symbrachydactyly group included bony prominence at the distal aspect of the lengthened ray. The symbrachydactyly patients tended to be operated on at an earlier age, which they speculated to be the reason that bone growth was seen after lengthening.

Seitz et al. reported on the long-term outcomes of distraction lengthening of over 400 individual bones in 141 patients [51]. Patients were evaluated postoperatively by their therapist regarding multiple outcome measures. Eighty-eight percent of patients reported no difficulty in performing functional activities of daily living and only 5 % reported inability to carry out activities of daily living. Ninety-seven percent of patients reported never having significant pain. Ninety-two percent of patients were satisfied with their outcome from surgery. Static two-point discrimination was unchanged when compared to the contralateral limb in all cases. When asked if the surgery and aftercare were worth it, 98.5 % of patients reported that they would undergo the procedure again. Major complications including the need for supplemental bone grafting (6 %), premature consolidation (0.7 %), soft tissue compromise (0.7 %), digital tip necrosis, angular deformity, pin loosening, joint stiffness, joint subluxation, regenerate fracture or infection occurred in 9 %. Five percent of the major complications required reoperation. Minor complications occurred in 45 % and consisted entirely of pin tract infections, treated with oral antibiotics.

Indications and Patient Selection

In the symbrachydactyly hand, distraction lengthening is indicated for digits lacking sufficient length to generate pinch and prehension. Adequate bone stock (bone length of at least 10 mm [48]) must be present to allow for lengthening to occur. If adequate bone stock is not present, lengthening of transferred toe phalanges can be performed 6 months post-transfer [51]. Patient and family selection is of utmost importance with these procedures. Patients and their families must be educated about the procedure and be able to understand and comply with the extensive aftercare program, including frame adjustments, pin site care, frequent appointments with the surgeon, long duration of treatment, and the high likelihood of complications.

Surgical Technique

Seitz et al. published their technique for lengthening nonvascularized toe phalangeal transfers in symbrachydactyly in 2010 [51]. The goal of lengthening was to provide prehension and improved mechanical advantage. The toe phalanges were harvested using a similar technique as previously discussed. Early reconstruction of a first web space is advantageous. In hands with significantly hypoplastic index finger rays, resections of the index metacarpal and Z-plasty web space deepening were performed at the same time as toe phalangeal transfers. The resected metacarpal can be used as bone graft for lengthening other rays. Six months after the phalangeal transfer, lengthening can be started. Two 2-mm self tapping half pins are placed on each side of the osteotomy, which is made using an osteotome in older children and a Beaver blade in younger children after circumferential periosteal elevation. The periosteum and skin are closed with absorbable suture. The lengthening program begins 5 days after surgery and consists of four lengthenings of 0.25 mm each per day. Showers are permitted at 2 weeks postoperatively. The consolidation phase lasts for two to three times the lengthening period. Seitz highlights the complicated nature of the treatment for children as well as their families.

Limitations

The main limitation of distraction osteogenesis is that it only provides function through increased digital length, and is complicated by frequent pin tract infections.

Microsurgical Toe-to-Hand Transfer

The next step in the evolution of treatment for transverse deficiency and symbrachydactyly, particularly for its more severe types III and IV, is microsurgical toe-to-hand transfers.

The first report of a microsurgical toe-to-hand transfer for a congenital hand difference was by O'Brien et al. who in 1978 [52] performed two toe-to-thumb transfers for congenital absence of the thumb. Gilbert [53] reported a series of 21 second toe-to-hand transfers for congenital hand anomalies, 4 of which were transferred to the thumb. Active motion of the toe was mainly determined by the motion of the native metacarpal. Toe transfers in children with amniotic band syndrome were technically easier due to more normal anatomy compared with children with aplasia. He felt that the best timing for a toe transfer was 16 months of age. Gilbert reported on a more extensive series of 49 toe transfers to 38 hands [54]. Eleven of these children had two toes transferred, one from each foot. One toe transfer failed in a 16-month-old child with aplasia and 10 of 85 epiphyseal plates closed prematurely.

Lister described 12 second toe transfers to reconstruct thumbs in cases of transverse arrest, constriction ring syndrome, and symbrachydactyly [55]. The average age at transfer was 3 years old, with the youngest child only 10 months old. Similar to Gilbert, he found that anatomical variations were always seen in cases of transverse arrest and symbrachydactyly. Only three transfers demonstrated interphalangeal motion at final follow-up, but 11 of the children regained good sensation.

Shvedovchenko [56] reported on the transfer of 103 toes in 66 children for diagnoses including brachydactyly, ectrodactyly, adactyly, hypoplasia, and after trauma. Forty-nine children had congenital hand differences. Distraction osteogenesis was performed to lengthen three of the transferred toes. Vilkki [57] performed toe-to-hand transfers in 30 children with congenital hand differences, 14 of whom had aplasia of all the fingers and 4 had reconstruction of a thumb.

Kay [58] reported a series of 66 toe transfers in 40 children, 85 % of whom had congenital differences. Fourteen children had two toes transferred at the same operation. There were no failures, but 75 % required secondary surgeries to improve function or appearance. Kay emphasized the benefit of the simultaneous transfer of two toes. Growth of the transferred toes was found to be at an average of 91 % of the contralateral toe. All children recovered protective sensation and the majority demonstrated adequate light touch perception.

Van Holder et al. [59] described 14 children with congenital hand differences including transverse failure of formation, constriction ring syndrome, and symbrachydactyly who underwent staged double second toe transfers. Foucher et al. [60] reported 65 toe transfers in 58 children, 51 of whom had a diagnosis of symbrachydactyly. Two toe transfers failed when only one artery was anastomosed and other complications included lateral instability of the transferred metatarsophalangeal joint. The average range of motion was reported to be 38° and the average two-point discrimination was 5 mm.

Richardson et al. [61] reported 18 toe transfers in 13 children with symbrachydactyly, and Jones et al. [62] reported 82 toe transfers in 68 children with diagnoses including symbrachydactyly, transverse deficiencies, and constriction ring syndrome.

Indications

Despite success rates of over 95 % in most reported series of microsurgical toe-to-hand transfers, the procedure remains rarely performed in children. Hand surgeons may be unwilling to risk the loss of a toe transferred in children who already have a congenital hand difference. Secondly, some hand surgeons feel that children with unilateral digital absence adapt well to their impairment over time. Finally, it can be very difficult for parents to make a decision to proceed with a complicated surgery that may potentially result in the loss of a toe with no benefit despite the surgery on the hand.

It can be helpful to show parents photographs and videos of other children who have undergone toe transfers to help them appreciate the benefits that can be achieved through such surgery. The senior author's practice is to introduce the parents of a candidate child for a toe transfer to the parents of a child who has previously undergone a toe transfer for a congenital hand difference. This allows the parents to discuss their concerns with other parents who have had to make a similar decision. It also affords them the opportunity to see a child with a toe transfer in person and obtain a better understanding of the appearance and function of a toe transfer.

Jones and Kaplan [63] suggest that the morphologic and radiographic appearance of a congenital hand difference, rather than its embryological etiology, should dictate the indications for a toe transfer, based on analysis of 100 toe transfers performed for reconstruction of children born with congenital absent digits. For a child with a hand missing a thumb, it seems intuitive to reconstruct a thumb to restore opposition. Similarly, for a child born with a thumb but no fingers, it makes sense to reconstruct a finger or even two fingers to restore opposition and pinch.

In children with an absent thumb, Jones and Kaplan [63] believe that there are three indications for microsurgical reconstruction. The first indication is an isolated absence of the thumb distal to the carpometacarpal joint with a remnant of a thumb metacarpal and thenar musculature as well as four normal or nearly normal fingers, the R1U4 hand, usually due to a transverse deficiency. Microsurgical toe transfers provide superior outcomes when compared to nonvascularized toe phalangeal bone grafting, index finger pollicization, and distraction osteogenesis, because they provide greater length and preserve the potential for growth as well as the full complement of fingers. The second indication is an absent thumb together with absence of the index, middle, (and ring fingers) but with one or two fingers remaining on the ulnar side of the hand, R3U2 and R4U1 hands, usually seen in the old "atypical" cleft hand. The absent thumb can be reconstructed with a second toe transfer with minimal donor site morbidity. In older children, a "trimmed" great toe can be considered since it provides a functional digit that is very similar in appearance and size to the contralateral normal thumb [64]. On rare occasions when there is an associated cleft foot, an abnormal great toe may be transferred to reconstruct the absent thumb [65]. The third indication is absence of all five digits, classified as a R5 hand.

There is a distinct difference between children only missing a thumb and children missing a thumb as well as missing the index, middle, and ring fingers. The former group of children has three reconstructive options available to them: pollicization of the index finger, distraction lengthening, or microsurgical reconstruction with a toe-to-thumb transfer. The only reconstructive option for children in the latter group is a toe-to-thumb transfer.

Jones and Kaplan [63] suggest that there are two indications for toe transfers to reconstruct absent fingers. The first indication is the absence of all four fingers but with a normal thumb, the U4R1 hand, usually due to monodactylic type III symbrachydactyly. A single second toe transfer can restore pinch and grip when placed in the ring or small finger position. Alternatively, two second toes can be transferred into the middle and small finger positions to restore chuck grip, performed either simultaneously or as sequential staged transfers. The second indication is to reconstruct a child's hand with complete absence of all five digits, the R5 hand, usually due to adactylic type IV symbrachydactyly . Usually, one second toe can be transferred into the thumb position first. Then a subsequent second toe transfer can be placed in the ring or small finger position. Performing these two transfers sequentially, rather than simultaneously allows the second toe transfer toe to be placed in the optimum position relative to the new "thumb."

Consequently, there are four specific indications for considering microsurgical toe-to-hand transfers for reconstruction of children born with transverse failure of formation or symbrachydactyly:

1. Transverse failure of formation of the thumb, distal to the CMC joint: **R1U4** phenotype (Fig. 11.14).
2. Central absence type of symbrachydactyly, the old "atypical" cleft hand, with absence of the thumb, index, middle, (and possibly) the ring fingers: **R3U2** or **R4U1** phenotypes.
3. Transverse failure of formation or monodactylic type III symbrachydactyly, with absence of all four fingers distal to the base of the proximal phalanges: **U4R1** phenotype (Figs. 11.15, 11.16, and 11.17).
4. Peromelic or adactylic type IV symbrachydactyly, with absence of all five digits: **R5** phenotype (Figs. 11.18 and 11.19).

Timing of Surgery

The optimal age for toe transfers is debatable. Generally, the earlier a transfer can be performed, the faster that the child will adapt to the new digit. The true limiting factor in toe transfers is the size of the donor and recipient vessels, which must be of adequate diameter to allow for anastomoses. The senior author typically performs his transfers at approximately 24 months of age. Both Gilbert [53, 54] and Lister [66] have performed toe transfers as early as 6–12 months of age. In general, toe transfers for congenital constriction ring syndrome can be performed at an earlier age, because the proximal recipient structures in the hand are more likely to be normal. Children with unilateral congenital hand differences should be reconstructed at an earlier age before use of the contralateral hand dominates.

Preoperative Evaluation

In order to evaluate the skeletal foundation for a toe transfer, plain radiographs are obtained of the hands and feet. Some hand surgeons routinely obtain preoperative angiograms of the donor foot and the recipient hand, but the senior author does not obtain preoperative angiograms. Immediately preoperatively, a pencil 8-mHz ultrasound Doppler probe is used to map the dorsal and plantar arterial anatomy in the foot.

Surgical Technique

Ideally, toe transfer surgery is carried out using two surgical teams who work simultaneously on the hand and foot, both under tourniquet control. Dissection of the hand should precede dissection of the foot to ensure that adequate recipient structures are present in the hand. If vessels in the hand are insufficient for microsurgical anastomoses, vein grafts can be used to reach suitable vessels in the forearm.

Triangular skin flaps on the dorsal and plantar surface of the foot are used to harvest the toe. On the dorsum of the

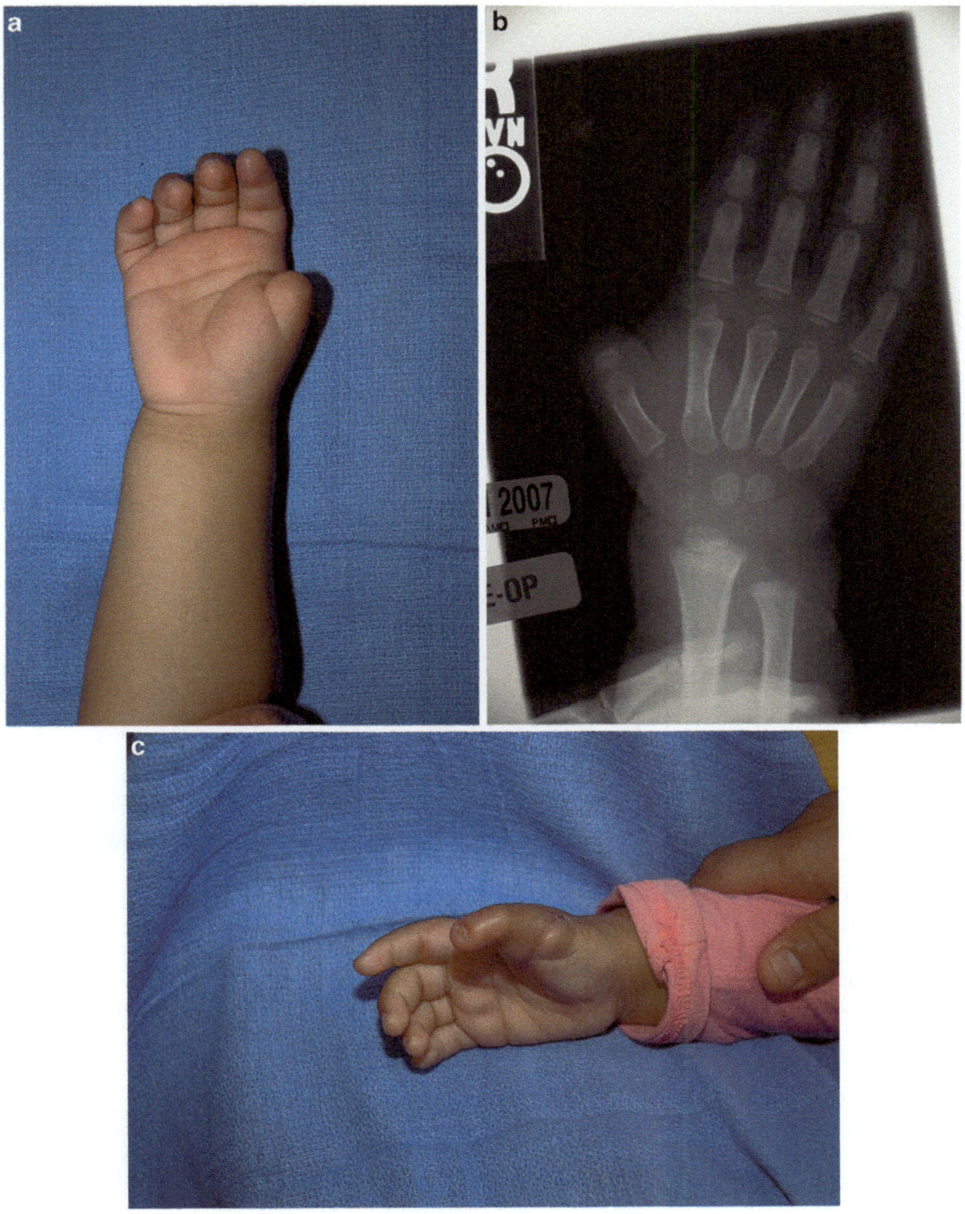

Fig. 11.14 Three-year-old girl with transverse failure of formation of her right thumb at the level of the base of the proximal phalanx (**a**, **b**). She underwent a left second toe-to-thumb transfer and was subsequently able to oppose to the tips of all four fingers (Kapandji stage 5) (**c**). Published with kind permission of Neil F. Jones ©2014. All rights reserved

foot, the venous drainage of the great toe or second toe is traced proximally to a large branch of the greater saphenous vein at the level of the ankle. The arterial supply of the great toe or second toe can be dissected either in a proximal-to-distal or a distal-to-proximal direction. The first dorsal metatarsal artery (FDMA) can be dissected proximal-to-distal from its origin from the dorsalis pedis artery. An alternative approach is to identify the FDMA in the dorsum of the great toe-second toe webspace and trace it proximally. The arterial anatomy of the toes is highly variable [67]. In an ideal situation, the FDMA lies superficially, but it can also lie within or deep to the interosseous muscle. The first plantar metatarsal artery (FPMA) can be used if the FDMA is absent. The FDMA is present in 66 % of patients, and the FPMA is present in 34 % of cases [67].

The extensor tendons to the toe to be transferred are identified and dissected in a distal-to-proximal direction. The digital nerves are then identified in the subcutaneous fat on the palmar aspect of the webspace. Because they are shorter than the digital nerves in the hand, intraneural dissection of the common digital nerve must be carried out to gain length. In some cases, a branch of the deep peroneal nerve can be identified and included in the harvest of the toe. Division of the transverse intermetacarpal ligament allows for further dissection of the flexor aspect of the toe. The flexor digitorum longus and brevis tendons are isolated proximal to the tendon sheath. It is important to determine the length of flexor tendon needed prior to transection of the tendons. An osteotomy is then performed usually at the metaphyseal flare for a second toe harvest.

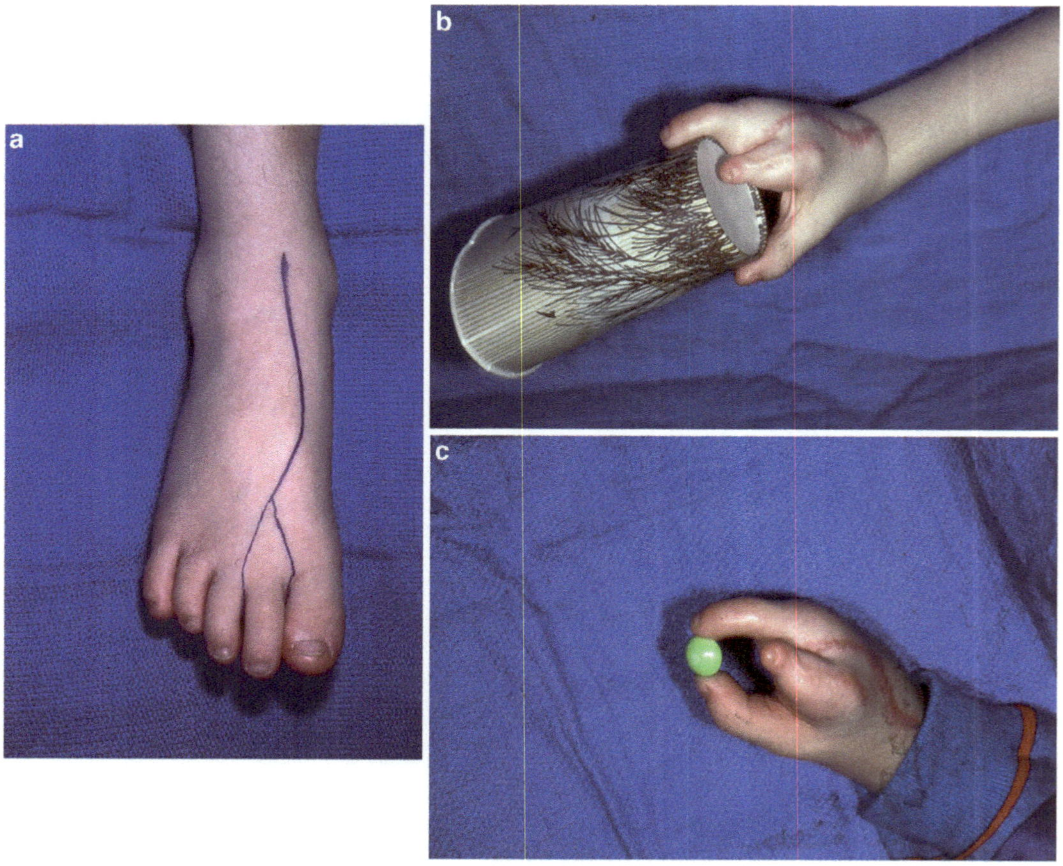

Fig. 11.15 The parents of the 1-year-old boy shown in Fig. 11.11a with monodactylic type III symbrachydactyly of his right hand, who had previously undergone a nonvascularized toe phalangeal bone graft to his right index finger, subsequently agreed to a microsurgical toe transfer (**a**). One year postoperatively, he had excellent grasp and pinch between the thumb and the second toe transfer in the middle finger position (**b, c**). The index finger reconstructed with the nonvascularized toe phalangeal bone graft was then completely excluded from functional activities. Published with kind permission of Neil F. Jones ©2014. All rights reserved

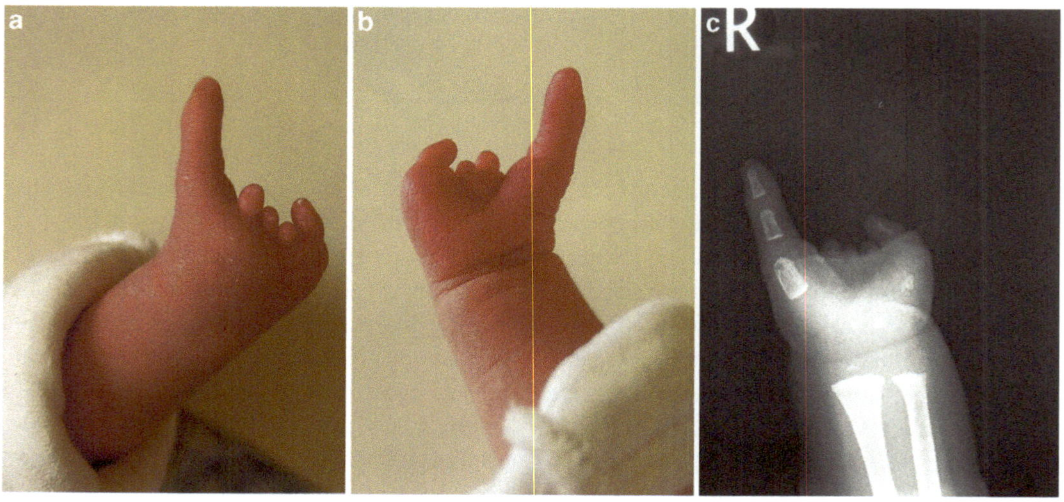

Fig. 11.16 (**a–c**) Dorsal and palmar photographs and radiograph of a 6-month-old girl with oligodactylic type III symbrachydactyly of her right hand. This would be classified as a U4R1 hand. Published with kind permission of Neil F. Jones ©2014. All rights reserved

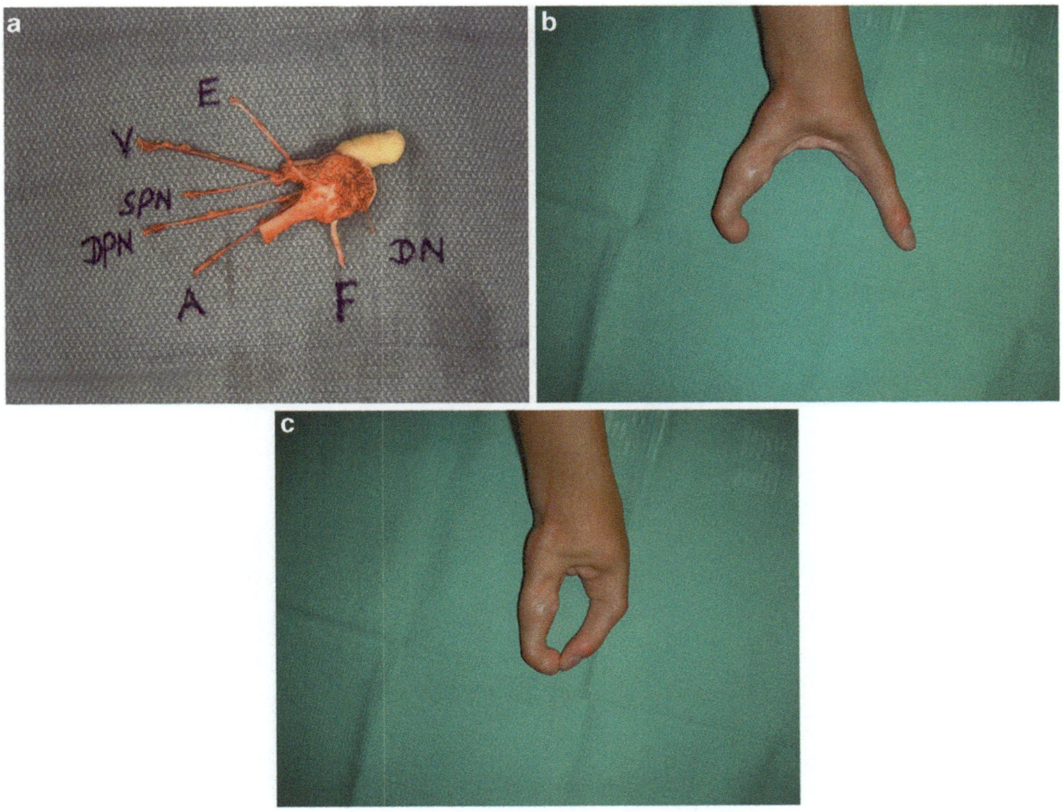

Fig. 11.17 At age 2, she underwent a second toe-to-small finger transfer (**a**). Seven years postoperatively, she has excellent grasp of large objects and precise pinch between the thumb and toe transfer (**b, c**). Published with kind permission of Neil F. Jones ©2014.

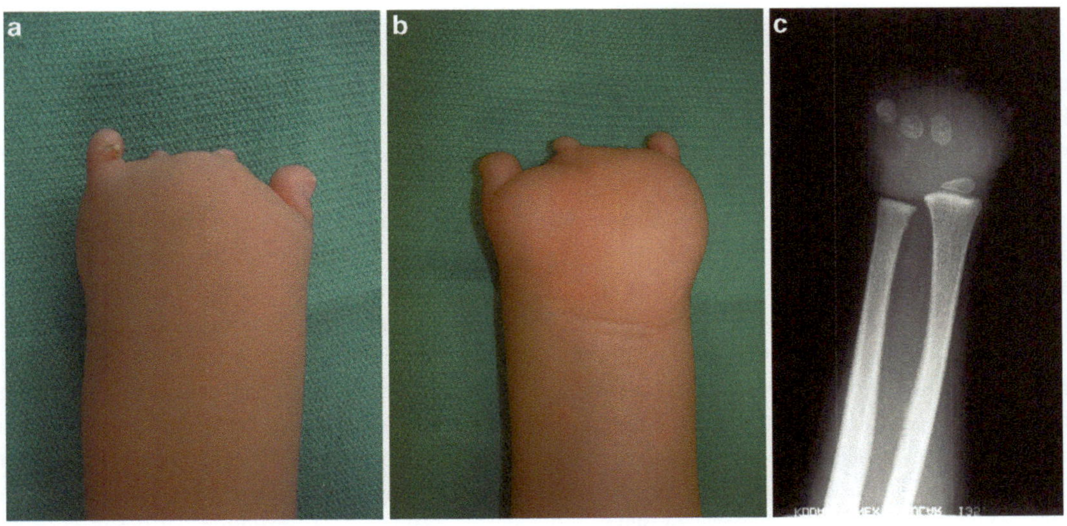

Fig. 11.18 (**a–c**) Dorsal and palmar photographs and radiograph of a 2-year-old boy with adactylic type IV symbrachydactyly affecting all five digits of his left hand. The digits are missing from the level of the metacarpal bases; classified as an R5 hand. Published with kind permission of Neil F. Jones ©2014.

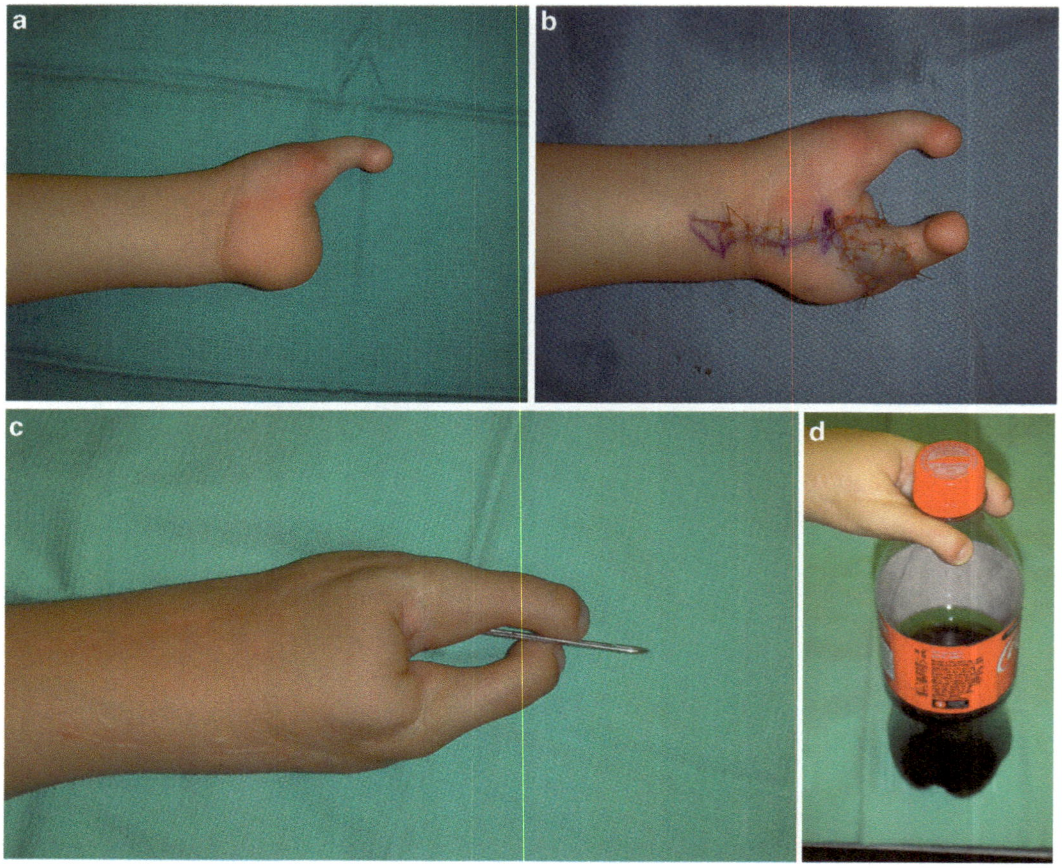

Fig. 11.19 The child underwent staged second toe transfers, firstly into the thumb position (**a**) and 6 months later into the small finger position (**b**). Six years postoperatively, the child demonstrates excellent ability to pick up small objects by side-to-side pinch between the two second toe transfers (**c**) and strong grasp to lift up a heavy bottle (**d**).

Once dissection of the foot has been completed, the tourniquet is released allowing reperfusion of the toe. After satisfactory perfusion of the toe on a single artery and vein is confirmed, the artery and vein are then ligated. The foot wound is closed primarily after repair of the intermetatarsal ligament. Skin grafting may be required to close the donor site if a great toe is harvested. A posterior splint is applied to the foot and leg.

The toe is then transferred to the previously dissected incision in the hand. Resection of the metatarsal is performed to achieve the correct length of the toe in either the thumb or finger position. If the toe is being used to reconstruct the thumb, the toe is rotated 120°. Bony fixation can be performed with 90–90 interosseous wires, K wires, or plates and screws, but special care should be taken to avoid injury to the epiphyseal plate. The flexor and extensor tendons are repaired. Tendon grafts may be required, especially in reconstruction of aplastic hands. The digital nerves of the toe transfer are coapted to appropriate digital nerves in the hand. Nerve grafts or even nerve transfers may be necessary. A branch of the deep peroneal nerve may be coapted to a branch of the superficial radial nerve. Finally the arterial and venous anastomoses are performed under the operating microscope using standard microsurgical techniques using 10–0 microsutures. Vascular anastomoses are typically end-to-end but end-to-side anastomoses can also be used.

The hand is then dressed in a large bulky dressing with a portion of the transferred toe left visible for clinical observation. Vascular checks including color and capillary refill are performed every hour by the nursing staff. A variety of objective monitoring techniques of digital perfusion including surface temperature, tissue pH, transcutaneous PO_2, and laser Doppler flowmetry have been proposed but the senior author uses a continuous oxygen saturation probe (pediatric pulse oximetry). Continuous differential pulse oximetry seems to be superior to laser Doppler flowmetry and surface temperature measurement [68] and allows almost immediate detection of thrombosis of either the arterial or venous anastomoses. Intravenous dextran-40 is used for 5 days postoperatively and the child is maintained on aspirin for 1 month postoperatively. The child is typically discharged on postoperative day 7.

Outcomes

Jones and Kaplan [69] compared 15 children who underwent microsurgical toe-to-hand transfers, 12 of whom had congenital hand differences, to age-matched children using the Pediatric Outcomes Data Collection Instrument (PODCI). The PODCI is an 86-question survey that evaluates six dimensions including upper extremity function, basic mobility and transfers, sports and physical function, pain and comfort, happiness, and global function. In this study, survey results from 15 parents, 10 adolescents, and normative data for age-matched children were compared. There was no statistically significant difference between the toe transfer patients and the normal pediatric population in 13 of the 18 groups. The adolescents' scores were significantly lower in upper extremity function and transfer/mobility, but adolescents self-reported higher scores than their parents in sports/physical function and happiness. The toe transfer adolescents also reported a significantly higher level of happiness than the general pediatric population.

Summary

It is difficult to prove definitively the superiority of microsurgical toe-to-hand transfers over other more conventional reconstructive techniques, but it is impossible to deny the satisfaction of seeing a child make normal use of a hand reconstructed with toe-to-hand transfers.

References

1. Flatt AE. The care of congenital hand anomalies. St. Louis: Mosby; 1977.
2. Swanson AB. A classification for congenital limb malformations. J Hand Surg Am. 1976;1(1):8–22.
3. Kay HW, Day HJ, Henkel HL, Kruger LM, Lamb DW, Marquardt E, et al. The proposed international terminology for the classification of congenital limb deficiencies. Dev Med Child Neurol Suppl. 1975;34:1–12.
4. Manske PR, Oberg KC. Classification and developmental biology of congenital anomalies of the hand and upper extremity. J Bone Joint Surg Am. 2009;91 Suppl 4:3–18.
5. Oberg KC, Feenstra JM, Manske PR, Tonkin MA. Developmental biology and classification of congenital anomalies of the hand and upper extremity. J Hand Surg Am. 2010;35(12):2066–76.
6. Tonkin MA, Tolerton SK, Quick TJ, Harvey I, Lawson RD, Smith NC, Oberg KC. Classification of congenital anomalies of the hand and upper limb: development and assessment of a new system. J Hand Surg Am. 2013;38(9):1845–53.
7. Pol R. 'Brachydaktylie'—'Klinodaktylie'—Hyperphalangie und ihre Grundlagen: Form und Entstehung der meist unter dem Bild der Brachydaktylie auftretenden Variet¨aten, Anomalien und Mißbildungen der Hand und des Fußes. Virchows Arch Pathol Anat. 1921;229:388–530.
8. Blauth W, Gekeler J. Morphology and classification of symbrachydactylia. Handchirurgie. 1971;3(4):123–8.
9. Sugiura Y, Kaneko M, Kataoka O, Nagira F, Ueke T, Tajima T, Asai T. Bone changes of unknown etiology affecting phalanges of fingers in children: report of eight cases. Pediatr Radiol. 1976;4(4):243–50.
10. Ogino T, Minami A, Kato H. Clinical features and roentgenograms of symbrachydactyly. J Hand Surg Br. 1989;14:303–6.
11. Yamauchi Y. Symbrachydactyly in Buck-Gramcko D (ed): Congenital malformations of the hand and forearm. London: Churchill Livingstone; 1998. p. 149–57.
12. Jones NF, Kaplan J. A new documentation system for congenital absent digits. Hand. 2012;7(4):391–9.
13. Buck-Gramcko D. Symbrachydactyly: a clinical entity. Tech Hand Up Extrem Surg. 1999;3:242–58.
14. Buck-Gramcko D. Cleft hands: classification and treatment. Hand Clin. 1985;1:467–73.
15. Manske PR. Symbrachydactyly instead of atypical cleft hand. Plast Reconstr Surg. 1993;91:196.
16. Kay SP, McCombe DB, Kozin SH. Deformities of the hand and fingers. In: Wolfe SW, Pederson WC, Hotchkiss RN, Kozin SH, editors. Green's operative hand surgery. 6th ed. Philadelphia: Churchill Livingstone; 2010. p. 1303–69.
17. Swanson AB, Swanson GD, Tada K. A classification for congenital limb malformation. J Hand Surg Am. 1983;8(5 Pt 2):693–702.
18. Patterson RW, Seitz Jr WH. Nonvascularized toe phalangeal transfer and distraction lengthening for symbrachydactyly. J Hand Surg Am. 2010;35(4):652–8.
19. Kallemeier PM, Manske PR, Davis B, Goldfarb CA. An assessment of the relationship between congenital transverse deficiency of the forearm and symbrachydactyly. J Hand Surg Am. 2007;32(9):1408–12.
20. Miura T, Suzuki M. Clinical differences between typical and atypical cleft hand. J Hand Surg Br. 1984;9(3):311–5.
21. Ogino T. Clinical features and teratogenic mechanisms of congenital absence of digits. Dev Growth Differ. 2007;49(6):523–31.
22. Knight JB, Pritsch T, Ezaki M, Oishi SN. Unilateral congenital terminal finger absences: a condition that differs from symbrachydactyly. J Hand Surg Am. 2012;37(1):124–9.
23. Bavinck JN, Weaver DD. Subclavian artery supply disruption sequence: hypothesis of a vascular etiology for Poland, Klippel-Feil, and Möbius anomalies. Am J Med Genet. 1986;23(4):903–18.
24. Kanauchi Y, Takahara M, Harada M, Ogino T. Growth of severely hypoplastic phalanges and metacarpals in symbrachydactyly: an experimental study in mice. J Hand Surg Am. 2008;33(9):1589–96.
25. Wolff H. Diskussion zu Lexer: Gelenktransplantation. Verhandlungender Deutschen Gesellschaft für Chirurgie, 39. Kongress, Berlin: 105; 1910.
26. Wolff H. Auswechselung von Finger und Zehenknochen: Beitrag zur Autoplastik. Münchener Medizinische Wochenschrift. 1911; 58:578.
27. Entin MA. Reconstruction of congenital abnormalities of the upper extremities. J Bone Joint Surg Am. 1959;41-A(4):681–701.
28. Carroll RE, Green DP. Proceedings of the American Society for Surgery of the Hand. J Bone Joint Surg Am. 1975;57-A(5):727.
29. Goldberg NH, Watson HK. Composite toe (phalanx and epiphysis) transfers in the reconstruction of the aphalangic hand. J Hand Surg Am. 1982;7(5):454–9.
30. Buck-Gramcko D, Pereira JA. Proximal toe phalanx transplantation for bony stabilization and lengthening of partially aplastic digits. Ann Chir Main Memb Super. 1990;9(2):107–18.
31. Radocha RF, Netscher D, Kleinert HE. Toe phalangeal grafts in congenital hand anomalies. J Hand Surg Am. 1993;18(5):833–41.
32. Cavallo AV, Smith PJ, Morley S, Morsi AW. Non-vascularized free toe phalanx transfers in congenital hand deformities—the Great Ormond Street experience. J Hand Surg Br. 2003;28(6):520–7.

33. Gohla T, Metz C, Lanz U. Non-vascularized free toe phalanx transplantation in the treatment of symbrachydactyly and constriction ring syndrome. J Hand Surg Br. 2005;30(5):446–51.
34. Unglaub F, Lanz U, Hahn P. Outcome analysis, including patient and parental satisfaction, regarding nonvascularized free toe phalanx transfer in congenital hand deformities. Ann Plast Surg. 2006;56(1):87–92.
35. Bourke G, Kay SP. Free phalangeal transfer: donor-site outcome. Br J Plast Surg. 2002;55(4):307–11.
36. Garagnani L, Gibson M, Smith PJ, Smith GD. Long-term donor site morbidity after free nonvascularized toe phalangeal transfer. J Hand Surg Am. 2012;37(4):764–74.
37. Jones NF. Nonvascularized toe phalangeal bone grafts for congenital anomalies of the hand. J Am Soc Surg Hand. 2004;4(1):27–34.
38. Netscher DT, Richards WT. Rational treatment for multiple digit congenital absence: case report of nonvascularized toe phalangeal transfers and distraction lengthening for symbrachydactyly. Ann Plast Surg. 2006;56(2):211–5.
39. Codivilla A. On the means of lengthening, in the lower limbs, the muscles and tissues which are shortened through deformity. J Bone Joint Surg Am. 1905;s2-2:353–69.
40. Matev IB. Thumb reconstruction after amputation at the metacarpophalangeal joint by bone lengthening. J Bone Joint Surg. 1970;52A:957–65.
41. Kessler I, Baruch A, Hecht O. Experience with distraction lengthening of digital rays in congenital anomalies. J Hand Surg Am. 1977;2(5):394–401.
42. Wenner SM. Angulation occurring during the distraction lengthening of digits. Orthop Rev. 1986;15(3):177–9.
43. Seitz Jr WH, Froimson AI. Callotasis lengthening in the upper extremity: indications, techniques, and pitfalls. J Hand Surg Am. 1991;16(5):932–9.
44. Seitz Jr WH, Froimson AI. Digital lengthening using the callotasis technique. Orthopedics. 1995;18(2):129–38.
45. Ogino T, Kato H, Ishii S, Usui M. Digital lengthening in congenital hand deformities. J Hand Surg Br. 1994;19(1):120–9.
46. Pensler JM, Carroll NC, Cheng LF. Distraction osteogenesis in the hand. Plast Reconstr Surg. 1998;102(1):92–5.
47. Hülsbergen-Krüger S, Preisser P, Partecke BD. Ilizarov distraction-lengthening in congenital anomalies of the upper limb. J Hand Surg Br. 1998;23(2):192–5.
48. Dhalla R, Strecker W, Manske PR. A comparison of two techniques for digital distraction lengthening in skeletally immature patients. J Hand Surg Am. 2001;26(4):603–10.
49. Miyawaki T, Masuzawa G, Hirakawa M, Kurihara K. Bone-lengthening for symbrachydactyly of the hand with the technique of callus distraction. J Bone Joint Surg Am. 2002;84-A(6):986–91.
50. Matsuno T, Ishida O, Sunagawa T, Ichikawa M, Ikuta Y, Ochi M. Bone lengthening for congenital differences of the hands and digits in children. J Hand Surg Am. 2004;29(4):712–9.
51. Seitz Jr WH, Shimko P, Patterson RW. Long-term results of callus distraction-lengthening in the hand and upper extremity for traumatic and congenital skeletal deficiencies. J Bone Joint Surg Am. 2010;92 Suppl 2:47–58.
52. O'Brien BM, Black MJ, Morrison WA, MacLeod AM. Microvascular great toe transfer for congenital absence of the thumb. Hand. 1978;10(2):113–24.
53. Gilbert A. Toe transfers for congenital hand defects. J Hand Surg Am. 1982;7(2):118–24.
54. Gilbert A. Reconstruction of congenital hand defects with microvascular toe transfers. Hand Clin. 1985;1(2):351–60.
55. Lister G. Microsurgical transfer of the second toe for congenital deficiency of the thumb. Plast Reconstr Surg. 1988;82(4): 658–65.
56. Shvedovchenko IV. Toe-to-hand transfers in children. Ann Plast Surg. 1993;31(3):251–4.
57. Vilkki SK. Advances in microsurgical reconstruction of the congenitally adactylous hand. Clin Orthop Relat Res. 1995;314: 45–58.
58. Kay SP, Wiberg M. Toe to hand transfer in children. Part 1: technical aspects. J Hand Surg Br. 1996;21(6):723–34.
59. Van Holder C, Giele H, Gilbert A. Double second toe transfer in congenital hand anomalies. J Hand Surg Br. 1999;24(4):471–5.
60. Foucher G, Medina J, Navarro R, Nagel D. Toe transfer in congenital hand malformations. J Reconstr Microsurg. 2001; 17(1):1–7.
61. Richardson PW, Johnstone BR, Coombs CJ. Toe-to-hand transfer in symbrachydactyly. Hand Surg. 2004;9(1):11–8.
62. Jones NF, Hansen SL, Bates SJ. Toe-to-hand transfers for congenital anomalies of the hand. Hand Clin. 2007;23(1):129–36.
63. Jones NF, Kaplan J. Indications for microsurgical reconstruction of congenital hand anomalies by toe-to-hand transfers. Hand. 2013; 8:367–74.
64. Wei FC, Chen HC, Chuang CC, Noordhoff MS. Reconstruction of the thumb with a trimmed-toe transfer technique. Plast Reconstr Surg. 1988;82(3):506–15.
65. Chang J, Jones NF. Simultaneous toe-to-hand transfer and lower extremity amputations for severe upper and lower limb defects: the use of spare parts. J Hand Surg Br. 2002;27(3):219–23.
66. Lister G. Reconstruction of the hypoplastic thumb. Clin Orthop Relat Res. 1985;195:52–65.
67. Villen GM, Julve GG. The arterial system of the first intermetatarsal space and its influence in toe-to-hand transfer: a report of 53 long-pedicle transfers. J Hand Surg. 2002;27B:73–7.
68. Jones NF, Gupta R. Postoperative monitoring of pediatric toe-to-hand transfers with differential pulse oximetry. J Hand Surg Am. 2001;26(3):525–9.
69. Kaplan JD, Jones NF. Outcome measures of microsurgical toe transfers for reconstruction of congenital and traumatic hand anomalies. J Pediatr Orthop. 2014;34(3):362–8.

Dorsal–Ventral Deficiency

12

Mohammad M. Al-Qattan

Introduction

The limb bud develops into an upper limb by complex interactions between the ectoderm and mesoderm. There are three axes of limb development: the proximal-distal axis mediates the outgrowth of the limb, the anterior-posterior axis mediates the differentiation of radial and ulnar elements of the forearm/hand, and the dorsal–ventral axis mediates the differentiation of dorsal and ventral structures in the hand only [1]. Differentiation of dorsal–ventral structures in the arm and forearm also occurs but the mediators for such a differentiation are yet to be identified. This chapter deals with dorsal–ventral abnormalities within the hand only.

Embryology of the Dorsal–Ventral Axis of Development

Figure 12.1 shows a cross section of the limb bud. The ventral ectoderm expresses the transcription factor "ENGRAILED 1" (EN-1). EN-1 is essential for the normal development of ventral structures in the hand such as the thick hairless palmar skin, the pulp of the fingers, the palmar creases, and the flexor tendons. EN-1 will also restrict the "wingless" protein WNT7A to the dorsal ectoderm. Ectodermal WNT7A will induce the expression of a "LIM" transcription factor called LMX1B in the dorsal mesoderm. The normal expression of WNT7A and LMX1B in the dorsal ectoderm and mesoderm, respectively, leads to the normal development of dorsal structures of the hand such as the nails, the thin hairy dorsal skin, and the extensor tendons. WNT7A also acts as a "maintainer" of Sonic Hedgehog (SHH) activity within the zone of polarizing activity in the posterior mesoderm [2]. SHH is the key modulator of the anterior-posterior axis including the development of the ulnar ray and the induction of fibroblast growth factor 4 (FGF4) in the nearby posterior part of the apical ectodermal ridge (AER). FGF4 helps the ectodermal FGF8 to maintain the outgrowth of the limb along the proximal-distal axis; and FGF4 also helps to maintain SHH activity. This reciprocal relationship between SHH and FGF4 is known as the SHH-FGF4 loop [3, 4]. In other words, the two key proteins of the dorsal–ventral axis (EN-1 and WNT7A) interact with each other as well as with the mesoderm (via LMX1B induction). The dorsal–ventral axis also interacts with the anterior-posterior axis (via SHH maintenance) and the proximal-distal axis (via the SHH-FGF4 loop). EN-1 also contributes to the induction of the AER.

The ENGRAILED-1 Pathway and Dorsal Dimelia

Al-Qattan [2] defined the ENGRAILED-1 pathway (Fig. 12.2). In this pathway, EN-1 is a "transcription factor." In other words, it is expressed following the action of a "ligand" on a "receptor." The "ligands" are Bone Morphogenetic Proteins 4 and 7 (BMP4, 7) that act on the receptor BMPR1A. This results in the expression of EN-1 in the ventral ectoderm. EN-1 will have three main functions: induction of the AER, development of ventral structures of the hand, and restriction of WNT7A to the dorsal ectoderm. Disruption of this pathway will result in the lack of EN-1 functional expression in the ventral ectoderm. Ventral structures will not develop; and the unrestricted WNT7A will be expressed in the dorsal as well as the ventral ectoderm. Ectopic ventral WNT7A will induce the ectopic expression of LMX1B in the ventral mesoderm. The end result is "dorsal dimelia," which is a hand with dorsal structures on the ventral aspect.

M.M. Al-Qattan, M.B.B.S. (✉)
Department of Surgery, King Saud University, Riyadh, Saudi Arabia
e-mail: moqattan@hotmail.com

D.R. Laub Jr. (ed.), *Congenital Anomalies of the Upper Extremity: Etiology and Management*, DOI 10.1007/978-1-4899-7504-1_12, © Springer Science+Business Media New York 2015

Dorsal Dimelia in Experimental Animals

Experimental dorsal dimelia is induced by disruption of the EN-1 pathway. It is important to note that these animals will show dorsal dimelia of all digits in the fore- and hind-feet. In other words, each digit will show a double nail: one normal dorsal nail and another ectopic ventral nail. Experimental dorsal dimelia was induced in *Bmpr1a* conditional knockout animals [6], null mutations of *En-1* [7], mis-expression of *Wnt7a* in the ventral ectoderm [8], and mis-expression of *Lmx1b* in the ventral mesoderm [9].

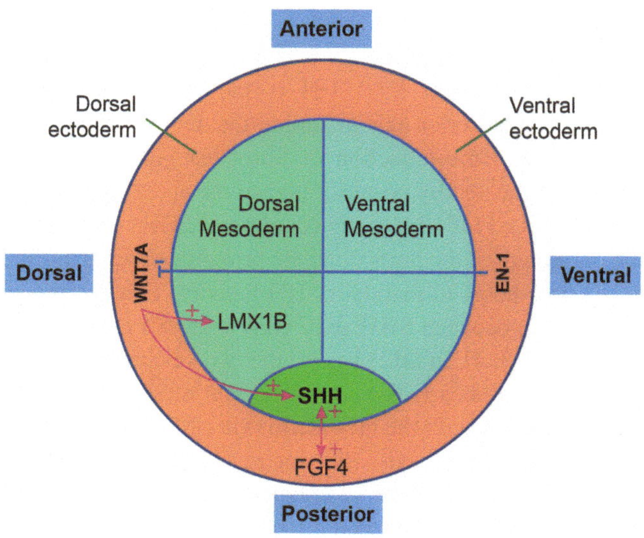

Fig. 12.1 A cross section of limb a bud showing the interactions of the two key players of the dorsal–ventral axis: EN-1 (ENGRAILED-1) and WNT7A

Dorsal Dimelia in Humans

Dorsal dimelia in humans may be classified into two main groups: distal dorsal dimelia and proximal dorsal dimelia [10].

Proximal Dorsal Dimelia in Humans

Al-Qattan et al. [11] described one Egyptian family with isolated dorsalization of the skin of the proximal palm and the instep of the sole of the foot. Inheritance was autosomal dominant. Fingers and toes were completely normal. Hand function and gait were also normal. The proximal palm had a subcutaneous hamartoma with hyperpigmented hairy skin. Linkage analysis/exome sequencing showed an R584w variant in the *GLE1* gene. *GLE1* is involved in mRNA export; and RNA in situ hybridization showed a high *Gle-1* expression in mouse embryo ventral cells and somites.

Distal Dorsal Dimelia in Humans

Distal dorsal dimelia is characterized by dorsalization of the distal palm and digits [12]. When fully expressed, the digit will have an ectopic palmar nail (the palmar and dorsal nails meet at the tip) (Fig. 12.3), the palmar skin of the digit and distal palm will show thin hyperpigmented skin, digital flexion is lacking, and the X-ray will show a tapering distal phalanx. The fully expressed phenotype is also known in the literature as “congenital palmar nail syndrome” [13, 14]. This fully expressed phenotype has amazing resemblance to the conjoined nail of Siamese “tripus” twins [15]. The twins have three lower limbs (hence the term tripus). Each twin has one normal lower limb on one side of the body. On the other side, the two adjacent lower limbs are fused into one. The conjoined feet will have eight separate toes, whereas the two

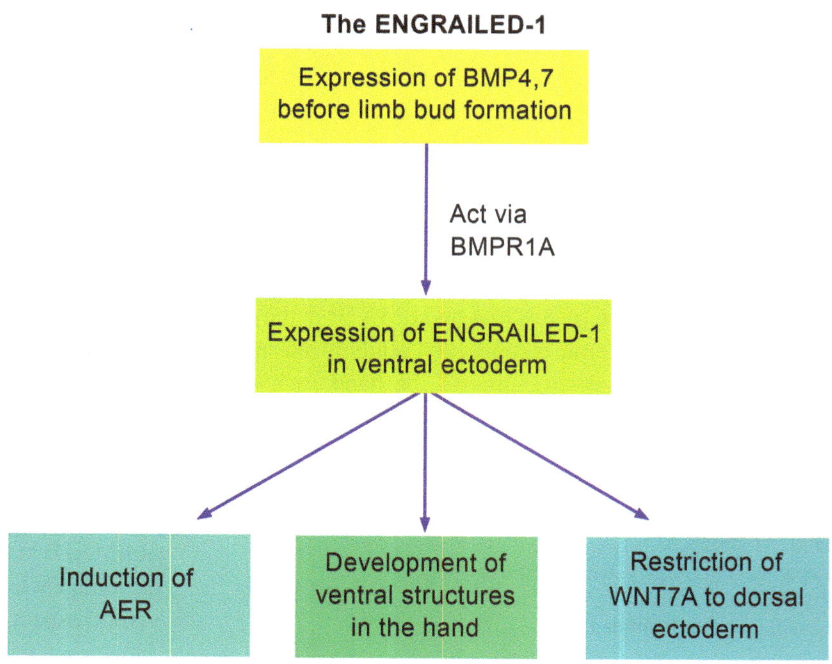

Fig. 12.2 The EN-1 pathway

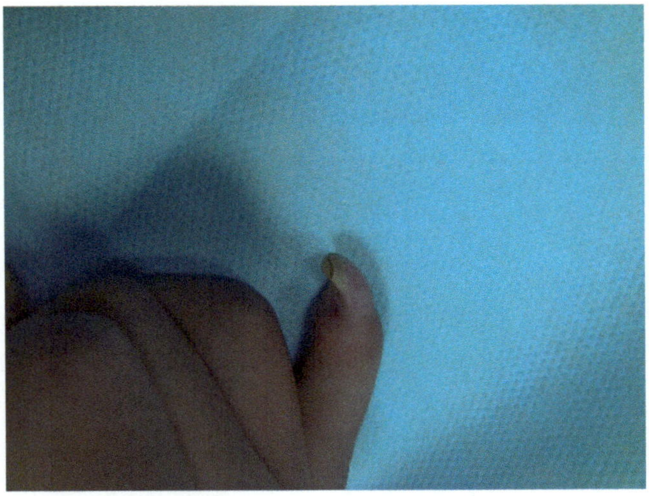

Fig. 12.3 Dorsal dimelia. Note the dorsal and ventral nails meeting at the tip of the little finger

big toes are fused into one digit. This digit will have all the features of "palmar nail syndrome."

Al-Qattan et al. [5] stressed that the clinical picture of distal dorsal dimelia in humans may not always be fully expressed. Hence, some cases may have isolated palmar nail while others may have isolated dorsalization of the palmar skin.

Al-Qattan and Kfoury [12] reviewed all cases of distal dorsal dimelia in humans and categorized them into three groups: syndromic, familial, and sporadic. Bilateral little finger dimelia has been described in syndromic patients with partial deletion the long arm of chromosome 6 [16] and Patau syndrome (trisomy 13) [17]. One case with *DLX5* mutation and split-hand–split-foot malformation (also known as lobster-claw deformity) had dorsal dimelia of all digits [18]. The latter is the only human case with involvement of all digits. In all other human cases, dorsal dimelia involves either the ulnar or radial digits. Familial cases may have a family history of dorsal dimelia [19, 20] or ulnar ray deficiency [13, 21]. This is interesting because it links dorsal dimelia to SHH activity. In fact, several sporadic cases occurred in patients with ulnar ray deficiency [22, 23] or ulnar-sided cleft hand [5, 10, 24]. As expected, all these patients with ulnar defects showed dorsal dimelia in the ulnar digits.

However, several sporadic cases involving the ulnar digits occurred in patients with negative family history and no other concurrent anomalies [25–28]. Al-Qattan et al. [5] screened several sporadic cases with dorsal dimelia involving the ulnar digits for candidate genes such as loss-of-function mutations of BMP4, *BMP7*, *BMPR1A*, and *EN-1*, as well as gain-of-function mutations of *WNT7A* and *LMX1B*. However, the genetic analysis did not show any mutations. It was concluded that sporadic dorsal dimelia is probably a stochastic developmental error that is commonly seen with other concurrent hand malformations. In support of the latter statement, the author reported 3 cases of dorsal dimelia involving the radial digits; and in all cases there was radial-sided malformations such as thumb polydactyly [12], or radial ray deficiency [29, 30].

Management of Dorsal Dimelia

Proximal dorsal dimelia requires no treatment. In contrast, patients with distal dorsal dimelia may have cosmetic (the palmar nail) and functional (the lack of flexion) concerns. Options of management include conservative treatment (observation only) or surgery in the form of excision of the palmar nail along with pulp reconstruction or amputation of the distal phalanx [28]. Affected digits are usually held in extension with no active or passive flexion because of symphalangism. Osteotomy and fixation of the proximal interphalangeal joint in a more functional position is an option but no such procedure has been reported in the literature in patients with dorsal dimelia.

Dorsal dimelia of the index finger may occur in patients with absent thumb [29]. This poses a problem when there is need to pollicize the affected index finger. Anatomically, the affected finger has cartilaginous symphalangism of the interphalangeal joints. There is also a mirror-image flat extensor tendon on the palmar and dorsal aspects of the finger with no intrinsic muscle attachments. More important, there are two neurovascular bundles: one dorsal and one palmar. Al-Qattan and Kfoury reported these anatomical findings in a patient who had amputation of a duplicated digit with dorsal dimelia [12]; and these findings have obvious implications in the pollicization procedure.

The WNT7A Pathway and Ventral Dimelia

Figure 12.4 shows the WNT7A pathway. WNT7A (which is normally expressed in the dorsal ectoderm) acts at the cellular level by stimulation of specific receptors and the activation of two different pathways [2]: the calcium-mediated pathway and the beta-catenin (canonical) pathway. The former pathway leads to the expression of LMX1B in the dorsal mesoderm that will result in the normal development of dorsal structures in the hand. The latter pathway is responsible for maintaining SHH activity. As mentioned before, SHH is responsible for the development of the ulnar ray and the induction of FGF4 in the posterior part of the AER. The beta-catenin pathway also maintains the expression of another protein called ISLET 1. ISLET 1 is a major contributor to the initiation/outgrowth of the vertebrate hind limb and pelvis [31].

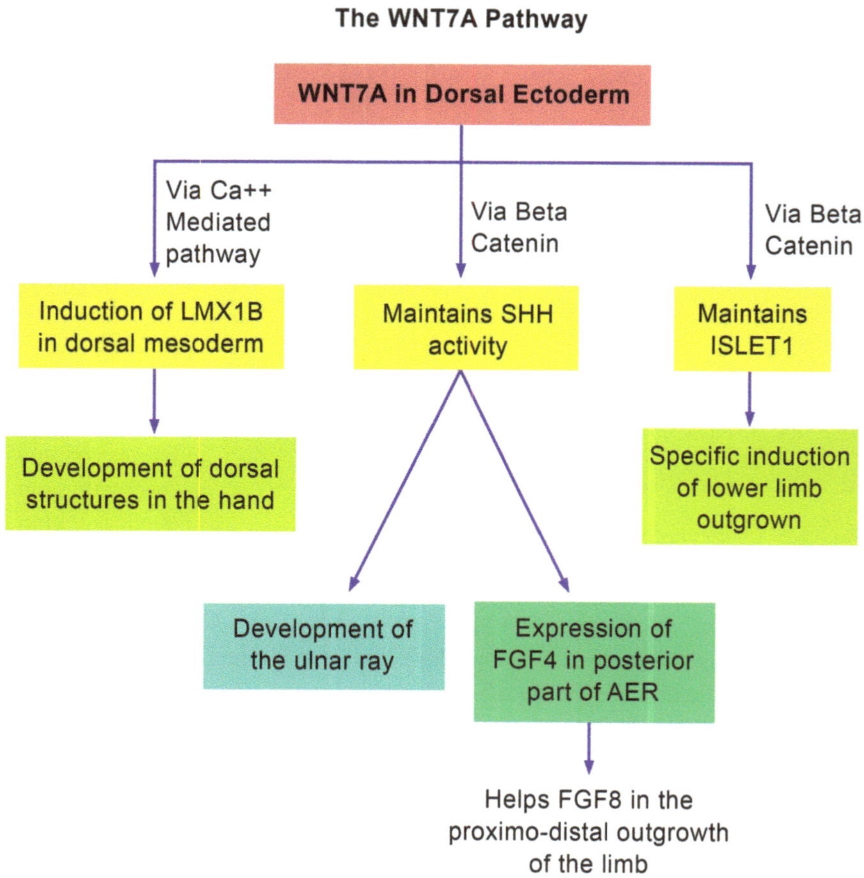

Fig. 12.4 The WNT7A pathway

Looking at the WNT7A pathway, one can speculate the phenotypes of syndromes associated with loss-of-function mutations of *WNT7A*: (1) the loss of LMX1B will result in ventralization of the dorsum of the hand; (2) the loss of SHH activity will result in a variable degree of ulnar ray deficiency as well as short upper limbs; and (3) the loss of ISLET1 maintenance will result in truncated lower limbs and pelvic dysplasia. The end result is a triad of ventral dimelia, ulnar ray deficiency, and truncated lower limbs.

Ventral Dimelia in Experimental Animals

Parr and McMahon [32] studied the effects of loss of function of *Wnt7a* in mice. The knockout mouse models showed ventral dimelia and ulnar ray deficiency but without truncation of the hind limbs. This may indicate that Wnt7A (beta-catenin)–ISLET 1 interactions are more functional in humans than mice.

Ventral Dimelia in Humans

Al-Qattan [10] classified ventral dimelia into three groups according to the severity of the phenotype. The classification was supported by the genetic basis of each group. The mildest phenotype is the nail-patella syndrome that is caused by *LMX1B* mutations. Features of nail-patella syndrome include hypoplastic/aplastic nails, absent patella, and renal defects. The second group has partial loss-of-function mutations of *WNT7A* leading the triad of ventral dimelia, mild ulnar ray deficiency, and truncated lower limbs. In the genetics literature, this is known as Fuhrmann syndrome. Two *WNT7A* mutations are known to be associated with the Fuhrmann phenotype: the R222W [33] and the A109T [34] mutations. The third group has complete loss of function of *WNT7A*; and as expected, this group has the most severe phenotype: severe ventral dimelia, severe ulnar ray deficiency, and frequently absent lower limbs. In the genetics literature, this severe phenotype is known as Al-Awadi syndrome. Three *WNT7A* mutations are known to be associated with Al-Awadi syndrome: the E72K [35], the R292C [34], and the G204S [36, 37] mutations (Fig. 12.5).

Management of Ventral Dimelia

The hand function in nail-patella syndrome is excellent and requires no specific treatment. In Fuhrmann syndrome, the ulnar ray deficiency is mild and hence poses no functional

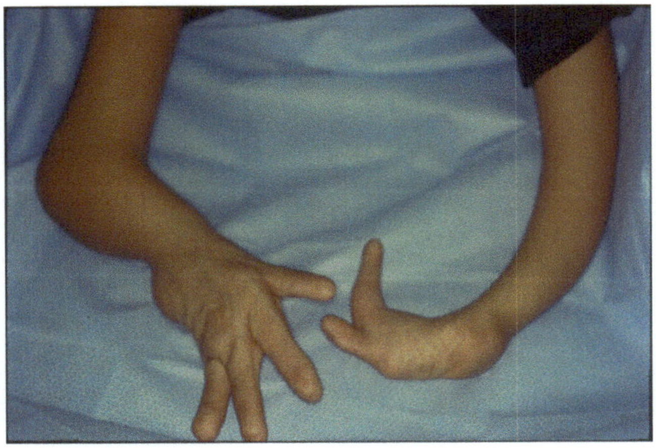

Fig. 12.5 Ventral dimelia. Note the absent nails and the variable degrees of ulnar ray deficiency. The lower limbs are truncated at the knees

problems. The main problem is the lack of interphalangeal joint flexion. However, patients manage very well in daily activities. In Al-Awadi syndrome, the ulnar ray deficiency is severe and should be treated accordingly with special attention to thumb/first web space reconstruction. These patients also frequently have radio-humeral synostosis and may have hand-in-flank deformity and hence osteotomies are indicated [38, 39]. The severe lower limb deficits in both Fuhrmann and Al-Awadi syndromes make rehabilitation of the limb/limbs an essential part of the management.

Acknowledgement The College of Medicine Research Center, Deanship of Scientific Research, King Saud University, Riyadh, Saudi Arabia, supported research by the author on the topic.

References

1. Al-Qattan MM, Yang Y, Kozin SH. Embryology of the upper limb. J Hand Surg Am. 2009;34:1340–50.
2. Al-Qattan MM. WNT pathways and upper limb anomalies. J Hand Surg Eur. 2011;36:9–22.
3. Laufer E, Nelson CE, Johnson RL, Morgan BA, Tabin C. Sonic hedgehog and Fgf-4 act through a signaling cascade and feedback to integrate growth and patterning of the development of limb bud. Cell. 1994;79:993–1003.
4. Niswander L, Jeffrey S, Martin GR, Tickle C. A positive feedback loop coordinates growth and patterning in the vertebrate limb. Nature. 1994;37:609–12.
5. Al-Qattan MM, Al-Mazyed M, Shamseldin H, Al-Kuraya FS. Dorsal dimelia: report of two cases with an emphasis on the variation of phenotype expression and a search for candidate genes. J Hand Surg Eur. 2010;35:715–20.
6. Ahn K, Mishina Y, Hanks MC, Behringer RR, Crenshaw EB. BMPR-1A signaling is required for the formation of the apical ectodermal ridge dorsal-ventral patterning of the limb. Development. 2001;128:4449–61.
7. Loomis CA, Harris E, Michand J, Wurst W, Hanks M, Jayver A. The mouse engrailed-1 gene and ventral limb patterning. Nature. 1996;382:360–3.
8. Riddle R, Ensini M, Nelson C, Tsuchida T, Jessel TM, Tabin C. Induction of the LIM homeobox gene Lmx1 by wnt7a establishes dorsal ventral pattern in the vertebrate limb. Cell. 1995;83:631–40.
9. Vogel A, Rodriguez C, Warnken W, Izpisna-Belmonte JC. Dorsal cell fate specified by chick Lmx1 during vertebrate limb development. Nature. 1995;387:716–20.
10. Al-Qattan MM. Classification of dorsal and ventral dimelia in humans. J Hand Surg Eur. 2013;38(9):928–33. doi:10.1177/1753193413484671 [Epub ahead of print].
11. Al-Qattan MM, Shamseldin HE, Al-Kuraya FS. Familial dorsalization of the skin of the proximal palm and the instep of the sole of the foot. Gene. 2012;500:216–9.
12. Al-Qattan MM, Kfoury H. Dorsal dimelia of a thumb. J Plast Reconstr Aesthet Surg. 2011;64:e177–80.
13. Rider MA. Congenital palmar nail syndrome. J Hand Surg Br. 1992;17:371–2.
14. Al-Qattan MM, Hassanain J, Hawary MB. Congenital palmar nail syndrome. J Hand Surg Br. 1997;22 674–5.
15. Al-Qattan MM, Al-Rabeeah A. Similarities between a conjoined nail and the palmar nail syndrome. J Hand Surg Br. 2000;25:8–10.
16. Kalisman M, Goldferg R, Ship AG. Dorsal skin and fingernail on the volar aspect of the hand: an unusual anatomic deformity. Plast Reconstr Surg. 1982;69:694–6.
17. Fattah A, Pickford MA. Dorsal dimelia in patau syndrome: a case report. J Hand Surg Eur. 2007;32:534–6.
18. Shamseldin HE, Faden MA, Al-Ashram W, Al-Kuraya FS. Identification of a novel DLXS mutation in a family with autosomal recessive split hand and foot malformation. J Med Genet. 2012;49:16–20.
19. Egawa T. Congenital claw-like fingers and toes. Case report of two siblings. Plast Reconstr Surg. 1977;59:569–72.
20. Miura T. Two families with congenital nail anomalies: nail formation in ectopic areas. J Hand Surg Am. 1978;3:348–51.
21. Corona-Rivera JR, Corona-Rivera E, Fragoso-Herrera R, Nuno-Arana I, Loera-Castaneda V. Probable new syndrome in a Mexican family with congenital palmar polyonychia and post-axial limb defects. Am J Med Genet A. 2004;125:205–9.
22. Alves GF, Poon E, Joh J, Salamao PR, Griffiths WA. Circumferential finger nail. Br J Dermatol. 1999;140:960–2.
23. Kiryu M, Huzita S, Saitou O. Congenital hypoplasia of the little finger associated with nail anomaly. Jpn J Plast Reconstr Surg. 1978;21:216–21.
24. Miura T. Cleft hand involving only the ring and small fingers. J Hand Surg Am. 1988;13:530–5.
25. Keret D, Ger E. Double fingernails on the small fingers. J Hand Surg Am. 1987;12:608–10.
26. Kikuchi I, Ono T, Ogata K. Ectopic nail: case reports. Plast Reconstr Surg. 1978;61:781–3.
27. Kinoshita Y, Kojima T, Uchida M, Kurimoto S. Calm nail deformity of the little finger. Plast Reconstr Surg. 1993;91:158–61.
28. Thoma A, Alexopoulou I. Circumferential little finger nail plate. Can J Plast Surg. 1995;3:161–2.
29. Al-Qattan MM. Dorsal dimelia of the index finger in a patient with absent thumb and radial club hand. Ann Plast Surg. 2011;67:90–1.
30. Al-Qattan MM. Fanconi anemia with concurrent thumb polydactyly and dorsal dimelia. A case report with discussion of embryology. Ann Plast Surg. 2013;70:116–8.
31. Kawakami Y, Marti M, Kawakami H, Itou J, Quach T, Johnson A, et al. Islet 1 mediated activation of the ß-catenin pathway is necessary for hind limb initiation in mice. Development. 2011;138:4465–73.
32. Parr BA, McMahon AP. Dorsalizing signal WNT7A required for normal polarity of D-V and A-F axes of mouse limb. Nature. 1995;374:350–3.

33. Kantaputra PN, Mundle S, Spirathomsawat W. A novel homozygous Arg 222 TRP missense mutation in WNT7A in two sisters with severe Al-Awadi/Raas-Rothschild/Schinzel phocomelia syndrome. Am J Med Genet A. 2010;152:2832–7.
34. Woods CG, Sticker S, Seeman P, Stern R, Cox J, Sherridan E, et al. Mutations in WNT7A cause a range of limb malformations, including Fuhrmann syndrome and Al-Awadi/Raas-Rothschild/Schinzel phocomelia syndrome. Am J Hum Genet. 2006;79:402–8.
35. Garavelli L, Wischeiyer A, Rosato S, Gelmini C, Reverberi S, Sassi S, et al. Al-Awadi-Raas-Rothschild (Limb/pelvis/uterus-hypoplasia/aplasia) syndrome and WNT7A mutations: genetic homogenecity and nasological delineation. Am J Med Genet A. 2011;155:332–6.
36. Al-Qattan MM, Al-Balwi M, Eyaid W, Al-Abdulkarim I, Al-Turki S. Congenital duplication of the palm syndrome: gene analysis and the molecular basis of its clinical features. J Hand Surg Eur. 2009;34:247–51.
37. Eyaid W, Al-Qattan MM, Fetaini N, Al Balwi M. A novel homozygous missense mutation (CGLOG>A, P.Gly 204 Ser) in the WNT7A gene causes tetra-amelia in two Saudi families. Am J Med Genet A. 2011;155:599–604.
38. Al-Qattan MM. Congenital duplication of the palm in a patient with multiple anomalies. J Hand Surg Br. 2003;28:276–9.
39. Al-Qattan MM, Eyaid W, Al-Balwi M. Congenital duplication of the palm syndrome. Ann Plast Surg. 2007;59:341–3.

Part III

Failure of Hand Plate Formation/Differentiation

13 Syndactyly

Daniel J. Jordan, Emma Snashall, and Sandip Hindocha

Epidemiology

Syndactyly is defined as the fusion of adjacent digits. The commonest of congenital hand deformities, it has an incidence of approximately 1 in 2,000 live births, is twice as common in males, as well as in the Caucasian population [1–4].

Syndactyly can involve union of the soft tissues only, but is also seen with varying amounts of bone involvement. It predominantly occurs due to the failure of differentiation between adjacent digits caused by the absence of programmed cell apoptosis in the interdigital mesenchyme, which normally occurs during the seventh and eighth weeks of gestation [1, 5]. In decreasing frequency the third, fourth, second, and first web spaces are affected, with around 57 % of cases occurring in the third web space [2, 3, 6]. The condition presents bilaterally in up to half of cases [2, 6].

Commonly presenting in a sporadic fashion, syndactyly involves a family history in 10–40 % of cases [2, 7]. Inheritance is thought to be through an autosomal dominant pattern with variable penetrance and expressivity, and this possibly explains the male predominance [1, 2].

Syndactyly can be found as an isolated finding or seen with other anomalies such as acrosyndactyly, clinodactyly, synostosis, cleft hand and polydactyly. It is also seen as part of congenital defect syndromes including Poland's, Pfeiffer, Holt–Oram, and Apert. The latter is discussed in detail in specific chapters elsewhere in this volume.

D.J. Jordan, M.B.Ch.B. • S. Hindocha, M.D., M.B.Ch.B. M.Phil, M.R.C.S. (✉)
Plastic Surgery, Whiston Hospital, Warrington Road, Liverpool L355DR, UK
e-mail: Jord_ls@Hotmail.Com; hindocha2001@yahoo.com

E. Snashall, M.B.ChB.
Burns and Plastic Reconstruction Unit, Whiston Hospital, Flat 1, 6 Parkfield Road, Aigburth, Liverpool L178UH, UK
e-mail: emmasnashall@googlemail.com

Development of the Human Limb

Before discussing the specifics related to each syndactyly, it is useful to understand how the malformation is believed to develop. The authors do not aim to explore the molecular biology of the human limb formation in detail, but aim to summarize the current findings in a systematic approach, discussing the multiple genes and vast number of encoding proteins which are so far believed to be key to vertebrate limb growth.

Control of Limb Growth

Arising from the main trunk, or body, the limb buds and consequent upper and lower limbs are formed between the fourth and eighth weeks of gestation. The limb bud is initially directed along three axes, along which the mesodermal cells grow and later become fixed. These axes include running along the shoulder to finger direction, the proximal-distal axis; the dorsal ventral axis, from the dorsum to the palm of the hand; and the anterior–posterior axis from thumb to little finger. The latter axis appears to be the most important in digit formation. The final and specific limb architecture resulting in the aesthetic limb normally involves cell proliferation, cell fate determination, cell differentiation, and apoptosis [8, 9].

The control of the human limb structure and positional identity appears to originate from two distinct signal centers: the apical ectodermal ridge (AER) which is key for limb growth and the zone of polarizing activity (ZPA) [10–12]. The ZPA appears to identify the position and overall patterning in relation to the anterior–posterior axis. Each center is dependent on the other [13].

By the 44th day the ZPA begins to regress, at which time the formation of the metacarpophalangeal joints and proximal phalanges begins. Chondrification of the middle phalanges occurs towards day 48, followed by the distal bones by day 51 and on day 54 digit separation has normally occurred.

D.R. Laub Jr. (ed.), *Congenital Anomalies of the Upper Extremity: Etiology and Management*,
DOI 10.1007/978-1-4899-7504-1_13, © Springer Science+Business Media New York 2015

Genetic and Molecular Pathways

Encoding proteins influence the processes described above. In particular, the hedgehog pathways, fibroblast growth factors (FGF), bone morphogenetic proteins (Bmp), and cartilage-derived morphogenetic protein have been found to be instrumental in relation to limb formation [14].

Syndactyly and polydactyly appear to both have a relationship with the Hedgehog (Hh) family of intercellular signalling proteins. These have a predominant function related to cell fate, with most research directed towards the Sonic hedgehog (Shh) pathway [15]. Shh has particular relevance as it is expressed in the ZPA overseeing anterior–posterior limb patterning [16]. In Mice, Shh appears to be a secreted molecule, related to the Drosophila Hh, which regulates the balance of Gli3 repressor and activator and through these its target genes.

Indian hedgehog (Ihh) is biologically akin to Shh and has been seen to play a key role in a pathway which is involved in regulating the rate of chondrocyte differentiation [17]. Ihh appears to be repressed by FGF receptor (FGFR) 3 [18, 19] and has been seen to play a role in bone ossification [20]. Multiple papers have suggested a role for the Ihh pathway, particularly in the later development of syndactyly as well as in other congenital abnormalities [21, 22].

The ZPA positioning, and its involvement with Shh, is determined in the main by transcription factors including dHand, Gli3, Alx4, and several Bmp antagonists, namely Formin and Gremlin. Changes involving any of these molecular components or pathways have been found to lead to -dactyly malformations (brachy-, syn-, and poly-) [23–27].

The FGF family (in particular FGF8) have been seen to influence the latter stages of mesenchymal ossification [28] and are discussed again later in the chapter. These growth factors are expressed at a similar time as members of the wingless-type MMTV integration site (WNT) family, which have a relationship with the region 2q35. This is a locus hypothesized as the source of syndactyly type 1 [29].

WNT6 and WNT10B have both been described as possible avenues of further research due to their expression in the developing mouse limb bud, as well as their role in cell apoptosis [30, 31]. Cell death along anterior, posterior, and finally interdigital necrotic zones leads to the familiar profile of the hand as the last stage of digit formation [32, 33]. This apoptotic period appears to coincide with restriction of FGF8 expression and downregulation of Gremlin in these regions [32, 34–37].

The number of phalanges has been shown to be influenced by several signalling molecules, including the Bmp's and their antagonist Noggin (Nog), all having a role in apoptosis [38–44]. Blockade of their signalling pathway has been shown to result in syndactyly [45–47].

The final digit distinctiveness appears dependant on the interdigital mesenchyme. Dahn and Fallon [48] found removal of this in chickens resulted in loss of digit identity, and it appears this is related to both the Shh and Gli3 pathways [23, 24]. Metalloproteases are similarly under scrutiny for their involvement in the formation of normal hand architecture, and appear to have a role independent of the Bmp for interdigital web regression [49].

Other areas requiring further research as they appear to induce soft tissue syndactyly in mice include N-Myc and several zinc finger transcription factors [50–52]. A recent study states a wide range of phenotypes can occur with only a Gli3 mutation, ranging from non-syndromic to syndromic syndactyly [53]. Also linked to digital anomalies are the Xq25 loci, with associated developmental delay [54] and defects in cholesterol metabolism [55]. ROR2 [56], nidogen [57], GAS [58], and MBOAT [59] genes have been shown to be related to limb and digit formation in animal and patient groups, likewise mutations in Jagged [60], Serrate [61], and MSX [62] genes appear to cause syndactyly amongst other congenital abnormalities.

Governing the end point in body patterning, are a whole host of transcription factors, all encoded by the Homeobox (HOX) gene family. Within the human genome, 39 HOX genes have so far been discovered which, as in most vertebrates, organize themselves into four clusters. These play an essential role in the development of the axial skeleton, central nervous system as well as the gastrointestinal and urogenital tracts, and our main interest, the limbs. Limb abnormalities have been seen with deletions of some of these HOX clusters (-A and -D) and in mutations affecting one or more HOX genes [63]. The specific HOX genes involved in syndactyly will be discussed in the non-syndromic section of this chapter.

Anatomical Classification

The classification of syndactyly is often described in respect to the anatomical findings. In this way, the syndactyly can be either simple or complex, and complete or incomplete. Simple syndactyly involves only the soft tissues, whereas complex includes side-to-side bony fusion with an origin both dorsal to and palmar to the neurovascular structures lying along the digits border.

When the adjacent digits are fused to the fingertip it is described as complete syndactyly, whilst incomplete refers to only partial union, with fusion ceasing at some point along the length of the digits involved. Distal growth of the digits can cause a lateral angulation to the normally longer digit, causing joint abnormalities as well as gross deformity up to the point of the distal separation of the fusion.

The most severe presentation, complex-complicated syndactyly, involves skeletal deformity accompanied by tendon and neurovascular abnormalities, the incidence of which rises as the complexity of the syndactyly increases [2].

Phenotypical Classification

Since its first description in the literature, syndactyly has also been classified by its phenotype. The simple and complex, and complete and incomplete descriptions are an easier reference for discussion amongst colleagues, whereas the phenotypical classification is more specific in terms of the digits involved, as well as the majority having a genetic source. This has led to syndromic and non-syndromic syndactylies being described. The genetic links related to syndactyly have allowed them to be incorporated into the Mendelian Inheritance in Man (MIM) database [64].

In 1978, Temtamy and McKusick [65] concluded, from information gathered from both the literature and their own experience, that there were at least five phenotypically different types of syndactyly involving the hands, with or without foot involvement. The majority of these appeared to be inherited as autosomal dominant traits. Within each pedigree there is uniformity of the type of syndactyly, allowing for the variation characteristic seen in dominant traits. These genetic forms of syndactyly are required to be analyzed separate to syndactyly related to congenital amniotic bands for which currently, there is little or no evidence of a genetic basis. This chapter focuses on the current understanding of the genetic and molecular causes of syndactyly. It will also discuss the varying clinical presentations as well as highlighting its management.

The non-syndromic syndactylies appear to only involve digit and appendage malformation, and have since been expanded to nine phenotypes, named syndactyly I to IX, although some are more commonly known by their synonyms [66–68] (Table 13.1, and Figs. 13.1, 13.2, 13.3, 13.4, 13.5, 13.6, 13.7, 13.8, and 13.9) [68].

Syndromic syndactyly describes syndactyly discovered alongside additional malformations of the body.

Table 13.1 The nine non-syndromic syndactyly phenotypes

Syndactyly (MIM) [64]	Sub-groups	Gene	Loci	Phenotype
SD1/Zygodactyly		–	2q34-q36	Syndactyly of the third + fourth finger web space and/or the web between the second and third toes
(MIM 185900)	Zygodactyly 1	–	3p21.31	Foot zygodactyly without hand or bony involvement
	Zygodactyly 2	–	–	Bilateral cutaneous and/or bony hand and foot involvement
	Zygodactyly 3	–	–	Specific bilateral webbing, cutaneous or bony, of the third + fourth finger
	Zygodactyly 4	–	–	Bilateral cutaneous webbing of the fourth + fifth toe
SD2/synpolydactyly (MIM 185900)	SPD 1	Homeobox D 13	2q31.1	Syndactyly of the third + fourth fingers associated with polydactyly of all components or of part of the fourth finger in the web. Foot polydactyly of the fifth toe included in a web of syndactyly of the fourth + fifth toes
	SPD 2	Fibulin 1	22q13.31	Syndactyly of the third/fourth finger web space and synostosis of the metacarpal and metatarsal bones
	SPD3		14q11.2-q12	Third and fourth finger syndactyly with varying degrees of polydactyly of the fourth finger web space. There is also polydactyly of the fifth toe commonly
SD3 (of the ODDD spectrum) (MIM 186100)		Gap Junction Protein Alpha 1	6q21-q23.2	Complete/bilateral, generally soft tissue syndactyly between the fourth and fifth fingers. The fifth finger is short with absent or rudimentary middle phalanx
SD4/Haas type (MIM 186200)		LMBR1	7q36	Complete syndactyly, bilateral with polydactyly, generally six metacarpals and six digits
SD5 (MIM 186300)		Homeobox D 13	2q31-q32	Soft tissue syndactyly usually affects the third and fourth fingers and second and third toes with associated metatarsal and metacarpal fusion (fourth and fifth or the third and fourth)
SD6/Mitten Hand (MIM n/a)		–	–	Unilateral syndactyly of digits 2–5

(continued)

Table 13.1 (continued)

Syndactyly (MIM) [64]	Sub-groups	Gene	Loci	Phenotype
SD7/Cenani–Lenz (MIM 212780)		LRP4	11p11.2	Severe shortening of the ulna and radius with fusion, fusion of the metacarpals and "disorganization" of phalangeal development including syndactyly
SD8 (MIM n/a)		MF4	? Xq26	Fusion of the fourth and fifth metacarpals
SD9/Mesoaxial Synostotic (MIM 609432)		–	17p13.3	Complete syndactyly and synostosis of the third and fourth fingers with severe bone reduction in the proximal phalanges, hypoplasia of the thumbs and halluces, aplasia/hypoplasia of the middle phalanges of the second and fifth fingers, and complete or partial soft tissue syndactyly of the toes

Reprinted from Jordan D, Hindocha S, Dhital M, Saleh M, Khan W. The epidemiology, genetics and future management of syndactyly. Open Orthop J. 2012;6:14–27. Copyright © Jordan et al.; Licensee Bentham Open

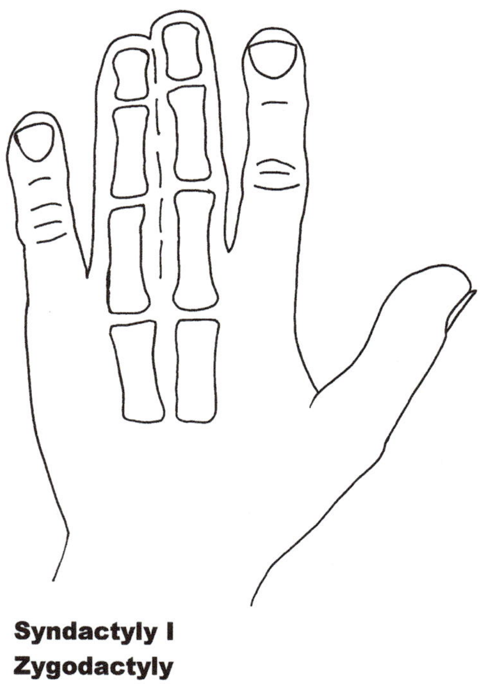

Fig. 13.1 Syndactyly 1. Reprinted from Jordan D, Hindocha S, Dhital M, Saleh M, Khan W. The epidemiology, genetics and future management of syndactyly. Open Orthop J. 2012;6:14–27. Copyright © Jordan et al.; Licensee Bentham Open

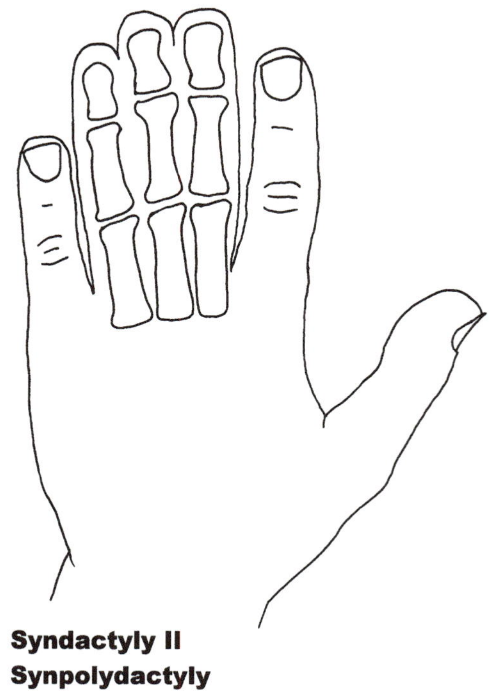

Fig. 13.2 Syndactyly 2. Reprinted from Jordan D, Hindocha S, Dhital M, Saleh M, Khan W. The epidemiology, genetics and future management of syndactyly. Open Orthop J. 2012;6:14–27. Copyright © Jordan et al.; Licensee Bentham Open

This list is extensive and continues to expand as syndactyly is discovered alongside other abnormalities, the majority of which appear to develop at a time during the fetal development alongside the digit anomaly formation. In this chapter, we will note some of the more well-known syndromes and review their currently known associated traits and the genes suggested as being causative.

Syndactyly: Non-syndromic Forms [68]

Syndactyly, in this and syndromic form, is seen to have an autosomal dominant transmission with variable expression and penetrance [1–4]. This is best represented with the increased prevalence in male offspring, possibly due to reduced penetrance in females. Occasionally skipping

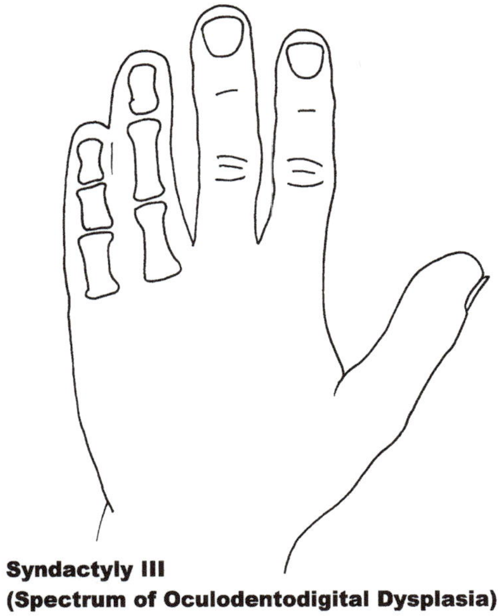

Fig. 13.3 Syndactyly 3. Reprinted from Jordan D, Hindocha S, Dhital M, Saleh M, Khan W. The epidemiology, genetics and future management of syndactyly. Open Orthop J. 2012;6:14–27. Copyright © Jordan et al.; Licensee Bentham Open

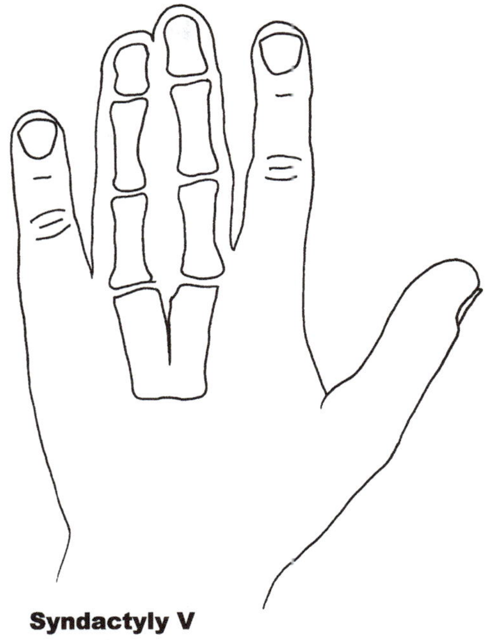

Fig. 13.5 Syndactyly 5. Reprinted from Jordan D, Hindocha S, Dhital M, Saleh M, Khan W. The epidemiology, genetics and future management of syndactyly. Open Orthop J. 2012;6:14–27. Copyright © Jordan et al.; Licensee Bentham Open

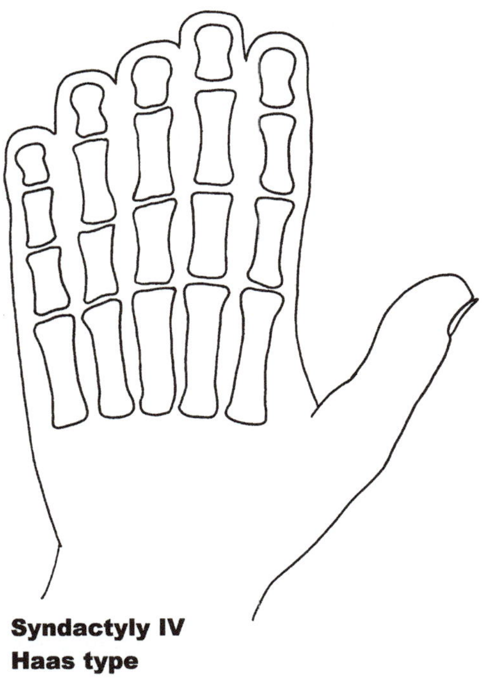

Fig. 13.4 Syndactyly 4. Reprinted from Jordan D, Hindocha S, Dhital M, Saleh M, Khan W. The epidemiology, genetics and future management of syndactyly. Open Orthop J. 2012;6:14–27. Copyright © Jordan et al.; Licensee Bentham Open

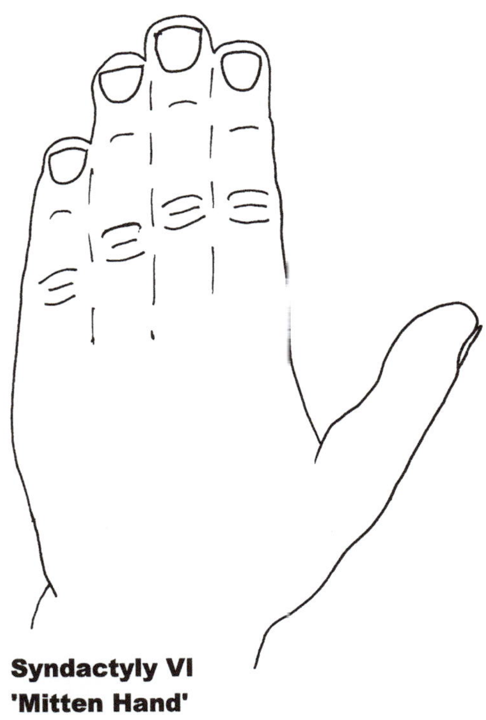

Fig. 13.6 Syndactyly 6. Reprinted from Jordan D, Hindocha S, Dhital M, Saleh M, Khan W. The epidemiology, genetics and future management of syndactyly. Open Orthop J. 2012;6:14–27. Copyright © Jordan et al.; Licensee Bentham Open

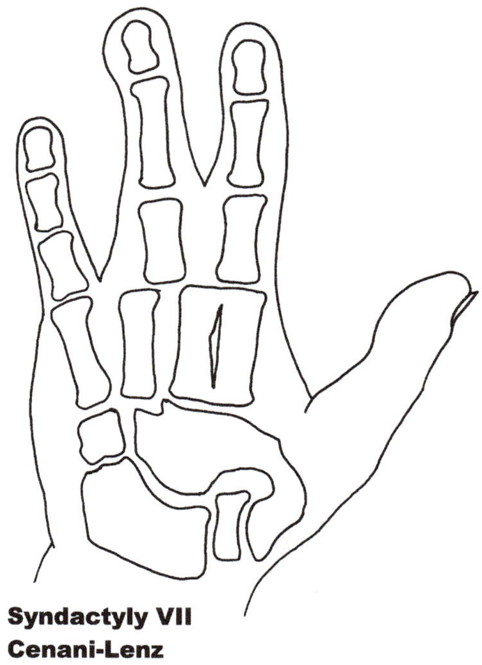

Fig. 13.7 Syndactyly 7. Reprinted from Jordan D, Hindocha S, Dhital M, Saleh M, Khan W. The epidemiology, genetics and future management of syndactyly. Open Orthop J. 2012;6:14–27. Copyright © Jordan et al.; Licensee Bentham Open

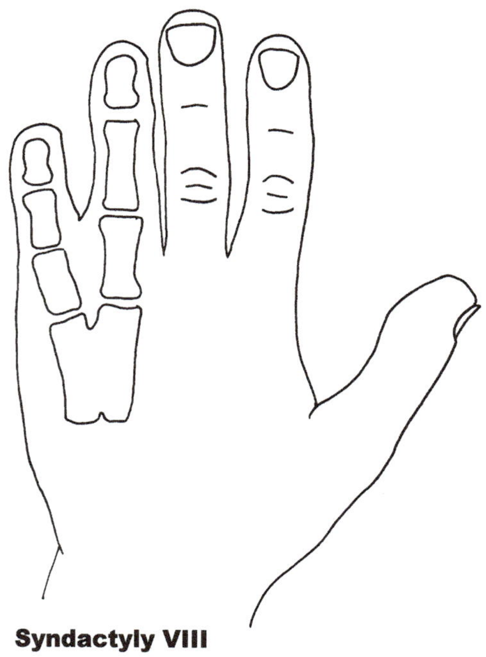

Fig. 13.8 Syndactyly 8. Reprinted from Jordan D, Hindocha S, Dhital M, Saleh M, Khan W. The epidemiology, genetics and future management of syndactyly. Open Orthop J. 2012;6:14–27. Copyright © Jordan et al.; Licensee Bentham Open

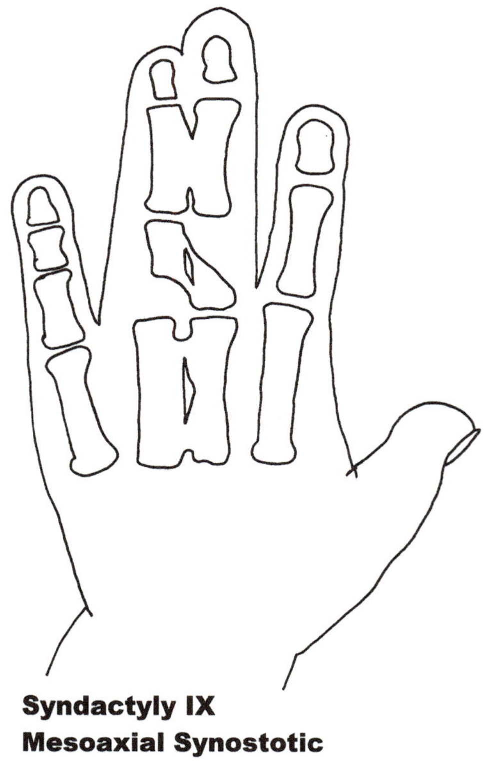

Fig. 13.9 Syndactyly 9. Reprinted from Jordan D, Hindocha S, Dhital M, Saleh M, Khan W. The epidemiology, genetics and future management of syndactyly. Open Orthop J. 2012;6:14–27. Copyright © Jordan et al.; Licensee Bentham Open

generations, it can present in a reduced form indicating variable phenotype.

The non-syndromic forms of syndactyly which are genetically distinct have been expanded from five to nine since the first discussion of syndactyly phenotypes by Temtamy and McKusick [65] and are summarized individually below.

Syndactyly Type I (SD1)

SD1 is characterized by involvement of the third and fourth finger web space and/or the web between the second and third toes. The most common non-syndromic presentation of syndactyly, it has been described with involvement of other digits and the underlying bones [69]. It is also known under the name zygodactyly.

The phenotype of zygodactyly has been seen to vary. It has been seen to affect the upper or lower limb, both simultaneously and independently. SD1 appears to be inherited only as an autosomal dominant trait. Initial genetic studies localized the 2q34-q36 region of the second chromosome, mapped during studies involving both a large German and a non-related Iranian family [70, 71]. This locus has also been linked to a Philadelphia type of craniosynostosis with associated syndactyly [72, 73].

Mouse studies have shown a chemically induced mutation on the chromosome 6 causes syndactyly of digits 2 and 3 of the hind legs (Sndy Jrt/Sndy +). This varies from simple complete to incomplete phenotype, and although sparing the front limbs appears to correlate well with the characteristics of SD1. The homologous region of this chromosomal mutation in humans would be found on 3p25.1 [74].

Malik et al. [75] postulated that SD1 can be further divided into four subtypes:

Subtype 1: Foot zygodactyly without hand or bony involvement

Subtype 2: Bilateral cutaneous and/or bony hand and foot involvement

Subtype 3: Specific bilateral webbing, cutaneous or bony, of the third and fourth finger

Subtype 4: Bilateral cutaneous webbing of the fourth and fifth toe

They designated the 3p21.31 locus to be specific for this first subtype and named it zygodactyly 1 (ZD1). This appeared to be a new locus for the same phenotype previously described in the German family by Bosse et al. [70].

Syndactyly Type II (SD2)

Synpolydactyly (SPD) is, in terms of both genetic and clinical terms, one of the most heterogeneous malformations of the non-syndromic syndactyly types. It appears to lack penetrance within SPD-affected families, with its typical signs including third and fourth finger syndactyly associated with varying degrees of polydactyly of the fourth finger web space. Polydactyly of the fifth toe is often seen.

SPD has been categorized several times in the literature. There is agreement that SPD is inherited in an autosomal dominant manner. Subtypes have been constructed as new genetic sources have been found.

The Homeobox family of genes were the first group to be acknowledged in relation to Synpolydactyly. Located on the 5′ region of the A- and D-clusters of human chromosomes 7 and 2, respectively, several distinct genes have been recognized [39]. These genes appear to influence limb patterning and of particular interest is the Homeobox D gene (HOXD), and precisely that related to the loci at 2q31 [76].

Following this theory, research into the HOXD13 gene found in one family a relation to polyalanine expansion [77–81]. Specifically, the N terminal region of the protein, involved in binding to DNA, is disturbed. With this there appears to be a correlation between expansion size and the appearance and severity of the SPD phenotype in affected patients, with a greater number of limb involvement seen with increasing expansion size [82]. It has correspondingly been found that minimal duplication does not seem to cause the phenotypical deformity [83]. Since its finding, HOXD13 has been linked with multiple limb deformities including SD5, brachydactyly, and several syndromic forms of syndactyly [84, 85].

The HOXD13 gene link has been supplemented by the discovery that a translocation between Chromosomes 12 and 22 resulting in a defect in the Fibulin gene, normally located on the latter, was found to cause SPD [86, 87]. Debeer and Schoenmakers team published further papers examining this translocation within the FBLN1 gene and localized specific involvement of an area represented by EST R72964, as well as ruling out several previously characterized genes [88].

This finding initially complicated the SPD phenotype, and resulted in the commonly recognized classification SPD 1–3. With this description, SPD 3 correlates to the more classical presentation of SPD and has been linked to the 14q11.2-q12 loci [89].

Likewise, the grouping of phenotype to gene of SPD 2 to the Fibulin 1 gene on Chromosome 12 (MIM 608180) and SPD 1 with Homeobox D13 (MIM 186000) is now widely accepted. SPD2 is generally thought to include synostosis of the metacarpal and metatarsal bones.

A more recent paper [90] has stated that SPD should be sub-classed more specifically relating to phenotype, stating genotype–phenotype correlation is weak when looking only at the HOXD13 mutation. They propose the phenotypic variant being classed as (1) typical SPD features, (2) minor variants, and (3) unusual phenotypes.

A further SPD subtype is described by one paper [91] where a new distinct clinical form involving a complicated and distinctive hypoplastic synpolydactyly was found. This currently does not appear to have been investigated on a genetic basis, and further research into this will help define this new phenotype as a new or mixed entity.

Continuing research has led to other genes being suggested as causative in SPD, although all of these have been found to involve the Shh pathway on one level or another [92].

Syndactyly Type III (SD3)

In syndactyly type III, the typical and first described phenotype involves complete and bilateral syndactyly between the fourth and fifth fingers. This is a soft tissue syndactyly but has been seen with the distal phalanges fused. An absent or rudimentary middle phalanx results in an often seen shorter fifth digit. The feet are generally not affected. Johnston and Kirby [93] presented a family which was one of the largest fully described pedigrees, involving seven affected males and seven affected females over five generations in a pattern compatible with an autosomal dominant inheritance [65].

Other papers to describe SD3 as a single entity, as opposed to as being part of a syndrome include De Smet et al. [94].

Isolated SD3 appears to be in a disease spectrum that includes oculodentodigital dysplasia (ODDD; MIM 164200), which commonly involves digit as well as craniofacial dysmorphia and neurological degeneration [95]. ODDD has complete penetrance but a varying phenotype. Gene research has led to the locus 6q21-q23 being associated with SD3, with significant crossover of the locus 6q22-q24, linked to ODDD, and in particular the Connexin 43 (Cx43) gene and its involvement with the gap junction protein, alpha 1 (GJA1) [96–98].

With six types, it has been found the Connexin family are key in forming gap junctions allowing small molecule and ion passage, with Cx43 being expressed in the developing limb bud and in particular relating to digit and cartilage condensation [99]. Further studies into both the phenotype and genetic regions above have found localized missense mutations causative for ODDD, of which over eight have been described, as well as tested in animal studies [100–104].

Dobrowolski et al. [105] have described ODDD phenotype in specific mutations (131M and G138R) whilst mutations at other points appear to result in no syndactyly (H194P) or solely facial abnormality (G143S). This has led to a belief that increased hemi-channel activity may strengthen ODDD phenotype in Cx43 gap junction deficient patients. Other studies have also confirmed a highly variable phenotype of Cx43 mutations which includes ODDD [106–108].

Syndactyly Type IV (SD4)

With only four reports in the literature, syndactyly type IV is rare [109–112].

Haas [109] was first to describe this phenotype, referred to as Haas type polysyndactyly, with the syndactyly described as complete, affecting the fingers of both hands, with associated polydactyly, generally involving six metacarpals and six digits. Flexion of the fingers results in the hands forming a cup shape. In contradistinction to the type of syndactyly in Apert syndrome, there is no bone fusion. In the reports, there is no mention of SD4 affecting the feet, with descriptions noting there were no associated malformations.

Following an autosomal dominant inheritance trait, 7q36 has been mapped as a locus for SD4 [110]. Shh regulation mutations have been found to be key in SD4 [113, 114], with one paper showing an involvement of an area on the limb region 1 (LMBR1) gene being causative [115].

Syndactyly Type V (SD5)

Another rare form of syndactyly, SD5 is as a rule characterized by the presence of an associated metacarpal and metatarsal fusion. The fourth and fifth, or third and fourth, metacarpals and metatarsals are most commonly fused, with soft tissue syndactyly usually affecting the third and fourth fingers and the second and third toes. In this form, the syndactyly tends to be more extensive and complete. In 1932, Kemp and Ravn [116] described this anomaly in five generations of a family from the island of Seeland. Other descriptions without metatarsal fusion have been documented, but these are usually seen with other foot abnormalities [117].

Syndactyly type V has an autosomal dominant trait but has been described as X-linked recessive. Research has linked SD5 to the locus at 2q31-q32 as well as mutations in the HOXD13 gene, including the pathogenicity of a c.950A→G (p.Q317R) mutation [84]. In this paper, the authors called for a genotype classification of HOXD13 limb morphologies, again confusing the genotype-phenotype boundaries of the syndactylies.

Interestingly, as in SPD, evidence of HOXD13 polyalanine expansion has been found in the Seeland family [118].

Syndactyly Type VI (SD6)

Also known as mitten hand syndactyly, this form consists of unilateral syndactyly of digits 2–5 [65]. One family has been described with this anomaly, where an autosomal dominant inheritance, but with variable expression and incomplete penetrance, is likely. Tentamy and McKusick included this phenotype in their initial classification but, even since their description, due to its rarity it remains the least researched non-syndromic syndactyly.

Syndactyly Type VII (SD7)

In 1967 two brothers with an Apert syndrome-like form of syndactyly were described by Cenani and Lenz [119]. They noted however, that additional features including severe shortening of the ulna and radius with fusion, as well as fusion of the metacarpals and "disorganization" of phalangeal development were present. The feet of both brothers were less severely affected. They identified similar cases reported by Liebenam [120], Borsky [121], and Yelton [122].

Cenani–Lenz syndrome, named after the pair's description, is a very rare phenotype and has been reported to show an autosomal recessive inheritance. There have been accounts of varying phenotypes, including a description of a patient with features consistent with Cenani–Lenz type but also displaying a severe form of SPD1 [69].

The LRP4 gene has been linked to syndactyly in cattle [123, 124], and it is reported with multiple mutations on Chromosome 11p12-p11.2 to be the causative factor in SD7 [125]. In the study group, two families did not exhibit LRP4 mutations, suggesting further gene involvement. Bachelli et al. found that this is unlikely to be related to the pathways involving Formin or Gremlin expression [126]. A more recent paper suggests a mutation involving the loci of these bmp antagonists can result in a phenotype similar to Cenani–Lenz syndrome [127].

Within the Cenani–Lenz syndactyly group, there appears to be two grossly variant phenotypes: one involving a spoon hand type, and the other an oligodactyly type [128].

Syndactyly Type VIII (SD8)

Fusion of the fourth and fifth metacarpals is an uncommon presentation of syndactyly. First described by Orel in 1928 [129], it was thought to have an X-linked recessive trait, which has been supported by later papers [130, 131].

An autosomal dominant inheritance has been suggested by Lerch [132] after he found a family with male–male transmission as well as female member being affected.

Xq26 has been suggested as a starting point for analysis, a known mapped area for split-hand/foot malformation (SHFM2), with the gene allocated as MF4 (MIM 309630), although there is general consensus that this syndactyly needs further research before its relationship is fully understood [133].

Syndactyly Type IX (SD9)

Type IX, mesoaxial synostotic syndactyly (MSSD) has been described only in two families. The characteristic features consist of complete syndactyly and synostosis of the third and fourth fingers with severe bone reduction in the proximal phalanges, hypoplasia of the thumbs and halluces, aplasia/hypoplasia of the middle phalanges of the second and fifth fingers, and complete or partial soft tissue syndactyly of the toes. Percin initially believed, with family members known to have SD1 trait, this to be a severe form of SD1 having a possible homozygous origin [134].

Malik et al. [135] found similar findings in another family, with an autosomal recessive trait, and ruled out genome candidates at 2q34-q36, 2q31, and 6q22-q23. The previous family had also had HOXD13 and the genome associated with 2q31 disproved as causative by Percin et al. Merging the two families into one study has revealed a likelihood of a causal gene being mapped to chromosome 17p13.3 [67].

Syndactyly: The Syndromic Forms

Syndactyly often presents as part of a syndrome, usually with other congenital abnormalities. Some of the more common syndromes are reviewed as follows.

Acrosyndactyly describes syndactyly associated with congenital constriction bands. It appears to lack a genetic basis, with Tentamy and McKusick [65] being first to find little or no evidence of a clear or simple genetic link. The formation of syndactyly in this syndrome is thought to be as a result of inflammatory changes resulting in scar formation fusing the digits [136–138]. This is reinforced by the appearance of dorsal to palmar epithelium lined sinuses lying proximal to the scar fusion site in these patients.

The ischemic insult after initial digit formation causes digit deformity although Patterson [137] has also noted the high incidence of deformity in other anatomical regions and raises the possibility of a molecular tissue defect. However, it is noted that any deformity is not usually seen to be symmetrical in the opposite limb pointing away from a genetic source.

Dependant on the degree of bone involvement, acrosyndactyly can be described as mild, moderate, or severe [139–141]. Mild deformity involves normal metacarpal structure with three well-formed digits, meaning three phalanges and two joints, whereas there is loss of a phalangeal bone resulting in one joint in the moderate form. The severe form relates to little or no digit presence with only small phalanges present, and occasionally metacarpal involvement. The variance in acrosyndactyly, as opposed to the other forms of syndactyly tends to involve no extra-skeletal parts and the fusion involving a scar lying either side-to-side or an on-top position.

Poland's syndrome (MIM 173800) presents with unilateral hypoplasia or absence of pectoralis muscle with ipsilateral hand and digit anomalies. The syndrome is named after Alfred Poland, who reported on George Elt's absent pectoralis major [142]. Patrick Clarkson later described the syndrome, including its hand anomalies [143]. As of yet no gene or loci has been implicated in its origin. It is believed that there may be a causative source in a disruption sequence related to the brachiocephalic arterial system [144–146].

The radial fingers are more typically involved in Poland's syndrome and hypoplasia of the digits is frequent. Breast hypoplasia, in varying degrees, is often a common presentation as well as involvement of the latissimus dorsi, deltoid and/or serratus anterior muscles [147]. Poland syndrome has also been reported with evidence of dextrocardia and sternal deformity. Karnak et al. described a bilateral Poland syndrome [148]; however, most presently agree that Poland syndrome is solely a unilateral disease.

Acrocephalosyndactyly (ACS), a condition involving syndactyly and craniosynostosis, where there is a premature fusion of one or more of the fibrous suture lines of the skull. Five types have been described, each having variances on the hand and skull deformity. There is confusion where the distinction between the ACS group and the syndromes involving craniosynostosis, syndactyly, and polydactyly (ACPS), which incorporates a different four syndromes into a further five types, ends. The main ACS/ACPS syndromes are commented on below.

Apert syndrome (MIM 101200) ACS type I is synonymous with the term acrocephalosyndactyly. Associated with the FGFR2 gene, and the loci 10q26, includes midface hypoplasia, foot and hand syndactyly with a trend for distal bony fusion [149].

A subgroup of the Crouzon syndrome linked to FGFR2 is termed ACS type 2. Although Crouzon syndrome usually involves only a craniofacial dysostosis, Crouzon type 2 also involves mild soft tissue syndactyly.

Saethre–Chotzen syndrome, ACS type III (MIM 101400), involves syndactyly of the second and third fingers, as well as the third and fourth toes, as well as eyelid anomalies and cranial abnormalities. It has been linked to the loci 7p21.2 and 10q26 involving the TWIST 1 and FGFR2 genes, respectively [150, 151].

ACS type V, also known as Pfeiffer syndrome (MIM 101600) has been linked to the FGFR 1 and 2 genes [152, 153]. This is likewise classified as ACPS 5, and has since had Noack syndrome, previously ACPS 1, grouped with it.

ACPS 2, Carpenter syndrome (MIM 201000), has been linked to RAB23 gene originating from 6p11, with malformations including foot and hand syndactyly/brachydactyly and acrocephaly [154]. ACPS 4 was known as Goodman syndrome (MIM 201020) but is thought now to be a variant of type II [155].

Other syndromes and chromosomal location include Acropectorevertebral dysplasia (MIM 102510) and 2q36 and Fraser syndrome (MIM 219000) associated with both the sites 4q21 and 13q13, involving the FRAS1 and FREM2 basement membrane genes, respectively [156, 157], which have also been shown to be linked to fin deformity in zebrafish [158].

Greig cephalopolysyndactyly (MIM 175700) is an autosomal dominant disorder associated with haplo-insufficiency of GLI3. This appears to be caused by deletions, truncations, or point mutations of the associated Gli3 gene. Similarly the zinc finger domain of Gli3 has been found to be causative in Pallister Hall syndrome whose phenotype includes central nervous system and craniofacial deformities, as well as anal defects [52].

Research into the individual phenotypes appears to complicating phenotypical classification as new genes are found both linked, and not linked, to each malformation.

This has been noted by several researchers [159, 160], and attempts have been made to simplify the current classifications although these are yet to be recognized across all specialities.

Environmental Influence on Limb Formation

It should be noted that sporadic distinct syndactyly with no familial history has been documented. In utero environmental factors that predispose the fetus to syndactyly and other congenital hand abnormalities have been evaluated. Man conducted a study that reports a probable association with these conditions and maternal smoking [161], and there are suggestions that syndactyly occurrence is associated with lower nutritional and economic status, including increased meat and egg intake whilst pregnant, although more research is required before suggesting that these are causative factors [162].

Anatomy and Management

The normal position of the web commissure lies at the midpoint of the proximal phalanx if looked at from a lateral view. From a distal view the space appears to be shaped like an hourglass with a larger area within the second and fourth web space when compared to the third. The web space appears to normally slope, towards this distal view, from the dorsal aspect of the hand at an angle of 45° (Figs. 13.10 and 13.11).

The mainstay of treatment for syndactyly remains surgical. Indications for operative intervention run along the same principles as that of all hand anomalies:

- Function—to allow hand function and the development of normal grip
- Cosmesis—to improve the aesthetic appearance of the hand to minimize the psychological and social effects of the deformity

The timing of the surgical intervention needs to be optimized in order to reduce long-term complications and improve outcome. Many centers begin corrective surgery by 12–18 months of age and aim to complete reconstruction by the time the child reaches school, helping social and functional tasks at this time. It is thought that there is less risk of scar contracture in comparison to younger age groups. However, it is imperative that patients be assessed on an individual basis and reconstruction tailored as to the complexity of the syndactyly. Some forms of syndactyly are operated on at 6 months of age [163] or earlier [164].

Involvement of border digits, complex syndactyly, and flexion contractures are all indications for early repair. The aim of early intervention is to reduce the loss of function associated with the deformity and provide normal grip development.

On the contrary, Kettlekamp and Flatt [165] found that surgery performed at less than 18 months of age was associated with a higher complication rate and poorer aesthetic outcome, particularly in relation to the web commissure. Timing of surgery, therefore, is often down to individual surgeon preference.

Multiple-digit syndactyly should be corrected as part of a multistage procedure. Release should be performed on only one side of a digit at a time so as not to risk necrosis, particularly in those supplied by only one artery [166]. As a rule, border digits should be released first followed by a second procedure performed at least 4 months later [167].

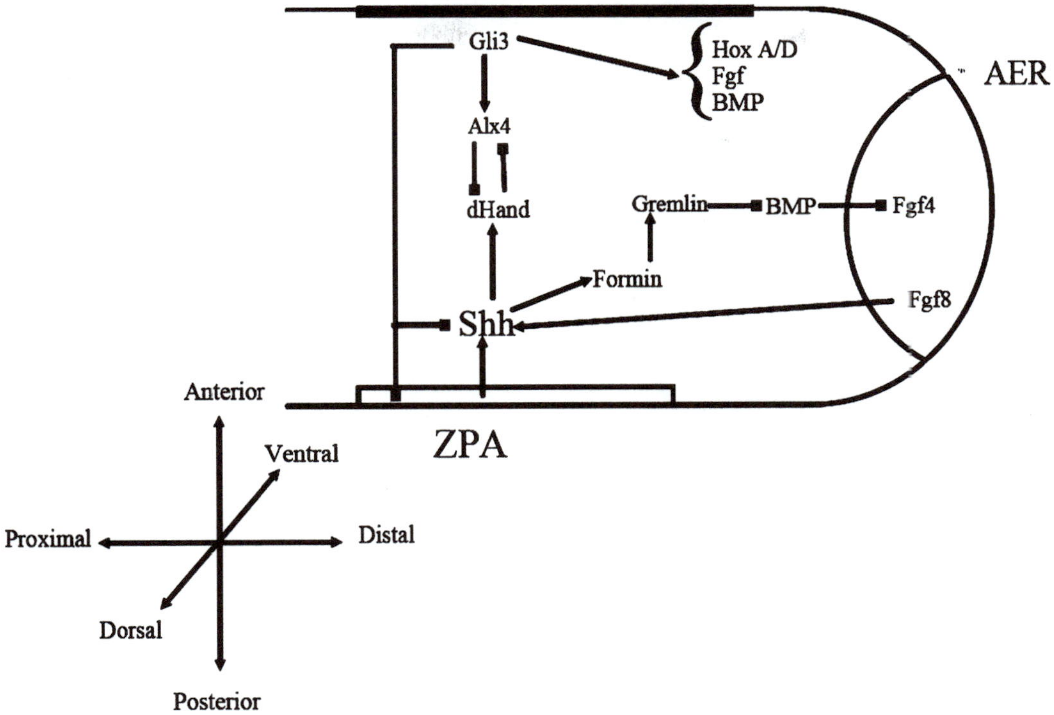

Fig. 13.10 Showing lateral view of interdigital web space. Note 45° dorsal to palmar fall finishing at midpoint of the proximal phalanx

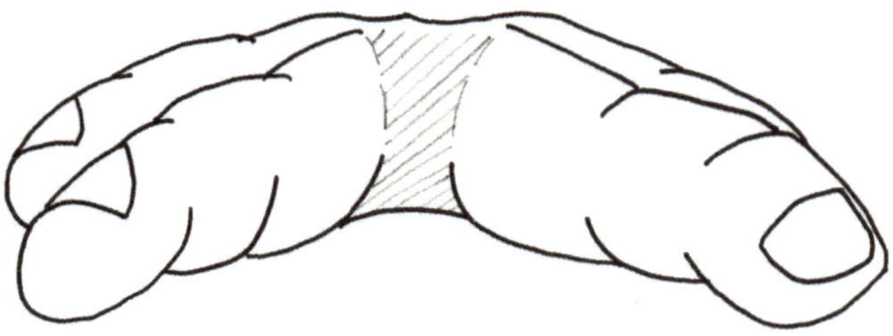

Fig. 13.11 Hourglass shape of interdigital space

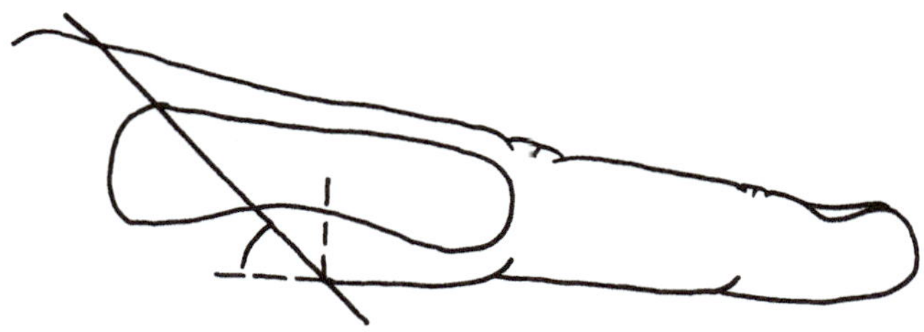

Fig. 13.12 Showing lateral view of interdigital web space. Note 45° dorsal to palmar fall finishing at midpoint of the proximal phalanx

Surgical Technique

Surgical correction of syndactyly requires the separation of digits and the creation of a new web space. The main concern with syndactyly is the greater surface area encountered on separation of the digits, with a circumference of approximately 1.4 times the preoperative state. Technique for repair therefore, must provide a means for adequate resurfacing.

Over the last two centuries, techniques for syndactyly repair have evolved significantly [163]. Many successful methods are described in the literature. Most employ a variant of the procedure described below (Figs. 13.12, 13.13, 13.14, 13.15, 13.16, 13.17, 13.18, 13.19, and 13.20):

1. A zigzag incision for the separation of digits
2. A dorsal flap for the creation of a web commissure
3. A skin graft to resurface raw areas

Skin grafts are associated with various complications: graft loss, hair growth from donor sites, scar contracture, web creep as well as general surgical risks including donor site infection. In general, full thickness grafts are used for resurfacing. Split thickness grafts have been shown to have higher complications from scar contracture [168] and have therefore fallen out of favor. Full thickness grafts may be taken from the dorsum, hypothenar region, antecubital fossa, and the groin. Although widespread use of the groin as a donor site, it has been recommended that more medial areas are avoided so as to avoid excessive hair growth on the hand [169].

Another consideration with the use of skin grafts is the problems associated with graft management in patients of a young age, mainly due to difficulties with immobilization. Recently, Kamath et al. [170] describe the use of a mini

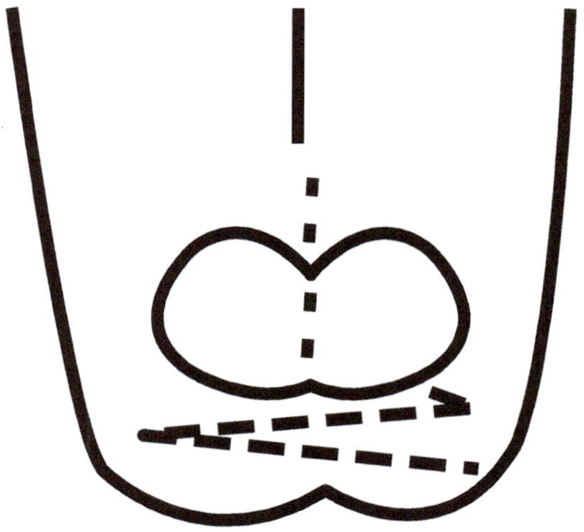

Fig. 13.13 Buck Gramcko nail fold creation

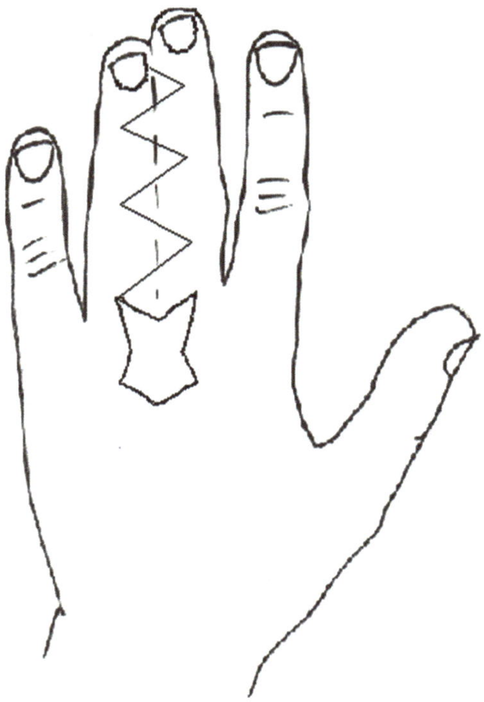

Fig. 13.14 Dorsal Island flap

external fixator to facilitate the maintenance of the neo-web space by allowing accurate positioning of the graft and make dressing changes easier and pain free.

Complications associated with graft use have led to the development of flaps that aim to minimize the surface area required for grafting. More recently, there has been a trend towards syndactyly repair without skin grafts. The goals of this technique involve the careful redistribution of available skin to allow direct closure. Various techniques have been described. The procedure is based upon a local flap to recreate the web commissure, whilst lateral finger defects are closed directly. Modifications of this design include the use of a transposition flap [171], a V-Y advancement flap originating from a distal subcutaneous pedicle [172] and more

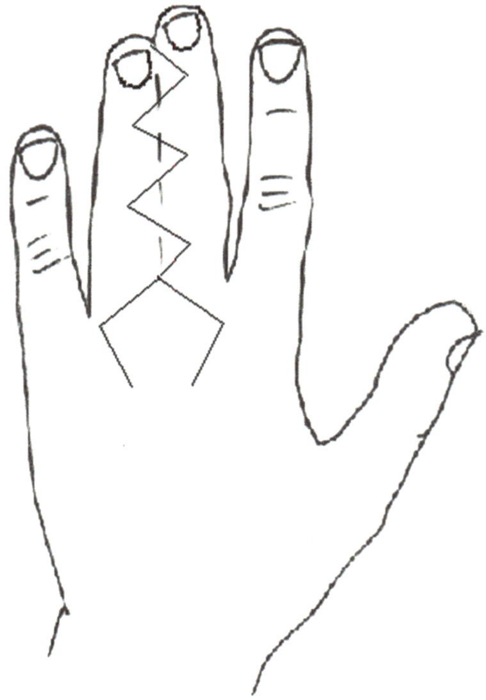

Fig. 13.15 Dorsal pentagonal flap

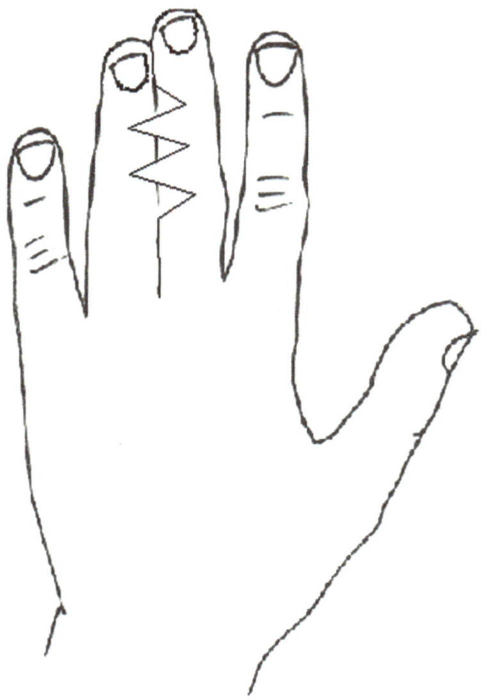

Fig. 13.16 Dorsal view of Jose et al. flap

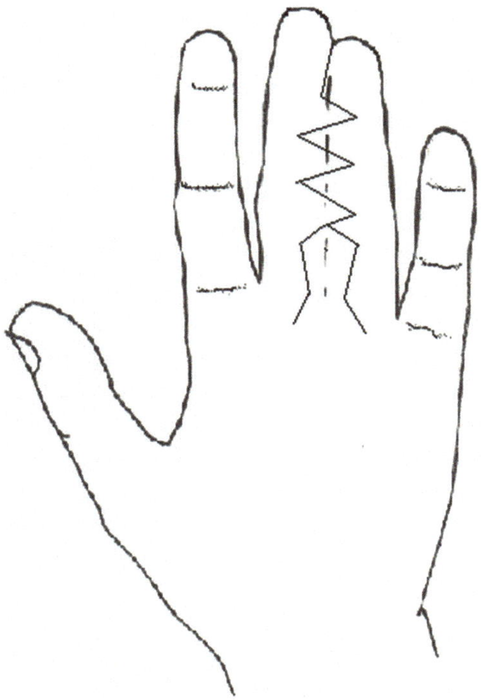

Fig. 13.17 Palmar view of palmar-shaped flap

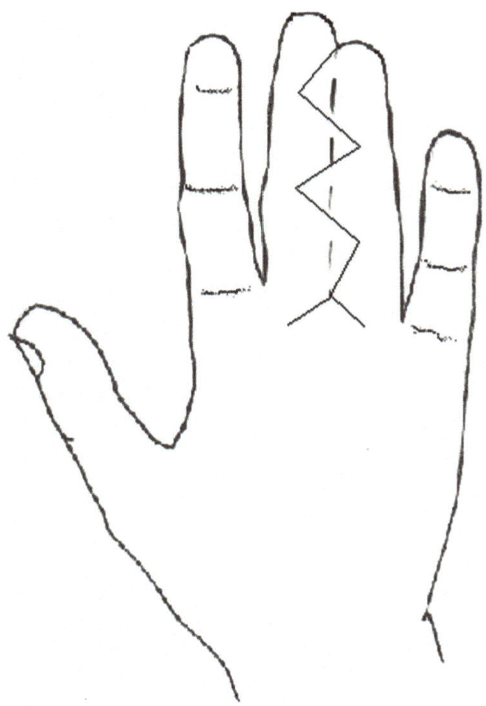

Fig. 13.18 Volar zigzag approach to release

recently a local dorsal pentagonal flap based on perforators from the dorsal metacarpal artery [173]. Although reliable in terms of resurfacing, these methods are associated with aesthetically displeasing scarring on the dorsum of the hand, which could potentially be avoided using other methods.

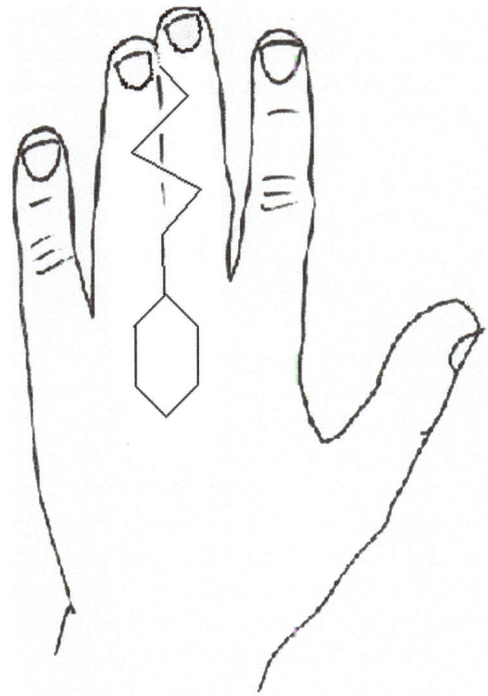

Fig. 13.19 Diagram of V-Y advancement flap for release

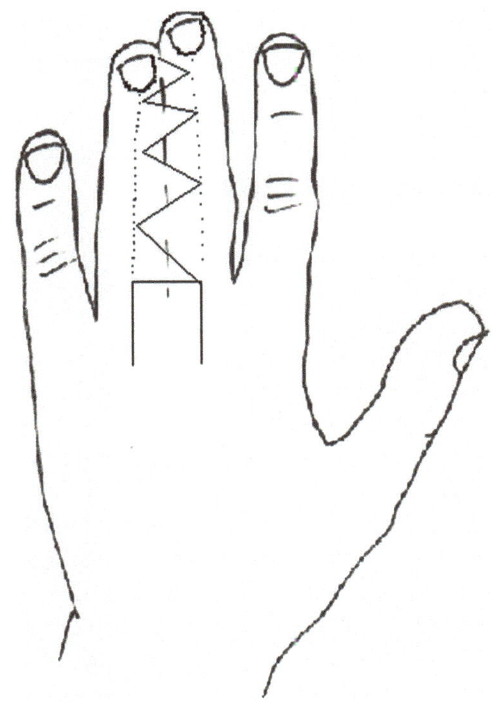

Fig. 13.20 Zigzag dorsal flap

Island flaps have been designed to reduce scarring to the socially visible dorsal aspect of the hand. The harvesting of island flaps has been described in the literature by various different means. Yao et al. [174] advocated that the flap be pedicled upon subcutaneous tissue and deep fascia to incorporate known perforators, where other authors have encouraged the direct isolation of the arterial feeding branch to the web flap [175]. Both methods detail excellent outcome in terms of vascularization.

For closure to be successful in most non-graft techniques, extensive "defatting" of the tissue is performed [176], with any small areas left to heal by secondary intention. There has been concern that the debulking technique employed in these procedures is associated with vascular injury and therefore increased risk of tissue necrosis [177]. It has also been recognized that these techniques can only be used in simple syndactylies, as the available surface on the dorsum of the hand would not be sufficient for extensive resurfacing.

Jose et al. [178] proposed a combination of techniques to reconstruct syndactyly in response to the problems associated with dorsal flaps (scarring) and dorsal metacarpal island flaps (restricted to simple syndactylies only). A palmar flap is used to recreate the web commissure, where lateral digit defects are closed via narrow-based V-flaps and full thickness grafts. Retrospective review of 176 procedures yielded low complication rates (Figs. 13.13, 13.14, 13.15, 13.16, 13.17, 13.18, 13.19, and 13.20).

For syndactyly involving the nail, the nail must first be split before creating a new nail fold from triangular flaps based laterally on the distal pulp. Most repairs involving the nail are variations of the Buck-Gramcko technique (see Fig. 13.13) [179].

Complications and Outcome

The most common acute complications of syndactyly correction include infection, necrosis, graft failure, and scar contracture. Long-term complications include web creep, keloid scarring, and joint deformity which all can result in a reduction of function. All of the listed complications may result in a secondary operative procedure.

Simple syndactyly repairs are often associated with good functional and cosmetic outcome [169, 179]. Many studies however have noted poorer outcome with complex syndactyly [159, 180], most likely due to the challenging nature of the reconstruction. Goldfarb et al. [181] found significantly higher rates of joint deformity amongst complex repairs and a high likelihood of abnormal nail appearance. Overall reoperation rates are quoted as 10 % [164] but are up to 50 % higher in those with polysyndactyly [181]. It is imperative that follow up should be continued until skeletal maturity to detect complications, particularly joint deformity, which may require arthrodesis.

There have been concerns that graft-free repairs may be associated with a higher incidence of web creep, thought to be related to increased tension leading to scar contractures. Niranjan et al. [179], however, published long-term outcome data of "graft-free" repairs with a mean follow up time of 6.6 years, and found superior cosmetic results and good functional outcome.

It is thought that an increased incidence of web creep is seen in dorsal rectangular flaps due to linear scar contracture along the palmar border. Miyamoto et al. [182] performed an analysis of scar stress and web creep using CT reconstructions and found that the dorsal rectangular flap was associated with greater stresses than those seen in palmar rectangular or dorsal V-shaped flaps. The authors advocated that a palmar break should be incorporated into any syndactyly repair to reduce scar contracture in the linear palmar scar and thus reduce the incidence of web creep.

Despite the abundance of techniques available for syndactyly reconstruction, it remains unclear as to which procedure is superior in terms of various outcomes and more data is needed to assess this.

Future Management Options

In view of the development of genetic and perinatal investigation for syndactyly, future management could be aimed at in utero intervention. The role of gestational ultrasound scans has allowed early diagnosis of upper limb anomalies and can now be supplemented with genetic review of those likely to be carriers. An animal study has observed that amniotic constriction bands can be released in utero to allow limb development to continue in a more anatomical manner [183].

Husler et al. [184] report seven cases of fetoscopic release of amniotic bands resulting in limb anomalies in the human fetus, but with few resulting in functional improvement. Incidence of premature rupture of membrane was high, and with one case of intrauterine death. Currently, the risks of complications in fetoscopic intervention do not outweigh the proposed benefits, particularly as the underlying condition described is nonfatal.

References

1. Canale ST, Beaty JH. Campbell's operative orthopaedics, vol. 4. 11th ed. Philadelphia, PA: Mosby Elsevier; 2008. p. 4403–4.
2. Green DP, Hotchkiss RN, Pederson WC, Wolfe SW. Green's Operative Hand Surgery, vol. 2. 5th ed. Philadelphia, PA: Mosby Elsevier; 2005. p. 1381–2.
3. Burke FD, McGrouther DA, Smith PJ. Principles of hand surgery, Chapter 15. Edinburgh: Churchill Livingstone; 1989. p. 256.
4. Eaton CJ, Lister GD. Syndactyly. Hand Clin. 1990;6(4):555.
5. Kozin SH. Syndactyly. J Am Soc Surg Hand. 2001;1:1–13.
6. Benson MKD, Fixen JA, Macnicol MF, Parsch K. Children's orthopaedics and fractures. 2nd ed. Edinburgh: Churchill Linigston; 2002. p. P306–7.

7. Netscher DT, Baumholtz MA. Treatment of congenital upper extremity problems. Plast Reconstr Surg. 2007;119(5):101e–29.
8. Hogan BL. Morphogenesis. Cell. 1999;96:225–33.
9. Oligny LL. Human molecular embryogenesis: an overview. Pedatr Dev Pathol. 2001;4:324–43.
10. Mariani FV, Martin GR. Deciphering skeletal patterning: clues from the limb. Nature. 2003;423:319–25.
11. Saunders JW. The proximo-distal sequence of origin of the parts of the chick wing and the role of the ectoderm. J Exp Zool. 1948;108(3):363–403.
12. Saunders JW, Gasseling, MT. Ectodermal-mesodermal interactions in the origin of limb symmetry. Epithelial-Mesenchymal Interactions. Eds., R.E. Fleischmajer and R. Billingham. Baltimore, Maryland: Williams & Wilkins. 1968;78–97.
13. Todt WL, Fallon JF. Posterior apical ectodermal ridge removal in the chick wing bud triggers a series of events resulting in defective anterior pattern formation. Development. 1987;101(3):501–15.
14. Manouvrier-Hanu S, Holder-Espinasse M, Lyonnet S. Genetics of limb anomalies in humans. Trends Genet. 1999;15(10):409–17.
15. Ingham PW, McMahon AP. Hedgehog signalling in animal development. Genes Dev. 2001;15:3059–87.
16. Riddle RD, Johnson RL, Laufer E, Tabin C. Sonic hedgehog mediates the polarizing activity of the ZPA. Cell. 1993;75(7):1401–16.
17. Vortkamp A, Lee K, Lanske B, Segre GV, Kronenberg HM, Tabin CJ. Regulation of rate of cartilage differentiation by Indian hedgehog and PTH-related protein. Science. 1996;273(5275):613–22.
18. Naski MC, Omitz DM. FGF signalling in skeletal development. Front Biosci. 1998;3:D781–94.
19. Ohbayashi N, Shibayama M, Kurotaki Y, Imanishi M, Fujimori T, Itoh N, et al. FGF18 is required for normal cell proliferation and differentiation during osteogenesis and chondrogenesis. Genes Dev. 2002;16:870–9.
20. Chung UI, Schipani E, McMahon AP, Kronenberg HM. Indian Hedgehog couples chondrogenesis to osteogenesis in endochondral bone development. J Clin Invest. 2001;107:295–304.
21. Klopocki E, Lohan S, Brancati F, Koll R, Brehm A, Seemann P, et al. Copy-number variations involving the IHH locus are associated with syndactyly and craniosynostosis. Am J Hum Genet. 2011;88(1):70–5. Epub 2010 Dec 17.
22. Gofflot F, Hars C, Illien F, Chevy F, Wolf C, Picard JJ, et al. Molecular mechanisms underlying limb anomalies associated with cholesterol deficiency during gestation: implications of Hedgehog signalling. Hum Mol Genet. 2003;12(10):1187–98.
23. Litingtung Y, Dahn RD, Yina L, Fallon JF, Chiang C. Shh and Gli3 are dispensable for limb skeleton formation but regulate digit number and identity. Nature. 2002;418:979–83.
24. Welscher P, Zuniga A, Kuijper S, Drenth T, Goedemans HJ, Meijlink F, et al. Progression of vertebrate limb development through Shh-mediated counteraction of Gli3. Science. 2002;298(5594):827–30.
25. Chiang C, Litingtung Y, Harris MP, Simandl BK, Li Y, Beachy PA, et al. Manifestation of the limb prepattern: limb development in the absence of sonic hedgehog function. Dev Biol. 2001;236:421–35.
26. Kraus P, Fraidenraich D, Loomis CA. Some distal limb structures develop in mice lacking Sonic hedgehog signalling. Mech Dev. 2001;100:45–58.
27. Drossopoulou G, Lewis KE, Sanz-Ezquerro JJ, Nikbakht N, McMahon AP, Hofmann C, et al. A model for anteroposterior patterning of the vertebrate limb based on sequential long and short range Shh signalling and Bmp signalling. Development. 2000;127:1337–48.
28. Kawakami Y, Capdevilla J, Buscher D, Itoh T, Rodríguez Esteban C, Izpisúa Belmonte JC. WNT signals control FGF-dependent limb initiation and AER induction in the chick embryo. Cell. 2001;104:891–900.
29. Rankin J, Strachan T, Lako M, Lindsay S. Partial cloning and assignment of WNT6 to human chromosome band 2q35 by in situ hybridization. Cytogenet Cell Genet. 1999;84:50–2.
30. Parr BA, Shea MJ, Vassileva G, McMahon AP. Mouse WNT genes exhibit discrete domains of expression in the early embryonic CNS and limb buds. Development. 1993;119(1):247–61.
31. Khan S, Basit S, Zimri F, Ali N, Ali G, Ansar M, et al. A novel homozygous missense mutation in WNT10B in familial split-hand/foot malformation. Clin Genet. 2012;82(1):48–55. doi:10.1111/j1399-0004.2011.01698.x.
32. Mori C, Nakamura N, Kimura S, Irie H, Takigawa T, Shiota K. Programmed cell death in the interdigital tissue of the fetal mouse limb is apoptosis with DNA fragmentation. Anat Rec. 1995;242:103–10.
33. Nishii K, Tsuzuki T, Kumai M, Takeda N, Koga H, Aizawa S, et al. Abnormalities of developmental cell death in Dad1-deficient mice. Genes. 1999;4(4):243–52.
34. Salas-Vidal E, Valencia C, Covarrubias L. Differential tissue growth and patterns of cell death in mouse limb autopod morphogenesis. Dev Dyn. 2001;220:295–306.
35. Merino R, Rodriguez-Leon J, Macias D, Gañan Y, Economides AN, Hurle JM. The BMP antagonist Gremlin regulates outgrowth, chondrogenesis and programmed cell death in the developing limb. Development. 1999;126:5515–22.
36. Crocoll A, Herzer U, Ghyselinck NB, Chambon P, Cato AC. Interdigital apoptosis and downregulation of BAG-1 expression in mouse autopods. Mech Dev. 2002;111:149–52.
37. Heymer J, Rüther U. Syndactyly of Ft/+mice correlates with an imbalance in bmp4 and fgf8 expression. Mech Dev. 1999;88(2):173–81.
38. Schwabe GC, Mundlos S. Genetics of congenital hand anomalies. Handchir Mikrochir Plast Chir. 2004;36:85–97.
39. Francis PH, Richardson MK, Brickell PM, Tickle C. Bone morphogenetic proteins and a signalling pathway that controls patterning in the developing chick limb. Development. 1994;120:209–18.
40. Lyons KM, Hogan BL, Robertson EJ. Colocalization of BMP 7 and BMP 2 RNAs suggests that these factors cooperatively mediate tissue interactions during murine development. Mech Dev. 1995;50:71–83.
41. Laufer E, Dahn R, Orozco OE, Yeo CY, Pisenti J, Henrique D, et al. Expression of Radical fringe in limb-bud ectoderm regulates apical ectodermal ridge formation. Nature. 1997;386:366–73.
42. Ganan Y, Macias D, Duterque-Coquillaud M, Ros MA, Hurle JM. Role of TGF beta s and BMPs as signals controlling the position of the digits and the areas of interdigital cell death in the developing chick limb autopod. Development. 1996;122:2349–57.
43. Zuzarte-Luis V, Hurle JM. Programmed cell death in the developing limb. Int J Dev Biol. 2002;46:871–6.
44. Guha U, Gomes WA, Kobayashi T, Pestell RG, Kessler JA. In vivo evidence that BMP signalling is necessary for apoptosis in the mouse limb. Dev Biol. 2002;249(1):108–20.
45. Yokouchi Y, Sakiyama J, Kameda T, Iba H, Suzuki A, Ueno N, et al. BMP 2/4 mediate programmed cell death in chicken limb buds. Development. 1996;122:3725–34.
46. Zou H, Niswander L. Requirement for BMP signalling in interdigital apoptosis and scale formation. Science. 1996;272:738–41.
47. Arteaga-Solis E, Gayraud B, Lee SY, Shum L, Sakai L, Ramirez F. Regulation of limb patterning by extracellular microfibrils. J Cell Biol. 2001;154(2):275–81.
48. Dahn RD, Fallon JF. Interdigital regulation of digit identity and homeotic transformation by modulated BMP signalling. Science. 2000;289:438–41.
49. McCulloch DR, Nelson CM, Dixon LJ, Silver DL, Wylie JD, Lindner V, et al. ADAMTS metalloproteases generate active ver-

sican fragments that regulate interdigital web regression. Dev Cell. 2009;17(5):687–98.
50. Talamillo A, Delgado I, Nakamura T, de-Vega S, Yoshitomi Y, Unda F, et al. Role of Epiprofin, a zinc-finger transcription factor, in limb development. Dev Biol. 2010;337(2):363–74.
51. Ota S, Zhou ZQ, Keene DR, Knoepfler P, Hurlin PJ. Activities of N-Myc in the developing limb link control of skeletal size with digit separation. Development. 2007;134(8):1583–92.
52. Vortkamp A, Gessler M, Grzeschik KH. GLI3 zinc-finger gene interrupted by translocations in Greig syndrome families. Nature. 1991;352:539–40.
53. Johnston JJ, Sapp JC, Turner JT, Amor D, Aftimos S, Aleck KA, et al. Molecular analysis expands the spectrum of phenotypes associated with GLI3 mutations. Hum Mutat. 2010;31(10):1142–54.
54. Ricks CB, Masand R, Fang P, Roney EK, Cheung SW, Scott DA. Delineation of a 1.65 Mb critical region for hemihyperplasia and digital anomalies on Xq25. Am J Med Genet A. 2010;152A(2):453–8.
55. Schmidt K, Hughes C, Chudek JA, Goodyear SR, Aspden RM, Talbot R, et al. Cholesterol metabolism: the main pathway acting downstream of cytochrome P450 oxidoreductase in skeletal development of the limb. Mol Cell Biol. 2009;29(10):2716–29.
56. Lv D, Luo Y, Yang W, Cao L, Wen Y, Zhao X, et al. A novel single-base deletion in ROR2 causes atypical brachydactyly type B1 with cutaneous syndactyly in a large Chinese family. J Hum Genet. 2009;54(7):422–5.
57. Böse K, Nischt R, Page A, Bader BL, Paulsson M, Smyth N. Loss of nidogen-1 and -2 results in syndactyly and changes in limb development. J Biol Chem. 2006;281(51):39620–9.
58. Liu Y, Liu C, Yamada Y, Fan CM. Growth arrest specific gene 1 acts as a region-specific mediator of the Fgf10/Fgf8 regulatory loop in the limb. Development. 2002;129(22):5289–300.
59. Dauwerse JG, de Vries BB, Wouters CH, Bakker E, Rappold G, Mortier GR, et al. A t(4;6)(q12;p23) translocation disrupts a membrane-associated O-acetyl transferase gene (MBOAT1) in a patient with a novel brachydactyly-syndactyly syndrome. Eur J Hum Genet. 2007;15(7):743–51.
60. Jiang R, Lan Y, Chapman HD, Shawber C, Norton CR, Serreze DV, et al. Defects in limb, craniofacial, and thymic development in Jagged2 mutant mice. Genes Dev. 1998;12(7):1046–57.
61. Sidow A, Bulotsky MS, Kerrebrock AW, Bronson RT, Daly MJ, Reeve MP, et al. Serrate2 is disrupted in the mouse limb-development mutant syndactylism. Nature. 1997;389(6652):722–5.
62. Hwang SJ, Beaty TH, McIntosh I, Hefferon T, Panny SR. Association between homeobox-containing gene MSX1 and the occurrence of limb deficiency. Am J Med Genet. 1998;75(4):419–23.
63. Goodman FR. Limb malformations and the human HOX genes. Am J Med Genet. 2002;112(3):256–65.
64. McKusick VA. www.usfca.edu/Library/databases/OMIM/ and Mendelian inheritance in man. 12th ed. Baltimore: Johns Hopkins University Press; 1998.
65. Temtamy SA, McKusick VA. The genetics of hand malformations. New York, NY: Alan R. Liss New York; 1978. p. 301–22.
66. Goldstein DJ, Kambouris M, Ward RE. Familial crossed polysyndactyly. Am J Med Genet. 1994;50:215–23.
67. Malik S, Percin FE, Ahmad W, Percin S, Akarsu NA, Koch MC, et al. Autosomal recessive mesoaxial synostotic syndactyly with phalangeal reduction maps to chromosome 17p13.3. Am J Med Genet A. 2005;134(4):404–8.
68. Jordan D, Hindocha S, Dhital M, Saleh M, Khan W. The epidemiology, genetics and future management of syndactyly. Open Orthop J. 2012;6:14–27.
69. Percin EF, Percin S. Two unusual types of syndactyly in the same family; Cenani-Lenz type and "new" type versus severe type I syndactyly? Genet Couns. 2003;14(3):313–9.
70. Bosse K, Betz RC, Lee YA, Wienker TF, Reis A, Kleen H, et al. Localization of a gene for syndactyly type 1 to chromosome 2q34-q36. Am J Hum Genet. 2000;67(2):492–7.
71. Ghadami M, Majidzadeh-A K, Haerian BS, Damavandi E, Yamada K, Pasallar P, et al. Confirmation of genetic homogeneity of syndactyly type 1 in an Iranian family. Am J Med Genet. 2001;104(2):147–51.
72. Robin NH, Segel B, Carpenter G, Muenke M. Craniosynostosis, Philadelphia type: a new autosomal dominant syndrome with sagittal craniosynostosis and syndactyly of the fingers and toes. Am J Med Genet. 1996;62:184–91.
73. Jain M, Wallis D, Robin NH, De Vrieze FW, Hardy JA, Ghadami M, et al. Locus homogeneity between syndactyly type 1A and craniosynostosis Philadelphia type? Am J Med Genet A. 2008;146A:2308–11.
74. Rossant J. ENU mutants from the Center of Modeling Human Disease. MGI Direct Data Submission. 2004;Accession ID MGI:3032560.
75. Malik S, Schott J, Ali SW, Oeffner F, Amin-ud-Din M, Ahmad W, et al. Evidence for clinical and genetic heterogeneity of syndactyly type I: the phenotype of second and third toe syndactyly maps to chromosome 3p21.31. Eur J Hum Genet. 2005;13:1268–74.
76. Sarfarazi M, Akarsu AN, Sayli BS. Localization of the syndactyly type II (synpolydactyly) locus to 2q31 region and identification of tight linkage to HOXD8 intragenic marker. Hum Mol Genet. 1995;4:1453–8.
77. Dai L, Heng ZC, Zhu J, Cai R, Mao M, Wang H, et al. Mutation analysis of HOXD13 gene in a Chinese pedigree with synpolydactyly. Zhonghua Yi Xue Yi Chuan Xue Za Zhi. 2005;22(3):277–80.
78. Wajid M, Ishii Y, Kurban M, Dua-Awereh MB, Shimomura Y, Christiano AM. Polyalanine repeat expansion mutations in the HOXD13 gene in Pakistani families with synpolydactyly. Clin Genet. 2009;76(3):300–2.
79. Muragaki Y, Mundlos S, Upton J, Olsen BR. Altered growth and branching patterns in synpolydactyly caused by mutations in HOXD13. Science. 1996;272(5261):548–51.
80. Akarsu AN, Stoilov I, Yilmaz E, Sayli BS, Sarfarazi M. Genomic structure of HOXD13 gene: a nine polyalanine duplication causes synpolydactyly in two unrelated families. Hum Mol Genet. 1996;5:945–52.
81. Goodman FR, Majewski F, Collins AL, Scambler PJ. A 117-kb microdeletion removing HOXD9-HOXD13 and EVX2 causes synpolydactyly. Am J Hum Genet. 2002;70:547–55.
82. Goodman FR, Mundlos S, Muragaki Y, Donnai D, Giovannucci-Uzielli ML, Lapi E, et al. Synpolydactyly phenotypes correlate with size of expansions in HOXD13 polyalanine tract. Proc Natl Acad Sci USA. 1997;94:7458–63.
83. Malik S, Girisha KM, Wajid M, Roy AK, Phadke SR, Haque S, et al. Synpolydactyly and HOXD13 polyalanine repeat: addition of 2 alanine residues is without clinical consequences. BMC Med Genet. 2007;8:78.
84. Zhao X, Sun M, Zhao J, Leyva JA, Zhu H, Yang W, et al. Mutations in HOXD13 underlie syndactyly type V and a novel brachydactyly-syndactyly syndrome. Am J Hum Genet. 2007;80(2):361–71.
85. Ghoumid J, Andrieux J, Sablonniere B, Odent S, Philippe N, Zanlonghi X, et al. Duplication of chromosome 2q31.1-q31.2 in a family presenting syndactyly and nystagmus. Eur J Hum Genet. 2011;19(11):1198–201. doi:10.1038/ejhg.2011.95.
86. Debeer P, Schoenmakers EF, Twal WO, Argraves WS, De Smet L, Fryns JP, et al. The fibulin-1 gene (FBLN1) is disrupted in a t(12;22) associated with a complex type of synpolydactyly. Med Genet. 2002;39(2):98–104.

87. Debeer P, Schoenmakers EF, De Smet L, Van de Ven WJ, Fryns JP. Co-segregation of an apparently balanced reciprocal t(12;22)(p11.2;q13.3) with a complex type of 3/3'/4 synpolydactyly associated with metacarpal, metatarsal and tarsal synostoses in three family members. Clin Dysmorphol. 1998;7(3):225–8.
88. Debeer P, Schoenmakers EF, Thoelen R, Holvoet M, Kuittinen T, Fabry G, et al. Physical map of a 1.5 mb region on 12p11.2 harbouring a synpolydactyly associated chromosomal breakpoint. Eur J Hum Genet. 2000;8(8):561–70.
89. Malik S, Abbasi AA, Ansar M, Ahmad W, Koch MC, Grzeschik KH. Genetic heterogeneity of synpolydactyly: a novel locus SPD3 maps to chromosome 14q11.2-q12. Clin Genet. 2006;69(6): 518–24.
90. Malik S, Grzeschik KH. Synpolydactyly: clinical and molecular advances. Clin Genet. 2008;73(2):113–20.
91. Kuru I, Samli H, Yucel A, Bozan ME, Turkmen S, Solak M. Hypoplastic synpolydactyly as a new clinical subgroup of synpolydactyly. Hand Surg Br. 2004;29(6):614–20.
92. Ikegawa M, Han H, Okamoto A, Matsui R, Tanaka M, Omi N, et al. Syndactyly and preaxial synpolydactyly in the single Sfrp2 deleted mutant mice. Dev Dyn. 2008;237(9):2506–17.
93. Johnston O, Kirby VV. Syndactyly of the ring and little finger. Am J Hum Genet. 1955;7:80–2.
94. De Smet L, Mulier T, Fabry G. Syndactyly of the ring and small finger. Genet Couns. 1994;5:45–9.
95. Schrander-Stumpel CTRM, de Groot-Wijnands JBG, de Die-Smulders C, Fryns JP. Type III syndactyly and oculodentodigital dysplasia: a clinical spectrum. Genet Couns. 1993;4:271–6.
96. Gladwin A, Donnai D, Metcalfe K, Schrander-Stumpel C, Brueton L, Verloes A, et al. Localization of a gene for oculodentodigital syndrome to human chromosome 6q22-q24. Hum Mol Genet. 1997;6(1):123–7.
97. Paznekas WA, Boyadjiev SA, Shapiro RE, Daniels O, Wollnik B, Keegan CE, et al. Connexin 43 (GJA1) mutations cause the pleiotropic phenotype of oculodentodigital dysplasia. Am J Hum Genet. 2003;72:408–18.
98. Richardson R, Donnai D, Meire F, Dixon MJ. Expression of Gja1 correlates with the phenotype observed in oculodentodigital syndrome/type III syndactyly. J Med Genet. 2004;41(1):60–7.
99. Dobrowolski R, Hertig G, Lechner H, Wörsdörfer P, Wulf V, Dicke N, et al. Loss of connexin43-mediated gap junctional coupling in the mesenchyme of limb buds leads to altered expression of morphogens in mice. Hum Mol Genet. 2009;18(15):2899–911.
100. Fenwick A, Richardson RJ, Butterworth J, Barron MJ, Dixon MJJ. Novel mutations in GJA1 cause oculodentodigital syndrome. Dent Res. 2008;87(11):1021–6.
101. Amador C, Mathews AM, Del Carmen MM, Laughridge ME, Everman DB, Holden KR. Expanding the neurologic phenotype of oculodentodigital dysplasia in a 4-generation Hispanic family. J Child Neurol. 2008;23(8):901–5.
102. Debeer P, Van Esch H, Huysmans C, Pijkels E, De Smet L, Van de Ven W, et al. Novel GJA1 mutations in patients with oculo-dento-digital dysplasia (ODDD). Eur J Med Genet. 2005;48(4):377–87.
103. Jamsheer A, Wisniewska M, Szpak A, Bugaj G, Krawczynski MR, Budny B, et al. A novel GJA1 missense mutation in a Polish child with oculodentodigital dysplasia. Appl Genet. 2009;50(3):297–9.
104. Dobrowolski R, Sasse P, Schrickel JW, Watkins M, Kim JS, Rackauskas M, et al. The conditional connexin43G138R mouse mutant represents a new model of hereditary oculodentodigital dysplasia in humans. Hum Mol Genet. 2008;17(4):539–54.
105. Dobrowolski R, Sommershof A, Willecke K. Some oculodento-digital dysplasia-associated Cx43 mutations cause increased hemichannel activity in addition to deficient gap junction channels. J Membr Biol. 2007;219(1–3):9–17.
106. van Es RJ, Wittebol-Post D, Beemer FA. Oculodentodigital dysplasia with mandibular retrognathism and absence of syndactyly: a case report with a novel mutation in the connexin 43 gene. Int J Oral Maxillofac Surg. 2007;36(9):858–60.
107. Vreeburg M, de Zwart-Storm EA, Schouten MI, Nellen RG, Marcus-Soekarman D, Devies M, et al. Skin changes in oculo-dento-digital dysplasia are correlated with C-terminal truncations of connexin 43. Am J Med Genet A. 2007;143(4):360–3.
108. Wiest T, Herrmann O, Stögbauer F, Grasshoff U, Enders H, Koch MJ, et al. Clinical and genetic variability of oculodentodigital dysplasia. Clin Genet. 2006;70(1):71–2.
109. Haas SL. Bilateral complete syndactylism of all fingers. Am J Surg. 1940;50:363–6.
110. Sato D, Liang D, Wu L, Pan Q, Xia K, Dai H, et al. Syndactyly type IV locus maps to 7q36. J Hum Genet. 2007;52:561–4.
111. Rambaud-Cousson A, Dudin AA, Zuaiter AS, Thalji A. Syndactyly type IV/hexadactyly of feet associated with unilateral absence of the tibia. Am J Med Genet. 1991;40:144–5.
112. Gillessen-Kaesbach G, Majewski F. Bilateral complete polysyndactyly (type IV Haas). Am J Med Genet. 1991;38:29–31.
113. Wieczorek D, Pawlik B, Li Y, Akarsu NA, Caliebe A, May KJ, et al. A specific mutation in the distant sonic hedgehog (SHH) cis-regulator (ZRS) causes Werner mesomelic syndrome (WMS) while complete ZRS duplications underlie Haas type polysyndactyly and preaxial polydactyly (PPD) with or without triphalangeal thumb. Hum Mutat. 2010;31(1):81–9.
114. Sun M, Ma F, Zeng X, Liu Q, Zhao XL, Wu FX, et al. Triphalangeal thumb-polysyndactyly syndrome and syndactyly type IV are caused by genomic duplications involving the long range, limb-specific SHH enhancer. J Med Genet. 2008;45:589–95.
115. Wang ZQ, Tian SH, Shi YZ, Zhou PT, Wang ZY, Shu RZ, et al. A single C to T transition in intron 5 of LMBR1 gene is associated with triphalangeal thumb-polysyndactyly syndrome in a Chinese family. Biochem Biophys Res Commun. 2007;355(2):312–7.
116. Kemp T, Ravn J. Ueber erbliche Hand-und Fussdeformitaeten in einem 140-koepfigen Geschlecht, nebst einigen Bemerkungen ueber Poly-und Syndaktylie beim Menschen. Acta Psychiatr Neurol Scand. 1932;7:275–96.
117. Robinow M, Johnson GF, Broock GJ. Syndactyly type V. Am J Med Genet. 1982;11:475–82.
118. Kjaer KW, Hansen L, Eiberg H, Utkus A, Skovgaard LT, Leicht P, et al. A 72-year-old Danish puzzle resolved—comparative analysis of phenotypes in families with different-sized HOXD13 polyalanine expansions. Am J Med Genet. 2005;138A:328–39.
119. Cenani A, Lenz W. Totale Syndaktylie und totale radioulnare Synostose bie zwei Bruedern. Ein Beitrag zur Genetik der Syndaktylien Ztschr Kinderheilk. 1967;101:181–90.
120. Liebenam L. Ueber gleichzeitiges Vorkommen von Gliedmassend efekten und osteosklerotischer Systemerkrunkung. Ztschr Mensch Vererbungs-und Konstitutionslehre. 1938;21:697–703.
121. Borsky AJ. Congenital anomalies of the hand and their surgical treatment. Springfield, IL: Charles C Thomas; 1958.
122. Yelton CL. Certain congenital limb deficiencies occurring in twins and half siblings. Inter-Clinic Inform Bull. 1962;1:1–7.
123. Drögemüller C, Leeb T, Harlizius B, Tammen I, Distl O, Höltershinken M, et al. Congenital syndactyly in cattle: four novel mutations in the low density lipoprotein receptor-related protein 4 gene (LRP4). BMC Genet. 2007;8:5.
124. Simon-Chazottes D, Tutois S, Kuehn M, Evans M, Bourgade F, Cook S, et al. Mutations in the gene encoding the low-density lipoprotein receptor LRP4 cause abnormal limb development in the mouse. Genomics. 2006;87(5):673–7.
125. Li Y, Pawlik B, Elcioglu N, Aglan M, Kayserili H, Yigit G, et al. LRP4 mutations alter Wnt/beta-catenin signaling and cause limb

and kidney malformations in Cenani-Lenz syndrome. Am J Hum Genet. 2010;86(5):696–706.
126. Bacchelli C, Goodman FR, Scambler PJ, Winter RM. Cenani-Lenz syndrome with renal hypoplasia is not linked to FORMIN or GREMLIN. Clin Genet. 2001;59:203–5.
127. Dimitrov BI, Voet T, De Smet L, Vermeesch JR, Devriendt K, Fryns JP, et al. Genomic rearrangements of the GREM1–FMN1 locus cause oligosyndactyly, radio-ulnar synostosis, hearing loss, renal defects syndrome and Cenani–Lenz-like non-syndromic oligosyndactyly. J Med Genet. 2010;47(8):569–74.
128. Harpf C, Pavelka M, Hussl H. A variant of Cenani-Lenz syndactyly (CLS): review of the literature and attempt of classification. Br J Plast Surg. 2005;58(2):251–7.
129. Orel H. Kleine Beitrage zur Vererbungswissenschaft. Synostosis Metacarpi Quarti et Quinti Z Anat. 1928;14:244–52.
130. Lonardo F, Della Monica M, Riccardi G, Riccio I, Riccio V, Scarano G. A family with X-linked recessive fusion of metacarpals IV and V. Am J Med Genet. 2004;124A:407–10.
131. Holmes LB, Wolf E, Miettinen OS. Metacarpal 4-5 fusion with X-linked recessive inheritance. Am J Hum Genet. 1972;24: 562–8.
132. Lerch H. Erbliche Synostosen der Ossa metacarpalia IV und V. Z Orthop. 1948;78:13–6.
133. Faiyaz-Ul-Haque M, Zaidi SHE, King LM, Haque S, Patel M, Ahmad M, et al. Fine mapping of the X-linked split-hand/split-foot malformation (SHFM2) locus to a 5.1-Mb region on Xq26.3 and analysis of candidate genes. Clin Genet. 2005;67:93–7.
134. Percin EF, Percin S, Egilmez H, Sezgin I, Ozbas F, Akarsu AN. Mesoaxial complete syndactyly and synostosis with hypoplastic thumbs: an unusual combination or homozygous expression of syndactyly type I. J Med Genet. 1998;35(10):868–74.
135. Malik S, Arshad M, Amin-ud-Din M, Oeffner F, Dempfle A, Haque S, et al. A novel type of autosomal recessive syndactyly: clinical and molecular studies in a family of Pakistani origin. Am J Med Genet. 2004;126A:61–7.
136. Losch G, Duncker H. Acrosyndactylism. Transactions of the International Society of Plastic and Reconstructive Surgeons, 5th Congress. Melbourne: Butterworth Pty; 1971.
137. Patterson T. Congenital ring constrictions. Br J Plast Surg. 1961; 14:1–31.
138. Torpin R, Faulkner A. Intrauterine amputation with the missing member found in the fetal membranes. JAMA. 1966;198:185–7.
139. Upton J. Congenital anomalies of the hand and forearm. In: McCarthy JG, May Jr JW, Littler JW, editors. The hand, vol 8 plastic surgery. Philadelphia, PA: WB Saunders; 1990. p. 5213–398.
140. Acrosyndactyly WR. A study of 27 patients. Clin Orthop. 1970; 71:99–111.
141. Maisels D. Acrosyndactyly. Br J Plast Surg. 1962;15:166–72.
142. Poland A. Deficiency of the pectoral muscles. Guy's Hosp Rep. 1841;VI:191–3.
143. Clarkson P. Poland's syndactyly. Guy's Hosp Rep. 1962;111: 335–46.
144. Bouvet J, Leveque D, Bernetieres F, Gros JJ. Vascular origin of Poland syndrome: a comparative rheographic study of the vascularisation of the arms in eight patients. Eur J Pediatr. 1978;128:17–26.
145. Fraser FC, Ronen GM, O'Leary E. Pectoralis major defect and Poland sequence in second cousins: extension of the Poland sequence spectrum. Am J Med Genet. 1989;33:468–70.
146. Bouwes-Bavinck J, Weaver D. Subclavian artery supply disruption sequence: hypothesis of a vascular etiology for Poland, Klippel-Feil, and Mobius anomalies. Am J Med Genet. 1986; 23:903–18.
147. Wilson M, Louis DS, Stevenson TR. Poland's syndrome: variable expression and associated anomalies. J Hand Surg Am. 1988;13:880–2.
148. Karnak I, Tanyel FC, Tunçbilek E, Unsal M, Büyükpamukçu N. Bilateral Poland anomaly. Am J Med Genet. 1998;75(5): 505–7.
149. Wilkie AOM, Slaney SF, Oldridge M, Poole MD, Ashworth GJ, Hockley AD, et al. Apert syndrome results from localized mutations of FGFR2 and is allelic with Crouzon syndrome. Nat Genet. 1995;9:165–72.
150. Howard TD, Paznekas WA, Green ED, Chiang LC, Ma N, Ortiz de Luna RI, et al. Mutations in TWIST, a basic helix-loop-helix transcription factor, in Saethre-Chotzen syndrome. Nat Genet. 1997;15:36–41.
151. Paznekas WA, Cunningham ML, Howard TD, Korf BR, Lipson MH, Grix AW, et al. Genetic heterogeneity of Saethre-Chotzen syndrome, due to TWIST and FGFR mutations. Am J Hum Genet. 1998;62:1370–80.
152. Muenke M, Schell U, Hehr A, Robin NH, Losken HW, Schinzel A, et al. A common mutation in the fibroblast growth factor receptor 1 gene in Pfeiffer syndrome. Nat Genet. 1994;8:269–74.
153. Rossi M, Jones RL, Norbury G, Bloch-Zupan A, Winter R. The appearance of the feet in Pfeiffer syndrome caused by FGFR1 P252R mutation. Clin Dysmorphol. 2003;12:269–74.
154. Jenkins D, Seelow D, Jehee FS, Perlyn CA, Alonso LG, Bueno DF, et al. RAB23 mutations in Carpenter syndrome imply an unexpected role for hedgehog signaling in cranial-suture development and obesity. Am J Hum Genet. 2007;80:1162–70. Note: Erratum: Am. J. Hum. Genet. 81: 1114 only, 2007.
155. Cohen DM, Green JG, Miller J, Gorlin RJ, Reed JA. Acrocephalopolysyndactyly type II—Carpenter syndrome: clinical spectrum and an attempt at unification with Goodman and Summitt syndromes. Am J Med Genet. 1987;28:311–24.
156. McGregor L, Makela V, Darling SM, Vrontou S, Chalepakis G, Roberts C, et al. Fraser syndrome and mouse blebbed phenotype caused by mutations in FRAS1/Fras1 encoding a putative extracellular matrix protein. Nat Genet. 2003;34:203–8.
157. Shafeghati Y, Kniepert A, Vakili G, Zenker M. Fraser syndrome due to homozygosity for a splice site mutation of FREM2. Am J Med Genet. 2008;146A:529–31.
158. Carney TJ, Feitosa NM, Sonntag C, Slanchev K, Kluger J, Kiyozumi D, et al. Genetic analysis of fin development in zebrafish identifies furin and hemicentin1 as potential novel fraser syndrome disease genes. PLoS Genet. 2010;6(4):e1000907.
159. Malik S, Ahmad W, Grzeschik KH, Koch MC. A simple method for characterising syndactyly in clinical practice. Genet Couns. 2005;16:229–38.
160. Winter RM, Tickle C. Syndactylies and polydactilies: embryological overview and suggested classification. Eur J Hum Genet. 1993;1:96–104.
161. Man LX, Chang B. Maternal cigarette smoking during pregnancy increases the risk of having a child with a congenital digital anomaly. Plast Reconstr Surg. 2006;117(1):301–8.
162. Luo JY, Fu CH, Yao KB, Hu RS, Qy D, Liu ZY. A case-control study on genetic and environmental factors regarding polydactyly and syndactyly. Zhonghua Liu Xing Bing Xue Za Zhi. 2009; 30(9):903–6.
163. Lorea P, Coessens BC. Evolution of surgical techniques for skin release. Eur J Plast Surg. 2001;24:275–81.
164. Oda T, Pushman AG, Chung KC. Treatment of common congenital hand conditions. Plast Reconstr Surg. 2010;126(3):121e–33.
165. Kettelkamp DB, Flatt AE. An evaluation of syndactylia repair. Surg Gynecol Obstet. 1961;113:471–8.
166. Dao K, Shin AY, Billings A. Surgical treatment of congenital syndactyly of the hand. J Am Acad Orthop Surg. 2004;12:39–48.
167. Hutchinson DT, Frenzen SW. Digital syndactyly release. Tech Hand Up Extrem Surg. 2010;14(1):33–7.
168. Deunck J, Nicolai JP, Hamburg SM. Long-term results of syndactyly correction: full-thickness versus split-thickness skin grafts. J Hand Surg Br. 2003;28(2):125–30.

169. Lumenta DB, Kitzinger HB, Beck H, Frey M. Long-term outcomes of web creep, scar quality and function after simple syndactyly surgical treatment. J Hand Surg Am. 2010;35(8): 1323–9.
170. Kamath JB, Vardhan H, Naik DM, Bansal A, Rai M, Kumar A. A novel method of using mini external fixator for maintaining web space after the release of contracture and syndactyly. Tech Hand Up Extrem Surg. 2013;17(1):37–40.
171. Aydin A, Ozden BC. Dorsal metacarpal island flap in syndactyly treatment. Ann Plast Surg. 2004;52(1):43–8.
172. Sharma RK, Tuli P, Makkar SS, Parashar A. End-f-skin grafts in syndactyly release: description of a new flap for web resurfacing and primary closure of finger defects. Hand. 2009;4(1):29–34.
173. Gao W, Yan H, Zhang F, Jiang L, Wang A, Yang J, et al. Dorsal pentagonal local flap: a new technique of web reconstruction for syndactyly without skin graft. Aesthetic Plast Surg. 2011;35(4):530–7.
174. Yao JM, Shong JL, Sun H. Repair of incomplete simple syndactyly by a web flap on a subcutaneous tissue pedicle. Plast Reconstr Surg. 1997;99:2079–81.
175. Tadiparthi S, Mishra A, Mcarthur P. A modification of the Chinese island flap technique for simple incomplete syndactyly release. J Hand Surg Eur Vol. 2009;34(1):99–103.
176. Greuse M, Coessens BC. Congenital syndactyly: defatting facilitates closure without skin graft. J Hand Surg Am. 2001;26:589–94.
177. Jose RM, Timoney N, Vidyadharan R, Lester R. Syndactyly correction: an aesthetoc reconstruction. J Hand Surg Eur Vol. 2010;35(6):446–50.
178. Buck-Gramcko D. Congenital malformations: syndactyly and related deformities. In: Higst H, Buck-Gramcko D, Millesi H, et al., editors. Hand surgery. New York, NY: Thieme Medical Publishers; 1988.
179. Niranjan NS, Azad SM, Fleming ANM, Liew SH. Long-term results of primary syndactyly correction by the trilobed flap technique. Br J Plast Surg. 2005;58:14–21.
180. Vekris MD, Lykissas MG, Soucacos PN, Korompilias AV, Beris AE. Congenital syndactyly: outcome of surgical treatment in 131 webs. Tech Hand Up Extrem Surg. 2010;14:2–7.
181. Goldfarb CA, Steffen JA, Stutz CM. Complex syndactyly: aesthetic and objective outcomes. J Hand Surg Am. 2012;37: 2068–73.
182. Miyamoto J, Nagasao T, Miyamoto S. Biomechanical analysis of surgical correction of syndactyly. Plast Reconstr Surg. 2010; 125(3):963–8.
183. Cromblehome TM, Dirkes K, Whitney TM, Alman B, Garmel S, Connelly RJ. Amniotic band syndrome in fetal lambs: I. Fetoscopic release and morphometric outcome. J Pediatr Surg. 1995;30:974.
184. Husler MR, Wilson RD, Horri SC, Bebbington MW, Adzick NS, Johnson MP. When is fetoscopic release of amniotic bands indicated? Review of outcome of cases treated in utero and selection criteria for fetal surgery. Prenat Diagn. 2009;29:457–63.

Syndactyly: Apert Syndrome

14

Brian C. Pridgen, Arhana Chattopadhyay, and James Chang

Introduction

History and Brief Description of Clinical Features

Apert syndrome is a rare congenital disorder characterized by premature craniosynostosis, midface hypoplasia, and bilateral syndactyly of the hands and feet, as well as a constellation of more variable findings in other organ systems [1]. Treating Apert patients requires a specialized team of clinicians who can provide close monitoring, carefully timed surgical interventions, and management of chronic symptoms.

In the late nineteenth century, there were a series of case reports, primarily in the French literature, describing what would come to be known as Apert syndrome. The initial description was by Robert Troquart in 1886 [2]. Eugene Apert made his initial observation in 1896 while working as an intern at Hôpital des Enfants-Malade, the children's hospital in Paris, where he saw a patient with a constellation of findings that he would later term acrocephalosyndactyly. In 1906 he described the syndrome of acrocephalosyndactyly based on eight case reports dating to 1886 with a cluster of malformations similar to the patient he saw as an intern [3]. Apert characterized acrocephalosyndactyly by both a tall skull that is flat in the back and sides but protruding abnormally in the front, resembling a French firefighter's helmet, and symmetrical syndactyly of the four limbs. He also described associated symptoms including cleft palate, ankylosis of the elbows, synonychia, and a spared trunk and proximal limbs. Apert's initial clinical descriptions remain accurate and have been complemented by advances in imaging that have expanded the morphological characterization of the disease.

In addition to characterizing the morphology of acrocephalosyndactyly anomalies, Apert also proposed potential etiologies. He theorized that a hereditary cause was unlikely because cases were isolated within families. One cause he proposed was polyhydramnios, which could cause amniotic compression of the fetus and, thus, deform the skull. He expressed skepticism, however, that this was the sole cause because amniotic compression generally caused both irregular deformities in the skull and congenital amputation of the digits accompanying the syndactyly, both of which were not consistent with his findings in acrocephalosyndactyly. He also admitted that his theory did not explain the highly uniform craniofacial features and symmetric syndactyly that were characteristic of the disease he observed [2].

Apert's critical look at his own theories paved the way for future researchers to search for the cause of acrocephalosyndactyly. A 1920 study by Park and Powers contested Apert's theory that acrocephalosyndactyly was a single disorder with a single etiology due to the great variability in its clinical presentation [4]. They cited the evidence that in several cases of acrocephalosyndactyly patients did not exhibit complete bilateral syndactyly. However, Blank resolved this discrepancy in 1959 with 54 case reviews, 34 of which he observed firsthand [5]. In this landmark study, he divided his cases into two subtypes—typical acrocephalosyndactyly with complete bilateral syndactyly as described by Apert (Type I) and atypical acrocephalosyndactyly with partial syndactyly (Type II). He proposed that Type I and Type II acrocephalosyndactyly were likely unrelated but that Type I syndrome was caused by a mutation of a single gene. Blank referred to typical Type I acrocephalosyndactyly as "Apert syndrome," thereby coining the term.

Because genetic theory had been developed by 1959, Blank had an advantage over his predecessors in describing the cause of Apert syndrome. He suggested that sporadic instances of Apert, which constituted the majority of cases, resulted from mutations in parental germ cells and that there

B.C. Pridgen, M.D. • A. Chattopadhyay, B.A.
J. Chang, M.D. (✉)
Division of Plastic and Reconstructive Surgery, Stanford University Medical Center, 770 Welch Road, Suite 400, Palo Alto, CA 94304, USA
e-mail: jameschang@stanford.edu

D.R. Laub Jr. (ed.), *Congenital Anomalies of the Upper Extremity: Etiology and Management*,
DOI 10.1007/978-1-4899-7504-1_14, © Springer Science+Business Media New York 2015

was a significant relationship between incidence of Apert syndrome and advanced paternal age [5]. However, the precise cause of Apert syndrome remained elusive until Wilkie et al. discovered a molecular basis involving two highly specific genetic mutations in fibroblast growth factor receptor 2 (*FGFR2*) [6]. Thereafter, studies using modern biochemical techniques continued to elucidate the molecular mechanisms underlying Apert syndrome, as will be discussed in the "Molecular etiology" section later in this chapter.

Prior to the discovery of the molecular basis of Apert syndrome, much of the work on the disease focused on the surgical management of the multiple associated anomalies [2]. An early focus of surgical intervention was to manage increased intracranial pressure in patients exhibiting craniosynostosis. Skull decompression and reconstruction techniques, including strip, linear, and circular craniectomies, were utilized until craniofacial skeletal advancement techniques were developed. Paul Tessier in particular considered Apert syndrome a prototype for other craniofacial deformities [7]. His methods for correcting hypertelorism and midface retrusion found in Apert patients pioneered the field of craniofacial surgery.

Correction of complex bilateral syndactyly was another area of emphasis for surgeons. In 1970, Hoover published the first study focusing specifically on surgical techniques for the Apert hand, as will be discussed later in this chapter [8].

Genetics and Embryology

Molecular Etiology

Apert syndrome can be inherited in an autosomal dominant pattern, but de novo mutations of paternal origin are the most common cause [9]. Ninety-eight percent of cases are due to two missense cytosine to guanine base substitutions in FGFR2: Pro253Arg and Ser252Trp [6]. *FGFR* is a member of the tyrosine kinase receptor family and is involved in normal limb bud patterning and connective tissue development during embryogenesis. Pro253Arg and Ser252Trp disrupt the linking region between the second and third immunoglobulin domains in FGFR2.

Of the 98 % of Apert cases caused by the two canonical FGFR2 mutations, the Pro253Arg mutation constitutes one-third of cases, and the Ser252Trp mutation constitutes two-thirds of cases [9]. Patients with a Pro253Arg missense mutation generally present with more severe forms of syndactyly and more impaired cognitive function than patients with a Ser252Trp mutation; however, the incidence of cleft palate is more common in patients with the Ser252Trp mutation [10].

Biochemical and structural studies of mutant FGFR2 provide potential mechanisms linking genetic mutations and patient phenotype. During normal embryonic development, the FGFR2b isoform is expressed in epithelial tissue and is activated by mesenchymal FGF ligand. The FGFR2c isoform is expressed in mesenchymal tissue and is activated by epithelial FGF ligand [11]. In Apert syndrome, Ser252Trp and Pro253Arg mutations are thought to induce the FGFR2b and FGF2Rc isoforms to lose ligand specificity. Ser252Trp and Pro253Arg disrupt the linking region between the second and third immunoglobulin domains in FGFR2c so that mesenchymal FGF7 and FGF10 ligands become capable of activating mesenchymal FGFR2c. Thus, FGFR2c becomes abnormally susceptible to autocrine signaling, which is thought to result in Apert pathology.

Ibrahimi et al. theorize that clinical variability can arise from differential degrees of FGFR2 gain-of-function [12]. They suggest that more severe forms of syndactyly occur in Pro253Arg mutation patients through increased autocrine signaling. This is based on the prediction that mesenchymal Pro253Arg FGFR2c has a higher affinity for mesenchymal FGF7 and FGF10 than both wild type and Ser252Trp FGFR2c do. They further suggest that the increased incidence of cleft palate in Ser252Trp patients as compared to Pro252Arg patients occurs via enhanced activation of normal FGF signaling. This is based on the crystal structure prediction that mesenchymal Ser252Trp FGFR2c has a higher affinity for epithelial FGF2 than mesenchymal Pro253Arg FGFR2c does.

An alternate genetic mechanism for a minority of Apert patients is a de novo Alu element insertion either upstream or within exon C of FGFR2, which can cause ectopic expression of FGFR2b in the mesenchyme along with normal expression of FGFR2c [13].

Historically, the advanced age of fathers of Apert children has suggested that Apert syndrome, like achondroplasia, is influenced by the Paternal Age Effect (PAE) [5]. The PAE posits that the incidence of certain genetic disorders increases with increasing paternal age due to an increased number of accumulated germline mutations and an increased mutation rate in the sperm of older males [14]. However, the combined effect of the linear increase in cell divisions and the increased mutation rate was insufficient to explain the exponential increase in Apert birth incidence with increasing paternal age. Goriely et al. suggested that the Ser252Trp mutation may confer a selective advantage to sperm stem cells, leading to increased clonal expansion of mutant sperm [15]. This mechanism could more fully explain the increased incidence of Apert births to older fathers.

Prenatal Diagnosis

Suspected Apert syndrome is confirmed prenatally by amniocentesis [16]. However, screening for Apert syndrome remains challenging because the pathognomonic facial and skeletal changes of Apert syndrome are difficult to visualize through ultrasound before the third trimester. David et al. report cases in which craniofacial and extremity abnormalities detected in the second trimester through careful 2D and 3D ultrasound examination were later confirmed as prenatal signs of Apert syndrome by amniocentesis [17]. Quintero-Rivera et al. point to fetal CNS abnormalities, such as agenesis of the corpus callosum (ACC) and ventriculomegaly, as early indicators of Apert syndrome that can be detected through MRI before pathognomonic morphologies can be discerned [16]. Thus, the algorithm for prenatal diagnosis is, after suspected Apert based upon detection of mild ventriculomegaly or ACC upon ultrasound, to follow up with an MRI and 3D ultrasound and confirmation using amniocentesis.

Epidemiology

Apert syndrome is a rare disorder that historically has been challenging to track, as most cases occur due to spontaneous mutations rather than due to familial inheritance; only 11 Apert patients have been documented to have had children [18]. It also has been difficult to distinguish Apert infants from patients with other craniosynostosis disorders or with multiple birth defects due to the great variability in clinical presentation [19]. Diagnosis and documentation of Apert syndrome has improved with the development of better birth defect surveillance systems and greater awareness of the disorder in the medical community. Cohen et al. published the first extensive multi-site epidemiological study of Apert syndrome in 1992 in which they defined an Apert case as a patient exhibiting craniosynostosis, midface hypoplasia, and symmetric syndactyly of hands and feet [19]. Based on data from seven sites, they calculated an Apert birth prevalence of 15.5 cases per million live births. They also estimated Apert syndrome to constitute 4.5 % of all craniosynostosis cases.

A more recent study that drew samples from the California Birth Defects Monitoring Program (CBDMP) calculated an Apert birth prevalence of 12.4 cases per million births [18]. Prevalence was found to be highest among Asians and lowest among Hispanics with approximately equal numbers of affected males and females. In almost half of tracked cases, the age of the father was 35 or older, supporting the theory of the PAE and the association of Apert syndrome with mutations in paternal rather than maternal alleles.

Clinical Features

Apert syndrome is clinically diagnosed based on the presence of craniosynostosis, midface hypoplasia, bilateral syndactyly, and specific genetic mutations. As mentioned previously, patients also present with a highly variable collection of features that affect multiple organ systems. The pathogenetic mechanisms underlying many of these features remain largely unknown. Clinical features associated with Apert syndrome can be broadly categorized into craniofacial, CNS, visceral, skeletal, and dermatological pathologies.

Craniofacial Anomalies

The skulls of Apert syndrome patients are characterized by a large cranial volume, increased height, and decreased rostral-caudal head length [20]. Fearon and Podner categorize Apert skulls into type I skulls, which have a split metopic suture without anterior turricephaly and soft nonbulging dura; type II skulls, which have a closed metopic suture with moderate turribrachycephaly; and type III skulls, which are Pfeiffer-type and exhibit severe turricephaly [21]. In type I skulls, which are most common, the coronal suture is fused at birth, but other sutures and fontanels are patent. Patients are born with a wide midline calvarial defect formed from the metopic and sagittal sutures extending from the glabella to the posterior fontanel. Bony islands form and coalesce to close the defect by age 2–4 [1]. This defect allows some early growth of the brain [21]. In contrast, the midline defect closes earlier in type II skulls, leading to constriction of anterior skull growth and turricephaly. The rare type III skulls have pansutural fusions, leading to a towering skull that presents like the skulls of Pfeiffer syndrome patients.

The primary goals for craniofacial surgical treatment of Apert patients are to preempt preventable developmental delays, minimize the number and risks of procedures, and help to improve aesthetic appearance by the time of skeletal maturity [21]. When optimizing timing and extent of cranial vault remodeling for each skull type, clinicians must weigh the benefits of intracranial decompression and improved appearance with the risks of causing iatrogenic skull growth inhibition. Fearon and Podner advocate a guiding principle of later surgery for less severe type I skulls (15 months) and earlier intervention for type II (9–12 months) and type III (6 months) skulls.

In addition, patients frequently present with a cleft palate and maxillary hypoplasia [22]. A cleft palate or bifid uvula may result in frequent otitis media. Shallow orbits and ocular proptosis predispose Apert patients to injury to unprotected eyes, exposure keratitis, and corneal abrasions. Patients may exhibit exotropia, hyperopia, or astigmatism. Increased ocular pressure can lead to blindness [23].

CNS Abnormalities

Several CNS anomalies are associated with Apert syndrome. Most patients exhibit corpus callosum and limbic structure malformation [24]. Cohen and Kreiborg also reported frequent occurrence of gyral abnormalities, cerebral white matter hypoplasia, and heterotopic grey matter.

Cognitive function among Apert patients ranges widely. The impact of timing of the first surgical intervention on Intelligence Quotient (IQ) is contested. Renier et al. found that initial skull surgery before age 1 was the main factor that caused increased IQ, with some contribution from septum pellucidum morphology [25]. However, Fearon and Podner did not find a significant correlation between IQ and timing of surgery, severity of turricephaly, type of genetic mutation, or corpus callosum and septum pellucidum morphology [21]. Similarly Yacubian et al. did not find significant correlations between IQ and timing of surgery or intervention via strip craniectomy, and instead attribute differences in mental development to family environment and parents' education level [26].

Visceral Anomalies

Apert patients can present with cardiac, genitourinary, and, less frequently, respiratory and gastrointestinal pathologies [27]. Cohen and Kreiborg report up to 10 % of autopsied Apert patients presented with various, often concurrent, congenital heart abnormalities such as atrial and ventricular septal defects, dextrocardia, and pulmonic stenosis. Complex heart defects were associated with early mortality. They also report that 9.6 % of patients presented with genitourinary anomalies, including cryptorchidism in males and hydronephrosis.

Cohen and Kreiborg report a much lower frequency of respiratory (1.5 %) and gastrointestinal (1.5 %) symptoms. The most serious lower respiratory defect was a completely or partially solid cartilaginous trachea that restricted tracheal distensibility and caused respiratory insufficiency. Upper respiratory problems stemmed from nasopharyngeal and oropharyngeal space constraints due to craniofacial bone displacement and resulted in sleep apnea, cor pulmonale, and sudden death in patients [1].

Skeletal Abnormalities

Apart from changes in the skull and bony skeleton of the hands and feet, Apert patients can also exhibit cervical spine fusion, with 68 % of cases presenting with a fusion of vertebrae C5 and C6 [1]. Cohen and Kreiborg report cases of progressive limitation of shoulder, elbow, and knee joint mobility; pectus excavatum; irregular pelvic girdles; subacromial and elbow dimpling; winged scapulae; and abnormally short humeri.

Dermatological Anomalies

Skin anomalies such as dimples in the knuckles of Type I hands, increased sweat and sebaceous glands, oily skin, and acneiform lesions can be found in Apert patients [28]. Other symptoms include hypopigmentation, wrinkling of the forehead, and hyperhidrosis; mothers of Apert patients frequently report that the children sweat excessively while crying, breastfeeding, or even sleeping.

Upper Extremity Anomalies

Upper extremity involvement of Apert syndrome includes a short thumb with radial clinodactyly; involvement of the first web space with varying degrees of syndactyly between the thumb and index finger; complex syndactyly between the index, long, and ring fingers typically at the level of the distal interphalangeal joints or beyond; and variable degrees of syndactyly between the ring and small fingers. Additional findings include aberrant anatomy of the intrinsic muscles, extrinsic tendon insertions, neurovascular bundles, and absent proximal interphalangeal joints with the only functional interphalangeal joint typically being the distal interphalangeal joint of the small finger [29]. Van Heest and Reckling proposed a classification system based on the radiographic appearance of hands in Apert syndrome patients [30]. However, the more widely used classification system was described by Upton and includes three types of hands [29]. Type I hands, or "spade" hands, are defined by a complex syndactyly between the index, long, and ring fingers, and a simple syndactyly between the ring and small fingers. The thumb and index finger are separated, although the first web space may be shallow. Type II hands, or "spoon" or "mitten" hands, are defined by the features of Type I hands plus a partial or complete simple syndactyly between the thumb and index finger and a more complete simple syndactyly between the ring and small fingers. Type III hands, or "rosebud" hands, are defined by a complex syndactyly between the thumb, index, long, and ring fingers, and a complete simple syndactyly between the ring and small fingers. The Type III deformity is often so severe that it can be difficult to distinguish the thumb from the index finger. Table 14.1 shows the reported incidence of each of the Upton type hands in several groups' series.

Treatment

Reconstruction of the hand in patients with Apert syndrome is an evolving technique that presents a significant challenge to hand surgeons, and the treatment of the

Table 14.1 Reported incidence of each of the Upton type hands in several groups' series

Reference	Number of patients	Type I Number (percent)	Type II Number (percent)	Type III Number (percent)
Upton [29]	68	28 (41 %)	24 (35 %)	16 (24 %)
Cohen and Kreiborg [31]	44	20 (45 %)	18 (39 %)	6 (16 %)
Holten et al. [32]	45	29 (64 %)	10 (22 %)	6 (13 %)
Chang et al. [33]	10	5 (50 %)	1 (10 %)	4 (40 %)
Fearon [34]	17	11 (65 %)	2 (12 %)	4 (24 %)
Guero [35]	52	11 (21 %)	19 (37 %)	22 (42 %)
Totals	236	104 (44 %)	74 (31 %)	58 (25 %)

numerous hand anomalies encountered in Apert syndrome requires a complex operative plan with multiple stages through childhood and into adolescence. There has been a lively discussion in the literature over the past 20 years, adding to the prior body of literature, in which a variety of reconstructive plans have been outlined and modified. Although there are several common goals of each of these reconstructive plans, each author or group has their own preferences and biases. Several factors account for the lack of a clear consensus on the management of these patients, including the rarity of this syndrome, the presentation of each patient with a unique cluster of anomalies with varying degrees of severity, the role of surgeon preference and surgeon comfort in determining a reconstructive plan, and the difficulty in having the long-term follow-up needed to evaluate the durability of the reconstruction. Despite this lack of consensus, the common goals between most of the proposed reconstructive plans include minimizing the number of procedures, maximizing the functional outcome of the hand, and providing a favorable cosmetic result, which includes preserving as many digits as possible through judicious use of amputations.

It should be noted that in the past, there was some question about the utility of offering hand reconstruction to Apert syndrome patients due to mental impairment that can be quite severe. However, we feel and want to echo the sentiment of other authors [8, 35] who also specifically have emphasized the point that, regardless of the degree of mental impairment of the patient, the functional gains and cosmetic improvements following reconstruction offer significant quality of life improvements, both for the patient and for the family, that should not be withheld from Apert syndrome patients.

The technical goals for reconstruction of the Apert hand address syndactyly and symphalangism, thumb radial clinodactyly, and later secondary deformities requiring revision. These goals have been organized by several authors into a reconstructive plan. Considerations that must be made in the formulation of a reconstructive plan include age of the patient at the time of the initial operation, timing and sequence of the release of border digits, creating skin flaps and providing soft tissue coverage, need for digital amputation, thumb lengthening and straightening, and secondary revisions.

Patient Age

Ideally, patients with Apert syndrome should be referred shortly after birth to a center with the multidisciplinary expertise necessary to treat the hand and craniofacial anomalies associated with Apert syndrome. However, due to a variety of reasons, including patients who were born in parts of the world without the multidisciplinary teams available for reconstruction, Apert syndrome patients are often seen well after infancy. This can present a challenge and requires modifications to the reconstructive sequence in these patients.

The age of the patient is particularly relevant to the decision of whether both hands are operated on simultaneously or whether the same operation for each hand is delayed in a staged manner. Following each reconstruction, the patients are typically placed in casts or splint, which is variable from group to group. In patients who require bilateral upper extremity restraints, this can cause significant distress for the patient, depending how independent and interactive he or she is, and place a significant burden on the parents, again, depending on how dependent the patient is on the parents for assistance with basic tasks of daily care. The age below which operations are performed on bilateral extremities simultaneously varies from 12 [33, 35, 36] to 18 [37] to 24 months [8] among authors who specified. In patients who underwent the same procedure on each hand individually, the delay between procedures on each hand ranged from as short as 2 weeks [35] up to 3 [33] to 6 months [35, 36] to allow time for the contralateral hand to heal and become more functional.

Another consideration for timing, though mentioned in only one paper, was discussed by Hoover et al., who recommended waiting 6–9 months before operating on the same hand to allow time for adequate revascularization [8]. However, many authors do not wait this long and have not reported increased complications due to vascular compromise.

Syndactyly, Symphalangism, and Border Digits

Timing of release of the border digits is a source of controversy. Some authors suggest that postponing separation of the digits will lead to angular growth deformities due to differential growth of each of the digits [8, 29, 38], while others state that in their experience this is not the case [34]. Another consideration in the timing of the release of the digits is to provide early mobility to promote earlier motor development. Earlier release of the thumb and the small finger, the border digits, allows the patient to begin development of a grasp. Hoover recommends performing a border digit release by 1 year of age [8]. Fearon, however, did not observe these problems in his patients that did not undergo early border digit release [34].

For those authors that prioritize the release of the border digits in Upton Type II and III hands, two additional procedures are required to release the remaining syndactylies. This is the case because the remaining syndactylies after release of the border digits are the index-long and long-ring finger syndactylies. Releasing both of these syndactylies in the second and third web spaces requires operating on both sides of the long finger. Operating on both sides of the long finger during the same operation theoretically risks compromising the vascular supply to the long finger and having a shortage of flap skin [30, 34, 36]. To minimize this risk, the long finger syndactyly release is typically staged as two separate operations, which increases to three the number of operations a patient must undergo and increases the time spent by a patient without full release of all of his or her fingers. To reduce the number of operations, most surgeons release alternating web spaces, including releasing one side of the long finger syndactyly during the first operation while neglecting one of the two border digit syndactylies during the first operation [34].

As just mentioned, the concern for vascular compromise dictates operative staging and forces surgeons to choose either prioritizing border digit release or limiting the number of operations to two. Even with careful consideration of the vascular supply to the digits, the aberrant anatomy of the neurovascular bundles increases the risk of inadvertent disruption of the blood supply to the digits. To address these problems, Harvey et al. examined the role of CT angiogram to assist with mapping of the vascular supply to each digit [39]. This imaging was done concurrently with CT imaging performed for operative planning for craniofacial reconstruction. After mapping the vascular supply to the hand and planning the surgical approach, they attempted to perform a single-stage syndactyly release paying careful attention to the vascular anatomy based on the CT angiogram findings. In both hands of all five patients in this study, they were able to perform successfully a single-stage syndactyly release without any major complications.

We have not adopted this approach because another problem with release of adjacent fingers is the shortage of dorsal skin that can be used for dorsal flap coverage of the webs. Therefore, we feel that the risks and limitations of adjacent finger release outweigh the benefit of a single-stage approach.

Separation of the syndactyly in the fingers is typically performed with a zigzag incision. This results in interdigitating triangular flaps along the sides of the newly released digits. The purpose of this pattern is to avoid a straight-line scar along the sides of the fingers due to the concern for scar contracture leading to deviation of the finger or limitation of function. Syndactyly release in Apert syndrome is different because the fingers have some degree of symphalangism, with resultant stiff joints that will not deviate with scarring of the skin incisions [34]. Straight-line syndactyly release incisions will prevent the zigzag incisions from extending onto the dorsal and volar surface of the fingers and will allow application of one piece of skin graft to each side of the finger (Fig. 14.1) Upton suggests the small finger should be treated with extra caution with regard to the use of straight-line incisions.

Because many syndactylized fingers in Apert syndrome are complex (involving bone at the tip), two specific operative maneuvers are critical. Zigzag fingertip flaps, attributed to Buck-Gramcko, are useful for recreating the nail folds [40] (Fig. 14.2). Also, intraoperative fluoroscopy is used to visualize the bony fusion prior to osteotomy. A fine gauge needle is placed slightly off center to the proposed longitudinal osteotomy, and the osteotome is slid on top of the needle to allow precise sectioning of the bone (Fig. 14.3).

Several flaps have been described for reconstruction of the second, third, and fourth, web spaces. Barot and Caplan describe a dorsal rectangular flap that they inset into a volar T-incision [36]. Guero describes an omega-shaped dorsal flap [35]. Other authors perform a similar long dorsal flap for reconstruction of the web space. Fearon, however, uses equal length triangular dorsal and volar flaps [34]. This results in a length-to-width ratio that provides more favorable blood supply to the distal tip of the flap and better healing. He attributes this technique as the reason for his very low reported rate of 3 % for secondary syndactylies requiring reoperation. He designs the base of his dorsal flap proximal to the base of the volar flap to recreate the normal slope of the web space. In Upton's commentary on Fearon's article, Upton agrees with the Fearon's triangular flaps, but he cautions that the second web space may require a future secondary release due to increased metacarpal growth [34]. To accommodate for this, Upton recommends considering a wide rectangular flap being used initially, which can then more easily be advanced again if needed later in life. This is the flap design that we usually choose to use (Fig. 14.4).

For areas along the fingers that are not covered by the skin flaps raised during release of the syndactyly, full thickness

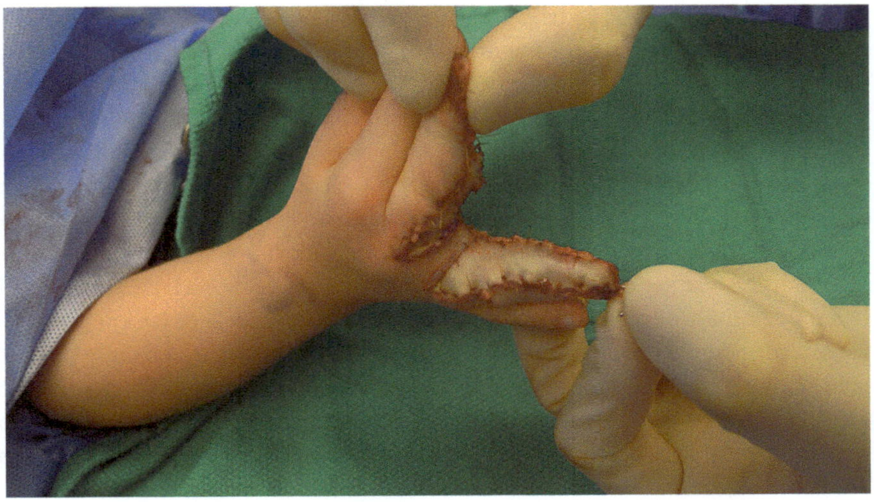

Fig. 14.1 Full thickness skin grafting after straight-line syndactyly release

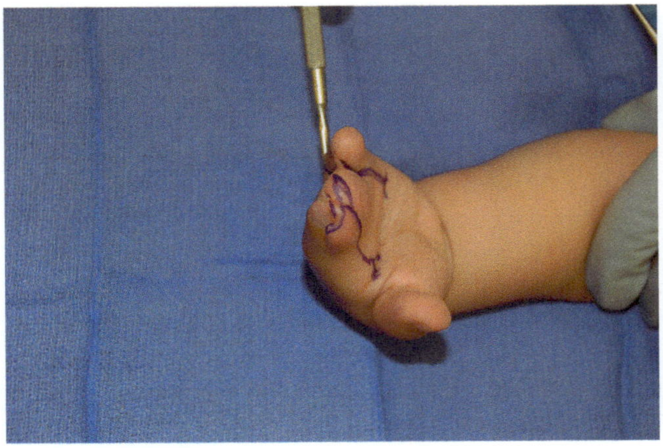

Fig. 14.2 Markings for zigzag fingertips for recreating the nail folds

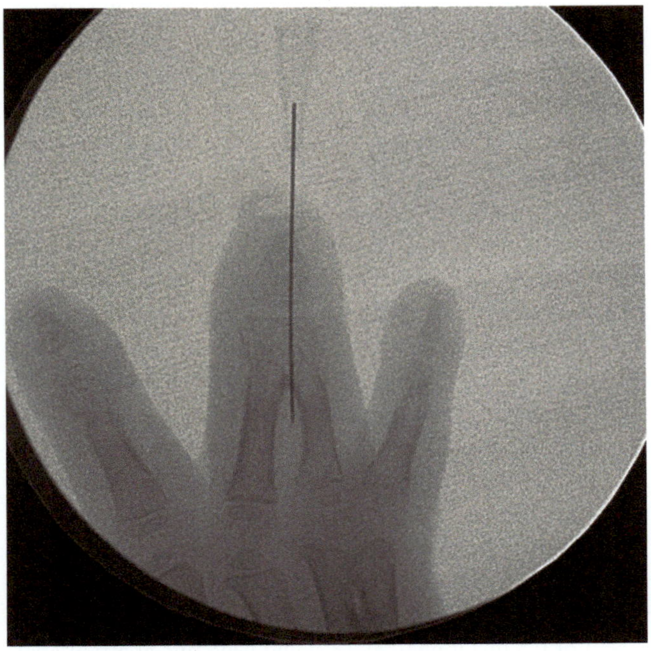

Fig. 14.3 Fluoroscopy image demonstrated needle positioning used to guide longitudinal osteotomy

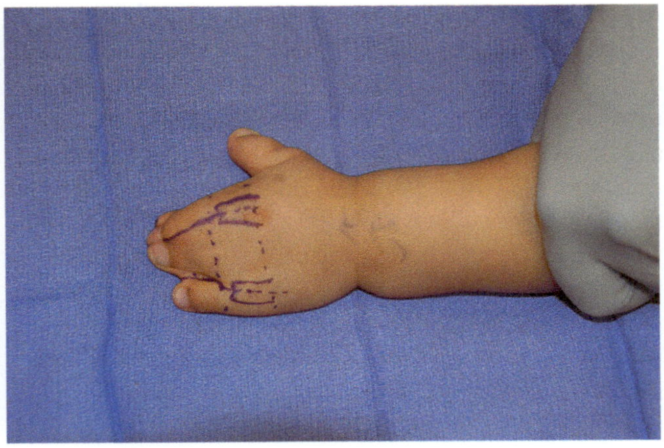

Fig. 14.4 Rectangular dorsal advancement flaps for web space reconstruction

skin grafts are typically applied. Split thickness skin grafts are rarely used due to graft contraction leading to decrease in size of the web space and due to the risk of recurrence of syndactyly. Full thickness skin grafts are typically harvested from the groin crease, avoiding the future hair-bearing skin, or occasionally from the antecubital crease. Skin harvested from circumcisions should never be used due to darkening of the harvesting skin with time, which provides a poor cosmetic result that patients often request to be revised. In cases with small areas of exposed bone without overlying vascularized tissue in the distal half of the released digits, Fearon did not provide coverage with skin grafts or tissue flaps [34]. This reduced the need for full thickness skin graft tissue but without increasing wound healing complications. In addition to skin grafts, several other techniques of increasing complexity have been suggested for providing soft tissue coverage, including pedicle groin flaps [38], tissue expanders, and silastic sheets [41]. Although these were not used in the more recent large series, the reconstructive surgeon should remain mindful of these techniques should additional soft tissue coverage be needed.

The techniques for the pedicle groin flap and tissue expansion are rather evident, but the use of silastic sheets warrants further discussion. This technique was described by Stefansson and Stilwell for use in cases in which extensive bone and soft tissue remains exposed after separation of complex syndactyly [41]. They developed this technique for cases in which they were concerned that the exposed bed of bone and cartilage would be poorly suited to a full thickness skin graft. After separating the digits, they interposed a 1-mm thick sheet of silastic along the exposed bone and cartilage and then closed the skin flaps in their original positions, leaving the silastic sheet in place. The silastic sheet was removed 1 month later, at which time they noticed a well-formed capsule covering the previously exposed bone. They then applied a full thickness skin graft from the groin, which survived. This is not usually necessary as small areas of exposed bone can be covered by skin grafts.

The role of digital amputation is a controversial topic with multiple practices described in the literature. Hoover recommended routine amputation of the long finger to provide additional soft tissue for coverage of the remaining index and ring fingers [8]. However, since Hoover's work in 1970, further discretion and nuance has been applied when deciding whether to amputate a digit. Guero attempts to achieve a five-digit hand in Upton Type I and Type II hands and only plans for a fourth ray amputation in Upton Type III hands with radiographic evidence of severe deformities including synostosis between the fourth and fifth metacarpals or misalignment between the third and fourth metacarpals [35]. Chang et al., too, recommended routine amputation only in Upton Type III hands, and if one digit was markedly smaller than the others [33]. Van Heest et al. created a new classification system for hands in Apert syndrome based on the radiographic appearance of the hands [30]. One of their justifications for the new classification system was to guide hand surgeons in determining if an amputation is necessary and, if so, which ray should be resected. Details of the classification system can be found in their paper, but their recommendations for amputation, briefly, are amputation of the third ray for complex syndactyly of the index, long, and ring fingers; amputation of the second ray for marked pronation and apex radial angulation of the index finger; and amputation of the fourth ray for marked supination and apex ulnar angulation of the ring finger. In general, all attempts should be made to achieve a five-digit hand, even in Upton III hands.

First Web Space Release, Thumb Radial Clinodactyly, and Short Thumb

In addition to releasing the small finger, which is typically the most normal and functional finger, reconstructing the thumb to allow opposition is one of the most important aspects of reconstructing the hand of an Apert patient. The anomalies of the thumb include a contracted first web space and syndactyly with the index finger, particularly in Upton Type II and III hands, thumb radial clinodactyly, and a shortened thumb. Ensuring patients have an adequate first web space allows maximal function from a shortened and radially deviated thumb. Preferred management of this first web space includes a four-flap z-plasty, a dorsal rotation-advancement flap for more severe syndactylies, or full thickness skin grafting for severe Type III hands in which local flaps do not provide adequate soft tissue coverage [34, 35]. Zucker et al. also describe the contribution of restrictive bands of palmar fascia across the first web space and a contracted adductor pollicis muscle that may also need to be released to achieve a more mobile first web space [38].

Upton, in his commentary on Fearon's article, describes his preferred method for facilitating thumb to small finger opposition [34]. He performs an open-wedge osteotomy of the thumb, which can be performed through a radial z-plasty to address the shortening and the radial clinodactyly. He then excises the fourth–fifth metacarpal synostosis in order to mobilize the small finger. To prevent the frequent refusion between the metacarpal bases, he has tried various methods including interposition of a palmaris longus tendon graft or silicone sheeting, though without much success. Instead, he has found that fascia lata, whether autologous or allogeneic, wrapped around the fifth metacarpal works well to prevent refusion. Guero prefers to interpose interosseous muscles [35]. The excised bone from the synostosis may be used to fill an opening wedge osteotomy defect. Chang et al., alternatively, suggested using bone harvested from the ulna as an alternative if digital bone is not available [33].

Fereshetian and Upton emphasized the importance of creating an adequate first web space during the first year of life to prevent delays in musculoskeletal and coordination development [37]. They felt that the first web space should be released during the first 6 months of life but that the radial clinodactyly does not need to be treated with an opening wedge osteotomy until age 4–7. In describing their technique for releasing the first web space, they noted several anatomic abnormalities, including an extensive and restrictive palmar aponeurosis, tight fascial connections between the metacarpals, distal branching of the princeps pollicis artery, and aberrant anatomy of several intrinsic muscles.

A significant departure from the paradigm of treating the thumb radial clinodactyly and shortening was described by Dao et al. [42]. The radial clinodactyly of the thumb had been attributed to a delta phalanx of the thumb [36] and a longitudinally bracketed diaphysis [29]. However, Dao took note of Fereshetian and Upton's description of an anomalous insertion of the abductor pollicis brevis (APB) onto the radial aspect of the distal phalanx [37] and used this aberrant anatomy as an explanation for the thumb anomalies in Apert syndrome. They cite Fereshetian and Upton's observation that thumb radial angulation recurs with growth in some patients [37]. They postulated that the recurrence of the thumb radial clinodactyly following a closing wedge or opening wedge osteotomy is not primarily a result of a delta phalanx or a longitudinally bracketed diaphysis but, rather, due to the abnormal radial force of the APB tendon that persists following a wedge osteotomy.

Dao et al. review the technique for APB release in detail in their paper [42]. They had only two patients in their series, whom they saw for follow-up for 1.5 and 5.6 years. Both patients had excellent results without recurrence of radial angulation at the end of follow-up. In their practice they perform the APB release concurrently with other reconstructive procedures, as the release is performed extraosseously and avoids the physis. This means that the APB release can be performed at a very early age before the deforming effects of the anomalous APB insertion have a chance to take effect. Upton, in his review of Fearon's paper, commented that he now favors Dao et al.'s approach and has changed his practice based on their work [34].

Oishi and Ezaki expanded on Dao et al.'s work to describe additional techniques in the management of the Apert thumb [43]. They note a paucity of skin along the radial aspect of the thumb that is typically addressed by a z-plasty by other groups, although they believe this leads to a soft tissue defect and a concave appearance. Instead, they described a V-to-Y and Y-to-V flap design encircling the thumb, which is nicely illustrated in their paper. They feel this offers improved mobilization of the skin for better exposure and a more aesthetic result. They agree with Dao et al.'s management of the anomalous APB insertion. Lastly, they perform an osteotomy of the proximal phalanx to address any radial angulation. This may be necessary in their series because they prefer to wait until after 4 years of age, by which time the anomalous insertion of the APB has had time to have a deforming effect. They typically perform an opening wedge osteotomy to preserve length in the thumb because it is usually short.

Secondary Revisions

Patients with Apert syndrome develop progressively stiff interphalangeal joints. Fearon addressed this deformity with phalangeal osteotomies [34]. At the age of 9–12, he performs an opening phalangeal osteotomy on the dorsal surface of the fingers at the midpoint of the fused proximal and middle phalanges where the proximal interphalangeal joint typically would be. He initially attempted to do the phalangeal osteotomies at age 7–9, but he observed that this was associated with lateral scissoring of the digits.

Additional secondary revisions include excision of pigmented skin at sites of skin grafting, readvancement of the first web space flap, release of recurrent syndactyly, performing longitudinal ostectomy for widened digits, and correction of deviated digits that may occur with growth.

Postoperative Care and Complications

Immobilization

The importance of postoperative immobilization has been emphasized by many groups due to the risk for recurrent syndactyly or wound breakdown. Upton observed that patients with a persistent or recurrent syndactyly often had been splinted for only a short period or had their cast or splint come off prematurely [37]. The recommended duration for postoperative splinting ranges from 2 to 3 weeks [33, 34, 36]. The goal for each of these immobilization regimens is to minimize motion and friction at the sites of grafts and flaps while balancing this against the risks of maceration from prolonged splinting and the inconvenience from prolonged splinting in young children.

Hyperhidrosis

Most patients with Apert syndrome have hyperhidrosis [44]. The excessive sweating can lead to maceration. This is of particular concern along fresh sutures lines, which may be disrupted with excessive maceration, possibly leading to a secondary syndactyly. Several authors go so far as to avoid reconstructive hand operations in Apert patients in the warm summer months to avoid the effects of excessive sweating [35, 37].

Secondary Syndactyly

"Web space creep" and recurrence of syndactyly is reported in most authors' series. This often requires revision at a later date ranging from 3 to 40 % in different authors' series [33, 34, 36]. Most cases of recurrent syndactyly have been attributed to insufficient postoperative immobilization. Thus, careful attention should be paid to splinting postoperatively.

Outcomes

Quantifiable outcomes have been difficult to measure in Apert syndromes patients due to the ranging functional status of these patients, the young age at which they receive

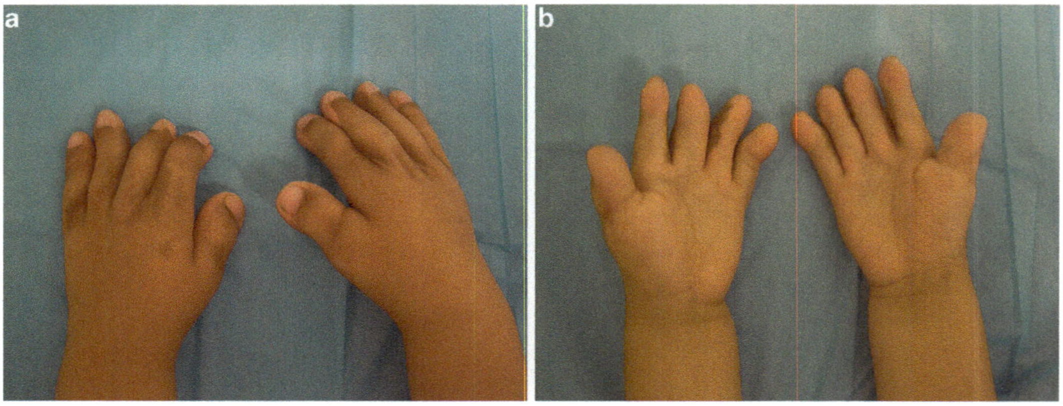

Fig. 14.5 Dorsal and volar views of a patient with a Type II Apert hand, 5 years after Apert syndactyly release and skin grafting

their reconstruction, and the unreliable follow-up that they receive. There are multiple anecdotal reports from authors describing variable functional improvements after reconstruction, although most patients do achieve opposition between the thumb and the most ulnar digit. With regard to the aesthetic outcomes, parents and patients are generally satisfied with the appearance of their hands in most authors' series and rarely request further operations in late adolescence and early adulthood (Fig. 14.5).

References

1. Cohen Jr MM, Kreiborg S. An updated pediatric perspective on the Apert syndrome. Am J Dis Child. 1993;147:989–93.
2. Perlyn CA, Nichols C, Woo A, Becker D, Kane AA. Le premier siècle: one hundred years of progress in the treatment of Apert syndrome. J Craniofac Surg. 2009;20:801–6.
3. Apert E. De l'acrocephalosyndactlie. Bull Mem Soc Med Hop Paris. 1906;23:1310.
4. Park EA, Powers GF. Acrocephaly and scaphocephaly with symmetrically distributed malformations of the extremities: a study of the so-called "acrocephalosyndactylism". Am J Dis Child. 1920;20:235–315.
5. Blank CE. Apert's syndrome (a type of acrocephalosyndactyly)-observations on a British series of thirty-nine cases. Ann Hum Genet. 1960;24:151–64.
6. Wilkie AO, Slaney SF, Oldridge M, Poole MD, Ashworth GJ, Hockley AD, et al. Apert syndrome results from localized mutations of FGFR2 and is allelic with Crouzon syndrome. Nat Genet. 1995;9:165–72.
7. Lee DS, Chung KC. Eugène Apert and his contributions to plastic surgery. Ann Plast Surg. 2010;64:362–5.
8. Hoover GH, Flatt AE, Weiss MW. The hand and Apert's syndrome. J Bone Joint Surg Am. 1970;52:878–95.
9. Au PKC, Kwok YKY, Leung KY, Tang LYF, Tang MHY, Lau ET. Detection of the S252W mutation in fibroblast growth factor receptor 2 (FGFR2) in fetal DNA from maternal plasma in a pregnancy affected by Apert syndrome. Prenat Diagn. 2011;31:218–20.
10. Lajeunie E, Cameron R, El Ghouzzi V, de Parseval N, Journeau P, Gonzales M, et al. Clinical variability in patients with Apert's syndrome. J Neurosurg. 1999;90:443–7.
11. Yu K, Herr AB, Waksman G, Ornitz DM. Loss of fibroblast growth factor receptor 2 ligand-binding specificity in Apert syndrome. Proc Natl Acad Sci U S A. 2000;97:14536–41.
12. Ibrahimi OA, Eliseenkova AV, Plotnikov AN, Yu K, Ornitz DM, Mohammadi M. Structural basis for fibroblast growth factor receptor 2 activation in Apert syndrome. Proc Natl Acad Sci U S A. 2001;98:7182–7.
13. Oldridge M, Zackai EH, McDonald-McGinn DM, Iseki S, Morriss-Kay GM, Twigg SR, et al. De novo alu-element insertions in FGFR2 identify a distinct pathological basis for Apert syndrome. Am J Hum Genet. 1999;64:446–61.
14. Glaser RL, Broman KW, Schulman RL, Eskenazi B, Wyrobek AJ, Jabs EW. The paternal-age effect in Apert syndrome is due, in part, to the increased frequency of mutations in sperm. Am J Hum Genet. 2003;73:939–47.
15. Goriely A, McVean GAT, Röjmyr M, Ingemarsson B, Wilkie AOM. Evidence for selective advantage of pathogenic FGFR2 mutations in the male germ line. Science. 2003;301:643–6.
16. Quintero-Rivera F, Robson CD, Reiss RE, Levine D, Benson C, Mulliken JB, et al. Apert syndrome: what prenatal radiographic findings should prompt its consideration? Prenat Diagn. 2006;26:966–72.
17. David AL, Turnbull C, Scott R, Freeman J, Bilardo CM, van Maarle M, et al. Diagnosis of Apert syndrome in the second-trimester using 2D and 3D ultrasound. Prenat Diagn. 2007;27:629–32.
18. Tolarova MM, Harris JA, Ordway DE, Vargervik K. Birth prevalence, mutation rate, sex ratio, parents' age, and ethnicity in Apert syndrome. Am J Med Genet. 1997;72:394–8.
19. Cohen Jr MM, Kreiborg S, Lammer EJ, Cordero JF, Mastroiacovo P, Erickson JD, et al. Birth prevalence study of the Apert syndrome. Am J Med Genet. 1992;42:655–9.
20. Rice DP. Clinical features of syndromic craniosynostosis. Front Oral Biol. 2008;12:91–106.
21. Fearon JA, Podner C. Apert syndrome: evaluation of a treatment algorithm. Plast Reconstr Surg. 2013;131:132–42.
22. Kreiborg S, Cohen Jr MM. Is craniofacial morphology in Apert and Crouzon syndromes the same? Acta Odontol Scand. 1998;56:339–41.
23. Oberoi S, Hoffman WY, Vargervik K. Craniofacial team management in Apert syndrome. Am J Orthod Dentofacial Orthop. 2012;141:S82–7.
24. Cohen Jr MM, Kreiborg S. The central nervous system in the Apert syndrome. Am J Med Genet. 1990;35:36–45.
25. Renier D, Arnaud E, Cinalli G, Sebag G, Zerah M, Marchac D. Prognosis for mental function in Apert's syndrome. J Neurosurg. 1996;85:66–72.

26. Yacubian-Fernandes A, Palhares A, Giglio A, Gabarra RC, Zanini S, Portela L, et al. Apert syndrome: factors involved in the cognitive development. Arq Neuropsiquiatr. 2005;63:963–8.
27. Cohen Jr MM, Kreiborg S. Visceral anomalies in the Apert syndrome. Am J Med Genet. 1993;45:758–60.
28. Cohen Jr MM, Kreiborg S. Cutaneous manifestations of Apert syndrome. Am J Med Genet. 1995;58:94–6.
29. Upton J. Apert syndrome. Classification and pathologic anatomy of limb anomalies. Clin Plast Surg. 1991;18:321–55.
30. Van Heest AE, House JH, Reckling WC. Two-stage reconstruction of apert acrosyndactyly. J Hand Surg. 1997;22:315–22.
31. Cohen Jr MM, Kreiborg S. Hands and feet in the Apert syndrome. Am J Med Genet. 1995;57:82–96.
32. Holten IW, Smith AW, Bourne AJ, David DJ. The Apert syndrome hand: pathologic anatomy and clinical manifestations. Plast Reconstr Surg. 1997;99:1681–7.
33. Chang J, Danton TK, Ladd AL, Hentz VR. Reconstruction of the hand in Apert syndrome: a simplified approach. Plast Reconstr Surg. 2002;109:465–70; discussion 471.
34. Fearon JA. Treatment of the hands and feet in Apert syndrome: an evolution in management. Plast Reconstr Surg. 2003;112:1–12; discussion 13–19.
35. Guero SJ. Algorithm for treatment of apert hand. Tech Hand Up Extrem Surg. 2005;9:126–33.
36. Barot LR, Caplan HS. Early surgical intervention in Apert's syndactyly. Plast Reconstr Surg. 1986;77:282–7.
37. Fereshetian S, Upton J. The anatomy and management of the thumb in Apert syndrome. Clin Plast Surg. 1991;18:365–80.
38. Zucker RM, Cleland HJ, Haswell T. Syndactyly correction of the hand in Apert syndrome. Clin Plast Surg. 1991;18:357–64.
39. Harvey I, Brown S, Ayres O, Proudman T. The Apert hand—angiographic planning of a single-stage, 5-digit release for all classes of deformity. J Hand Surg. 2012;37:152–8.
40. Golash A, Watson JS. Nail fold creation in complete syndactyly using Buck-Gramcko pulp flaps. J Hand Surg Br. 2000;25:11–4.
41. Stefansson GM, Stilwell JH. Use of silastic sheet in Apert's syndactyly. J Hand Surg Br. 1994;19:248–9.
42. Dao KD, Shin AY, Kelley S, Wood VE. Thumb radial angulation correction without phalangeal osteotomy in Apert's syndrome. J Hand Surg. 2002;27:125–32.
43. Oishi SN, Ezaki M. Reconstruction of the thumb in Apert syndrome. Tech Hand Up Extrem Surg. 2010;14:100–3.
44. Solomon LM, Fretzin D, Pruzansky S. Pilosebaceous abnormalities in Apert's syndrome. Arch Dermatol. 1970;102:381–5.

Central Deficiency (Cleft Hand)

15

Toshihiko Ogino

Definition

Central deficiency of the hand is called cleft hand, split hand, lobster-claw, or central oligodactyly. Barsky defined cleft hand as a form of congenital absence of one or more digits in which the central rays of the hand are affected [1]. According to his definition, there are two types of cleft hand, typical and atypical. Typical cleft hand is characterized by a deep V-shaped or funnel-shaped defect in the central part of the hand; atypical cleft hand is a more severe anomaly in which the three central rays are missing and is associated with various degrees of hypoplasia of the thumb and little finger. In atypical cleft hand there are often rudiments of the missing fingers along the web between the thumb and little finger (Fig. 15.1). Atypical cleft hand has the common characteristic features of other types of symbrachydactyly: all cases were unilateral; various degrees of hypoplasia existed not only in the affected finger but also in the adjacent fingers and in the proximal part of the limbs, and are associated with pectoral muscle absence [2, 3]. Atypical cleft hand is considered to be a moderate grade of symbrachydactyly, and the Congenital Committee of the International Federation of Societies for Surgery of the Hand (IFSSH) has urged not to use the term atypical cleft hand in order to prevent confusion of terminology [4]. This chapter only deals with typical cleft hand.

T. Ogino, M.D., Ph.D. (✉)
Hokushin-Higashi Hospital, Sapporo Hand Surgery and Congenital Hand Differences Center, 3-2, Fushiko 5-Jyou, 3-Choume, 3-2, Higashi-ku, Sapporo, Hokkaido 007-0865, Japan
e-mail: hand@ogino1.com

Incidence and Genetics

Birch-Jensen [5] estimated the ratio of occurrence of typical cleft hand as 1 in 90,000 births. The incidence of cleft hand among all anomalies of the upper extremity is 2.3 % of 1,476 patients in Flatt's Iowa series [6] and 2.6 % of 943 patients in Ogino's Sapporo series [7].

Regular autosomal dominant inheritance was evident in about 34 % of reported pedigrees. In other pedigrees, there are some different types of inheritance, such as lack of penetrance of autosomal dominant inheritance and markedly irregular dominant inheritance [8]. Vogel classified cleft hand into two types from the genetic aspect [9]. In type 1 pedigree affected members showed constant involvement of feet and had a consistent autosomal dominant inheritance. In type 2 pedigrees affected members showed variable involvement of feet and irregular inheritance.

Split hand/foot malformation (SHFM) is a congenital absence of the central rays of the hands and feet. Some authors use ectrodactyly to denote any absence deformity of the distal limbs and reserve SHFM for the typical malformation; others use ectrodactyly synonymously with SHFM [10]. The Human Genome Organization Nomenclature Committee determined in 1994 that split hand/foot malformation should be denoted SHFM. SHFM may present with syndactyly, median clefts of the hands and feet, as well as aplasia or hypoplasia of the phalanges, metacarpals, and metatarsals. In severe cases, the hands and feet have a lobster claw-like appearance [11]. However, the severity of SHFM is highly variable. In mildly affected patients, SHFM may be limited to syndactyly and several instances of non-penetrance have been documented. Clinical variability not only exists between patients, but also between limbs of a single individual [12]. The most common mode of inheritance is autosomal dominant with variable penetrance. Autosomal-recessive and X-linked forms occur more rarely and other cases of SHFM and may be caused by chromosomal deletions and duplications. Abnormality of six SHFM loci has been found [13, 14].

D.R. Laub Jr. (ed.), *Congenital Anomalies of the Upper Extremity: Etiology and Management*,
DOI 10.1007/978-1-4899-7504-1_15, © Springer Science+Business Media New York 2015

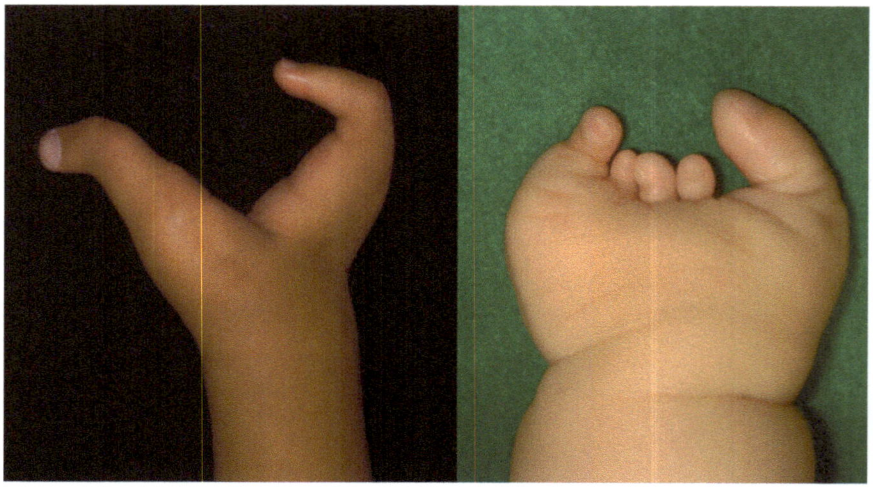

Fig. 15.1 Typical cleft hand (*left*) and atypical cleft hand (*right*)

Difference Between Cleft Hand and Other Types of Longitudinal Deficiency

The Swanson classification, which has been adopted as the IFSSH classification, has two major categories of congenital absence of digits [15, 16]: transverse deficiency (symbrachydactyly) and longitudinal deficiency. Atypical cleft hand is best classified as transverse deficiency or symbrachydactyly. In longitudinal deficiency, the congenital absence of digits is confined to the long axis of the upper limb and is classed as ulnar deficiency, radial deficiency, or central deficiency (cleft hand). In ulnar deficiency, there are various degrees of defects of ulnar fingers, such as the hypoplastic little finger, absence of the little finger, absence of the little and ring fingers, absence of the ulnar three digital rays, and absence of the ulnar four digital rays [17]. In radial deficiency, the mildest form of the hand deformity is hypoplasia of the thenar muscles and the most severe form is total absence of the thumb [18]. Non-opposable triphalangeal thumb, which is called five-fingered hand, is also one of the types of hypoplastic thumb. In some cases, the thumb and index finger are absent. In both radial and ulna deficiencies, there may be hypoplasia or aplasia of the forearm bones, and syndactyly and central polydactyly are not often seen.

Cleft hand is central deficiency, and the severe form is the absence of central three fingers, but in some cases thumb or little finger is also absent. The forearm bones are never involved, although defect or fusion of the carpal bones in distal carpal row may be seen in severe cleft hand. There are many cases in which central polydactyly, syndactyly, and cleft hand are associated in various combinations in an affected hand or in both hands of a patient [19, 20]. These anomalies also may occur in the members of the same family in various combinations. Manske [21] reported three cleft hands and one central polydactyly in four hands of identical twins. Satake et al. [22] reported a family of a mother with bilateral cleft hands, an elder daughter with the right cleft hand and the left central polydactyly, and young daughter with the left osseous syndactyly of the middle and ring fingers associated with cross bone between the middle and index fingers. There are some cases in which the middle finger is apparently missing but on X-ray, the middle and ring fingers are fused [23]. On the other hand, Müller (1936) [24] reported cases, which seemed to be cleft hands apparently, but skeletal changes were more consistent with a polydactyly of the middle finger. This issue has not been discussed in the literature for many years. Some authors reported that there were some cases in which the middle finger appears to be missing, but the metacarpus of the middle finger is duplicated [19, 25]. It is difficult or impossible to classify these cases into central polydactyly, syndactyly, or cleft hand. By these observations, cleft hand is seen to be an anomaly closely related to central polydactyly and syndactyly [19, 20, 26–29] (Fig. 15.2). When one looks at the radiographs of patients with osseous syndactyly between the middle and ring fingers, or polydactyly of the middle finger, if the defect occurs sufficiently proximal, then an appearance of cleft hand is seen (Figs. 15.3 and 15.4a, b) [28]. These observations support the concept that a common etiological mechanism is involved in the development of central polydactyly, cleft hand, and syndactyly. They also support that a common teratogenic mechanism might be the abnormal induction of finger rays in the process of formation of the fingers in the hand plate [20, 29]. From this point of view, cleft hand is one phenotype of abnormal induction of digital rays of the hand plate in which the central fingers are missing [29].

Teratogenic mechanisms of formation of cleft hand and other types of longitudinal deficiency:

In order to have a better understanding of the classification, it is necessary to clarify the development of longitudinal deficiency and cleft hand. The authors developed animal

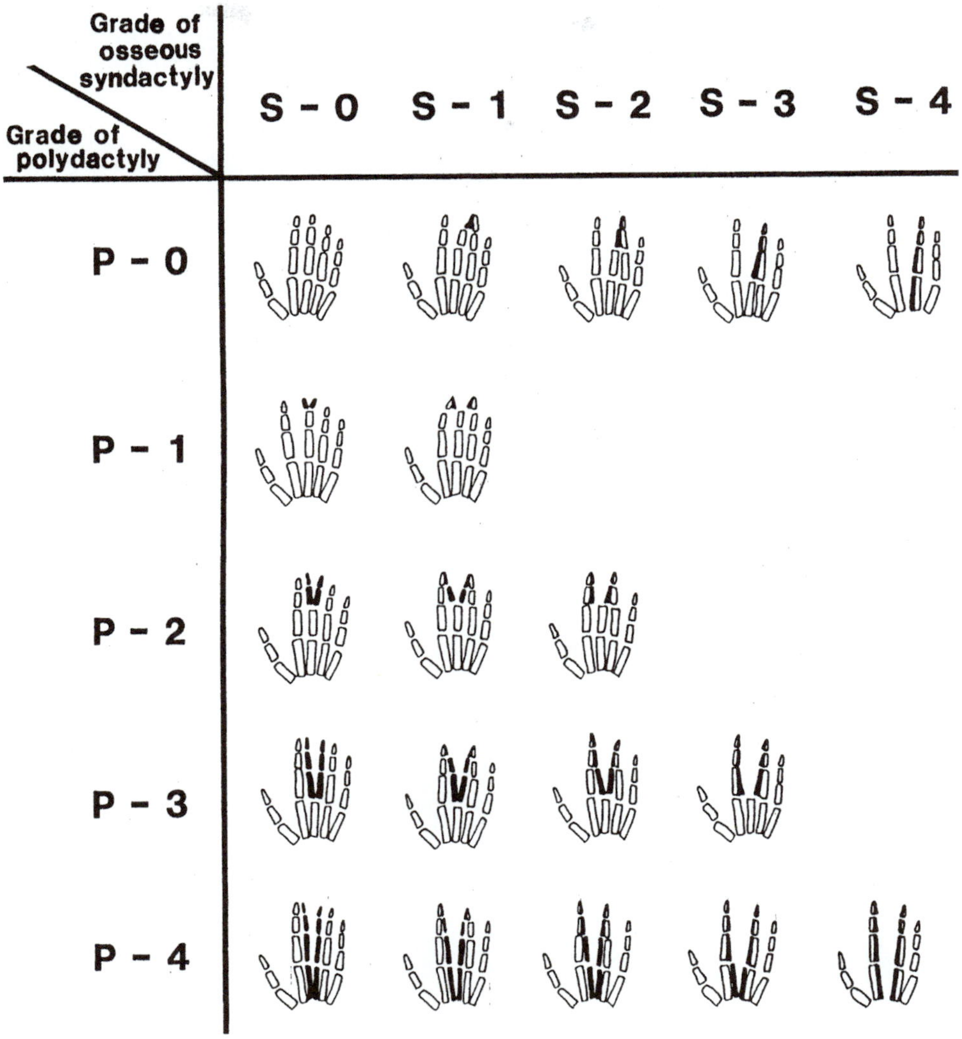

Fig. 15.2 Cleft hand formation processes from central polydactyly and/or osseous syndactyly. Reprinted with permission from Ogino T. A clinical and experimental study on teratogenic mechanism of the cleft hand, polydactyly and syndactyly. J Jpn Orthop Assoc.1979;53: 535–43

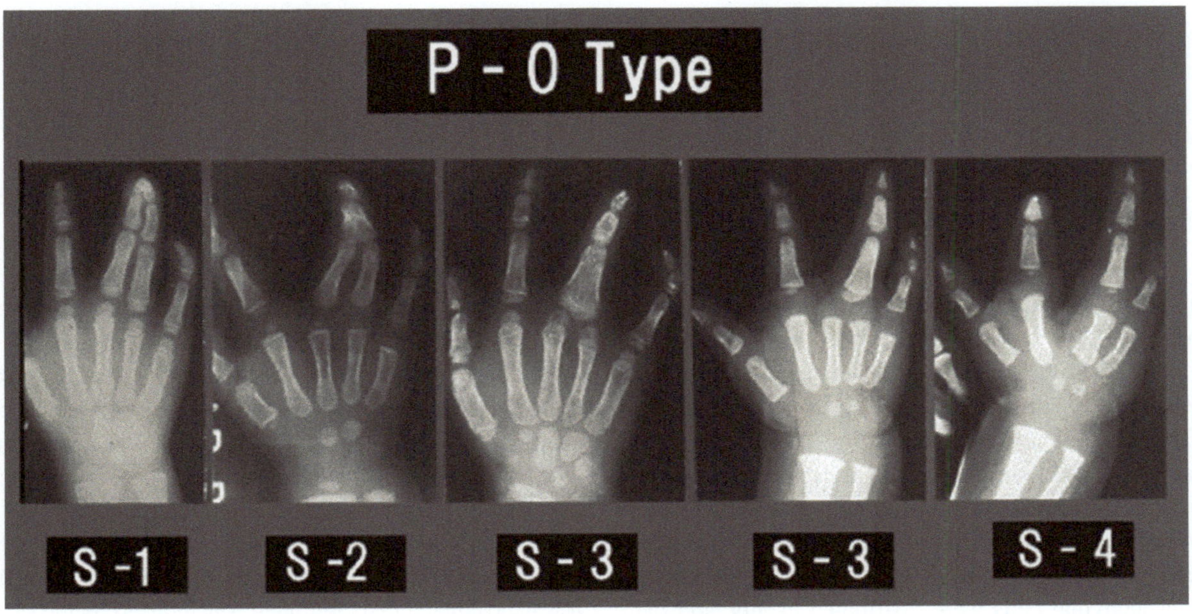

Fig. 15.3 The skeletal changes of P-0 type of anomalies in clinical cases. They seem to show that cleft hand formation proceeds from osseous syndactyly. Reprinted with permission from [28]

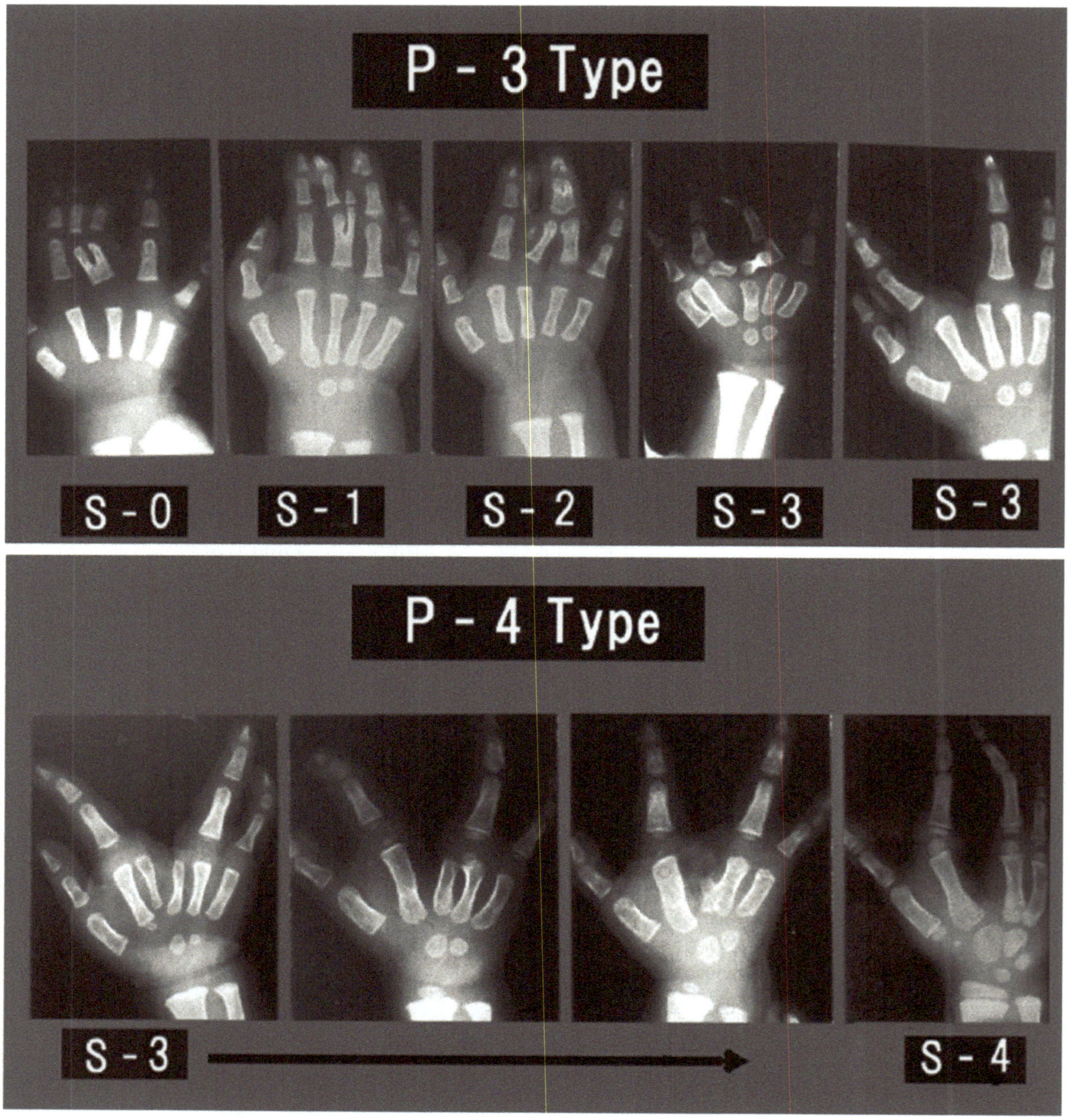

Fig. 15.4 (**a, b**) The skeletal changes of P-3 and P-4 types of polysyndactyly in clinical cases. They seem to show the cleft hand formation proceeds from central polydactylies. Reprinted with permission from [28]

models of these deformities using cleft foot as a model of cleft hand [17, 30–33]. The antineoplastic drug busulfan is given to pregnant rats, and radial deficiency and ulnar deficiency have been induced [19, 30]. The skeletal changes in busulfan-induced ulnar and radial deficiencies were similar to those of clinical cases. The critical period of ulnar deficiency in rats is about 1 day earlier than that of radial deficiency, and the critical period of radial deficiency in rats is just before limb buds appear [17, 30]. It was found that the dead mesenchymal cells were distributed evenly, and there was no localized cell deficiency inside the limb bud [33]. It was clear that the absence of digits in longitudinal deficiency was not caused by the localized deficiency of the limb bud.

A single cause affecting the limb bud in a certain receptive period of the development of the limb bud can induce central polydactyly, cleft hand, and syndactyly. When busulfan was given to rat fetuses at a critical period of these anomalies, later than that of longitudinal deficiency, cleft hand, central polydactyly, and osseous syndactyly were induced. The deformities were seen in varying stages of severity of osseous fusion. It was postulated that cleft hand was induced by the same etiology as osseous syndactyly and central polydactyly [29].

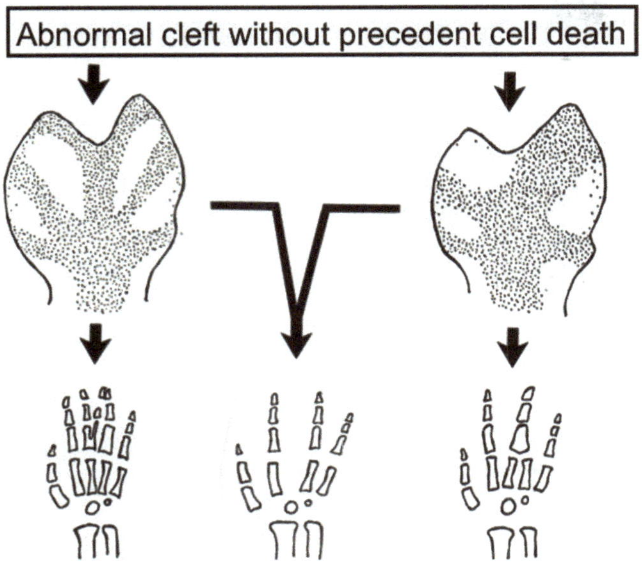

Fig. 15.5 Abnormal induction of digital rays. The early morphological changes leading to central polydactyly, syndactyly, and cleft hand were growth reduction and abnormal clefts in the central parts of the hand plates. The abnormal cleft was induced without precedent cell death and the cleft became deeper without cell death. If the abnormal cleft is induced on the edge of digital radiation, it might induce polydactyly or cleft hand. If the abnormal cleft is induced on the interdigital tissue, it might induce syndactyly or cleft hand. Reprinted with permission from Ogino T. Teratogenic mechanisms of congenital absence of digits. Locomotor System: Advances in Research, Diagnosis and Therapy 2011;18:173-93

In order to examine the underlying mechanism of busulfan-induced cleft hand, central polydactyly, and syndactyly, the authors evaluated localized apoptosis by Nile Blue staining and TdT-mediated dUTP nick end labeling (TUNEL) assays in treated rat embryos [34]. The authors further evaluated the potential disruption of major developmental pathways linked to digit number and syndactyly using Fgf8, Bmp4, and Shh as markers of these pathways. In busulfan-treated embryos, there was no difference of expression of Fgf8, BMp4, and Shh in the limb bud and footplate. The early morphological changes leading to central polydactyly, syndactyly, and cleft hand or foot were growth reduction and abnormal clefts in the central parts of the footplates. The abnormal cleft was induced without precedent cell death and the cleft became deeper also without cell death [34]. If the abnormal cleft were induced on the edge of digital radiation, it might induce polydactyly or cleft hand or foot. If the abnormal cleft were induced on the interdigital tissue, it might induce syndactyly or cleft hand or foot. The authors conclude that the abnormal cleft formation without precedent cell death was an early change leading to central polydactyly, syndactyly, and cleft hand or foot by a teratogen (Fig. 15.5 [35]). Abnormal cleft formation without precedent cell death might be caused by localized inactivation of the apical ectodermal ridge (AER) in the central part of the footplate [36].

Results of recent studies on split-hand/split-foot malformation (SHFM) using murine Dactylaplasia mutant (Dac) have shown that the central segment of the AER degenerates, leaving the anterior and posterior segments intact [37]. From this observation, it was suggested that localized failure of ridge maintenance activity was the fundamental developmental defect in Dac and it might also be suggested in SHFM [10]. Therefore, the teratogenic mechanism of formation of cleft hand/foot is the same both in drug-induced cleft hand in rats and in mutant mice with cleft hand.

Position of Cleft Hand in Japanese Modification of Swanson's Classification

Based on the clinical and experimental studies, the author modified the IFSSH classification in 1986 and added a fourth new category—abnormal induction of digital rays [38, 39]. In IFSSH classification, brachysyndactyly is classified into undergrowth and transverse deficiency into failure of formation of parts, and there is no item of cleft of the palm. However, analysis of clinical cases showed that brachysyndactyly, atypical cleft hand, or transverse deficiency seemed to be morphological variants of symbrachydactyly [2, 3]. Therefore, these deformities are included in a similar concept to transverse deficiency in failure of formation of parts in modified classification.

On the other hand, central polydactyly is classified as duplication, syndactyly as failure of differentiation of parts and typical cleft hand as failure of formation of parts in the IFSSH classification. However, these congenital deformities appear when the same teratogenic factor acts on embryo at the same developmental period. Because they have a similar causation, central deficiency, osseous syndactyly, central polydactyly, and cleft of the palm may be grouped together, and are included in the same category of abnormal induction of digital rays in modified classification [38, 39] (Table 15.1). Recent literature has reported that chromosome abnormality and also abnormalities of the positional gene may cause these anomalies [40–42].

The Japanese Society for Surgery of the Hand adopted our modification of the IFSSH classification in 1996 and it is now called the Japanese modification [43]. As a skin manifestation, there are syndactyly and cleft of the palm. As a skeletal manifestation, there are osseous syndactyly, central polydactyly, and absence of central finger rays (cleft hand), and triphalangeal thumb associated with cleft hand.

The author reviewed his own cases of abnormal induction of digital rays affecting 186 hands in 125 patients. Eighty-three cases were male and 42 female. The right side was affected in 47 cases, the left in 17 cases, and both in 61 cases. The deformities of the affected hand were expressed by the combination of cleft on the palm, cutaneous syndactyly,

Table 15.1 The Japanese Society for Surgery of the Hand Modification of the IFSSH classification revised by Ogino T. (2013)

I. Failure of formation of parts (arrest of development)
A. Transverse deficiency
1. Peripheral hypoplasia type
2. Short webbed finger type
3. Tetradactyly type
4. Tridactyly type
5. Didactyly type
6. Monodactyly type
7. Adactyly type
8. Metacarpal type
9. Carpal type
10. Wrist type
11. Forearm type
12. Above elbow type
B. Longitudinal deficiencies
1. Radial deficiencies:
(a) Dysplasia of the radius
(b) Deformities of the hand
(c) Dysplasia of the elbow
2. Ulnar deficiencies:
(a) Dysplasia of the ulna
(b) Deformities of the hand
(c) Dysplasia of the elbow
C. Phocomelia
D. Tendon or muscle dysplasia
E. Nail dysplasia
1. Aplapsia/hypoplasia of the nail
2. Nail defect with brachytelephalangia
II. Failure of differentiation of parts
A. Synostosis
B. Radial head dislocation
C. Symphalangism
D. Contracture
1. Soft tissue
(a) Arthrogryposis multiplex
(b) Webbed elbow (pterygium cubitale)
(c) Clasped thumb
(d) Windblown hand
(e) Camptodactyly
(f) Aberrant muscles
(g) Nail deformities:
(i) Nail deformity with clinodactyly
(ii) Nail deformity with hypoplasia of the distal phalanx
(iii) Nail deformity or palmar nail with hypoplastic digit and symphalangism
2. Bone
(a) Kirner deformity
(b) Delta bone (longitudinal epiphyseal brancket)
(c) Madelung deformity
3. Others
E. Tumorous conditions
III. Duplication
A. Thumb polydactyly
B. Central polydactyly (it should be category IV)
C. Polydactyly of little finger
D. Opposable triphalangeal thumb
E. Other hyperphalangism
F. Mirror hand
G. Dorsal and palmar duplication
1. Double dorsal limited in the digit
2. Double dorsal including the hand
3. Double palmar limited in the digit
4. Double palmar including the hand
IV. Abnormal induction of digital rays
A. Soft tissue:
(1) Cutaneous syndactyly, (2) Cleft of the palm
B. Bone:
(1) Osseous syndactyly, (2) Central polydactyly, (3) Absence of central finger ray(s), (4) Triphalangeal thumb with cleft hand
C. Ulnar cleft hand:
(1) Cleft of the fourth web space: (a) with absent ring finger, (b) without absent ring finger
(2) Stiff finger: (a) symphalangism; PIP and/or DIP joint, (b) partial ankylosis; PIP and/or DIP joint
(3) Nail deformity: (a) clam nail, (b) claw nail, (c) circumferential nail
D. Abnormal induction of digital rays with hypoplastic hand:
(1) polydactyly, (2) syndactyly, (3) central finger absence
V. Overgrowth
A. Macrodactyly
B. Hemihypertrophy
VI. Undergrowth
A. Microcheiria (hypoplastic hand)
B. Brachydactyly
C. Clinodactyly
VII. Constriction band syndrome
(1) Constriction ring, (2) Lymphedema, (3) Acrosyndactyly, (4) Amputation type
VIII. Generalized skeletal abnormalities and a part of syndrome
IX. Others (including unclassifiable cases)

osseous syndactyly, absence of central digit(s), which is absence of all phalanges of the digital ray(s), and central polydactyly. Of the 186 abnormal hands, a single deformity appeared in 86 hands: cutaneous syndactyly alone in 65 hands, osseous syndactyly alone in 17 hands, and cleft on the palm without absence of digit in 4 hands. In 100 hands, multiple deformities appeared in the same hand of a patient. Polydactyly and syndactyly were present in the same hand in 16 cases; a combination of cleft on the palm and syndactyly in six cases; a cleft, polydactyly, and syndactyly in one case; an absence of central digit and cleft on the palm in 37 cases; an absence of central digit, cleft on the palm, and syndactyly in 34 cases; an absence of central digit, cleft on the palm, and polydactyly in one case; and an absence of central digit, a cleft on the palm, central polydactyly, and syndactyly in five cases. In these cases there were eight hands with triphalangeal thumb associated with absence of the index finger, and there was one hand with a floating little finger. In bilaterally affected cases, same type of expression was evident in both the right and left hands in 47 cases. Different abnormalities occurred in the right and left hands in 14 cases. Hand deformities were expressed by combinations of cutaneous syndactyly, cleft on the palm, osseous syndactyly, central polydactyly, absence of central digit, and triphalangeal thumb with cleft hand with absence of the index finger. This review suggested that abnormal induction of digital rays may explain simultaneous occurrence of differing abnormalities within the same hand. The concept of abnormal induction of digital rays seemed useful for classification of congenital hand differences.

In this chapter, the author has revised the Japanese modification of the IFSSH (see Table 15.1). The abnormality of the nail has not been clearly classified, and the abnormalities of the dorso-ventral plane of the hand also have not been described in the previous Japanese modification. First, "E. Nail dysplasia" in I. Failure of formation of parts was subdivided into:

1. Aplapsia/hypoplasia of the nail.
2. Nail defect with brachytelephalangia.
3. Others.

Secondly, II. Failure of differentiation of parts had (g) Nail deformities added as a sub-category, and it is sub-classified into:

1. Nail deformity with clinodactyly
2. Nail deformity with hypoplasia of the distal phalanx
3. Nail deformity or palmar nail with hypoplastic digit and symphalangism (This is the same deformity observed in "ulnar cleft hand: VI. C")
4. Others

Thirdly, III. Duplication had "G. dorsal and palmar duplication" added and is sub-classified into:

1. Double dorsal limited in the digit
2. Double dorsal including the hand
3. Double palmar limited in the digit
4. Double palmar including the hand
5. Others

Fourthly, the categories IV. Abnormal induction of digital rays added the categories:

C. Abnormal induction of digital rays, ulnar cleft hand
D. Abnormal induction of digital rays with hypoplastic hand

After these changes, it becomes easier to differentiate true typical cleft hand described by Barsky and other cleft hand-like deformities.

Clinical Characteristics

Blauth and Falliner's reported incidence of cleft hand: they found bilateral involvement in 50 %, and in unilateral involvement, the ratio of right hand to left hand is 60 to 40 %. The ratio of male to female is 60 to 40 % [44]. In approximately one out of three cases of cleft hand there was associated cleft foot.

Defect of the central finger rays varies [45]: there are hands with deep cleft formation on the palm without absence of the finger rays. This is a type of central deficiency, and therefore a form of cleft hand (Type 0) [46]. There are cleft hands with one finger absent, two fingers absent, three fingers absent, or four digits absent. In one finger absence type (Type 1), the middle finger is most commonly absent. In that case, the ring finger often will have camptodactyly. This deformity is not actually true camptodactyly, but a claw finger deformity due to abnormal lumbrical or interosseus muscles. Most often, the affected ring finger has no joint contracture when the child is young. If the metacarpophalangeal joint of the ring finger is passively flexed to neutral, the patient can actively extend the PIP and DIP joints of the affected finger.

Some cases with mild excessive cleft and absence of the middle finger will have normal looking third metacarpal bone radiologically. However, in some cases the third metacarpal bone deviates ulnarly and has a common MP joint with the fourth metacarpal bone and proximal phalanx of the ring finger. Alternately, third metacarpal bone will deviate radially and have a common MP joint with the second metacarpal bone and proximal phalanx of the index finger. In the former case, the ring finger is wider than normal and in the later case the index finger is wider than normal. When middle finger ray including the third metacarpal is absent, the cleft is deeper than usual. The deeper the cleft is, the more often syndactyly of the first web space and the fourth web space occur. In some rare cases of deep cleft, hypoplasia of the little finger, or the fusion of the fourth and fifth metacarpals, is seen. In Type 1 cleft hand, the index finger or ring finger also may be absent [47, 48]. When the index finger is absent, the thumb is often triphalangeal and will deviate radially, in contrast to most triphalangeal thumbs, which deviate ulnarly. A "Y" shaped second metacarpal bone between the thumb and middle finger, or two thumb metacarpal bones may be seen on X-ray. When the ring finger is absent, the little finger is small and stiff, and this may be called "ulnar cleft hand." When the finger is not absent and the cleft is in the forth web apace, this is often associated with stiffness of the IP joints, palmar nail, and the dorsal skin on the palmar side of the little finger. This may be called "double dorsal deformity of the finger." The etiology of this deformity is considered to be different from other types of cleft hand (see below).

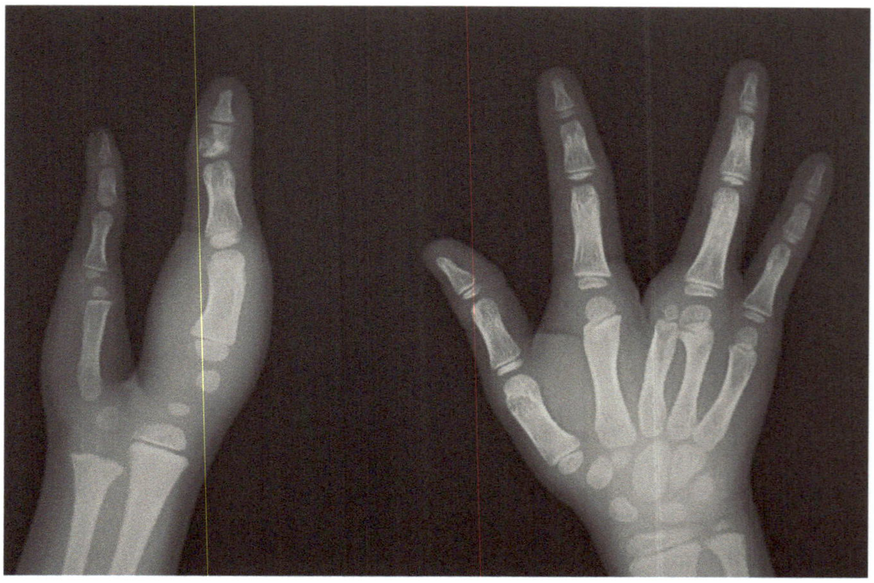

Fig. 15.6 Different degree of absence of the fingers associated in both hand of a patient. *Left*: type 3 cleft hand with central three-finger absence and triphalangeal thumb with radial deviation of the IP joint. *Right*: type 1 cleft hand with absence of the middle finger

In two-finger absence type (Type 2), the index and middle fingers are absent more commonly than the middle and ring fingers. When the index and middle fingers are absent, the thumb is usually triphalangeal. In three-finger absence type (Type 3), if the thumb is opposable then pinch is possible between the thumb and the little finger. If the thumb is in the plane of the hand however, pinch between the thumb and little finger is impossible [49]. In four-digit absence type (Type 4), the radial four digits are absent in most commonly, but very rarely the ulnar four digits will be absent and only the thumb remains [46]. In radial-four-digits absence type, the metacarpals of the thumb and affected fingers are usually only partially absent or not involved.

A cross bone is a transverse or oblique bone lying in the base of the cleft. It is regarded as the displaced remnant of the metacarpal or proximal phalanx of the missing digit and it bridges between the end of the metacarpal bones of the missing digit and the proximal phalanx, MP joint, or the metacarpal bone of the adjacent finger. There may be two cross bones which might be duplicated proximal phalanges of the missing digit and are located between missing digit and adjacent fingers between the end of the metacarpal bones of the missing digit and the proximal phalanx, MP joint, or the metacarpal bone of the adjacent finger. There may be two cross bones, which might be duplicated proximal phalanges of the missing digit, and are located between missing digit and adjacent fingers. There may be solid bone union or cartilaginous continuity between the cross bone and the proximal phalanx of the adjacent finger in the skeletally immature patient. In some cases, the proximal phalanx of the adjacent finger will have a deltaphalanx (longitudinal epiphyseal bracket). X-ray films may show, two metacarpals supporting one digit, side-to-side fusion of the neighboring metacarpals, broad metacarpals, or duplicated metacarpals.

Surgical Classification of the Cleft Hand

Saito et al. [45] classified typical cleft hand into four types on the basis of the number of defective finger rays:

Type 1: deep cleft formation on the palm without missing finger.

Type 2: defect of a single finger ray.

Type 3: defect of two finger rays.

Type 4: defect of three finger rays.

Watari and Tsuge [27] classified typical cleft hand according to the same idea. In their classification there is no type without absence of the finger, but a type in which four finger rays are absent. They divided single ray defect type of cleft hand into proximal and distal types. In the proximal type all phalanges and the metacarpus are missing and in the distal type only phalanges are missing. The author modified these classifications as follows (Fig. 15.6):

Type 0: cleft hand without missing finger

Type 1: defect of a single finger ray

Type 2: defect of two finger rays

Type 3: defect of three finger rays

Type 4: defect of four digital rays

In every type, when the index finger is absent, the thumb is mostly triphalangeal and deviated radially.

Manske et al. [50] proposed surgical classification for cleft hand based on the characteristics of the thumb web space, because he thought the thumb web was more important to the function of the hand than the central deficiency. According to his report, cleft hand is classified into five types:

Type 1: normal first web

Type 2A: mildly narrowed first web

Type 2B: severely narrowed first web

Type 3: syndactylized first web
Type 4: merged web in which index ray suppressed, thumb web space is merged with the cleft
Type 5: absent web, in which thumb elements suppressed, ulnar rays remain and thumb web space no longer present

One benefit of sub-classification of the congenital hand deformities is that one can better picture the deformity of the hand, from description with the classification. For example, when told or read: "Type 4 thumb polydactyly in Wassel's classification [51]" or "Type 3 hypoplastic thumb in Blauth's classification [18]," one can clearly image the deformities of the hand and the possible associated deformities. Both hypoplastic thumb and thumb polydactyly may have the narrowing of the first web. This is an important factor not only when treating cleft hand, but also hypoplastic thumb and thumb polydactyly. Manske reported that the progressive narrowing of the thumb web correlated with progressive severity of the central defect. The author also observed the same findings and published it in 1977 [19]. Therefore, one can imagine the possible condition of the first web associated with cleft hand, using Saitou's classification based on the number of defective finger rays. Surgical treatment is not only directed to the first web, but also the deep or wide cleft. I feel that sub-classification should be valuable not only for the patient but also for communication of the people who are treating these deformities. Based on this viewpoint, Saitou's classification based on the number of defective finger rays seems more valuable for sub-classification of the cleft hand. If one uses Manske's classification [50], it would be more useful if combined with Satou's classification [45]. Falliner [52] classified cleft hand into three types as follows:

Radial cleft hand
- Hand deformities including osseous syndactyly of the thumb and index finger
- Absence of the index finger
- Absence of the thumb and index finger
- Absence of the radial three or four digits

Central cleft hand
- Central defect with absence of the middle finger
- Central defect with absence of the central two fingers
- Central defect with absence of the central three fingers
- Cleft hand with only the thumb and little finger present

Ulnar cleft hand
- Absence of the ring finger
- Absence of the ring and middle fingers, with or without of hypoplasia of the little finger

This classification seems to be too simple for clinical use. Moreover, ulnar cleft hand has characteristic clinical features such as deep cleft in the fourth web space, absence of the ring finger and/or hypoplastic little finger associated with stiffness of the PIP joint and palmar nail, and it is considered to differentiate it from other types of cleft hand. When one uses Japanese modification of the IFSSH classification [43], in abnormal induction of finger rays, the hand deformities are expressed with combination of the cleft, syndactyly, and other phenotypes. Therefore, if one describes deformities combined with the degree and the location, one can expresses the deformity of the cleft hand and other combined deformities precisely.

Cleft of the Fourth Web Space of the Hand

Cleft of the fourth web space of the hand is associated with or without absence of the ring finger. These deformities are called ulnar cleft hand [48]. However, its clinical features are different from various types of abnormal induction of digital rays including cleft hand. Moreover, characteristic clinical features of cleft of the fourth web space with absence of the ring finger are different from those without absence of the ring finger, although the little finger is hypoplastic in both conditions [47, 53]. There is no appropriate terminology and precise classification for the sequence of these congenital hand deformities. Ulnar cleft hand without absence of the ring finger is characterized with combination of various degrees of cleft of the ring and little finger, hypoplasia of the little finger, hypoplasia of hypothenar muscles, extension contracture or symphalangism of the little finger and clam nail, claw nail or circumferential nail deformity, and dorsal skin of the palmar little finger [53] (Fig. 15.7). In the opposite hand, the same deformity, polydactyly of the little finger, ulnar deficiency, or partial duplicated distal phalanx of the ring finger may be seen. In this anomaly, there are various associated deformities of the hand. Hand and nail deformities in this anomaly are similar to those of ulnar-mammary syndrome or Schinzel syndrome [54]. The teratologic sequence of the variety of hand deformities with ulnar cleft of the fourth web without absence of digits is most likely a different entity from abnormal induction of finger rays.

Abnormal Induction of Digital Rays (Including Cleft Hand) Associated with Hypoplastic Hand

Abnormal induction of digital rays in the hand plate means induction of abnormal number of the digital rays in the hand plate. Therefore, excessive or decreased number of induction of digital ray occurs, but nearly all of the hands with deformities of abnormal induction of digital rays do not seem to have hypoplasia of the hand. However, there are hand deformities, with combinations of syndactyly, cleft of the palm, central polydactyly, osseous syndactyly, or absence of the central fingers associated with hypoplasia of the affected hand. This deformity is most often unilateral.

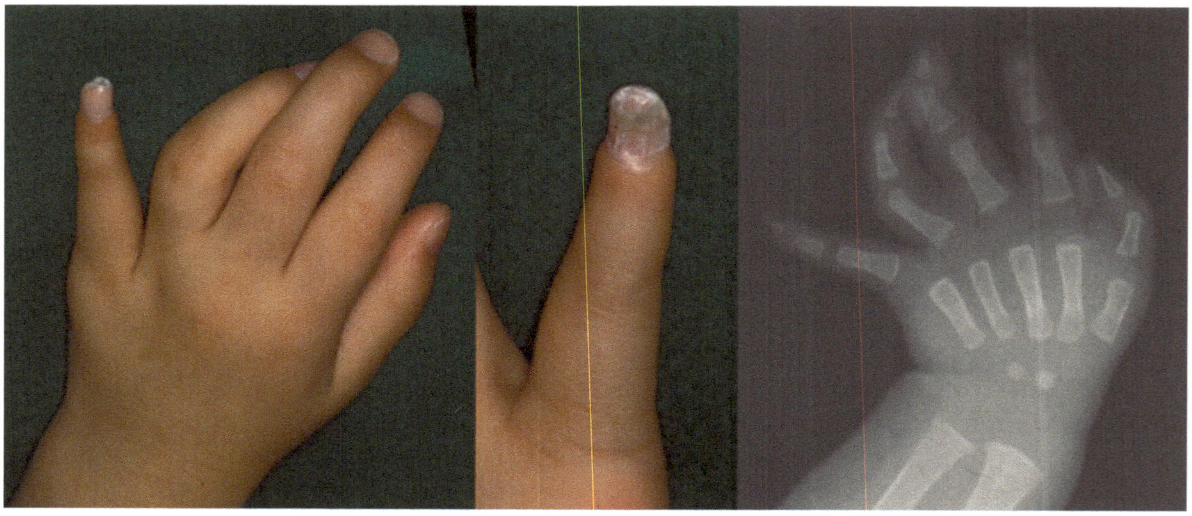

Fig. 15.7 Cleft of the fourth web space without absence of the finger. *Left*: cleft of fourth web space associated with stiff PIP joint (symphalangism) and hypoplastic little finger. *Center*: circumferential nail and dorsal skin on the palmar side of the little finger. *Right*: synchondrosis of the PIP joint of the little finger

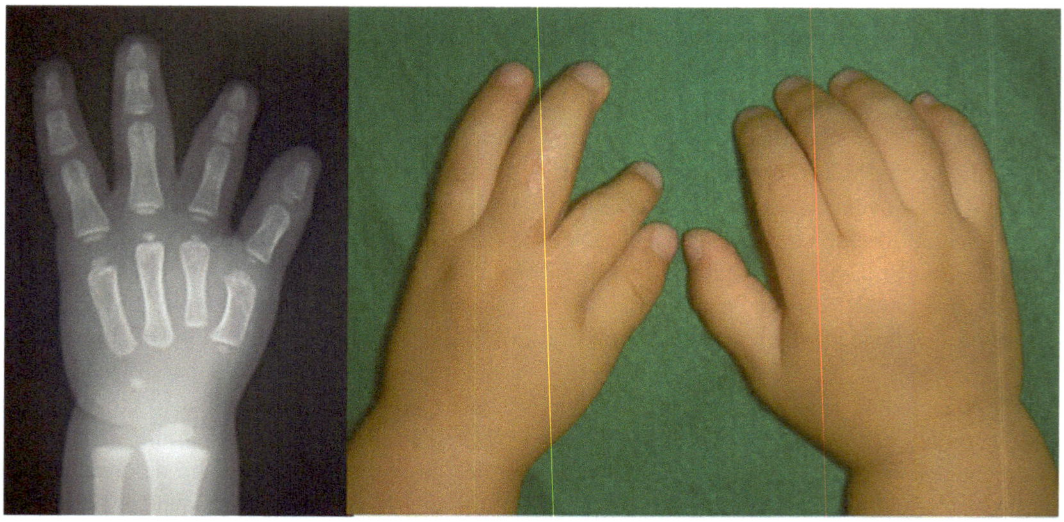

Fig. 15.8 Abnormal induction of the finger rays associated with hypoplasia of the affected hand. The characteristic features of this condition seem to be those of transverse deficiency, which are unilateral involvement and hypoplasia of the whole affected hand compared to the opposite hand, and those of abnormal induction of digital rays, which are that the hand has cleft of the palm, syndactyly, central polydactyly, osseous syndactyly, and/or absence of the central fingers. It is difficult to say which finger rays are missing in X-ray film

This condition seems to have both the characteristic features of transverse deficiency (hypoplasia of the affected hand and unilateral involvement) and those of abnormal induction of digital rays (central polydactyly, syndactyly, and cleft hand). This condition is not associated with polydactyly, syndactyly, and/or central deficiency of the opposite hand and the feet. In the affected hand, thenar and hypothenar muscles are relatively well formed and it is sometimes difficult to say which finger rays are missing in the central finger rays, although the thumb and the little finger are never absent [55, 56] (Fig. 15.8).

Associated Anomalies

As regional association, syndactyly of the thumb and index finger or that of the ring and little fingers, and brachydactyly of the little finger are most common. Triphalangeal thumb often occurs in cleft hand associated when the index finger is absent. Polydactyly of the thumb and side-to-side synostosis of the fourth and fifth metacarpals are rarely seen. Occasionally, some patients will be affected bilaterally in which there is a cleft hand on one side and on the other, another type of anomaly, such as cutaneous syndactyly, osseous syndactyly, or central polydactyly. The central deficiency in SHFM patients may also be accompanied by other distal limb anomalies including central polydactyly and/or syndactyly [57].

Foot deformities, such as cleft foot, syndactyly, central polydactyly, and tibial ray deficiency, are also associated with cleft hand.

Cleft hand appeared as a part of syndrome, such as, ectrodactyly–ectodermal dysplasia–clefting (EEC) syndrome, de Lange syndrome, split hand/split foot with mandibulo-facial dysostosis, split hand with perceptive deafness, split hand with congenital nystagmus, fundal changes and cataract, anonychia with ectrodactyly, and the acrorenal syndrome.

As mentioned above, split hand/foot malformation (SHFM), or central ray deficiency, can occur as an isolated malformation or as a part of syndrome, such as in the EEC syndrome. Rüdiger et al. in 1970 [58] named an anomaly complicated three malformations the EEC syndrome, based on their initials, namely, ectrodactyly, ectodermal dysplasia and clefting syndrome. The main clinical signs, in order of frequency observed in Rodini and Richieri-Costa [59] reported group, were ectodermal dysplasia (100 %), ectrodactyly (78 %), tear duct anomaly (71 %), cleft lip/plate (58 %), genito-urinary anomalies (15 %), deafness (9 %), and mental retardation (2 %). The clinical expression of the EEC syndrome is quite variable; any one of the above signs may be absent except ectodermal signs. Ectrodactyly may occur only in hands (25 %) or in both hands and feet (65 %). Ten percent of the patients had no limb involvement. Cleft hands and feet are characteristic anomalies of this syndrome, but syndactyly, polydactyly of the central digital ray may be associated with this syndrome [57, 60, 61]. Majewski and Küster [62] stated that ectrodactyly is not an obligatory symptom. Skin anomalies related to ectodermal dysplasia are fine, thine smooth skin, hyperkeratosis, and dermatoglyphic alterations. Trichodysplasia, dental defects, onychodysplasia, and dyshidrosis may be associated. In EEC syndrome, most cases have *p63* gene mutations. In contrast, *p63* mutations were detected in only a small proportion of patients with isolated SHFM [63].

Treatment of Cleft Hand

Indication and Timing of Surgery

Cleft hand has several associated deformities. The goals of surgical treatment for cleft hand may need to address:

- Reduction of the excessive deep or wide interdigital space
- Separation of syndactyly of the first web or the interdigital space between the ring and little fingers
- Correction of claw finger deformity of the ring finger
- Correction of the deviation of the thumb due to triphalangeal thumb
- Correction of the deviation of the index finger due to trapezoidal shape of middle phalanx

Many authors stated that surgery of cleft hand is mainly performed for esthetic reasons. Reduction of the interdigital space is in fact performed mainly for the cosmetic reasons in cleft hand without missing finger (Type 0) and cleft hand with defect of a single finger ray (Type 1). However, correction of thumb deformities including the first web contracture and that of the deviation of the thumb due to triphalangeal thumb gives significant functional improvement. Such procedures may be performed simultaneously in order to prevent multiple surgeries. Reduction of the interdigital space, separation of syndactyly of the first web space, correction of the deviation of the thumb and that of claw finger deformity of the ring finger are usually performed at initial surgery. Claw finger deformity of the ring finger is corrected by reconstruction of the MP joint flexor with FDS tendon of the missing finger as in lasso procedure. It is easily done at initial surgery, as the flexor tendons are exposed in the palm and it is easy to select the transferred tendon before the cleft is closed. Alternatively, this procedure may be performed later as a second stage surgery, if the deformity is not corrected spontaneously after closing the cleft. The combination of the surgical procedures is different in each case according to the associated deformities. Reduction of the interdigital space should not be performed for some kind of cleft hand that is cleft hand with missing index finger, that with missing index and middle fingers, and cleft hand with defect of central three finger rays (Type 4). If reduction of the interdigital space is performed in these cases, the patient will have difficulty in grasping a large object. On the other hand, in cleft hand with trapezoidal proximal phalanx of the ring finger, the proximal phalanx is a delta phalanx and the ring finger has ulnar deviation. It may be corrected in some extent by physiolysis with free fat graft, if the surgery is performed in a young patient [64]. However, a secondary corrective osteotomy may be needed if satisfactory correction has not been achieved after physiolysis.

Closure of the excessive interdigital space (cleft) for cleft hand without missing finger (Type 0) or that with absence of a single finger (Type 1), separation of syndactyly between thumb and index finger and removal of the delta phalanx of the thumb, and correction of the claw finger deformity of the ring finger are performed at the age of 1 year. The author prefers to perform these surgeries simultaneously. Separation of syndactyly of the ring and little fingers is usually carried out at the second stage surgery, since the level of the interdigital web to be corrected can be more easily determined at that time. Separation of the side-to-side fusion of the metacarpals, and arthrodesis of the finger should be performed at a later stage as needed. Physiolysis with free fat graft should be performed around the age of 3–4 years. All necessary surgery should be completed by the time the child enters school at the age of 6 years.

Preoperative Care

Usually no preoperative care is needed. The author asks the parents to close the cleft of the hand manually by pushing the border digits at least one a day, when the simple closure of the cleft is indicated. If the cleft hand is associated with claw finger deformity of the ring finger, the author asks them also to prevent contracture of the finger with manual correction.

When the interdigital space is wide or deep and simple closure of the cleft is indicated, static splint may be applied in order to close the cleft until surgery. When we examine a patient, the first web contracture associated with cleft hand at the age of 1 or 2 years, sometimes the patient does not use the thumb for pinch but uses two fingers adjacent to the cleft for pinch. When the splint is applied to close the wide cleft soon after birth, the patient can learn normal pinch pattern. While the literature has generally not recommended splinting prior to surgery for cleft, the author believes that the splint may establish proper muscle balance in a corrected position and prevent secondary skeletal deformities in selected cases. Preoperative splinting facilitates correction of the deformity during surgery.

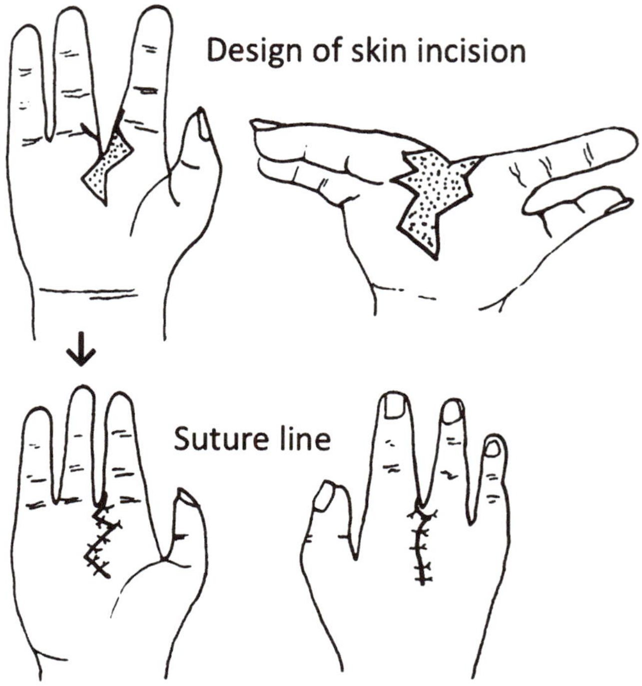

Fig. 15.9 Skin incision for reduction of the interdigital space using small triangular flap for the web. The *dotted area* of the skin will be excised

Closure of the Excessive Interdigital Space

In order to make natural slope of the interdigital web after closing the cleft, many procedures have been reported: Barsky [1] used a diamond-shaped flap based on one digit, Kelikian [65] used a rectangular flap from across the apex of the palmar cleft of the hand and Tsuge [66] used a triangular flap. The author prefers to use small triangular flap [46] (Fig. 15.9). Before skin incision, the second and fifth metacarpals are pushed toward each other and cleft is manually closed. The cleft can be closed easily, since the parents have been manually closing it for certain period before surgery. Then zigzag incisions may then be designed in expectation of an interdigitating closure. However, dorsal zigzag suture line may not give the best aesthetic result. In that case, the author uses dorsal straight incision instead of zigzag incision. An ulnar-based small triangular flap is raised by this incision. Excessive skin of a wide or deep interdigital space may then be removed. After necessary treatment of bone, tendon, and ligament, the skin incision is closed.

Treatment of Metacarpus and Cross Bone

There are different types of metacarpal bone deformities. In some cases, two metacarpals shift each other and support one digit. For example, in cleft hand with absent middle finger, the third metacarpal bone deviates ulnarwards and has common MP joint among fourth metacarpal bone and proximal phalanx of the ring finger or it deviates radial wards and has common MP joint among second metacarpal bone and proximal phalanx of the index finger. If the third metacarpal bone prevents to close the cleft manually in these types of deformities, the shortening or partial removal of the metacarpal shaft is indicated (Fig. 15.10a, b), but it was not necessary in most cases. There are also, side-to-side fusion of the neighboring metacarpals, broad metacarpus, and duplicated metacarpals. In the cleft hand with absent index finger, the Y-shaped second metacarpal bone is located between the thumb and middle finger, or two metacarpal bones exist in the thumb. These metacarpal deformities usually do not disturb hand function nor induce secondary deformities. Therefore, it is not necessary to treat them surgically.

On the other hand, many authors advocate removal of the cross bones and osteotomy of one or both of the adjacent metacarpals. Some authors thought that osteotomy is not essential. If the metacarpal remnants or cross bone prevent to draw the metacarpals together, these bone should be removed. If the second and fourth metacarpals could not be put into parallel after removing the third metacarpal, osteotomy of the second metacarpal or metacarpal transfer of the second metacarpal to the third one is recommended, but it is not essential. When these bones are removed, extensor hood and capsule of the metacarpophalangeal joint of the absent finger ray and/or adjacent finger ray must be incised. In such cases, repair of extensor hood

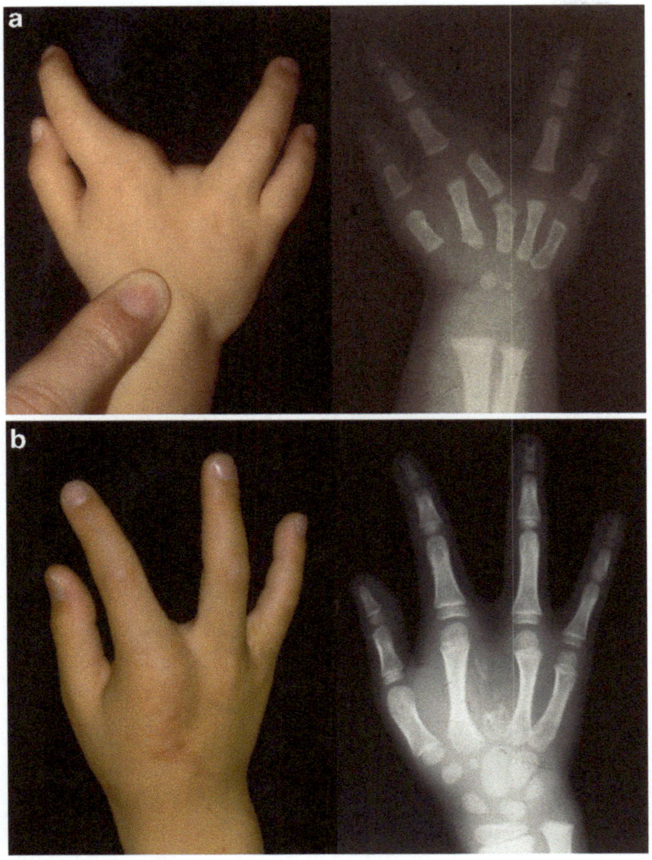

Fig. 15.10 Excision of the cross bone. (a) Preoperative appearance and roentgenogram. At the age of 1 year 2 months, the cross bone and the third metacarpal were resected. Osteotomy of the second metacarpal base was performed and the cleft was close. (b) Postoperative appearance and roentgenogram: after surgery, good alignment has been achieved

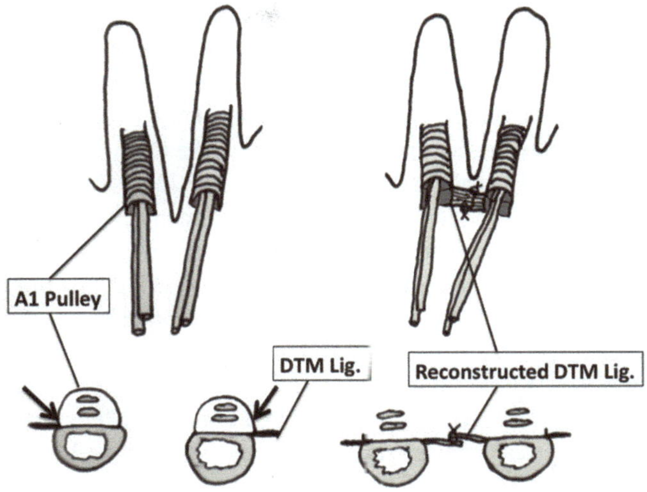

Fig. 15.11 Reconstruction of the deep transverse metacarpal ligament using flexor tendon sheath. Ligamentous flexor tendon sheaths are cut and ligamentous flaps are made. They are turned over and sutured each other

and joint capsule are necessary to prevent deformity after surgery. However, the tight soft tissue on the radial side does not allow the metacarpal to transfer ulnarward easily.

Reconstruction of the Deep Transverse Metacarpal Ligament

The deep transverse metacarpal ligament connects the anterior surfaces of the adjacent metacarpal heads. It normally blends with the volar plates of the metacarpophalangeal joints and prevents spreading of the fingers [67]. In cleft hand, the deep transverse metacarpal ligament is absent in the cleft where the finger is missing.

In order to obtain a satisfactory commissure and to prevent later spreading of the fingers, reconstruction of the deep transverse metacarpal ligament is necessary. Barsky makes two drill holes through both metacarpals adjacent to the cleft just proximal to the heads. Chromic catgut sutures are passed through these holes and tightened to approximate the diverging metacarpals on each side of the cleft. Flatt [6] used to fashion some sort of ligament out of the adjacent soft tissues, but he used also catgut or silk sutures in a technique similar to that reported by Barsky. Free tendon graft can be also used for tethering the adjacent metacarpals. However, one should know that excessive tethering of the metacarpals causes rotation of the metacarpals and cross over the fingers during grasping. Excessive force should be avoided to coapting the two metacarpal together. If excessive force is necessary to coapt the two metacarpal together, metacarpal osteotomy or metacarpal shift is recommended. In order to reconstruct the deep transverse metacarpal ligament, the author uses ligamentous flaps made out of the flexor tendon sheaths of the index and ring fingers (Fig. 15.11). The advantage of this method is that the reconstructed deep transverse metacarpal ligament is located in anatomical position and it is possible to avoid excessive tethering or rotation of the metacarpals. The index finger and ring finger are drawn together. If there is slackening of the extensor hood, it should be repaired by plication or tendon transfer. Then the deep transverse metacarpal ligament is reconstructed by flexor tendon sheath. If osteotomy or metacarpal shift is necessary, it should be carried out before reconstruction of the ligament.

Widening of the Thumb Web Space or Syndactyly Release of the Thumb and Index Finger

When the cleft of the hand is deep, the thumb web space is narrow. In this type of cleft hand, cleft closure and release of the adduction contracture of the thumb are necessary. Various procedures have been reported to treat the cleft and syndactyly simultaneously. In every procedure, a rotation flap fashioned from the skin of the cleft is used to separate the web between the thumb and index finger and ulnar transposition of the index finger is performed to close the cleft. Snow and Littler used a palmar-based flap from the cleft, Takahashi and Yabe [68] used dorsal and palmar flaps from the cleft. Miura et al. [69], Ueba [70, 71], and Upton and Taghinia [72] solved this problem by transposition of the index finger ray to the ulnar side of the cleft by using skin incision around the base of the index finger. In all these procedures, an osteotomy is performed at the base of the second metacarpal or the index finger metacarpal is transferred to an ulnar finger ray. In these procedures, care must be taken to preserve adductor pollicis muscle and prevent injury of the ulnar nerve to the adductor pollicis.

On the other hand, Foucher et al. [73] stated that none of surgical techniques reported previously is easily applied to the treatment of very deep clefts accompanied by a significant divergence of the metacarpal bones. In such cases, the results of current techniques are disappointing. They proposed a new technique of "Translocation in the Radial Direction of the Ulnar Finger(s)" (TRUF) by intracarpal osteotomy. The reported cases were limited. The TRUF operation allowed closing of the cleft, alignment of the metacarpal bones, and preservation of carpometacarpal mobility. They transfer the little finger or the little and ring fingers with carpometacarpal joint(s) and hamate radially after intracarpal osteotomy. They put the hamate and ulnar fingers on the capitate. The best indication of this procedure is in the case of good alignment of the second metacarpal with the radius and no stump of the middle metacarpal but divergence of the ulnar finger(s). If the second metacarpal has severe radial inclination, a closing wedge osteotomy of the ulnar base of the index metacarpal should be performed.

Previously, the author used a dorsally based flap from the cleft to widen the first web. The skin incision outlines the sides of the cleft on the palmar surface of the index and ring fingers forming a zigzag incision with a proximal V-shaped apex. At the sides of the adjacent metacarpal heads, a ulnarly based small triangular flap is raised by this incision. As the incisions curve back onto the dorsal aspect, they run almost parallel the index finger to the cleft side of the midline of the two fingers. Additional incision starts on the palm of the thumb and index web at the same level as the V-shaped cleft incision. It runs distally parallel with the index finger, curves back onto the dorsal aspect of the thumb–index web and runs proximally and across in an ulnar direction to meet the dorsal index cleft incision. Fibrous bands between the thumb and index finger and fascia of the adductor pollicis and first dorsal interosseus muscle have to be released. Care must be taken to avoid the injuries to the neurovascular bundles. The index finger and ring finger are drawn together and deep transverse metacarpal ligament is reconstructed by a flap of the flexor tendon sheath. Osteotomy of the metacarpal may be performed, if it is necessary. The flap raised from the cleft is transposed to the thumb–index web and wound is closed in layers. However, the dorsal zigzag scar is not esthetically acceptable and in some cases necrosis of the distal tip of the flap due to poor circulation occurred. The author has used palmar rotation flap from the cleft to widen the first web (Snow–Littler procedure) for the past 25 years. The procedure is nearly the same as dorsal rotation flap [74, 75] (Figs. 15.12 and 15.13a, b). The digital artery is not included in the flap, but necrosis of the distal tip of the flap has never occurred.

When the cleft is very deep or there is complete syndactyly between the thumb and index finger, the Snow–Littler procedure is not indicated, as it is not easy to adapt the rotation flap from the cleft to the first web and the created deep V-shaped first web is not as esthetically acceptable. If there is complete or nearly complete syndactyly between the thumb and index finger, a palmar rotation flap from the cleft can be used but usually is not enough to cover the raw surface of the first web and a full thickness skin graft is necessary. In such cases, dorsal and palmar triangular flaps from the first web with free skin graft are better than Snow–Littler procedure in order to obtain functionally and esthetically good first web.

Syndactyly Release Between Ring and Little Finger

Separation of syndactyly between ring and little fingers is carried out by using dorsal rectangular flap combined with free skin graft. This surgery is usually performed when the patient is about 2 years old. Sometimes author performs cleft closure and separation of syndactyly between the ring and little fingers simultaneously. In such cases, there is a benefit to be able to use skin removed from the cleft for the free skin graft, if rotation skin from the cleft to the first web is not needed. If cleft hand is associated with the fourth and fifth metacarpal fusion, and partial cutaneous syndactyly between the ring and little fingers, deepening of the web space improves the appearance and the length of the fingers. In such cases, syndactyly release is indicated electively.

Correction of the Deviation of the Thumb

Deviation of the thumb in cleft hand is often caused by triphalangeal thumb with a delta phalanx or rectangular extra phalanx [76]. Deviation of the thumb is corrected by remov-

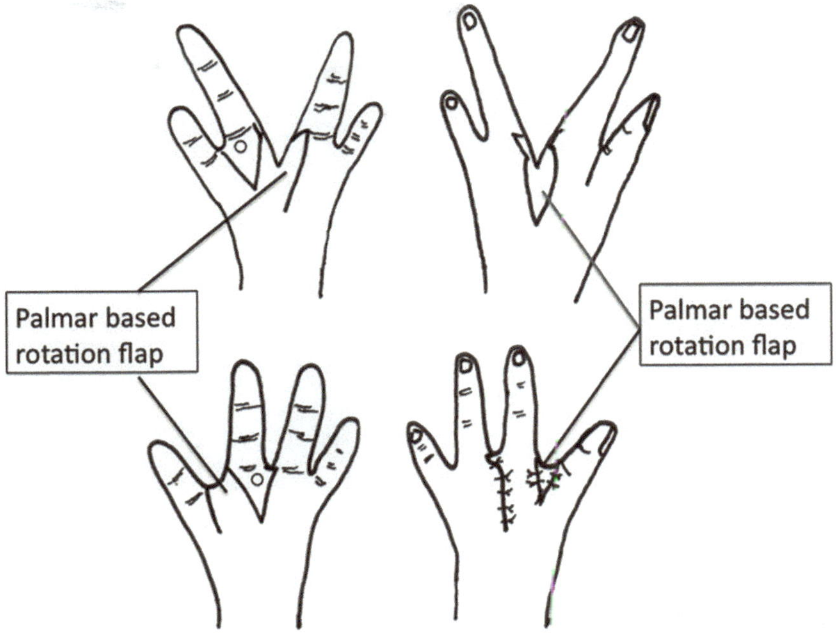

Fig. 15.12 Widening of the narrow first web by Snow–Littler procedure

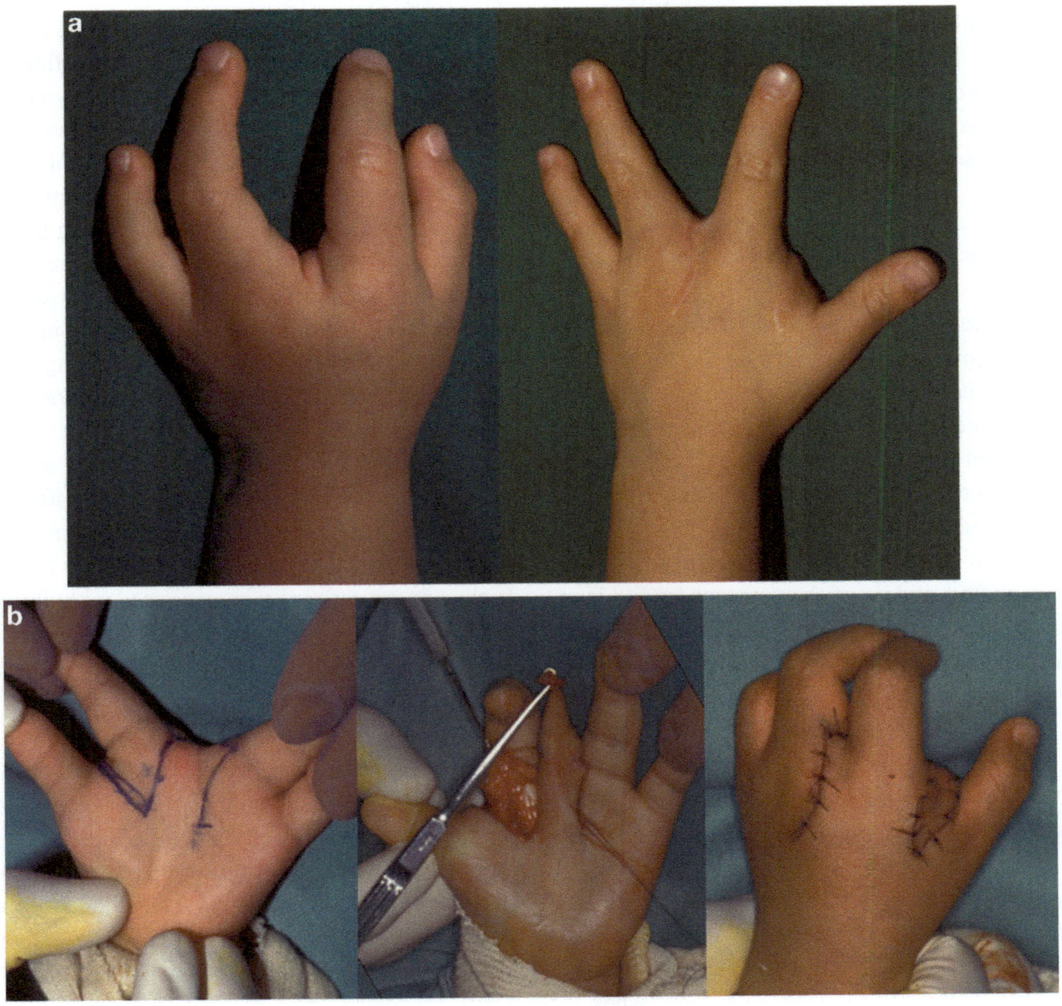

Fig. 15.13 (**a**) Snow–Littler procedure. *Left*: preoperative. *Right*: postoperative. (**b**) Snow–Littler procedure: during surgery. *Left*: design of skin incision. *Center*: palmar flap from the cleft. *Right*: transferred flap into the thumb web space and skin closure

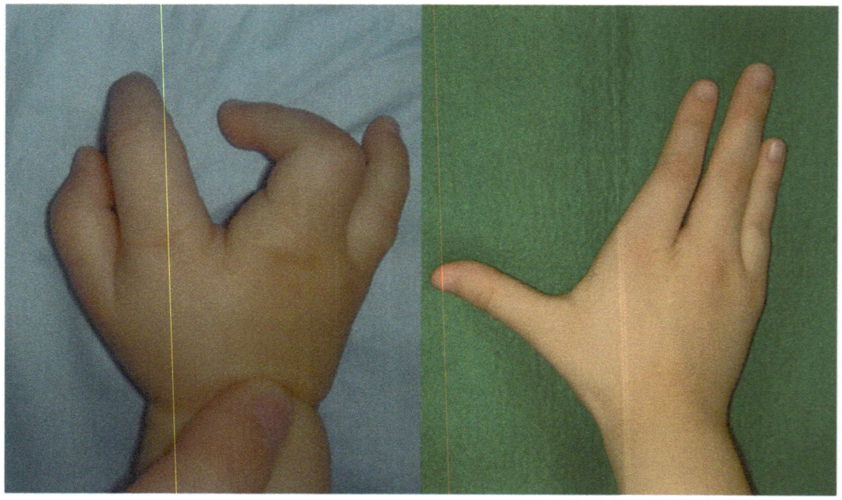

Fig. 15.14 Correction of the claw finger associated with cleft hand

ing the delta phalanx when the patient is less than 5 years. If the child is older than 5 years, the PIP joint or the DIP joint, where angulation occurs, is shortened and fused.

In removal of the delta phalanx, a short midlateral incision over the convex side of the thumb is used. The capsular structure including the collateral ligament is incised longitudinally and split. The delta phalanx is removed and the IP joint is fixed with a Kirschner wire for approximately 6 weeks. The collateral ligament is shortened and repaired, but the redundant skin is not excised, as it recovers spontaneously.

Correction of the Deviation of the Index Finger

Deviation of the index finger in cleft hand is caused by inclination of the DIP joint due to the rectangular middle phalanx. Most patients have no complaint due to this deformity. However, some patients will strongly desire correction of this deformity, when they reach adolescence. In such cases, corrective closing wedge osteotomy at the distal third of the middle phalanx is indicated.

Osteotomy of the phalanx: Longitudinal dorsal skin incision is carried out and middle of the extensor tendon is cut longitudinally. Closed wedge osteotomy is performed after subperiosteal exposure; fixation is carried out by crossed Kirschner wires or modified interosseous wiring.

Correction of Claw Finger Deformity of the Ring Finger

If the middle finger is absent, the ring finger may have a claw finger deformity. This deformity is described as camptodactyly associated with cleft hand in many papers. Flexion deformity of the PIP joint becomes rigid when the patients ages if passive correction of the PIP joint flexion deformity is not performed. This is not a true camptodactyly because the patient able to extend the PIP joint actively when the hyperextension of the MP joint of the affected finger is corrected to a neutral or slightly flexed position. Passive stretching and continuous splinting may correct this contracture. When cleft is closed around 1 year of age, spontaneous correction of the flexion deformity is sometimes observed, as hyperextension of the MP joint is usually corrected by the tension of the closed palmar skin. However, flexion deformity of the PIP joint or claw finger deformity should be corrected with tendon transfer at the initial surgery. In order to close a deep cleft, the structures including tendon and bone under the cleft are exposed. It is at this time that the surgeon has the best chance to select a tendon for transfer. In most cases of cleft hand, flexion of the PIP joint caused by the dysfunction of the intrinsic muscles. During surgery, we can often observe the extra flexor digitorum superficialis tendons of the ring finger or middle finger. One of them can be detached from the membranous insertion at the end of the stump of the missing finger. It is then transferred to the base of the proximal phalanx or the proximal end of the ligamentous flexor tendon sheath of the ring finger [77] (Fig. 15.14). If claw finger deformity is associated with divergence of the index and ring fingers, the detached flexor digitorum superficialis tendon may be divided into two slips. One slip is transferred to the radio-palmar periosteum of the base of the proximal phalanx of the ring finger and the other slip is transferred to the palmar periosteum of the ulnar base of the proximal phalanx of the index finger. The same type of procedure may be performed for extensor side. Extrinsic extensor tendon to the ring finger is transferred to the dorso-ulnar side of the expansion hood of the index finger and the extensor digitorum communis to the index finger is transferred to the dorso-radial side of the expansion hood of the ring finger. These procedures may prevent divergence deformity of the index and ring fingers when the fingers are extended.

Summary

Cleft hand is often associated with other deformities, which are phenotypes of abnormal induction of the finger ray numbers in the hand plate. When one classifies the congenital hand deformities, one has to face the problems how to classify the cases associated with cleft hand, central polydactyly, and syndactyly. It is easy to understand the association of these anomalies, once the concept of abnormal induction of the finger ray numbers in the hand plate has been accepted. The situation is the same as in congenital constriction band syndrome. One can easily understand the association among constriction band, acrosyndactyly, and amputation, if one has accepted the concept of congenital constriction band syndrome.

As I mentioned before, many authors think surgery of cleft hand is mainly performed for esthetic reasons, but some of the procedures have been performed for functional improvement. As in other congenital hand deformities, patient with cleft hand should use their hand skillfully when they become old, even if they have not surgically treated. Prof. P.C. Leung in Hong Kong, who is a respected hand surgeon and a person, delivered a lecture and told us as follows. Surgeons should be ambitious for treating the child with congenital hand problems. However, over ambitions may lead miserable surgeon and miserable patient. Surgery has its limitation and never forget "Don't make it worse!"

Acknowledgments I wish to thank Hiroyuki Kato, MD, Takuji Naruse, MD, and Miwako Ohtuji, MD, who worked hard to do animal experiments, and also to my wife, Tomoko Ogino, who supported all my studies for the past 40 years.

References

1. Barsky J. Cleft hand: classification, incidence, and treatments. J Bone Joint Surg. 1964;46A:1707–20.
2. Blauth W, Gekeler J. Symbrachydaktylien; Beitrag zur Morphologie, Klassifikation und Therapie. Handchirurgie. 1973;5:121–74 (in German).
3. Ogino T, Minami A, Kato H. Clinical features and roentgenograms of symbrachydactyly. J Hand Surg. 1989;14B:303–6.
4. Manske PR. Symbrachydactyly instead of atypical cleft hand. Plast Reconstr Surg. 1993;91:196.
5. Birch-Jensen A. Congenital deformities of the upper extremities. Copenhagen: Ejnar Munksgaart; 1949.
6. Flatt AE. The care of congenital hand anomalies. St. Louis: CV Mosby; 1977. p. 50.
7. Ogino T, Minami A, Fukuda K, Kato H. Congenital anomalies of the upper limb among the Japanese in Sapporo. J Hand Surg. 1986;11B:364–71.
8. Temtamy SA, McKusick V. The genetics of hand malformations. New York: Alan R Liss; 1978. p. 53.
9. Vogel IF. Verzogerte mutation bei menschen? Ann Hum Genet. 1957/1958;22:132 (in German).
10. Duijf PHG, van Bokhoven H, Brunner HG. Pathogenesis of split-hand/split-foot malformation. Hum Mol Genet. 2003; 12:51–60.
11. Elliott AM, Evans JA. Genotype-phenotype correlations in mapped split hand foot malformation (SHFM) patients. Am J Med Genet. 2006;140A:1419–27.
12. Elliott AM, Reed MH, Roscioli T, Evans JA. Discrepancies in upper and lower limb patterning in split hand foot malformation. Clin Genet. 2005;68:408–23.
13. Scherer SW, Poorkaj P, Massa H, Soder S, Allen T, Nunes M, et al. Physical mapping of the split hand/split foot locus on chromosome 7 and implication in syndromic ectrodactyly. Hum Mol Genet. 1994;3:1345–54.
14. Basel D, Kilpatrick MW, Tsipouras P. Research review. The expanding panorama of split hand foot malformation. Am J Med Genet. 2006;140A:1359–65.
15. Swanson AB. A classification for congenital limb malformations. J Hand Surg. 1976;1A:8–22.
16. Swanson AB, Swanson GG, Tada K. A classification for congenital limb malformations. J Hand Surg. 1983;8:693–702.
17. Ogino T, Kato H. Clinical and experimental studies on ulnar ray deficiency. Handchir Mikrochir Plast Chir. 1988;20:330–7.
18. Blauth W. Der hypoplastische Daumen. Arch Orthop Unfallchirur. 1967;62:225–46 (in German).
19. Ogino T, Ishii S, Minami M, Usui M, Muramatsu I, Miyake A. Roentgenological and clinical analyses of cleft hand, polydactyly of the middle finger. Seikeigeka. 1977;28:1508–11 (in Japanese).
20. Ogino T. A clinical and experimental study on teratogenic mechanism of the cleft hand, polydactyly and syndactyly. Nihon Seikeigeka Gakkai Zasshi. 1979;53:535–43 (in Japanese).
21. Manske PR. Cleft hand and central polydactyly in identical twins: a case report. J Hand Surg. 1983;8A:906–8.
22. Satake H, Ogino T, Takahara M, Kikuchi N, Muramatsu I, Muragaki Y, et al. Occurrence of central polydactyly, syndactyly, and cleft hand in a single family: report of five hands in three cases. J Hand Surg. 2009;34A:1700–3.
23. Miura T. Syndactyly and split hand. Hand. 1976;8:125–30.
24. Müller W. Die angeborenen Fehlbildungen der menschlechen Hand. Georg Thieme: Liepzig; 1937 (in German).
25. Jones NF, Kono N. Cleft hands with six metacarpals. J Hand Surg. 2004;29A:720–6.
26. Egawa T, Horiki A, Senrui H, Tada K. Characteristic anatomical findings of the cleft hand—its significance and classification. Handchirurgie. 1978;10:3–8 (in German).
27. Watari S, Tsuge K. A classification of cleft hands, based on clinical findings. Plast Reconstr Surg. 1979;64:381–9.
28. Ogino T. Teratogenic relation between central polydactyly, osseous syndactyly and cleft hand. J Hand Surg. 1990;15B:201–9.
29. Ogino T. Clinical features and teratogenic mechanisms of congenital absence of digits. Dev Growth Differ. 2007;49:523–31.
30. Kato H, Ogino T, Minami A, Ohshio I. Experimental study on radial ray deficiency. J Hand Surg. 1990;15B:470–6.
31. Ogino T, Kato H. Histological analysis of myleran induced oligodactyly of longitudinal deficiency in rats. Handchirurgie. 1988;20: 271–4.
32. Ogino T, Kato H. Clinical and experimental studies on teratogenic mechanisms of congenital absence of digits in longitudinal deficiencies. Congenit Anom. 1993;33:187–96.
33. Otsuji M, Takahara M, Naruse T, Guan D, Harada M, Zhe P, et al. Developmental abnormalities in rat embryos leading to tibial ray deficiencies induced by busulfan. Birth Defects Res A Clin Mol Teratol. 2005;73:461–7.
34. Naruse T, Takahara M, Takagi M, Ogino T. Early morphological changes leading to central polydactyly, syndactyly, and central deficiencies: an experimental study in rats. J Hand Surg. 2007;32A: 1413–7.

35. Ogino T. Teratogenic mechanisms of congenital absence of digits. Locomotor System. Adv Res Diagn Ther. 2011;18:173–93.
36. Naruse T, Takahara M, Takagi M, Oberg KC, Ogino T. Busulfan-induced central polydactyly, syndactyly and cleft hand or foot: a common mechanism of disruption leads to divergent phenotypes. Dev Growth Differ. 2007;49:533–41.
37. Ianakiev P, Kilpatrick MW, Toudjarska I, Basel D, Beighton P, Tsipouras P. Split-hand/split-foot malformation is caused by mutations in the p63 gene on 3q27. Am J Hum Genet. 2000;67:59–66.
38. Ogino T. Congenital anomalies of the upper limb in our clinic—an application of modified Swanson's classification. J Jpn Soc Surg Hand. 1986;2:909–16 (in Japanese).
39. Ogino T. Current classification of congenital hand deformities based on experimental research. In: Saffar P, Amadio CP, Foucher G, editors. Current practice in hand surgery. London: Martin Dunitz; 1997. p. 337–41.
40. Muragaki T, Mundlos S, Upton J, Olsen BR. Altered growth and branching pattern in synpolydactyly caused by mutations in HOXD 13. Science. 1996;272:548–51.
41. Debeer P, Bacchelli C, Scambler PJ, De Smet L, Fryns JP, Goodman FR. Severe digital abnormalities in a patient heterozygous for both a novel missense mutation in HOXD13 and a polyalanine tract expansion in HOXA13. J Med Genet. 2002;39:852–6.
42. Kjaer KW, Hedeboe J, Bugge M, Hansen C, Friis-Henriksen K, Vestergaard MB, et al. HOXD13 polyalanine tract expansion in classical synpolydactyly type Vordingborg. Am J Med Genet. 2003;110:116–21.
43. Congenital Hand Committee of the Japanese Society for Surgery of the Hand. Manual for classification of congenital hand anomalies. J Jpn Soc Surg Hand. 1996;13:455–67 (in Japanese).
44. Blauth W, Falliner AA. Zur Morphologie und Klassifikation von Spalthanden. Handchirurgie. 1986;18:161–95.
45. Saito H, Seki T, Suzuki Y, Fujino K. Operative treatments for various types of the cleft hand. Seikeigeka. 1978;29:1551–3 (in Japanese).
46. Ogino T. Cleft hand. Hand Clin. 1990;6:661–71.
47. Kato S, Ishii S, Ogino T, Shiono H. Anomalous hands with cleft formation between the fourth and fifth digits. J Hand Surg. 1983;8: 909–13.
48. Tonkin MA, Nanchahal J, Kwa S. Ulnar-sided cleft hand. J Hand Surg. 2002;27A:493–7.
49. Langer JS, Manske PR, Steffen JA, Hu C, Goldfarb C. Thumb in the plane of the hand: characterization and results of surgical treatment. J Hand Surg. 2009;34A:1795–801.
50. Manske PR, Halikis MN. Surgical classification of central deficiency according to the thumb web. J Hand Surg. 1995;20A:687–97.
51. Wassel HD. The result of surgery for polydactyly of the thumb, a review. Clin Orthop Relat Res. 1969;64:175–93.
52. Falliner AA. Analysis of anatomic variations in cleft hands. J Hand Surg. 2004;29A:994–1001.
53. Kikuchi N, Ogino T, Takahara M, Ito K, Kato Y. Cleft of the 4th web space of the hand without finger defect. J Jpn Soc Surg Hand. 2005;22:635–8 (in Japanese).
54. Schinzel A. Ulnar-mammary syndrome. J Med Genet. 1987;24: 778–81.
55. Ogino T, Minami A, Fukuda K, Nakazato T, Sakuma T, Kato H. Cleft hand complex with mirocheiria. J Jpn Soc Surg Hand. 1986;3:847–52 (in Japanese).
56. Buck-Gramcko D, Ogino T. Congenital malformation of the hand: non-classifiable cases. Hand Surg. 1996;1:45–61.
57. Küster W, Majewski F, Meinecke P. EEC syndrome without ectorodactyly? Clin Genet. 1985;28:130–5.
58. Rüdiger RA, Haase W, Passarge E. Association of ectrodactyly, ectodermal dysplasia and cleft lip-palate. Am J Dis Child. 1970;120:160–3.
59. Rodini ESO, Richieri-Costa A. EEC syndrome: report on 20 new patients, clinical and genetic considerations. Am J Med Genet. 1990;37:42–53.
60. Christodoulou J, McDougall P, Sheffield LJ. Choanal atresia as a feature of ectrodactyly-ectodermal dysplasia-clefting (EEC) syndrome. J Med Genet. 1989;26:576–89.
61. Fryns JP, Legius E, Dereymaeker AM, Van den Berghe H. EEC syndrome without ectrodactyly: report of two new families. J Med Genet. 1990;27:165–8.
62. Majewski F, Küster W. EEC syndrome sine sine? Clin Genet. 1988;33:69–72.
63. van Bokhoven H, Hamel BCJ, Bamshad M, Sangiorgi E, Gurrieri F, Duijf PH, et al. p63 gene mutations in EEC syndrome, limb–mammary syndrome, and isolated split hand split foot malformation suggest a genotype-phenotype correlation. Am J Hum Genet. 2001;69:481–92.
64. Vickers D. Clinodactyly of the little finger: a simple operative technique for reversal of the growth abnormality. J Hand Surg. 1987;12-B:335–42.
65. Kelikian H. Split hand complex. In: Congenital deformities of the hand and forearm. Philadelphia: WB Saunders Company; 1974. p. 467–95
66. Tsuge K, Sanada Y, Yamamoto M. Treatment of cleft hand. Seikeigeka. 1965;16:854–6 (in Japanese).
67. Al-Qattan MM, Robertson GA. An anatomical study of the deep transverse metacarpal ligament. J Anat. 1993;182:443–6.
68. Takahashi M, Yabe Y. Treatment for cleft hand with syndactyly; a case report of a new skin incision. Seikeigeka. 1978;29:1554–7 (in Japanese).
69. Miura T, Komada T. Simple method for reconstruction of the cleft hand with an adducted thumb. Plast Reconstr Surg. 1979; 64:65–7.
70. Ueba Y. Plastic surgery for the cleft hand. J Hand Surg. 1981; 6A:557–60.
71. Ueba Y. Cleft hand. In: Buck-Gramcko D, editor. Congenital malformation of the hand and foerarm. London: Churchill Livingstone; 1998. p. 199–215.
72. Upton J, Taghinia AH. Correction of the typical cleft hand. J Hand Surg. 2010;35A:480–5.
73. Foucher G, Lorea P, Hovius S, Pivato G, Medina J. Radial shift of the ulnar fingers: a new technique for special cases of longitudinal central deficiency. J Hand Surg. 2006;31:156–61.
74. Buck-Gramcko D. Cleft hands: classification and treatment. Hand Clin. 1985;1:467–73.
75. Rider MA, Grindel SI, Tonkin MA, Wood VE. An experience of the Snow-Littler procedure. J Hand Surg. 2000;25B:376–81.
76. Ogino T, Ishii S, Kato H. Opposable triphalangeal thumb, clinical features and results of treatment. J Hand Surg. 1994;19-A:39–47.
77. Zancolli EA. Structure and dynamic bases of hand surgery. 2nd ed. Philadelphia: JB Lippincott; 1978.

Camptodactyly and Clinodactyly

16

Raymond Tse and Karin Ljungquist

Camptodactyly

Camptodactyly is a non-traumatic progressive flexion deformity of the proximal interphalangeal (PIP) joint that typically involves one or both ulnar digits and is usually noted during infancy or adolescence [1] (Fig. 16.1). It is classified as a failure of differentiation of parts under the International Federation of Societies for Surgery of the Hand classification of congenital hand anomalies.

The term camptodactyly is Greek for "bent finger." Ever since Tamplin's description in 1846 [1], the definition, etiology, and treatment have varied in the literature. Almost every structure around the PIP joint has been implicated, and reconciliation of these pathologic observations has been debated.

Presentation

Camptodactyly affects less than 1 % of the population and is usually asymptomatic [2, 3]. The anomaly generally occurs sporadically; however, it can be inherited in an autosomal dominant pattern with variable expressivity and incomplete penetrance. Bilateral deformities occur in approximately two-thirds of cases and the little finger is almost always involved. Multiple digits can be affected, with less frequent involvement of the radial digits. The thumb is not involved. Metacarpophalangeal (MCP) joint hyperextension can accompany PIP flexion contractures.

R. Tse, M.D., F.R.C.S.(C.) (✉)
Pediatric Plastic Surgery, University of Washington, Seattle Children's Hospital, 4800 Sand Point Way NE, M/S OB.9.527, Seattle, WA 98105, USA
e-mail: raymond.tse@seattlechildrens.org

K. Ljungquist, M.D.
Bone and Joint Center, Department of Orthopaedics and Sports Medicine, University of Washington Medical Center, 4245 Roosevelt Way Northeast, Seattle, WA 98105-6920, USA
e-mail: kljun01@gmail.com

When the initial presentation is during infancy, males and females are equally affected. Females are more commonly affected when the initial presentation is during adolescence.

Benson classified patients into three types. Type I is an isolated anomaly of the little finger PIP joint that presents in infancy and can involve up to two fingers. Type II has the same clinical features but presents in adolescence. Type III is characterized by severe contractures, bilateral involvement, multiple digits, and other associated congenital anomalies. Type III camptodactyly presents at birth and is seen as a manifestation of a more generalized condition (Table 16.1).

The initial presentation of Type I and Type II camptodactyly at infancy and adolescence, respectively, may be related to growth spurts during which flexor–extensor imbalances manifest.

The PIP flexion deformity may be fixed or passively correctible, which has important treatment implications. Foucher proposed subclassifying Type I and II camptodactyly into "stiff" or "correctable" categories to guide his treatment approach [4].

Pathology

Abnormalities of almost every structure around the PIP joint have been described. Some believe all of these structures are involved but to varying degrees [4, 5]. Others believe that specific abnormalities of the flexor digitorum superficialis (FDS) or the intrinsic musculature [6–8] result in secondary changes with time and growth.

Early descriptions of camptodactyly have noted a tight, contracted, or underdeveloped FDS tendon [1, 9] and suggest that the deformity is the result of an imbalance of flexor and extensor forces. Aberrant FDS tendon origins in the absence of a normal muscle belly have been described and include the A2 pulley, palmar aponeurosis, flexor tendon sheath, and transverse carpal ligament [10].

Surgical explorations by Courtemanche and McFarlane have identified consistent abnormalities of lumbrical

D.R. Laub Jr. (ed.), *Congenital Anomalies of the Upper Extremity: Etiology and Management*,
DOI 10.1007/978-1-4899-7504-1_16, © Springer Science+Business Media New York 2015

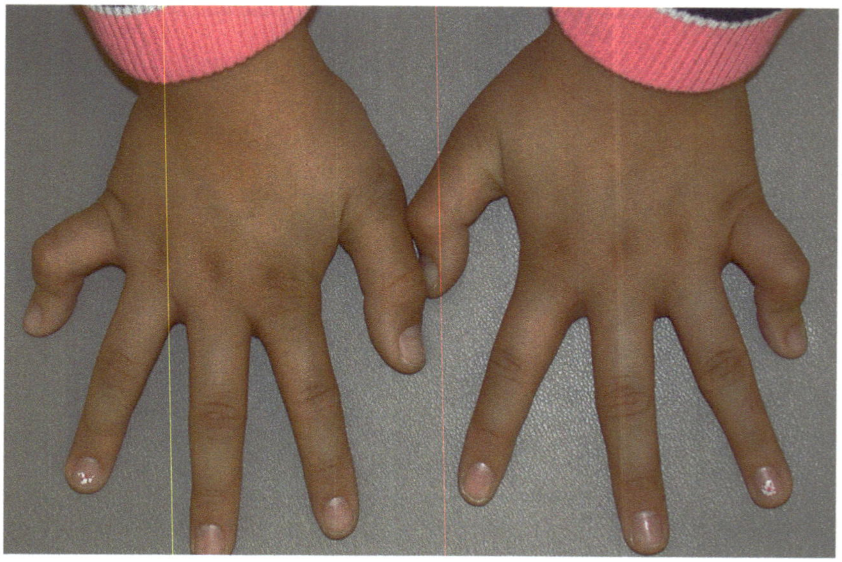

Fig. 16.1 Camptodactyly. Non-traumatic progressive flexion deformity typically involving the ulnar digit(s), often with an intrinsic minus posture

Table 16.1 Generalized conditions associated with camptodactyly

	Conditions
Craniofacial	Orofaciodigital syndrome
	Craniocarpotarsal dystrophy (Freeman–Sheldon syndrome)
	Oculodentodigital dysplasia
Chromosomal	Trisomy 13–15
Short Stature	Campomelic dysplasia I
	Mucopolysaccharidosis
	Facial–digital–genital (Aarskog–Scott syndrome)
Others	Osteo-onychodysostosis (Turner–Kieser syndrome)
	Cerebrohepatorenal (Zellweger's syndrome)
	Jacob-Downey syndrome

This table is adapted from Kozin SH, Kay SP, Griffin JR, Ezaki M. Congenital contracture. In: Green DP, Hotchkiss RN, Pederson WC, Wolfe SW, editors. Green's Operative Hand Surgery, 6th ed. Philadelphia: Elsevier Churchill Livingstone; 1507–26. Copyright Elsevier 2013

muscles, suggesting that these may be the primary etiology of camptodactyly [6–8]. An aberrant lumbrical origin from the flexor retinaculum [11] has also been described. More commonly, aberrant lumbrical insertions have been described and include the FDS tendon [6–8, 12, 13] and MCP joint capsule [6–8]. Inadequate lumbrical muscle function leads to an intrinsic-minus posture, which may lead to the deformity seen with camptodactyly.

Other soft tissue abnormalities include extensor incompetence, collateral ligament contracture, volar plate contracture, and volar skin deficiency [1, 4, 5]. Bony changes can be seen with long-standing deformities [1, 7] and are consistent with growth in the setting of a chronically flexed joint. The head of the proximal phalanx is narrowed in the dorsovolar plane with loss of the normal volar convexity. The articular surface of the middle phalanx base can have a shallow dorsal groove. Radiographic changes were seen in approximately 15 % of patients in McFarlane and Smith's series [1, 7]. Smith argues that all of these abnormalities are common to all cases of camptodactyly, but to varying degrees. McFarlane argues that aberrations of lumbrical muscle insertion are the unifying cause and all other changes occur secondary to chronic motor imbalance. He points out how previous anatomic studies have demonstrated that normal anatomic variations of the intrinsic muscles occur more frequently in the ulnar digits and that these are the same digits that are involved with camptodactyly.

Diagnosis

Differentiation of camptodactyly from other conditions is accomplished through careful history and physical examination. Camptodactyly is seen in the absence of trauma, inflammation, and palpable lesions. The deformity is slowly progressive and generally occurs in isolation. A trigger finger may be associated with a palpable click on extension. Juvenile palmar fibromatosis or Dupuytren's disease is associated with palpable subcutaneous nodules. A boutonniere deformity should be associated with antecedent trauma and swelling. Inflammatory arthridities manifest with inflammation and more generalized involvement. Symphalangism is characterized by no active or passive joint motion and an absence of skin creases. Arthrogryposis involves generalized muscular and skeletal deficiencies. Pterygium syndrome is usually associated with involvement of multiple joints.

Following a thorough examination of the upper extremity, active and passive range of motion of the PIP joint should be evaluated and the influence of adjacent joint positions should be noted. FDS tightness can be determined by tenodesis effect in which wrist and MCP extension places the FDS on stretch and results in further loss of passive PIP extension. Intrinsic motor deficiency can be assessed using the Bouvier maneuver, in which active PIP extension is tested with the MCP joint stabilized in flexion. Restoration of full PIP extension suggests that inadequate MCP flexion, via the intrinsic muscles, contributes to the deformity. Extensor competence can be tested using an extensor tenodesis test in which full flexion of the wrist and MCP places the extensor system on stretch. This should result in full PIP extension. Long-standing flexion deformities can result in attenuation of the central slip, in which case PIP extension would not occur with this test. Volar skin deficiency can be determined by testing passive PIP extension with the MCP in flexion and in extension. Blanching and loss of passive PIP extension when the MCP is extended suggests volar soft tissue deficiency.

Flexor digitorum profundus (FDP) and FDS function of each finger should be evaluated. Given that the FDP to each finger acts through a common muscle belly, in order to test isolated FDS function to an individual finger, all other digits must be held in extension while finger flexion of the digit of interest is evaluated. The ring and little finger FDS are conjoined in 30 % of people. If PIP flexion is not possible for the little finger, release of the ring finger should result in PIP flexion of both digits if their FDS is conjoined.

Treatment

Conservative management should be the first line of treatment. PIP contractures of less than 30° rarely have any functional impact, and greater contractures are often well tolerated.

Nonsurgical Management

Methods of nonsurgical treatment include passive stretching, static splinting, dynamic splinting, or any combination of these. Results often rely upon patient and family compliance, but can also vary with patient age and severity of the contracture.

Rhee et al. reported on the results of passive stretching for simple camptodactyly in children younger than 3 years of age [14]. They included 61 digits in 22 patients. Their stretching protocol involved 5 min of passive stretching 20 times per day until the deformity was corrected or the improvement "stabilized," followed by maintenance stretching 5–10 times per day. Children were stratified according to initial severity of contracture (<30°, 30–60°, >60°) and were found to have significant corrections: 20° to 1° for mild contractures, 39° to 12° for moderate contractures, and 75° to 28° for severe contractures. The mean follow-up was 26 months and the only correlation with degree of improvement was the initial flexion contracture. Although they demonstrated good results in a homogenous group of Korean children with Type I camptodactyly, their protocol is time intensive, requires considerable caregiver effort, and the long-term outcomes, especially regarding the risk of progression or recurrence as children move into adolescence, are unknown.

Benson et al. reported on the results of passive stretching combined with static splinting in patients with all types of camptodactyly. They treated 24 digits in 13 patients with Type I camptodactyly with static splints and daily passive stretching. The splints were initially worn for 15–18 h per day and slowly weaned after full passive motion was achieved. The average correction was −22.9° to −0.9° of passive extension with a mean follow-up of 36 months. They treated five digits in four patients with Type II camptodactyly who had experienced an overall worsening of the flexion contracture. They also treated 30 digits in five patients with Type III camptodactyly with overall improvement from −23° to −1° of passive extension. Most fingers were treated with splinting and the fingers that underwent surgery had significant improvements.

Hori et al. used dynamic splints to treat 34 digits in 24 patients. Treatment involved splinting for 24 h per day during the first few months until full correction was achieved, followed by use of the digit for 8 h per day. Fifteen patients were less than 5 years old and eight patients were older than 10 years of age; however, they did not report results according to camptodactyly type. The average correction of the contractures was 40° to 10° with average follow-up of 56 months (minimum 10 months). Miura et al. also used dynamic splints and found that the results were better in children younger than 5 years than in children who were older than 5 years [15].

Siebert et al. reported results of both nonsurgical and surgical treatment for simple camptodactyly. Nonsurgical treatment involved combinations of passive stretching, static splinting, and dynamic splinting. Although patients were not classified according to age of onset, most children who underwent nonsurgical treatment were close to adolescence. Their results were similar to those reported by Rhee when stratified according to initial contracture severity. The authors found that the overall results of surgical treatment were worse than nonsurgical treatment and suggest that surgery should only be considered with contractures of greater than 60°, after nonsurgical treatment has failed.

Surgical

Surgical treatment of camptodactyly should be reserved for severe cases in which all efforts towards nonsurgical management have failed. The results of surgery are inconsistent and the risk of PIP flexion loss needs to be weighed against the more limited gains in PIP extension. Flexion contractures of up to 60° in the ulnar digits are well tolerated and should not be treated surgically. Postoperative rehabilitation is key to treatment success and patient compliance should be confirmed prior to surgery. There currently is no consensus on indications for surgical treatment, as the relative risks and benefits of surgical and nonsurgical treatment continue to be debated.

If surgical treatment is elected, all of the pathologic changes of camptodactyly should be considered of these can be detected via clinical exam.

The initial skin incision should consider a potential volar soft tissue deficit following correction. A midline longitudinal approach with subsequent Z-plasties at closure can provide moderate length [6, 7] in most cases. Other approaches include zigzag Bruner incisions [3] or a large proximally based flap [3] that can incorporate a full thickness skin graft at closure if needed. A proximally based lateral finger transposition flap has also been proposed [16].

The incision extends from beyond the PIP joint to the proximal palm so that the distal edge of the transverse carpal ligament can be exposed. The FDS should be inspected from the carpal canal through its course under the A1 pulley. Proximal traction with the wrist in a neutral position should have the spring-like feel of a muscle belly. Lack of excursion may suggest a proximal fibrous origin. Distal traction should produce normal PIP flexion. Further exploration using windows in the annular ligaments may be necessary to find abnormal distal insertions.

The FDP should be identified and the lumbrical should be followed from origin to insertion. The lumbrical may insert abnormally into the MCP joint capsule, the FDS tendon, or the adjacent finger extensor system. If the lumbrical is found to have an abnormal insertion it can be released and reinserted into the extensor apparatus.

Resection of the FDS can result in significant loss of finger flexion. Unless the origin is abnormal, the FDS can be used in a tendon transfer. If the preoperative exam demonstrates that PIP extension can be restored with stabilization of the MCP in flexion, the FDS can be transferred to the A1 pulley as a “lasso” to produce MCP flexion (Fig. 16.2a). If the preoperative exam demonstrates that PIP extension cannot be restored with stabilization of the MCP in flexion, the FDS is transferred to the extensor system so that it can act as both an MCP flexor and PIP extensor (see Fig. 16.2b).

If the FDS has been found to act independently, it can be transferred without further dissection. If it is not independent, the FDS needs to be dissected and freed from the adjacent FDS. Alternatives for tendon transfer include an adjacent FDS [8] tendon or the extensor indicis proprius (EIP) re-routed volar to the intermetacarpal ligament [2, 17]. Gupta suggests that EIP transfer is only appropriate when stabilization of the MCP to prevent hyperextension allows full or near full active PIP extension.

When passive PIP extension cannot be restored after releasing the FDS insertion or anomalous intrinsic muscles, some authors perform releases of the volar plate, capsule, and/or ligaments. Any surgical release of the PIP joint results in considerable inflammation and scar and is likely an important factor in the loss of flexion noted in some series or case reports [4–7, 18, 19]. Siegert et al. reported poor results of surgical treatment [18] and McFarlane reported an average flexion to distal crease of palm of 1.8 cm [7]. In the latter series only 33 % of patients retained full flexion. McFarlane suggests that it is better to accept an incomplete correction of the flexion contracture rather than risking loss of flexion due to scarring about the PIP joint [6].

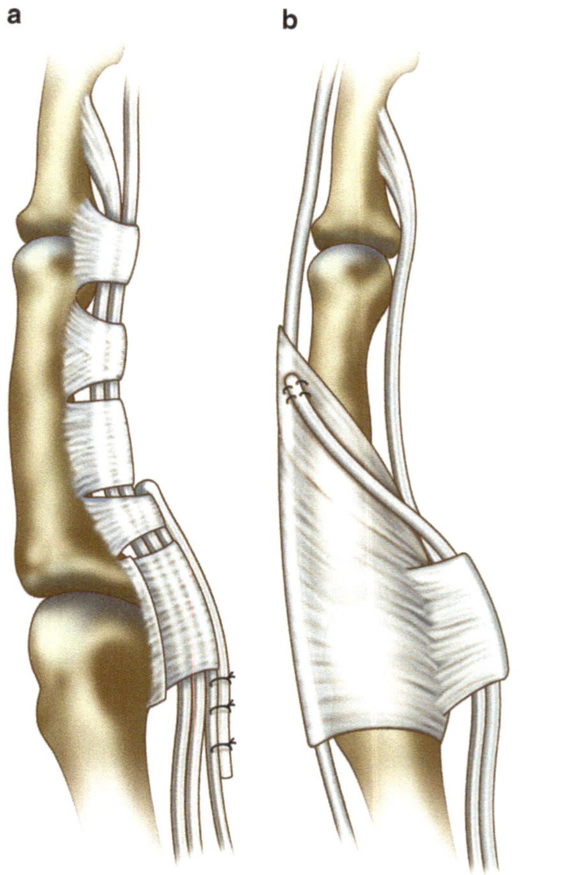

Fig. 16.2 (**a**) Zancolli lasso procedure. The FDS tendon is released from its insertion and sutured around the A2 pulley to act primarily as an MCP flexor. (**b**) Intrinsic transfer. The FDS tendon is re-routed to insert into the extensor apparatus to act as an MCP flexor and a PIP extensor

The results of surgery are variable and difficult to compare due to differences in methodology and incompatible formats of results reporting. A passively correctable PIP joint prior to surgery is generally favorable. In case reports where the PIP joint was not released there was no loss of flexion [12, 13, 17]. In case series where the PIP joint was rarely released, the loss of flexion was minimal and often less than 10° [4, 5]. Smith reported an improvement of 57° with surgery [5] and Foucher reported 68–88 % improvement depending upon the preoperative type [4].

Earlier case series reported unfavorable surgical results; however, these involved FDS tenotomy without a tendon transfer [1, 9]. Other case reports using this approach do not report whether there was any loss of flexion [10, 20].

In the case of severe flexion with significant bony changes, soft tissue reconstruction is unlikely to be successful. In these situations, the only alternative to accepting the deformity is a bony salvage procedure. An osteotomy does not increase the available range of motion; it only serves to reposition the arc of available motion [21]. Arthrodesis sacrifices all motion. Circumstances in which these salvage options are worthwhile are rare.

Summary

Treatment of camptodactyly remains controversial. Nonsurgical treatment is the first line and mainstay of management. The results of surgery are variable; however, more favorable results tend to be achieved with correctable deformities and a tendon transfer to restore intrinsic function. Loss of flexion remains a significant concern with surgical treatment. Given that the lack of full extension is better tolerated than loss of flexion, these risks must be considered when surgery is contemplated for severe deformities.

Clinodactyly

Clinodactyly (Greek; klinen = to bend, daktylos = finger) refers to digital angulation in the radioulnar plane distal to the MCP joint. It is classified as a failure of hand-plane formation and/or differentiation in Manske and Oberg's modification of the International Federation of Societies for Surgery of the Hand classification of congenital hand anomalies [22]. The earliest report of the condition is attributed to Smith, who described its radiographic appearance in 1896 [23]. Incidence of the condition is difficult to accurately assess, as the accepted parameters of normalcy vary. Minor angulation of the digits, especially the small finger, is very common and generally considered to be a normal variant. The stated upper limit of normal angulation varies between 10° and 15°; a considerable variation in incidence rates follows, with reports ranging from 1 % [24] to 20 % [25]. In North America incidence has been reported as 1 %, compared to 3–5 % in Japan [26].

Presentation

Clinodactyly typically presents as radial deviation of the little finger, is often bilateral, and is more common in males. The thumb and ring finger are the next most frequently affected digits. Involvement of the middle and index fingers is uncommon; that of the index finger tends to be unilateral [27]. Work by Dutta [24] and Hersh [28] has confirmed the mode of genetic inheritance to be autosomal dominant with variable penetrance. It is usually an isolated finding, but can be associated with a number of other hand differences and syndromes including trisomy 21 and trisomy 18 (Table 16.2). Apert and Rubinstein–Taybi syndromes [29, 30] are associated with bilateral thumb clinodactyly. The "kissing delta phalanx" deformity, Trevor disease, and Mohr–Wriedt brachydactyly are associated with index finger clinodactyly [27]. Clinodactyly can also be seen with polydactyly and macrodactyly. A genetic work-up should be considered if any additional abnormalities are noted during physical examination of a child presenting with clinodactyly. Most patients seek care due to cosmetic concerns or progressive deformity. Clinodactyly of the small finger is rarely functionally limiting, as any flexion impairment can typically be compensated for with increased digital abduction. Patients with thumb or central digit involvement may present with impaired flexion or pinch that is clinically significant.

Table 16.2 Causes and associated conditions of clinodactyly

	Conditions
Trauma	Phalangeal shaft malunion
	Frostbite injuries
	Salter–Harris I–V fractures
Chromosomal disorders	Down's syndrome
	Klinefelter's syndrome
	Turner's syndrome
	Trisomy 18
	Trisomy 21
	Cri du chat
	XXXXY
	XXXXX
Limb anomalies	Symphalangism
	Familial brachydactyly
Craniofacial disorders	Apert's syndrome
	Orodigital facial
	Orodigital palatal
	Oculodentodigital
	Treacher Collins
Miscellaneous	Silver's syndrome
	Prader–Willi
	Cornelia de Lange
	Seckel dwarfism
	Marfan's syndrome
	Myositis ossificans progressive
	Mohr's syndrome
	Goltz
	Freeman–Sheldon
	Laurence–Moon–Biedl
	Poland
	Holt Oram
	Fanconi anemia
	Nail patella syndrome

Adapted with permission from Burke F, Flatt A. Clinodactyly. A review of a series of cases. Hand 1979;11:269–280

Etiology

Clinodactyly is most commonly due to an abnormally triangular or trapezoidal shaped middle phalanx; the result of an anomalous, longitudinally oriented epiphysis running along the short side of the involved phalanx. The proximal physis is usually normal, whereas the distal physis may be aberrantly persistent [25]. Light and Ogden have further characterized this longitudinal epiphyseal bracket [31]. This abnormal tethering of the radial aspect of the phalanx results in progressive angulation of the digit towards the concave side. A very short triangular, "delta" phalanx is the result of early complete ossification of a C-shaped bracket and results in the most severe deformities [25]. Incomplete, or cartilaginous, brackets allow for some longitudinal growth. A trapezoidal phalanx develops and the angulation can be progressive [32]. The longitudinal epiphyseal bracket may not be visible radiographically until the age of 3–4 years because the physis is not yet ossified. Clinodactyly of the thumb associated with Apert's syndrome, while it shares a radially angulated presentation with classic clinodactyly, may be the result of a different etiology. There is continued debate regarding if the clinodactyly is the result of an anomalous insertion of the abductor pollicis brevis muscle onto the distal phalanx, or due to an abnormal bracketed physis [33, 34]. Clinodactyly can occur in association with a triphalangeal thumb; however, discussion of this entity is beyond the scope of this chapter. Clinodactyly may also occur as a result of a growth plate insult that produces asymmetric growth and physeal closure. Trauma, fractures, thermal injury, frostbite, inflammatory arthritis, and tumors can be responsible for such growth plate abnormalities.

Classification and Differential Diagnosis

Burke and Flatt grouped 50 patients with clinodactyly into three broad categories: familial, or classic, clinodactyly; clinodactyly associated with other congenital abnormalities; and clinodactyly due to epiphyseal injuries [35]. The third grouping refers to posttraumatic angular deformities resulting from various insults, not true congenital conditions. Although this classification is helpful for differential diagnosis, it is not as useful for directing treatment decisions.

Cooney proposed the most commonly utilized classification system, based upon tissue involvement and angulation. Simple forms involve bone only while complex forms involve both bone and soft tissue. If the angulation is greater than 45° the designation of complicated is added. Complex clinodactyly is typically associated with syndactyly, whereas complex complicated clinodactyly is often associated with polydactyly or macrodactyly [36]. More recently, Ali and Rayan proposed a simple classification based on severity of angular deformity. Group 1 referred to physiologic angulation, which they defined as <5°; group 2 defined as mild angulation between 5° and 10°; group 3 was defined as moderate deformity between 15° and 30°, and group 4 was defined as severe deformity of greater than 30° [37].

Treatment

Nonsurgical

The vast majority of patients with isolated clinodactyly present with cosmetic, rather than functional concerns. Observation alone is the appropriate course of action for such cases, as the possibility for significant scarring and loss of range of motion with surgical correction for the sole purpose of potentially improving the appearance of the finger represents an unacceptable risk. There is also no role for splinting or stretching of the digit, as it is completely ineffective [35].

Surgical

While nonoperative management is the mainstay of treatment for clinodactyly, and appropriate for most patients, surgical intervention is indicated for significant angulation that interferes with hand function. Correction requires either osteotomy of the phalanx or resection of the longitudinal epiphyseal bracket allowing the digital curvature to correct over time with longitudinal growth. A variety of surgical procedures have been described, including closing wedge osteotomy [37], opening wedge osteotomy [35, 38], reverse wedge osteotomy [39], a partial excision greenstick, or "PEG" osteotomy [40], distraction osteotomy [41], and physiolysis [42–45]. The common theme amongst all osteotomies is correction of the angular deformity of the digit. Each technique presents unique advantages and disadvantages.

Closing wedge osteotomy (Fig. 16.3a, b) is simple, technically straightforward, and reliable; however, it further shortens an already short digit and may slacken the extensor mechanism. Rayan reported on a series of 25 fingers in patients with an average age of 6 years, all treated with a closing wedge osteotomy that removed 2–3 mm of bone. Clinically, average angulation improved from 33° preoperatively to 9° postoperatively, a 79 % correction. Radiographically, the average correction was 29° preoperatively to 5° postoperatively. Patients were satisfied with the appearance of the finger in 96 % of cases. Range of motion was slightly decreased, with the loss of 3° of motion at the DIP joint and 1° at the PIP joint. No patients reported subjective loss of motion. The authors recommend this treatment for moderate (15–30°) and severe (>30°) deformities. Burke and Flatt in their review of 50 patients with clinodactyly advised waiting until skeletal maturity before performing a closing wedge osteotomy in order to achieve maximum length of the finger, thereby minimizing the risks of shortening and range of motion compromise [35].

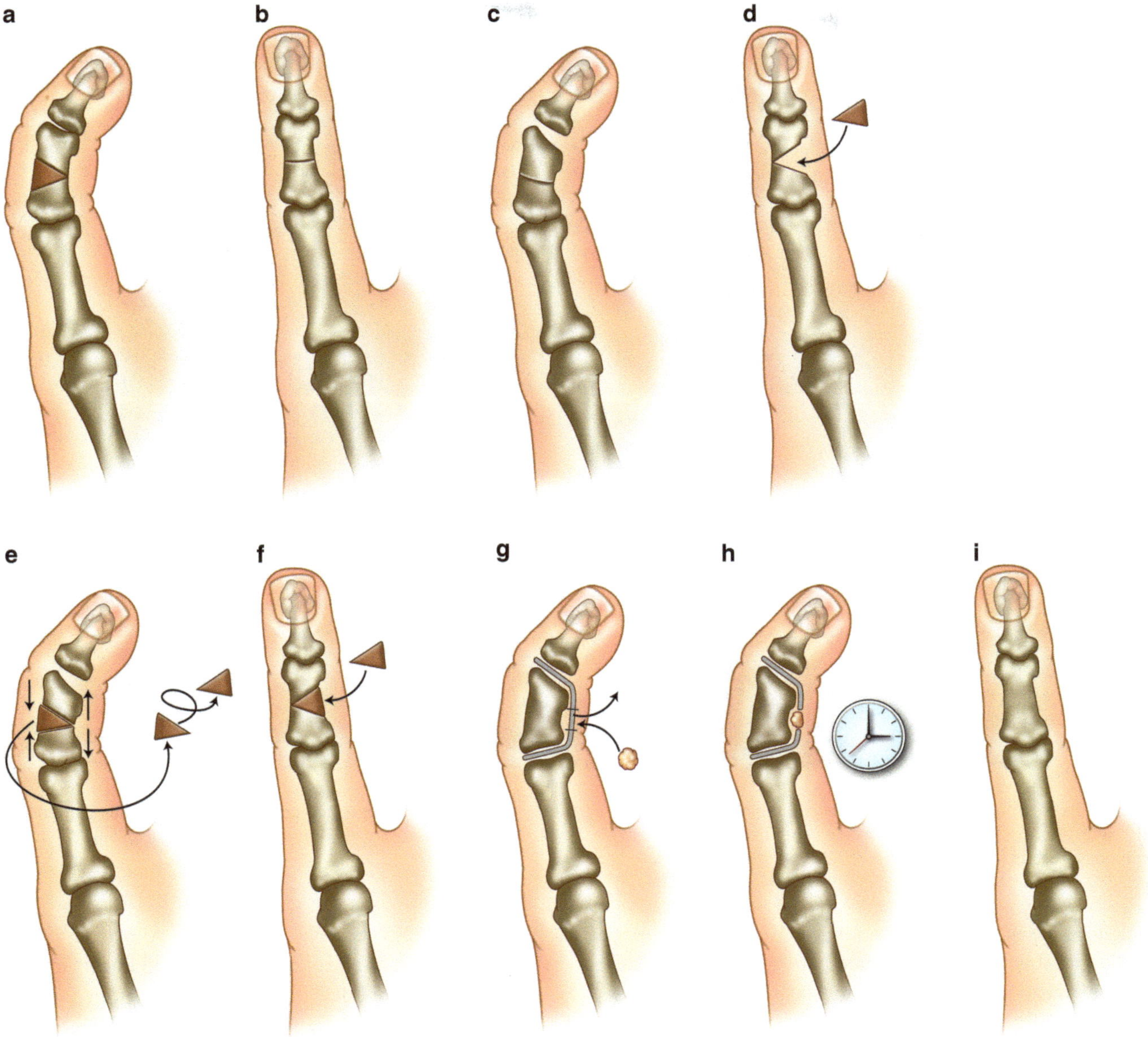

Fig. 16.3 (**a, b**) Clinodactyly treatment. Closing wedge osteotomy. (**c, d**) Clinodactyly treatment. Opening wedge osteotomy with bone graft. (**e, f**) Clinodactyly treatment. Reverse wedge osteotomy with autograft. (**g–i**) Clinodactyly treatment. Physiolysis

Opening (see Fig. 16.3c, d) and reverse wedge (see Fig. 16.3e, f) osteotomies offer the advantage of maintaining, or even increasing, length but are technically more demanding procedures. Additionally, the soft tissue envelope may need to be lengthened. This may be accomplished with a Z-plasty, although more severe cases may require a rotational flap or step advancement flap. Bone grafting is necessary in an opening wedge osteotomy, and donor site options are limited in small children. A reverse wedge osteotomy is made more difficult by the small caliper of a child's phalanx, and also exposes both sides of the digit to a surgical insult. Wood and Flatt described the use of an opening wedge osteotomy to treat congenital triangular bones in the hand, and Light and Ogden advocate opening wedge osteotomy with fat interposition [31, 35]. Recently, Tansley and Pickford described a modification of the opening wedge osteotomy in which they created a greenstick fracture, which required only interosseous wiring for fixation. They coined this partial excision greenstick (PEG) osteotomy, with the described advantages of minimizing the risk of soft tissue injury and improved rotational control [40]. Opening wedge osteotomy with the use of a distraction external fixator has also been described [41]. Carstam and Theander described a reverse wedge osteotomy in which a wedge of bone was excised from the non-bracketed side of the digit, reversed, and transfixed into the site of an opening wedge osteotomy on the

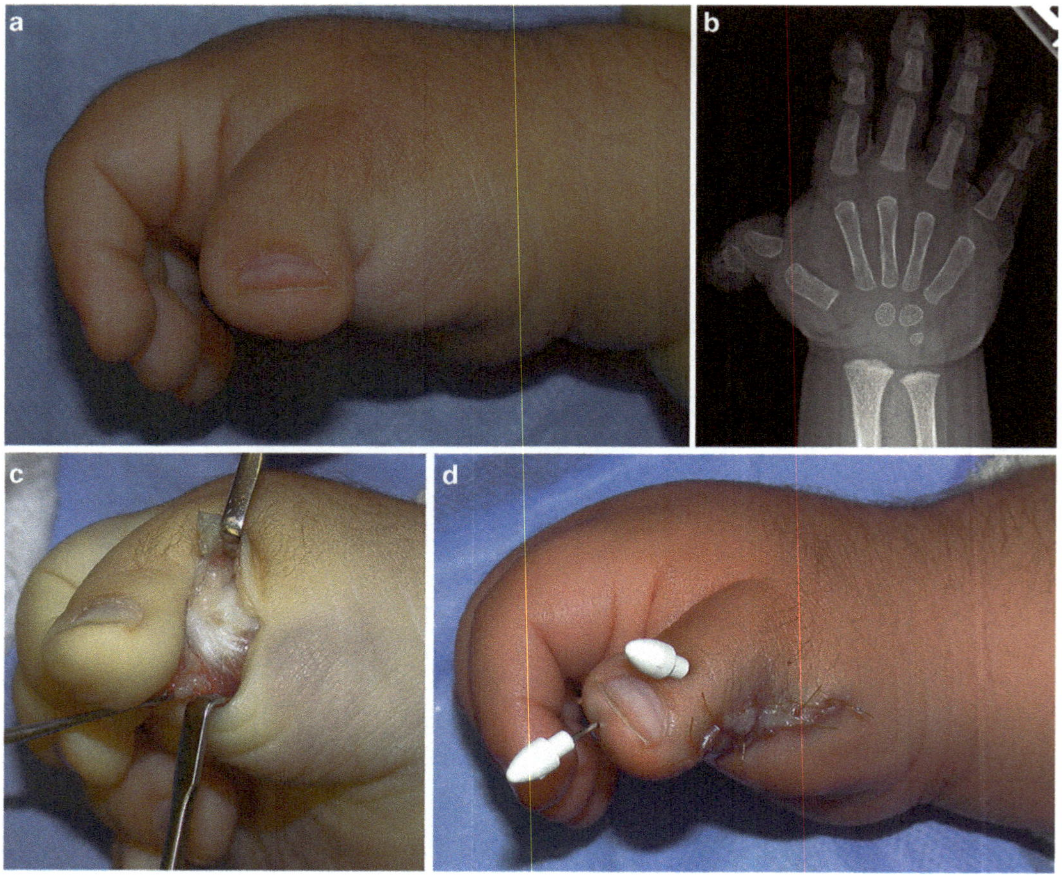

Fig. 16.4 (a, b) Thumb clinodactyly. Bilateral thumb deformities in a child with Rubenstein–Taybi syndrome. (c) Thumb clinodactyly. Abnormal abductor pollicis brevis (APB) tendon insertion into the base of the distal phalanx determined on exploration. (d) Thumb clinodactyly. Correction following APB release, osteotomy, and Z-plasty

bracketed side of the digit with a wire. They achieved good results with this technique in three patients with an average age of 14 years, reporting deformity correction to 10° or less in all cases [39].

Physiolysis addresses the angular deformity by excising the abnormal longitudinal epiphyseal bracket and interposing fat (see Fig. 16.3g–i). This allows the curved digit to straighten over time with longitudinal growth, as the concave side is no longer tethered. As this procedure requires growth potential to achieve angular correction, it is limited to patients with open growth plates and is best performed at an earlier age. Vickers described the results of physiolysis of 12 digits in six patients, with an average age of 9. He achieved good results, although one patient, aged 12 at the time of surgery, did require an osteotomy to correct residual deformity. While he felt the procedure was reasonable to perform as long as 3–5 years of growth remained, he considered the ideal time for surgery to be about 3 years of age [44]. Al-Qattan, in a review of sporadic clinodactyly of the index finger, echoed this recommendation for early surgery and advised a Vickers physiolysis as early as possible for patients presenting in the first 5 years of life [27]. Yamazaki et al. reported achieving an average 20° correction using Vickers's technique in a 5.5-year-old child [45]. A review of 23 children of an average age of 6.6 years with 35 fingers treated with physiolysis revealed an average correction of 11°. Improved correction (20° ± 9.7°) was obtained in fingers with greater deformity (>40°) preoperatively. Patients who had surgery before the age of 6 also had significantly better correction. Two patients had premature fusion of the physis on the operated aspect of the digit and required a closing wedge osteotomy after skeletal maturity, which was not complicated by the history of physiolysis [43]. More recently, Light et al. reviewed the literature and a case of a 2.5-year-old male with bilateral clinodactyly and drew the following conclusions: physiolysis is most commonly performed for children between the ages of 2 and 6 years with more than 30° of angulation and should be avoided in children older than 9 years; patients should be advised that while deformity will be improved, it may not be completely corrected, and persistent deformity may be treated with osteotomy [42].

Thumb clinodactyly seen with Apert or Rubinstein–Taybi syndrome may be associated with abnormally distal abductor pollicis brevis tendon insertions that need to be released and re-inserted more proximally in order to address a potentially primary deforming force (Fig. 16.4).

Summary

Clinodactyly is the congenital curvature of a digit in the radioulnar plane. The middle phalanx is often triangular or trapezoidally shaped. While clinically significant clinodactyly is rare, curvature of the small finger up to 10–15° is quite common and considered a normal variant. Nonoperative management is the appropriate treatment for the majority of cases. For the rare case where the curvature is severe enough to be functionally limiting, surgical options include physiolysis and various osteotomy techniques. Good corrections can be achieved with both techniques in properly selected patients. Physiolysis is best used in patients less than 6 years of age. Surgery should not be undertaken for cosmetic concerns alone.

References

1. Smith RJ, Kaplan EB. Camptodactyly and similar atraumatic flexion deformities of the proximal interphalangeal joints of the fingers. A study of thirty-one cases. J Bone Joint Surg Am. 1968;50(6):1187–203.
2. Burke FD. Camptodactyly. In: Gupta A, Kay SP, editors. The growing hand. London: Mosby; 2000. p. 293–6.
3. Kozin SH, Kay SP, Griffin JR, Ezaki M. Congenital contracture. In: Green DP, Hotchkiss RN, Pederson WC, Wolfe SW, editors. Green's operative hand surgery. 6th ed. Philadelphia: Elsevier Churchill Livingstone; 2013. p. 1507–26.
4. Foucher G, Lor AP, Khouri RK, Medina J, Pivato G. Camptodactyly as a spectrum of congenital deficiencies: a treatment algorithm based on clinical examination. Plast Reconstr Surg. 2006;117(6):1897–905.
5. Smith PJ, Grobbelaar AO. Camptodactyly: a unifying theory and approach to surgical treatment. J Hand Surg Am. 1998;23(1):14–9.
6. McFarlane RM, Curry GI, Evans HB. Anomalies of the intrinsic muscles in camptodactyly. J Hand Surg Am. 1983;8(5 Pt 1):531–44.
7. McFarlane RM, Classen DA, Porte AM, Botz JS. The anatomy and treatment of camptodactyly of the small finger. J Hand Surg Am. 1992;17(1):35–44.
8. Courtemanche AD. Campylodactyly: etiology and management. Plast Reconstr Surg. 1969;44(5):451–4.
9. Engber WD, Flatt AE. Camptodactyly: an analysis of sixty-six patients and twenty-four operations. J Hand Surg Am. 1977;2(3):216–24.
10. Ogino T, Kato H. Operative findings in camptodactyly of the little finger. J Hand Surg Br. 1992;17(6):661–4.
11. Minami A, Sakai T. Camptodactyly caused by abnormal insertion and origin of lumbrical muscle. J Hand Surg Br. 1993;18(3):310–1.
12. Maeda M, Matsui T. Camptodactyly caused by an abnormal lumbrical muscle. J Hand Surg Br. 1985;10(1):95–6.
13. Inoue G, Tamura Y. Camptodactyly resulting from paradoxical action of an anomalous lumbrical muscle. Scand J Plast Reconstr Surg Hand Surg. 1994;28(4):309–11.
14. Rhee SH, Oh WS, Lee HJ, Roh YH, Lee JO, Baek GH. Effect of passive stretching on simple camptodactyly in children younger than three years of age. J Hand Surg. 2010;35(11):1768–73.
15. Miura T. Non-traumatic flexion deformity of the proximal interphalangeal joint-its pathogenesis and treatment. Hand. 1983;15(1):25–34.
16. Glicenstein J, Haddad R, Guero S. [Surgical treatment of camptodactyly]. Ann Chir Main Memb Super. 1995;14(6):264–71.
17. Gupta A, Burke FD. Correction of camptodactyly. Preliminary results of extensor indicis transfer. J Hand Surg Br. 1990;15(2):168–70.
18. Siegert JJ, Cooney WP, Dobyns JH. Management of simple camptodactyly. J Hand Surg Br. 1990;15(2):181–9.
19. Kakinoki R, Duncan SF, Ohta S, Nakamura T. Simultaneous reconstruction of a palmar skin defect and the digital artery with an arterialized venous flap after correction of camptodactyly with severe flexion deformity. Hand. 2011;6(4):445–9.
20. Hoogbergen MM, Schuurman AH, Kon M. Camptodactyly caused by an anomalous origin of the flexor digitorum superficialis tendon. Case report. Scand J Plast Reconstr Surg Hand Surg. 1996;30(1):71–3.
21. Flatt AE. Crooked fingers. The care of congenital hand anomalies. St Louis: Quality Medical Publishing; 1994. p. 197–227.
22. Manske PR, Oberg KC. Classification and developmental biology of congenital anomalies of the hand and upper extremity. J Bone Joint Surg Am. 2009;91 Suppl 4:3–18.
23. Smith TT. Peculiarity in the shape of the hand in idiots of the mongol type. Paediatrics. 1896;2:315–20.
24. Dutta P. The inheritance of the radially curved little finger. Acta Genet Stat Med. 1965;15:70–6.
25. Jones GB. Delta phalanx. J Bone Joint Surg Br. 1964;46:226–8.
26. Fujita H, Iio K, Yamamoto K. Brachymesophalangea and clinodactyly of the fifth finger in Japanese children. Acta Paediatr Jpn. 1964;31:26–30.
27. Al-Qattan MM. Congenital sporadic clinodactyly of the index finger. Ann Plast Surg. 2007;59:682–7.
28. Hersh AH, DeMarinis F, Stecher RM. On the inheritance and development of clinodactyly. Am J Hum Genet. 1953;5:257–68.
29. Wood VE, Rubinstein JH. Surgical treatment of the thumb in the Rubinstein-Taybi syndrome. J Hand Surg Br. 1987;12:166–72.
30. Jain A, Rehman S, Smith G. Long-term results following osteotomy of the thumb delta phalanx in Rubinstein-Taybi syndrome. J Hand Surg Eur Vol. 2010;35(4):296–301.
31. Light TR, Ogden JA. The longitudinal epiphyseal bracket: implications for surgical correction. J Pediatr Orthop. 1981;1:299–305.
32. Ty JM, James MA. Failure of differentiation: part II (athrogryposis, camptodactyly, clinodactyly, Madelung deformity, trigger finger, and trigger thumb). Hand Clin. 2009;25:195–213.
33. Dao KD, Shin AY, Kelley S, Wood VE. Thumb radial angulation correction without phalangeal osteotomy in Apert's syndrome. J Hand Surg. 2002;27A:125–32.
34. Oishi SN, Ezaki M. Reconstruction of the thumb in Apert Syndrome. Tech Hand Surg. 2010;14:100–3.
35. Burke F, Flatt A. Clinodactyly. A review of a series of cases. Hand. 1979;11:269–80.
36. Cooney WP. Camptodactyly and clinodactyly. In: Carter P, editor. Reconstruction of the child hand. Philadelphia: Lea & Febiger; 1991.
37. Ali M, Jackson T, Rayan GM. Closing wedge osteotomy of abnormal middle phalanx for clinodactyly. J Hand Surg. 2009;34A:914–8.
38. Wood VE, Flatt AE. Congenital triangular bones in the hand. J Hand Surg. 1977;2:179–93.
39. Carstam N, Theander G. Surgical treatment of clinodactyly caused by longitudinally bracketed diaphysis ("delta phalanx"). Scand J Plast Reconstr Surg. 1975;9:199–202.
40. Tansley PDT, Pickford MA. The partial excision greenstick (PEG) osteotomy: a novel approach to the correction of clinodactyly in children's fingers. J Hand Surg Eur Vol. 2009;34(4):516–8.
41. Ravishanker R, Bath AS. Distraction: a minimally invasive technique for treating camptodactyly and clinodactyly. Med J Armed Forces India. 2004;60:227–30.
42. Bednar MS, Bindra RR, Light TR. Epiphyseal bar resection and fat interposition for clinodactyly. J Hand Surg. 2010;35A:834–7.
43. Caouette-Laberge L, Laberge C, Egerszegi EP, Stanciu C. Physiolysis for correction of clinodactyly in children. J Hand Surg. 2002;27A:659–65.
44. Vickers D. Clinodactyly of the little finger: a simple operative technique for reversal of the growth abnormality. J Hand Surg. 1987;12B:335–42.
45. Zhang G, Kato H, Yamazaki H. Physiolysis for correction of the delta phalanx in clinodactyly of the bilateral little fingers. Hand Surg. 2005;10:297–302.

Synostosis and Coalitions of the Hand and Wrist

17

Hilton Phillip Gottschalk and Terry R. Light

Carpal Coalition

Congenital carpal coalitions are uncommon. The incidence is variable; for example, the condition is more common in African Americans. Carpal coalitions can be either isolated or associated with a syndrome. Isolated carpal coalitions most frequently occur between the lunate and triquetrum; however, coalitions have been described between almost all adjacent carpal bones. When carpal coalitions are associated with a syndrome, multiple carpal bones can be involved. Most inter-carpal coalitions are asymptomatic. The condition is usually discovered as an incidental finding during radiographic evaluation following trauma. Patients with symptomatic carpal coalitions tend to have incomplete coalitions.

Embryology

Carpal coalitions are anatomic variations which are the result of failure of separation of the cartilaginous interzone of adjacent bones. Three distinct layers in the interzone have been described: a central loose layer, which gives rise to the synovium and intracapsular structures, and two denser zones, which form the articular cartilage of the two bones [1–3]. If the central layer does not develop appropriately or at all, then either a partial or complete coalition will result. For this reason, many authors prefer the term "incomplete coalition" when describing the lack of bony continuity across the carpal bones [3–5]. Thus, the term "fusion" should be avoided because the mechanism is a failure of segmentation of the cartilaginous precursors rather than the joining of two distinct structures [2].

The theory of failure of segmentation applies well to coalitions between adjacent bones in the same row, specifically the lunate and triquetrum. With respect to pisiform hamate coalitions, this theory is not well supported. O'Rahilly examined carpal anomalies in embryos, looking at articular interzones of future contiguous bone structures and observed that the pisiform and hamate are not united in cartilage during development [6, 7]. The coalition between the pisiform and hamate is hypothesized to occur as a consequence of ossification of the distal portion of the flexor carpi ulnaris or because the pisohamate ligament undergoes metaplasia, transforming into bone [6–11].

Incidence

Congenital coalitions occur in less than 1 % of the population [12]. The most frequent carpal coalition is between the lunate and triquetrum. The incidence varies by race, with a rate of 0.1 % in a Caucasian population compared to 1.6 % in African Americans and greater than 8 % in certain West African tribes [2, 8, 13, 14]. Lunatotriquetral coalitions are twice as common in females as in males. There appears to be a multifactorial inheritance pattern [13].

Classification

Carpal coalition was first described by Sandifort in 1779 with the first documented case report in 1908 by Corson [15]. Subsequent publications have been published describing many variations in carpal coalitions. In 1952 A. B. DeVilliers Minnaar [16] described 12 cases of congenital coalition of the lunate and triquetral bones in the South African Bantu and divided them into four types (Table 17.1). The four Minnaar subtypes of these coalitions are (1) incomplete fusion resembling a pseudarthrosis, (2) proximal osseous bridge with a distal notch of varying depth, (3) complete fusion of lunate and triquetrum alone, and (4) complete

H.P. Gottschalk, M.D. (✉)
Department of Pediatric Orthopaedics, Dell Children's Medical Center, 1301 Barbara Jordan Blvd., Ste 300, Austin, TX 78723, USA
e-mail: hpgottschalk@gmail.com

T.R. Light, M.D.
Department of Orthopaedic Surgery and Rehabilitation, Loyola University Stritch School of Medicine, 2160 South First Avenue, Maywood, IL 60153, USA
e-mail: tlight@lumc.edu

D.R. Laub Jr. (ed.), *Congenital Anomalies of the Upper Extremity: Etiology and Management*, DOI 10.1007/978-1-4899-7504-1_17, © Springer Science+Business Media New York 2015

fusion with other carpal anomalies [16]. Though this scheme has been used to describe other carpal coalitions, it has limitations. First, associated anomalies can be seen in Minnaar types I and II [17, 18]. Second, associated anomalies are not restricted to the hands alone and many may involve the feet or other parts of the skeleton as well. The Minnaar classification may be too narrow in scope [10, 17, 19]. Lastly, the Minnaar classification scheme does not adequately address the substantial variation in non-osseous coalitions. It has been observed that incomplete coalitions tend to be more symptomatic than their complete counterparts [2, 7, 10, 14, 20, 21]. In light of these limitations, Burnett [10] proposed a simplified classification scheme with two main types, non-osseous or osseous. He states that this "simplified terminology captures the two main variations in coalition appearance, which are likely to be associated with differences in clinical significance" [10].

Carpal coalitions can occur in isolation or associated with syndromes. Isolated coalitions have been described between all adjacent carpal bones [3, 7, 8, 13, 21–28]. More commonly, the non-syndromic coalitions involve only two bones (Fig. 17.1a, b), usually within the same carpal row, while syndrome-associated coalitions often include multiple bones (see Fig. 17.1c).

Table 17.1 Minnaar [16] classification of lunate triquetrum coalitions

Type I	Incomplete fusion resembling a pseudarthosis
Type II	Fusion with a notch of varying depth
Type III	Complete fusion of lunate and triquetrum alone
Type IV	Complete fusion associated with other carpal anomalies

Isolated Carpal Coalitions

The most common isolated carpal coalition is between the lunate and triquetrum [14, 29]. The majority of these coalitions are bilateral, asymptomatic, and incidental findings; most require no treatment. However, there is growing evidence that incomplete coalitions are more susceptible to injury and hence can become symptomatic [2, 5, 7, 14, 20]. Incomplete coalition is likely the result of a failure of separation during early fetal development, with the degree of cellular death dictating the type of coalition which will develop [5, 8, 13, 16]. Ritt et al. [14] believe that the incomplete coalitions are covered by a thin layer of articular cartilage that in time can wear down and lead to localized degenerative arthritis or be unusually susceptible to fracture. In patients who have symptomatic incomplete coalitions between the lunate and triquetrum, lunato-triquetrum (LT) fusion is recommended. LT fusion provides predictable improvement of symptoms, with little loss of motion [5, 12, 14, 20].

Less common is a coalition between the hamate and pisiform. The first case in the English literature was described by Cockshott as an isolated asymptomatic entity [9]. However, subsequent authors have reported ulnar side symptoms, including pain and/or parasthesias [7, 10, 11, 30, 31]. According to Burnett, ulnar neuropathy was more frequent in non-osseous hamate-pisiform coalitions compared to those displaying an osseous coalition [10, 31]. In addition, non-osseous coalitions may be more susceptible to degenerative arthritis given the abnormal joint mechanics and the thin cartilage surfaces between the affected carpals [10, 30]. The literature suggests that patients with an osseous hamate-pisiform

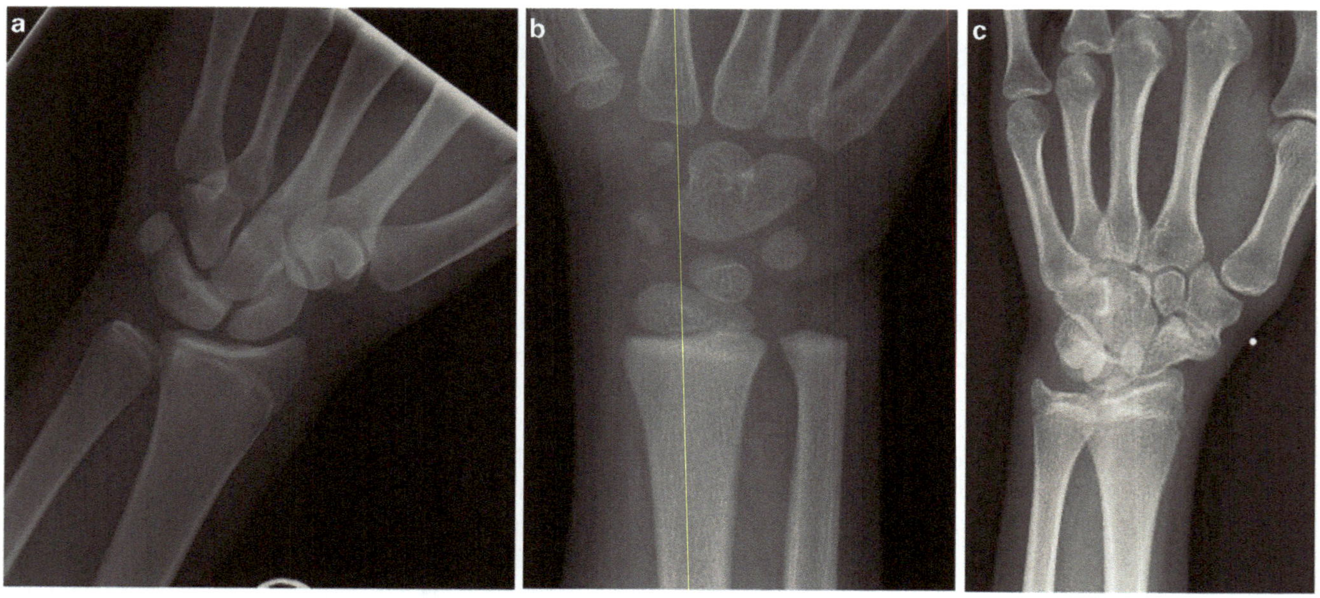

Fig. 17.1 (**a**) Incomplete coalition between lunate and triquetrum (Minnaar type II). (**b**) Incomplete coalition between capitate and hamate. (**c**) Multiple coalitions—capitate and hamate; scaphoid and trapezium

coalition are predisposed to fracture [7, 10, 30]. An acute symptomatic hamate-pisiform coalition should be initially treated by conservative therapy (typically immobilization). If immobilization does not resolve the pain, then treatment should consist of excision of the pisiform and accompanying coalition [7, 10, 11].

Syndromes Associated with Coalitions

Carpal coalitions are seen in patients with a variety of syndromes:

1. Arthrogryposis
2. Diastrophic dwarfism
3. Dyschondrosteosis
4. Ellis–Van Creveld syndrome
5. Hand-foot-genital syndrome
6. Fetal alcohol syndrome
7. Oto-palato-digital syndrome
8. Turner syndrome

Typically, the syndrome-associated coalitions involve multiple carpal bones, cross-carpal rows, and are often associated with other anomalies in the involved extremity as well as anomalies of other organ systems [5, 22, 29].

Ellis–van Creveld Syndrome

Also known as chondro-ectodermal dysplasia, Ellis–van Creveld syndrome is an autosomal recessive disorder with characteristics of disproportionate dwarfism, congenital heart disease, dysplastic nails and teeth, polydactyly, and other hand anomalies [22, 32–35]. The disorder has variable expression with genetic defects in the EVC1 and EVC2 genes, which are located on chromosome 4p16 [33, 35].

The incidence of Ellis–van Crevald Syndrome is estimated to be 1 in 60,000 live births, with boys and girls equally affected. The radiographic findings include delayed bone maturation and particularly involve the lateral tibial condyle, leading to genu valgum [35, 36]. Additional radiographic findings include shortened ribs, a trident acetabular roof, and premature ossification of the femoral heads. Although not specific for Ellis–van Creveld syndrome, findings on hand radiographs include coalition of the hamate and capitate, postaxial polydactyly, fusion of metacarpals, and clinodactyly of the small finger.

Treatment focuses on the congenital heart disease and respiratory changes secondary to the thoracic insufficiency. These children typically require early removal of neonatal teeth to help with feeding. The postaxial polydactyly is treated based on the physical findings [35]. No treatment is required for the carpal coalition.

Syndromes with Carpal and Tarsal Coalitions

The combination of carpal and tarsal coalitions can occur in several conditions, including: hand-foot-genital syndrome, symphalangism, and arthrogryposis.

Hand-Foot-Genital Syndrome

Hand-foot-genital syndrome (formerly hand-foot-uterus syndrome) was first described in 1970 in four generations of a single family [37]. Hand-foot-genital syndrome is an autosomal dominant disorder caused by a nonsense mutation in HOXA13 [38]. Both males and females can be affected. In females there may be duplication of the genital tract and other abnormalities involving the ureters and urethra. Males may present with hypospadias of variable severity [39, 40]. Abnormalities in the lower limb consist of small feet with short great toes and tarsal coalitions. The upper extremity includes shortened, somewhat stiff thumbs. Clinically the thumb is proximally placed with a hypoplastic thenar eminence; the index finger is ulnarly deviated, while the small finger often demonstrates clinodactyly and brachydactyly. Delayed ossification and coalition of the carpal bones, specifically the scaphoid and trapezium may be noted. Surgical intervention for the limb deformities is usually not necessary, but these patients do need urologic evaluation [40].

Symphalangism

Symphalangism is an uncommon condition characterized by fusion of the interphalangeal joints of the hands and feet [41, 42]. The term was first used by Harvey Cushing in 1916 to describe a family with ankylosis of the interphalangeal joints of the hand [43, 44]. Two types of symphalangism are recognized: proximal and distal. This refers to the proximal interphalangeal joint (most common) or the distal interphalangeal joint; either form is inherited in an autosomal dominant pattern [41, 42, 45]. Clinically, patients will have limited or no motion across the interphalangeal joint without flexion creases. Radiographs prior to skeletal maturity may suggest a joint space but as the cartilaginous bridge between phalanges ossifies as the skeleton matures, bony continuity across the joint will be apparent [42].

Flatt and Wood described three forms of symphalangism [45]:

1. True symphalangism without additional skeletal abnormalities
2. Symphalangism associated with symbrachydactyly
3. Symphalangism with syndactyly

The small finger is most commonly affected, followed by the ring, long, and index fingers [41, 45, 46].

Multiple additional skeletal abnormalities have been reported in association with symphalangism, including: brachydactyly, camptodactyly, clinodactyly, syndactyly, radiohumeral fusion, carpal coalitions, pes planus, bilateral hip dislocation, tarsal coalitions, cervical and thoracic spinal fusions [41, 42]. The most common carpal coalition occurring in association with symphalangism is triquetrum-hamate; capitate-hamate and capitate-trapezium, triquetrum-lunate, and scaphoid-trapezium coalitions have also been reported [22, 44, 47]. Despite the radiographic appearance, fusion of the phalanges in symphalangism rarely impairs hand function.

Arthrogryposis Multiplex Congenita

Arthrogryposis multiplex congenital encompasses several conditions of differing etiology and mixed clinical features. Common to each type are multiple congenital contractures in multiple body areas [48, 49]. The term "arthrogryposis" is more of a description of clinical findings than a specific diagnosis, with the overall prevalence being one in 3,000 live births [49, 50]. The etiology of arthrogrypotic syndromes is presumed to be multifactorial resulting in limitation of fetal movement. The resultant effect is loss of muscle mass with imbalance of muscle power across joints, which provokes a collagen response. This in turn leads to partial replacement of muscle volume and collagenous thickening of joint capsules and finally joint fixation [51].

Although tarsal coalitions can occur in arthrogryposis, carpal coalitions are more common [22]. The coalitions can be variable, with the proximal carpals involved first and then more extensive involvement between rows [22]. Newcombe et al. [52] reported that these carpal coalitions seen in arthrogryposis are likely acquired rather than congenital. They dissected specimens and found evidence of some remnants of joint space. Another theory is that the continued stretching and splinting in these patients causes fractures which lead to eventual coalitions.

The typical patient with arthrogryposis will have a flexed and ulnarly deviated wrist. Most of these patients will have a rigid flexion deformity and are resistant to nonoperative treatment. [53]. As these patients mature, the midcarpal joint can become obliterated from the multiple carpal coalitions. Coalition between the scaphoid and capitate is frequently observed. The presence of this coalition makes proximal row carpectomy impossible in these children [53]. Ezaki and Carter [53] describe a biplanar wedge resection of the carpus designed to extend the wrist and correct the ulnar deviation. Timing of surgery is recommended before the child reaches preschool age.

Isolated carpal coalitions are usually asymptomatic; however, when they form partial coalitions, they are more susceptible to injury. Partial coalitions, refractory to conservative treatment, can be either excised or fused (depending on their location) with good success. Syndrome-associated carpal coalitions tend to involve both carpal rows, though few require surgical intervention.

Metacarpal Synostosis

Metacarpal synostosis is an uncommon congenital hand malformation characterized by the coalescence of adjacent metacarpals [54]. It most often involves the ring and little finger metacarpals. The condition can be found in isolation or in association with other hand abnormalities, including: polydactyly, radial and ulnar deficiencies, cleft hand, and Apert syndrome [54–57]. Isolated metacarpal synostosis is most often sporadic, though cases have been described that suggest familial inheritance in either X-linked recessive [55, 58] or autosomal dominant patterns [59]. In patients with X-linked recessive inheritance, recent exome sequencing detected a nonsense mutation in exon 3 of FGF16, which is part of the Xq21.1 chromosome [58]. Jamsheer et al. [58] also concluded that FGF16 may play a role in fine tuning the human skeleton of the hand.

Physical Findings

The condition most commonly occurs between the ring and little finger metacarpals (Fig. 17.2). Typically the little finger is short, hypoplastic, with limited range of motion, and held in an abducted position. This awkward abducted position limits its digital dexterity and may disturb hand function, for example: getting the digit caught in pockets and other enclosed spaces [54, 55, 60]. In addition, some patients have noticed that small objects may fall through their hands, more commonly seen in middle-ring finger metacarpal synostosis [54].

Classification

Metacarpal synostosis may be partial or complete. Both forms represent a failure of differentiation. Two classification schemes have been described. Buck-Gramcko and Wood [55] identified three types of anatomic deformity based on the extent of the synostosis (Table 17.2) This type of classification is helpful in defining the extent of metacarpal involvement, but may not be as helpful in providing guidelines for treatment [54, 55].

Foucher et al. [56] described a system using letters of the alphabet (I, U, Y, k) and based the system on the shape of the synostosis, the degree of hypoplasia, direction of epiphyseal growth, and deformity of the finger distal to the synostosis.

Gottschalk et al. [54] attempted to quantify the extent of abduction deformity in patients with metacarpal synostosis. A posteroanterior radiograph should be taken with the patient's digits adducted as much as possible. For ring-small

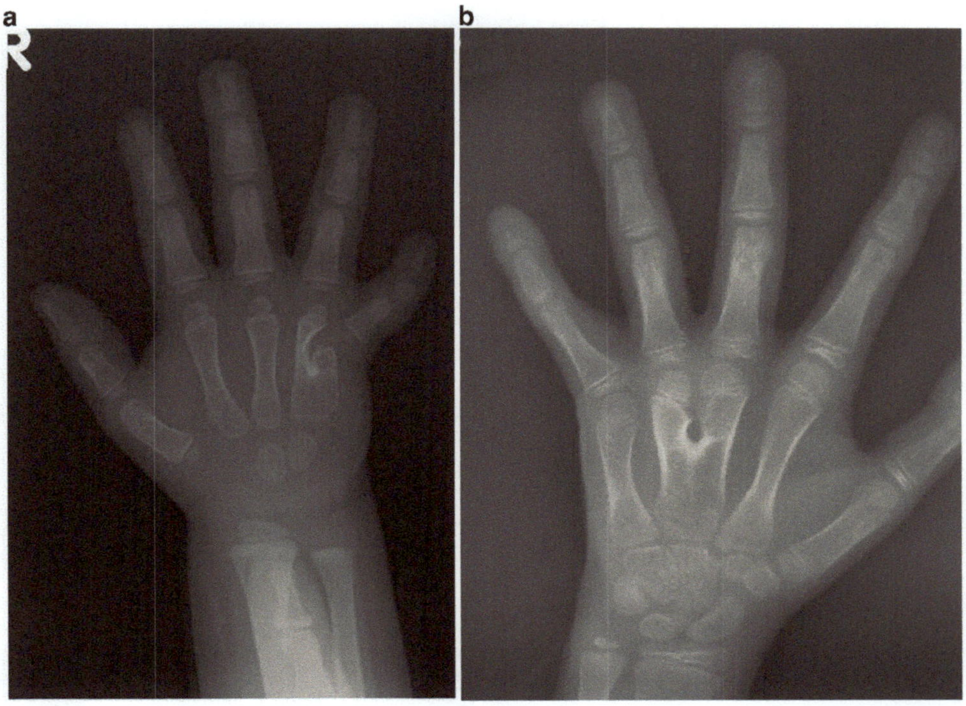

Fig. 17.2 (**a**) Radiograph of a ring-little metacarpal synostosis with abduction of the little finger. (**b**) Radiograph of a middle-ring metacarpal synostosis

Table 17.2 Buck-Gramcko and Wood [55] classification of metacarpal synostosis

Type I	Coalition only at the base of the metacarpal
Type II	Synostosis extends up to half the length of the metacarpal
Type III	Synostosis extends more than half the length of the metacarpal

finger metacarpal synostosis, the middle metacarpal is used as a reference point. The angle between the abducted small digit and the axis of the middle metacarpal is measured. In contrast, when the middle finger metacarpal is involved, the angle formed by the proximal phalanges is documented (Fig. 17.3). We recommend having the patient adduct the fingers as much as possible during the posteroanterior radiograph to give a uniform measurement of deformity.

Treatment

Not all metacarpal synostoses are the same, and treatment will vary. Most surgical techniques involve splitting the metacarpal synostosis and placing a spacer to hold the bones apart [54–57, 60, 61]. Our preferred spacer is a bone graft substitute, coralline hydroxyapatite (Interpore, Biomet, Parsippany, NJ), which mimics the porosity of cancellous bone. This limits donor site morbidity.

The technique is as follows: under tourniquet control, a longitudinal incision is made on the dorsum of the hand over the synostosis. The extensor tendons are retracted and a Keith needle is used to identify the midpoint of the coalition under fluoroscopy. The synostosis is split longitudinally and a lamina spreader is placed between the bones to assess the size of the spacer needed. As the lamina spreader is opened, the finger alignment begins to normalize. The graft is cut to size and placed at the osteotomy site. Care is taken to make sure that the graft is proximal to the growth plates (Fig. 17.4), to avoid creating a growth arrest. Transverse pins are placed through both metacarpals to secure the graft. We bury the pins under the skin, and a cast or splint is worn for at least 4 weeks. The pins remain buried until symptomatic.

Although the abduction deformity has been corrected, this specific procedure does not address the hypoplastic nature of the small finger. The decreased motion at the little finger metacarpophalangeal joint will persist [54, 55]. In addition, certain metacarpal synostoses are not amenable to this technique. Each case should be evaluated.

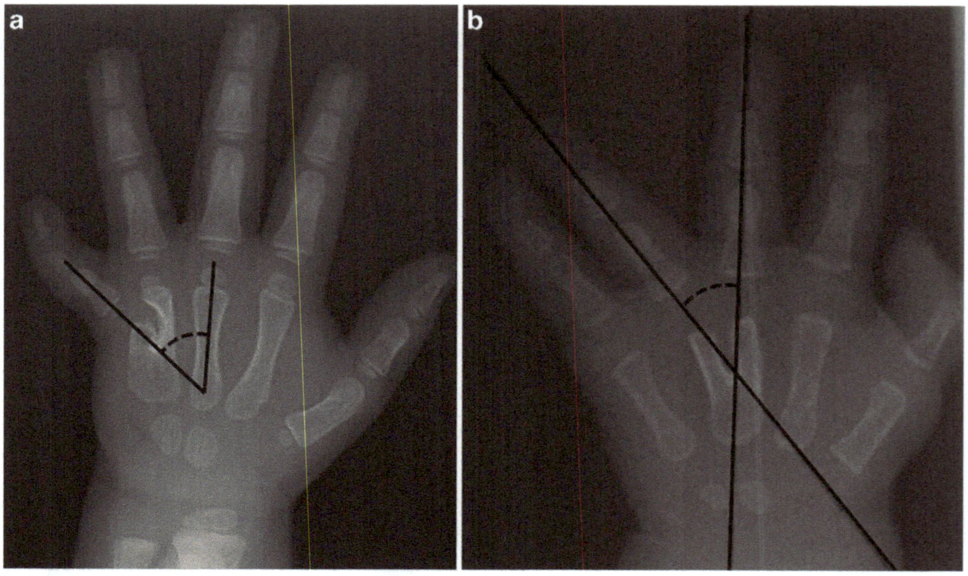

Fig. 17.3 (**a**) The angle between the abducted small digit and the axis of the middle metacarpal is measured in a ring-little metacarpal synostosis. (**b**) In a middle-ring metacarpal synostosis, the angle between the affected digits is calculated by using the longitudinal axes of both proximal phalanges

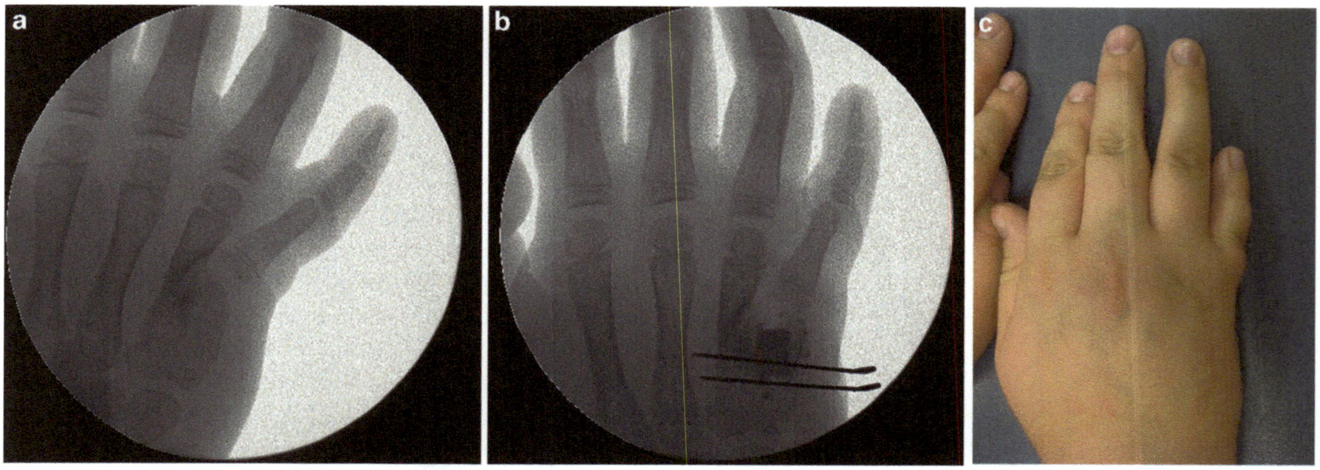

Fig. 17.4 (**a**) Fluoroscopic image of a ring-little metacarpal synostosis before correction. (**b**) Intra-operative image after placement of the bone graft substitute and pinning, with the graft well proximal to the growth plate of the ring metacarpal. (**c**) Clinical appearance 1 year after surgery. Note the improved adduction posture of the little finger; however, the finger remains hypoplastic

References

1. Sledge CB. Some morphologic and experimental aspects of limb development. Clin Orthop Relat Res. 1966;44:241–64.
2. Resnick CS, Grizzard JD, Simmons BP, Yaghmai I. Incomplete carpal coalition. AJR Am J Roentgenol. 1986;147:301–4.
3. Kennedy K, Waller CJ, Hartley RH. Congenital lunotriquetral and capitotrapezoid coalitions. J Hand Surg Eur Vol. 2010;35B:79–80.
4. Garn SM, Burdi AR, Babler WJ. Prenatal origins of carpal fusions. Am J Phys Anthropol. 1976;45:203–8.
5. Simmons BP, Mckenzie WD. Symptomatic carpal coalition. J Hand Surg Am. 1985;10A:190–3.
6. O'Rahilly R. A survey of carpal and tarsal anomalies. J Bone Joint Surg. 1953;35A:626–42.
7. Richterman IE, Kozin SH. Symptomatic pisiform hamate synchondrosis: a case report and review of the literature. J Hand Surg Am. 1996;21A:311–3.
8. Cockshott WP. Carpal fusions. Am J Roentgenol Radium Ther Nucl Med. 1963;89:1260–71.
9. Cockshott WP. Pisiform hamate fusion. J Bone Joint Surg. 1969;51A:778–80.
10. Burnett SE. Hamate-pisiform coalition: morphology, clinical significance, and a simplified classification scheme for carpal coalition. Clin Anat. 2011;24:188–96.
11. Kawamura K, Yajima H, Takakura Y. Pisiform and hamate coalition: case report and review of literature. Hand Surg. 2005;10:101–4.
12. Gross SC, Watson HK, Strickland JW, Palmer AK, Brenner LH. Triquetral-lunate arthritis secondary to synostosis. J Hand Surg Am. 1989;14A:95–102.
13. Garn SM, Frisancho AR, Poznanski AK, Schweitzer J, McCann MB. Analysis of tiquetral-lunate fusion. Am J Phys Anthropol. 1971;34:431–3.
14. Ritt MJ, Maas M, Bos KE. Minnaar type 1 symptomatic lunotriquetral coalition: a report of nine patients. J Hand Surg Am. 2001;26A:261–70.

15. Szaboky GT. Anomalous fusion between the lunate and triquetrum. J Bone Joint Surg. 1969;51A:1001–3.
16. DeVilliers Minnaar AB. Congenital fusion of the lunate and triquetral bones in the South African Bantu. J Bone Joint Surg. 1952;34B:45–8.
17. Hughes PC, Tanner JM. The development of carpal bone fusion as seen in serial radiographs. Br J Radiol. 1966;39:943–9.
18. Carlson DH. Coalition of the carpal bones. Skeletal Radiol. 1981;7:125–7.
19. Burnett SE, Case DT. Naviculo-cuneiform I coalition: evidence of significant differences in tarsal coalition frequency. Foot. 2005; 15:80–5.
20. Van Schoonhoven J, Prommersberger KJ, Schmitt R. Traumatic disruption of a fibrocartilage lunate-triquetral coalition—a case report and review of the literature. Hand Surg. 2001;6:103–8.
21. Peters S, Colaris JW. Carpal coalitions: symptomatic incomplete bony coalition of the capitate and trapezoid—case report. J Hand Surg Am. 2011;36A:1313–5.
22. Poznanski AK, Holt JF. The carpals in congenital malformation syndromes. Am J Roentgenol Radium Ther Nucl Med. 1971; 112:443–6.
23. Samir N, Al-Mahrezi A. Congenital fusion of the trapezium and trapezoid. Sultan Qaboos Univ Med J. 2010;10:405–6.
24. Wilson SM, Moreel P, Roulot E. Symptomatic congenital fusion of the scaphoid and the trapezium. J Hand Surg Am. 2006;31B:581.
25. Moreel P, Wilson SM, Descamps S, Roulot E. Bilateral congenital fusion of the scaphoid and the trapezium. A case report. Rev Chir Orthop Reparatrice Appar Mot. 2008;94:84–6.
26. Weinzweig J, Watson HK, Herbert TJ, Shaer JA. Congenital synchondrosis of the scaphotrapezio-trapezoidal joint. J Hand Surg Am. 1997;22A:74–7.
27. Ingram C, Hall RF, Gonzalez M. Congenital fusion of the scaphoid, trapezium, trapezoid and capitate. J Hand Surg Am. 1997;22B: 167–8.
28. Kahane S, Isaac SM, Wildin C. A new type of carpal coalition. J Hand Surg Eur Vol. 2012;37:581–2.
29. Delaney TJ, Eswar S. Carpal coalitions. J Hand Surg Am. 1992; 17A:28–31.
30. Ganos DL, Imbriglia JE. Symptomatic congenital coalition of the pisiform and hamate. J Hand Surg Am. 1991;16A:646–50.
31. Berkowitz AR, Melone CP, Belsky MR. Pisiform-hamate coalition with ulnar neuropathy. J Hand Surg Am. 1992;17A:657–62.
32. Ellis RW, Van Creveld S. Syndrome characterized by ectodermal dysplasia, polydactyly, chondro-dysplasia and congenital morbus cordis; report of three cases. Arch Dis Child. 1940;15:65–84.
33. Polymeropoulos MH, Ide SE, Wright M, Goodship J, Weissenbach J, Pyeritz RE, et al. The gene for the Ellis-van Creveld Syndrome is located on chromosome 4p16. Genomics. 1996;35:1–5.
34. Galdzicka M, Patnala S, Hirshman MG, Cai JF, Nitowsky H, Egeland JA, et al. A new gene, EVC2, is mutated in Ellis-van Creveld syndrome. Mol Genet Metab. 2002;77:291–5.
35. Muensterer OJ, Berdon W, McManus C, Oestreich A, Lachman RS, Cohen Jr MM, et al. Ellis-van Creveld syndrome: its history. Pediatr Radiol. 2013;43(8):1030–6. PMID: 23754541.
36. Caffey J. Chondroectodermal dysplasia (Ellis-Van Creveld disease); report on three cases. Am J Roentgenol. 1952;68:875–86.
37. Stern AM, Gall Jr JC, Perry BL, Stimson CW, Weitkamp LR, Poznanski AK. The hand-foot-uterus syndrome. A new hereditary disorder characterized by hand and foot dysplasia, dermatoglyphic abnormalities, and partial duplication of female genital tract. J Pediatr. 1970;77:109–16.
38. Goodman FR, Bacchelli C, Brady AF, Brueton LA, Fryns JP, Mortlock DP. Novel HOXA13 mutations and the phenotypic spectrum of hand-foot-genital syndrome. Am J Hum Genet. 2000;67:197–202.
39. Halal F. The Hand-Foot-Genital (Hand-Foot-Uterus) syndrome: family report and update. Am J Med Genet. 1988;30:793–803.
40. Innis JW. Hand-foot-genital syndrome. In: Pagon RA, Adam MP, Bird TD, editors. Gene reviews [internet]. Seattle: University of Washington; 1993–2013.
41. Letts M, Davidson D, Beaule P. Symphalangism in children: case report and review of the literature. Clin Orthop Relat Res. 1999;366:178–85.
42. Tuncay I, Akpinar F, Tosun N. Congenital true complete symphalangism of all proximal interphalangeal joints of hands with carpal anomalies: a case report. Hand Surg. 2001;6:223–6.
43. Cushing H. Hereditary anchylosis of the proximal phalangeal joints (Symphalangism). J Nerv Ment Dis. 1916;43:445.
44. Geelhoed GW, Neel JV, Davidson RT. Symphalangism and tarsal coalitions: a hereditary syndrome. J Bone Joint Surg. 1969;51B: 278–89.
45. Flatt AE, Wood VE. Rigid digits or symphalangism. Hand. 1975;7:197–213.
46. Dellon AL, Gaylor R. Bilateral symphalangism of the index finger. J Bone Joint Surg. 1976;58A:270–1.
47. Harle TS, Stevenson JR. Hereditary symphalangism associated with carpal and tarsal fusions. Radiology. 1967;89:91–4.
48. Kalampokas E, Kalampokas T, Sofoudis C, Deligeoroglou E, Botsis D. Diagnosing arthrogryposis multiplex congenital: a review. ISRN Obstet Gynecol. 2012;2012:264918.
49. Bamshad M, Van Heest AE, Pleasure D. Arthrogryposis: a review and update. J Bone Joint Surg. 2009;91 Suppl 4:40–6.
50. Bevan WP, Hall JG, Bamshad M, Staheli LT, Jaffe KM, Song K. Arthrogryposis multiplex congenital (Amyoplasia) an orthopaedic perspective. J Pediatr Orthop. 2007;27:594–600.
51. Swinyard CA, Bleck EE. The etiology of arthrogryposis (multiple congenital contracture). Clin Orthop Relat Res. 1985;194:15–29.
52. Newcombe DS, Abbott JL, Munsie WJ, Keats TE. Arthrogryposis multiplex congenital and spontaneous carpal fusion. Arthritis Rheum. 1969;12:345–54.
53. Ezaki MB, Carter PR. Carpal wedge osteotomy for the arthrogrypotic wrist. Tech Hand Up Extrem Surg. 2004;8:224–8.
54. Gottschalk HP, Bednar MS, Moor M, Light TR. Metacarpal synostosis: treatment with a longitudinal osteotomy and bone graft substitute interposition. J Hand Surg Am. 2012;37A:2074–81.
55. Buck-Gramcko D, Wood VE. The treatment of metacarpal synostosis. J Hand Surg Am. 1993;18A:565–81.
56. Foucher G, Navaro R, Medina J, Khouri RK. Metacarpal synostosis: a simple classification and a new treatment technique. Plast Reconstr Surg. 2001;108:1225–31.
57. Miura T. Congenital synostosis between the fourth and the fifth metacarpal bones. J Hand Surg Am. 1988;13A:83–8.
58. Jamsheer A, Zemojtel T, Kolanczyk M, Stricker S, Hecht J, Krawitz P, et al. Whole exome sequencing identifies FGF16 nonsense mutations as the cause of X-linked recessive metacarpal 4/5 fusion. J Med Genet. 2013;50(9):579–84. doi:10.1136/jmedgenet-2013-101659.
59. Temtamy D, McKusick V. The genetics of hand malformations (Chapter 8). In: Birth defects, Original article series. Vol. 14, No. 3. New York: Alan R. Liss; 1978.
60. Horii E, Miura T, Nakamura R, Nakao E, Kato H. Surgical treatment of congenital metacarpal synostosis of the ring and little fingers. J Hand Surg Am. 1998;23B:691–4.
61. Iwasawa M, Hayashi R, Matsuo K, Hirose T. The use of costal cartilage as a spacer in the treatment of congenital metacarpal fusion. Eur J Plast Surg. 1988;11:138–40.

18 Congenital Clasped Thumb

Hisham Abdel-Ghani and Mostafa Mahmoud

Definition

A persistent flexion of the thumb with lack of active extension after the age of 3 months of life has been variously termed congenital clasped thumb [1], pollex varus [2], infant's persistent thumb-clutched hand [3], thumb in palm deformity [4], and flexion adduction deformity of the thumb [5] (Fig. 18.1). This definition applies to simple form or isolated forms of clasped thumbs but complex cases with evident contractures, syndromes, or windblown deformity could be diagnosed at birth. It should be differentiated from the developmental spastic adduction deformity of the thumb associated with brain insults, including cerebral palsy, that is usually not congenital in nature.

Clinical Picture

Congenital clasped thumb has heterogeneous presentations. The main finding is lack of active extension of the metacarpophalangeal (MCP) joint of the thumb. Anderson and Breed suggested that the Moro reflex might be a useful way to detect congenital clasped thumb early. The thumb normally extends during the Moro reflex [6].

Lack of active extension may involve also the interphalangeal (IP) joint of the thumb (Fig. 18.2). There may be callosities on the dorsum of the IP joint secondary to grasping objects against that side of the thumb (see Fig. 18.2). The carpometacarpal (CMC) articulation may be mobile and show active extension or may be stiff, especially in cases of severe deformity or generalized disorders. Full passive range of movement of the thumb indicates absence of soft tissue contractures. Passive limitation of extension of the thumb with full wrist extension may reveal hidden shortening of the flexor pollicis longus (FPL) muscle. Limitation of passive extension of the thumb with the wrist in neutral position indicates the presence of palmar soft tissue contractures that may be associated with skin webbing at the level of MCP joint (see Fig. 18.1b). The first web space may show variable degrees of narrowing and skin deficiency (Fig. 18.3). The MCP joint may show variable degrees of instability that may become evident only after release of flexion contracture. In severe cases, the thumb may appear very short, stumpy, adducted, flexed, and externally rotated (see Fig. 18.3). The thenar muscles may show some degree of mild hypoplasia. Severe thenar muscle hypoplasia or aplasia points to the diagnosis of congenital hypoplastic thumb type III [7] with predominant deficiency of extrinsic extensor tendons rather than clasped thumb. Meticulous examination and analysis of deformities are mandatory to plan treatment accordingly.

Associated deformities of the hands with clasped thumb include abnormal skin creases (see Fig. 18.2), stiffness of the fingers with incomplete flexion (see Fig. 18.2), wrist extension deformity (see Fig. 18.3), camptodactyly (Fig. 18.4), radial deviation of index finger (Fig. 18.5), lack of extension of the index finger (Fig. 18.6), and ulnar drift hand (Fig. 18.7).

Ulnar drift hand is characterized by ulnar deviation of the fingers at the level of the MCP joints with or without flexion contracture of the MCP joints. Although ulnar deviation of the fingers is the most common feature of ulnar drift hand, webbing of the thumb to the palm is the most limiting disability [8].

Clasped thumb could be diagnosed in radial club hand in the presence of well-developed thenar muscles and flexed thumb (Fig. 18.8) [9].

Some cases show lack of extension or severe hypoplasia of index finger or index and middle fingers and the only active functioning fingers are the ring and little ones (see Fig. 18.6). After correction of thumb deformity, the patients continue to grasp with the thumb against the ulnar most fingers.

H. Abdel-Ghani, M.D. (✉) • M. Mahmoud, M.D.
Department of Orthopedics, Kasr Al Ainy University Hospital, Cairo University, Al-Saray Street, El Manial, Cairo, 11956, Egypt
e-mail: hishamghani@kasralainy.edu.eg; hishamortho@gmail.com; mostafa.mahmoud@kasralainy.edu.eg; dr.mostmah@gmail.com

D.R. Laub Jr. (ed.), *Congenital Anomalies of the Upper Extremity: Etiology and Management*, DOI 10.1007/978-1-4899-7504-1_18, © Springer Science+Business Media New York 2015

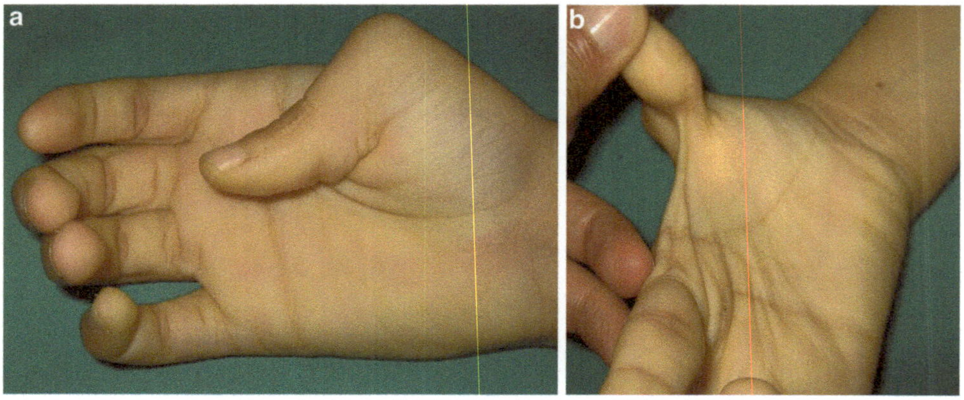

Fig. 18.1 (**a**) Congenital clasped thumb with lack of extension of MCP joint only and active extension of the IP joint. (**b**) Palmar contracture of the thumb

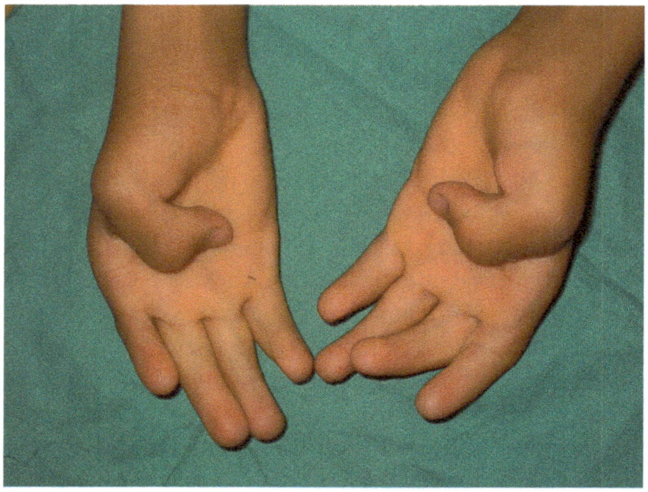

Fig. 18.2 Congenital clasped thumb with flexed IP joint indicating combined deficiency of both EPL and EPB. Callosities are evident on the dorsum of IP joint

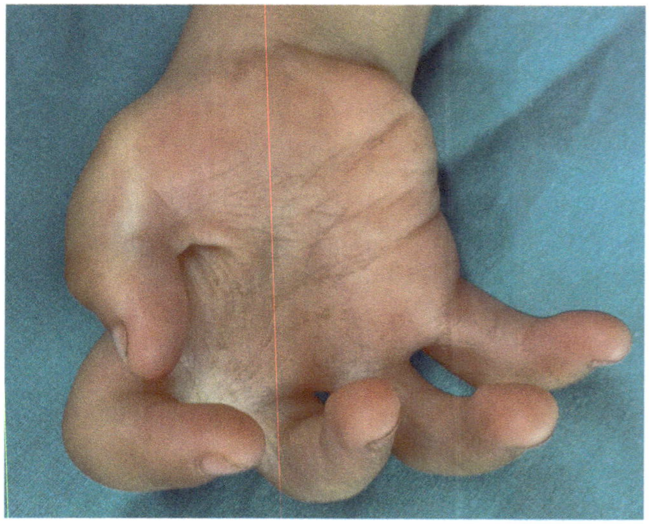

Fig. 18.4 Clasped thumb with camptodactyly of the four fingers

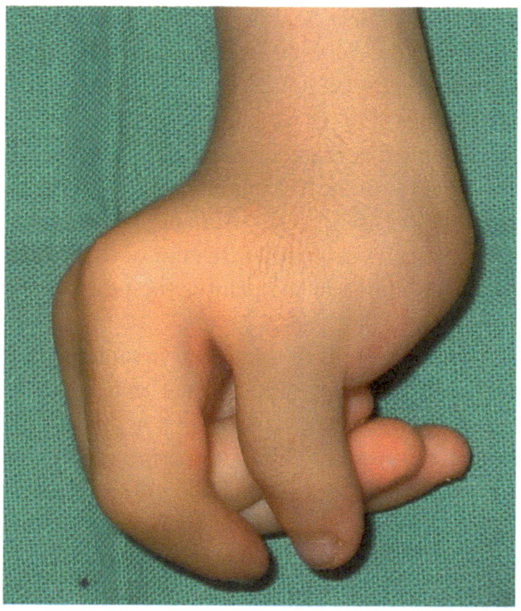

Fig. 18.3 Clasped thumb with severe narrowing of the web space and extension contracture of the wrist

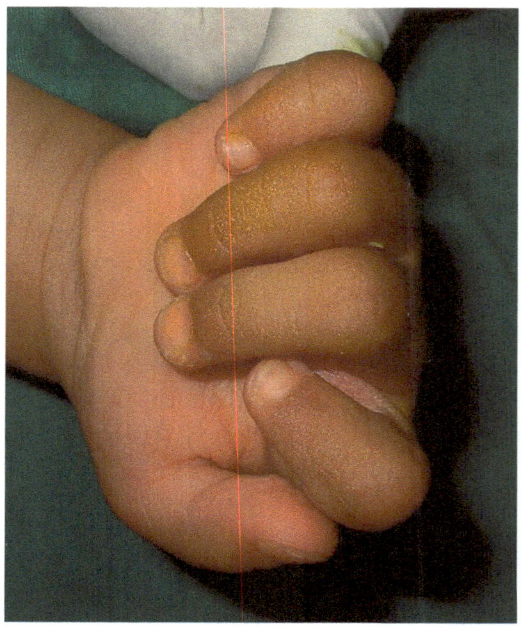

Fig. 18.5 Radial deviation of the index finger at the level of the MCP joint in association with clasped thumb

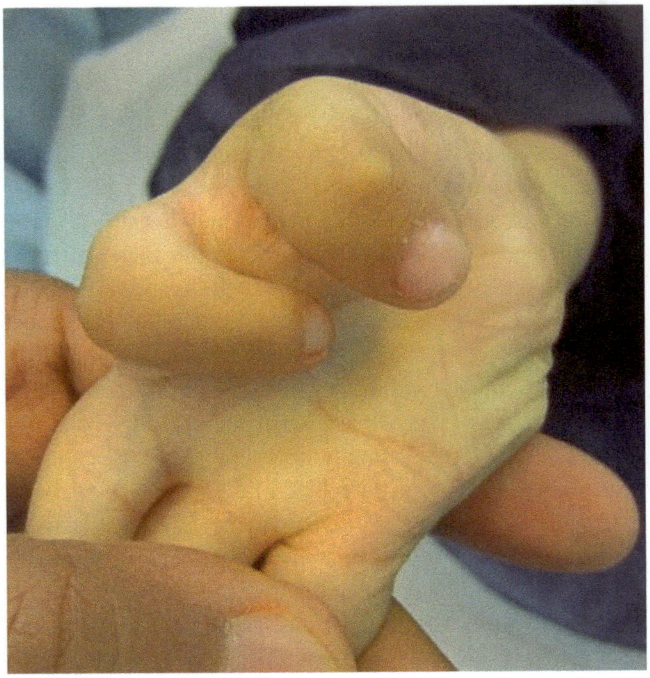

Fig. 18.6 Clasped thumb associated with deficient extensors of the index finger

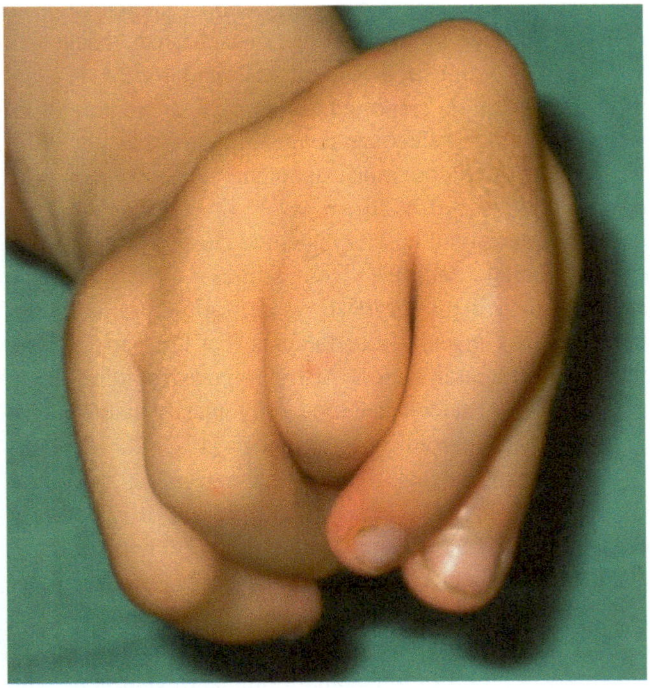

Fig. 18.7 Ulnar drift hand

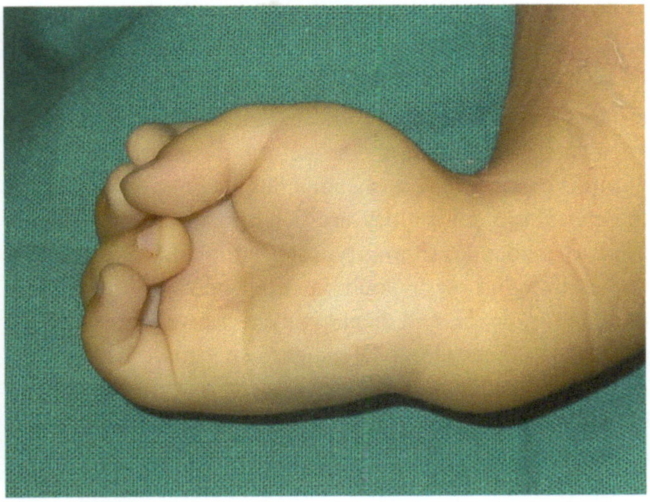

Fig. 18.8 Radial dysplasia with congenital clasped thumb evident by the presence of well-developed thenar muscles and flexed thumb

Congenital clasped thumb commonly manifests as part of generalized disorder especially multiple joint contractures syndromes collectively called arthrogryposis, which is a purely descriptive term [2, 9–12]. Arthrogryposis is defined as the presence of two or more joint contractures in multiple body areas [2]. Wood considered ulnar drift hand representing a conglomerate of syndromes and different anatomical causes. Probably all of these cases represent a forme fruste of arthrogryposis [8].

Arthrogryposis with CNS involvement includes chromosomal abnormalities and other syndromes [13].

Congenital clasped thumb should be differentiated from trigger thumb, where a palpable nodule of the flexor pollicis tendon is present at the level of the MCP joint. When locked, the IP joint is flexed with extension of the MCP joint and a palpable clunk is felt on unlocking the trigger thumb and extending the IP joint.

Pathoanatomy and Classification

Many authors have suggested that flexor extensor imbalance is central to the development of clasped thumb. The long extensor tendons are not totally absent, but vestigial strands or hypoplastic extensor tendons are always present [9, 10, 14–16]. Flatt [16] found that in the course of tendon transfer, the vestigial tendon narrows proximally and eventually ends in fibro fatty tissues rather than muscular tissue. Crawford et al. [15] found that on releasing the flexion contractures, all tissues were involved, including skin, subcutaneous fascia, and periarticular structures. They also found an increase in fibrous tissue present in the form of numerous subcutaneous strands in the digits, palm, and forearm, making dissection, mobilization, and transfer of the tendons more difficult than anticipated [15, 17].

Weckesser et al. [11] classified congenital clasped thumbs into four groups. Group I consisted of isolated clasped thumb. The extensor pollicis brevis (EPB) or extensor pollicis longus (EPL) muscles and tendons are either weak or attenuated. In addition to the deformities seen in group I, group II patients have associated flexion contractures of the fingers. These deformities are believed to be the result of mild to moderate arthrogrtyposis. Group III deformity is related to radial ray hypoplasia with findings of hypoplasia of extensor, flexor, and thenar muscles as well as associated osseous elements. Group IV patients are a miscellaneous category that include polydactyly. The authors believe that this classification includes cases that should not be considered as clasped thumbs.

McCarroll [10] classified congenital clasped thumbs into supple and complex types. The former is characterized by lack of active thumb extension with ability to fully reverse the deformity passively. The latter group may demonstrate soft tissue contractures, lax ligaments, and tight skin in addition to the lack of active thumb extension.

Tsuyuguchi et al. [12] designed a classification consisting of three groups: Group I: The supple clasped thumb, where the thumb is passively abductable and extendable against the resistance of thumb flexors, without other digital anomalies. Group II: The clasped thumb with hand contractures, where the thumb is not passively extendable and abductable, with or without other digital anomalies. Group III: The clasped thumb, which is associated with arthrogryposis or windblown hand.

The authors have not found any anatomical differences or different outcome between Tsuyguchi's types II and III, so we prefer using the McCarroll subtypes [9].

In complex cases, abnormal articular surface of the first MCP joint was described with hypoplasia of the volar aspect of the first metacarpal head. The dorsal capsule of the MCP joint may be adherent to the cartilage of the metacarpal head and sharp dissection was needed to separate it [9, 15]. The flexion contracture of the MCP joint is secondary to skin deficiency, abnormal subcutaneous fibrous tissue, and contracted periarticular structures including volar plate, collateral ligaments, and capsule [9, 10]. Shortening of the FPL may add to the flexion contracture. Narrowing of the web space is secondary to contracture of one or more of the following structures: palmar fascia, adductor pollicis, and first dorsal interosseous muscles [9]. The pathology of complex clasped thumb could be summarized as hypoplastic or attenuated thumb extensors, flexion contracture of MCP joint, ulnar collateral laxity or global instability of the MCP joint, adduction contracture of the CMC joint, and contracture of the first web space. We noted that the severity of these pathological findings is variable, and dependent on the age of the patient at the time of surgery [9, 16].

Prevalence and Etiology

Congenital clasped thumb occurs twice as often in males as in females and it is bilateral in more than 80 % [9, 11, 16, 18]. Positive family history of 32–36 % was reported [9, 11]. Positive consanguinity was reported as high as 60 % [9]. The high incidence of bilateral deformity implies that a defect is present in the zygote before the first cell division. In supple deformity, the very limited and specific nature of the defect also suggests that the cause is a genetic defect rather than some environmental influence on the zygote which would be much more likely to produce widespread defects. The familial occurrence of this anomaly in a number of cases adds to the evidence for genetic defect [9, 11].

The high incidence of defect in the EPB may have a phylogenetic basis in that this phylogenetically new muscle is found only in the gorilla and in man [11].

Most of the cases of congenital clasped thumbs are part of generalized disorders. Abdel-Ghani et al. [9] reported associated congenital malformation in 77.5 % of cases, incidence of 15 % of associated malformations of the hand [9, 19], and 68 % incidence of associated syndromes [9]. The most common associated anomalies are manifestations of congenital contractures: congenital hip dislocation, congenital knee dislocation, knee stiffness, congenital clubfeet, congenital vertical talus, scoliosis, elbow stiffness, and limited shoulder movement. Rarely reported associated anomalies were ventricular septal defect and congenital blindness [9]. There were no reported abdominal anomalies in association with clasped thumbs [9, 19, 20].

In the majority of cases, congenital clasped thumb is part of congenital multiple contractures loosely termed arthrogryposis. Arthrogryposis, as defined before, describes the multiple congenital contractures that are part of more than 200 different disorders. Arthrogryposis could be classified into three major categories: amyoplasia, distal arthrogryposis, and syndromic arthrogryposis [13].

Amyoplasia is also called arthrogryposis multiplex congenital (AMC) or classic arthrogryposis. It is the most common form, seen in approximately 1/3,000 live births [9], and has sporadic incidence with no genetic or hereditary predisposition [20].

The second group is distal arthrogryposis syndromes, which are a group of autosomal dominant syndromes with congenital contractures primarily involving the hands and feet, which often are associated with abnormal facies without primary neurological and/or muscle disease affecting limb function [13]. Many affected individuals present in an orthopedic setting. There are at least 10 different types of distal arthrogryposis that include a large number of syndromes [13, 21]. The most common distal arthrogryposis syndromes that are linked to clasped thumbs are Freeman–Sheldon syndrome, multiple pterygia syndrome, digitotalar dysmorphism, clasped thumb clubfoot syndrome, and congenital contractural arachnodactyly [21]. In amyoplasia and distal arthrogryposis, neurological examination is normal.

The third group of congenital multiple contractures include a great number of genetic syndromes and chromosomal anomalies. This group is characterized by abnormal neurological examination secondary to central nervous system or peripheral neuromuscular disorders. This group is a common cause of arthrogryposis and responsible for the most severe forms. Central nervous system disorders can be suspected on clinical examination if hyperreflexia, unilateral arthrogryposis, or cognitive deficits are present and can be anatomically localized by magnetic resonance imaging of the brain or spinal cord [13]. This group includes a great number of genetic syndromes and chromosomal anomalies. Examples from this group are COFS (cerebro-oculo-facio-skeletal) syndrome, congenital muscular dystrophy, Miller–Dieker (lissencephaly), lethal multiple pterygium syndrome, Pena-Shokeir phenotype, Potter syndrome, Zellweger syndrome, trisomy 8/mosaicism, trisomy 18, and many others. This group includes lethal syndromes and syndromes with severe disabilities due to central nervous system malfunction.

Mental retardation/CNS involvement is found in approximately 25 % of individuals with arthrogryposis [13, 22].

The features of these syndromes are described to allow diagnosis, establish prognosis, provide family counseling, and treatment. Increased recognition will lead to improved knowledge of the natural history [21].

Arthrogryposis appears to occur secondary to fetal akinesia (lack of movement), which is the common endpoint of several different in utero processes. The causes of arthrogryposis include conditions that are intrinsic to the fetus, such as neuromuscular disorders, skeletal dysplasias or aneuploidy, as well as those resulting from influences extrinsic to the fetus [23].

While the pathoanatomy and pathophysiology vary and continue to be investigated, it appears that the joints initially have full developmental potential but fail to form mobile articulations secondary to the absence of movement in utero. This theory has been supported by a number of chick embryo studies, in which paralytic agent were administrated during development, resulting in abnormal joint morphology and stiffness [24]. The lack of joint motion results in articular cartilage abnormalities, failure of joint cavitation, and secondary fusions.

Amyoplasia has an increased prevalence in twins and in extrinsic conditions that would lead to decreased limb movement, such as a bicornuate uterus, oligohydramnios, or intrauterine crowding [25]. Also it may be secondary to major vascular insult to the fetus [22].

Most of the cases of distal arthrogryposis are due to mutations in genes responsible for myofiber function, including TNNI2, TNNT3, TPM2, MYH3, AND MYH8 [26–31].

Treatment

Supple Clasped Thumb

Most of these cases respond to non-operative treatment. In young infants, especially those with shortening of FPL muscle, they respond well to manipulation by the mother. Manipulation entails bringing the thumb out of the palm and holding it in an extended position. Stretching exercises should be done while the wrist is in extension to effectively stretch the short FPL muscle. Mothers are instructed to do exercises with every feeding and diaper change.

Splinting is used if there is no active thumb extension after trial of manipulation. We find difficulty in applying splints in very young infants or small hands. Different forms of splints were used. We use a rigid splint that keeps the wrist in full extension and the thumb in full abduction and extension of the MCP joint. There is no solid protocol for splinting; almost similar protocols were followed by Weckesser et al. [1], McCarroll [10], Lipskeir and Weizenbluth [32], and Abdel-Ghani et al. [9]. Currently, we start exercises at the time of presentation if splinting cannot be started. Once we can use splints, full-time splinting is adopted until observing active thumb extension. This is followed by daily exercises and night splinting for further 6 months. Flatt [16] mentioned that if there is no improvement of the posture of the thumb or absolute lack of any active extension after 3 months of splinting, then it is reasonable to assume that the EPB is non-functional. He assumed that there is no harm in continuing splinting for further 3 months, but it is unlikely to have active thumb extension after this extra time of splinting [16].

Lin et al. [18] reported successful treatment of supple form with splinting in patients below 1 year of age. Tsuyuguchi et al. [12] and Abdel-Ghani et al. [9] reported excellent results of splinting in all patients with supple clasped thumbs in all their patients with an average time of splinting more than 3 months. In our practice, most of the patients presented early, before age of 6 months, with shortening of FPL respond well and restore full active thumb extension with proper stretching exercises.

The long-term results of treatment with corrective splinting have been shown to be good if the response to primary treatment was good. No adverse effects on growth of the hand have been noted [16].

Splinting was not as successful in treating those with volar side contracture, but it was superior to employing passive range of motion alone in these cases [9, 12].

Kozin mentioned that the goal of splinting is to prevent additional attenuation of the hypoplastic extensor mechanism and allow hypertrophy over time [33].

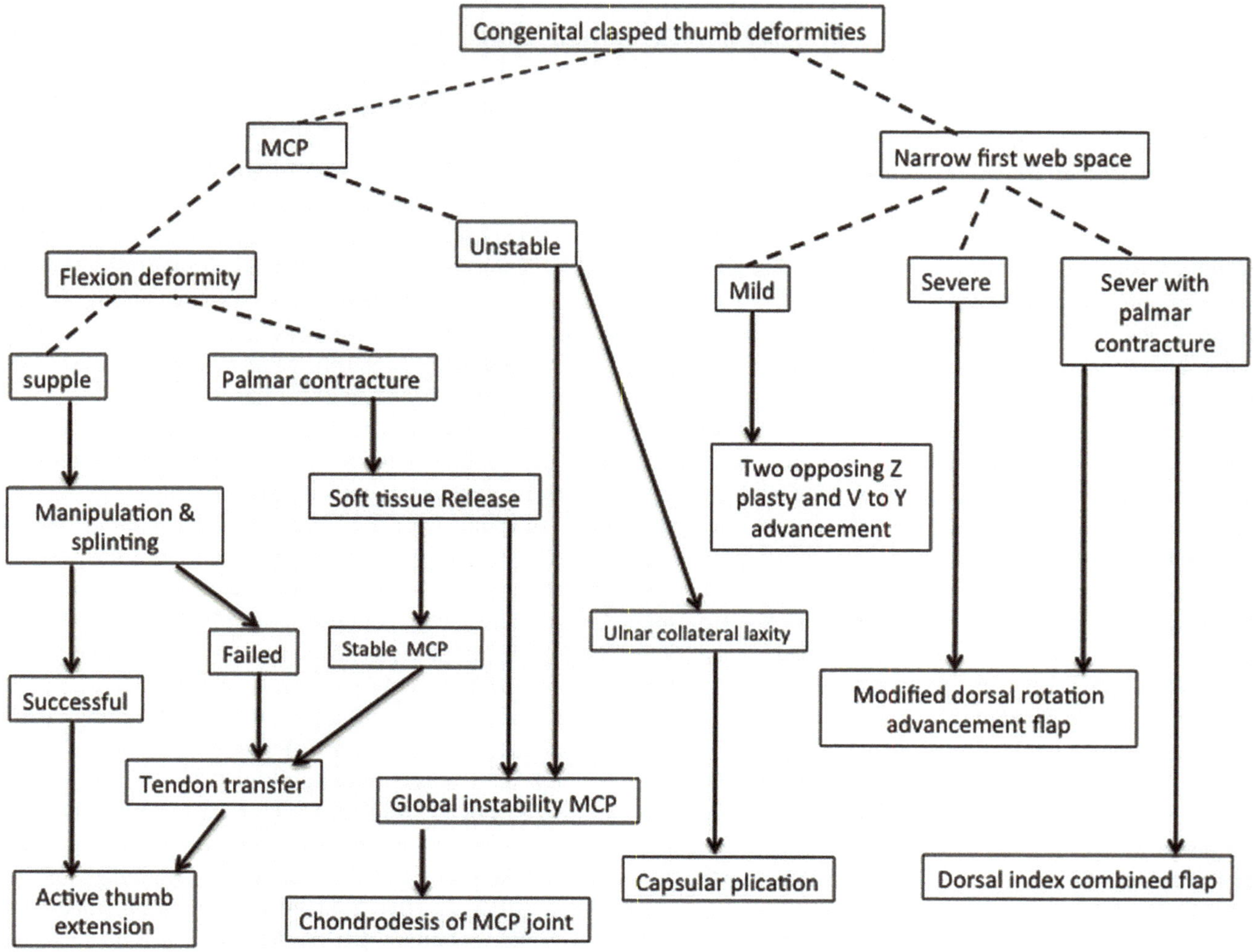

Fig. 18.9 Algorithm for management of congenital clasped thumb

We think that keeping the thumb in a splint allows growth of the child while the attenuated extensor tendons are kept unstretched. This allows differential growth of the bones and the extensor tendons, allowing stretching of the long thumb flexors and shortening of extensor tendons. This is why splinting is effective in young infants with rapid rate of growth and less effective in older children with slower rate of growth.

Complex Clasped Thumb

Early manipulation could be tried in all patients during the first few months of life. This may improve the deformity and contractures but will usually fail to correct it completely. A trial of night splinting may be used in selected cases but in severe deformities and marked laxity of the MCP joint, splints are not able to be applied, nor effective. Most of these cases will require surgical intervention.

Surgical Treatment

Surgery for clasped thumbs is a la carte; surgery is tailored according to the present deformities (Fig. 18.9). Reconstruction of clasped thumbs entails different combination of surgical procedures:

1. Restoration of active thumb extension
2. Release of thumb web space and palmar thumb contracture
   (a) Release of contracted tissues
   (b) Widening of the skin of web space and skin augmentation of the volar aspect of the thumb
3. Stabilization of MCP joint
4. Lengthening of FPL

Timing of surgery is variable; Senrui recommended surgery between the ages of 3 and 5 years [34]. In our experience, surgery is feasible after the age of 1.5 years without maximum limits. All surgeries are done under tourniquet control, and magnifying loupes are mandatory.

Restoration of Active Thumb Extension

Tendon transfer to restore active thumb extension is indicated in the presence of mobile and stable MCP joint. This is done in cases of supple deformities failing to respond to non-operative treatment or in complex cases after ligament reconstruction of the MCP joint and widening the web space. The most commonly used transfers are extensor indicis (EI) [5] or the ring finger flexor digitorum superficialis (FDS) [34]. The extensor digitorum communis (EDC) tendon to the index can also be used as a transfer, but only after demonstrating an effective EI [16]. Less commonly, the extensor carpi radialis longus transfer may be used [35]. In cases of absent EPL, the EI is usually absent [16]. Transfer is done to attenuated EPB or EPL tendons. Using either EI or ring finger FDS provides enough length for transfer, but if using any of the wrist extensors, tendon graft is mandatory.

Technique of EI Transfer [33]

Make a short transverse incision at the head of the index metacarpal and locate the EI tendon deeper and ulnar to the EDC tendon to index finger. Divide the tendon at its confluence with the extensor hood. Next make a short transverse incision over the dorsum of the wrist in line with the EI tendon and withdraw the tendon into this wound. Make a bayonet-shaped incision over the dorsoulnar aspect of the thumb centered over the MCP joint. Identify the attenuated thumb extensor tendons. Reroute the tendon of the EI. We do not use an osseous tunnel in the proximal phalanx for the EI tendon as originally described [33], and instead we suture it to the attenuated extensor tendons [16, 36].

Technique of FDS of the Ring Finger Transfer [34]

The tendon is divided proximal to the vincula longa through an oblique incision over the palmar aspect of the proximal interphalangeal joint and drawn into the forearm. It is drawn back under the abductor pollicis longus tendon into another small incision, which has been made at the radial side of the wrist and then attached to the vestigial tendons of the EPB or EPL.

We retrieve the tendon by a transverse incision at the level of A1 pulley; this provides enough length for the transfer without the need to go distal at the level of the proximal phalanx.

In the patients with arthrogryposis, this transfer may not be possible because of the lack of demonstrable FDS or flexor digitorum profundus function. Once it has been determined that a profundus tendon is present, the superficialis tendon may be harvested.

Release of Thumb Web Space and Palmar Thumb Contracture

Release of thumb web space and palmar thumb contracture entails release of contracted tissues and skin reconstruction and augmentation of the web and palmar aspect of the thumb.

Release of Contracted Tissues

Release of contracted tissues entails release of contractures of deeper tissues of the thumb web space and the palmar aspect of the thumb. This is usually done through the skin incisions used to reconstruct the skin of the web space and skin deficiency of the palmar aspect of the thumb.

Release of Thumb Web Space

Dissection is deepened through the skin incisions designed to widen the web to the underlying fascia over the intrinsic muscles, protecting the distal branches of the superficial radial nerve, the flexor tendon and neurovascular bundles to the index finger. The tight structures to be released are identified; the fascia of the first web space is the most common structure to require release. The origin of adductor pollicis muscle is the second most common structure to need release from the third metacarpus [9]. If necessary, the first dorsal interosseus muscle is elevated from the first metacarpus. The thumb is then manipulated into extension and abduction. If necessary, the CMC joint capsule is released. After achieving full release, the first metacarpus is maintained in full abduction with two crossed k-wires across the first web space [9].

Ezaki and Oishi prefer to release the thenar muscles from their origins at the base of the palm even through a separate incision. Also, they release both heads of the adductor pollicis through this palmar incision. If necessary, they leave the palmar incision to heal by secondary intention [37]. We did not find this release necessary, as we manipulate the thumb and stabilize it in full abduction and not just full extension, which does not necessitate this form of release of the thenar muscles.

Release of Palmar Contracture of the Thumb

Treatment of the MCP joint flexion contracture requires release of all thick subcutaneous fascial adhesions with preservation of the digital bundles. The flexor tendon sheath also may contribute to flexion contracture and may require release to allow full extension of the thumb. Extensive release of the volar plate or of the MCP joint capsule to achieve full extension may destabilize the joint and make it unsuitable for transfer. Sharp dissection is required to release the adherent capsule to the head of the metacarpus. After full release, the joint is manipulated to full extension. Transarticular pinning using one or two crossing Kirschner wires is used to hold the joint in full extension [9, 38].

Skin Reconstruction and Augmentation of the Web and Palmar Aspect of the Thumb

Different techniques of skin reconstruction of the web space are used according to the degrees of narrowing of the web. Random based skin flaps are the most common techniques used. The aim of skin reconstruction is to provide wide skin

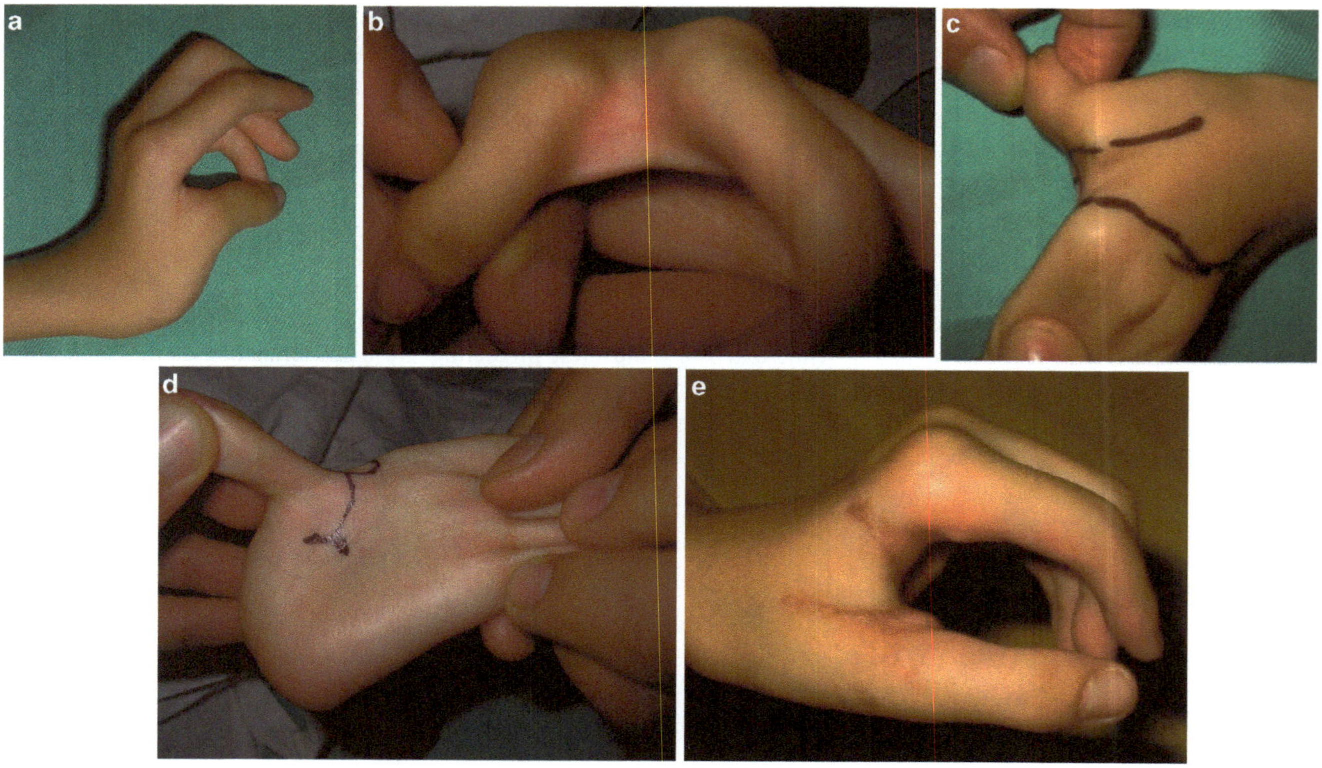

Fig. 18.10 (**a**) Clasped thumb. (**b**) Severe narrowing of the web space and marked instability of the MCP joint. (**c**) Drawing of the dorsal rotation advancement flap on the dorsum of the hand. (**d**) Drawing on the palmar aspect of the flap. (**e**) Result of surgery after widening of the web and chondrodesis of the MCP joint

flaps, without scarring along the edge of the web, avoid using full thickness skin graft as possible and closure without tension to avoid necrosis of the edges. The flap should extend beyond the edge of the web to avoid consequent recurrence of contracture after healing and with follow up. We found that simple Z-plasty is not useful because it deepens the web, transforming it into a slit with apparent lengthening of the thumb and poor cosmetic appearance [39]. For mild cases, four flap Z-plasty or double opposing Z-plasty with Y to V advancement [40] gives a natural appearance of the widened web space [39]. Ezaki and Oishi [37] described an index rotation flap that could be used either for widening the web space or for skin augmentation of palmar thumb contracture. This flap cannot address both deformities; however, they are commonly encountered together.

We currently use the modified dorsal rotation advancement flap described by the first author [41]. This flap provides a wide-tipped long flap that extends beyond the edge of the web to avoid recurrence of narrowing of the web after healing. In addition to widening of the web, it provides skin augmentation for the thumb palmar contracture.

In severe palmar thumb contracture, we use the dorsal index-combined flap described by Mahmoud et al.; this technique combines a dorsal index flap with a dorsal triangular flap and a palmar rectangular one to widen the web. These two flaps provide good skin augmentation and release of severe palmar contracture [17].

Modified Dorsal Rotation Advancement Flap Technique (Fig. 18.10) [41]

The flap is begun on the dorsum of the hand with a straight incision over the first metacarpal bone. The second, ulnar incision curves from the second to the fifth metacarpal bones, extending to the wrist level. The two lines are extended in rectangular shape to the edge of a narrow distal web (see Fig. 18.10c).

On the palmar aspect, either an inverted T-shaped incision or a Z-shaped incision is made 1–2 cm proximal to the level of the thumb MCP joint (see Fig. 18.10d). Meticulous technique of raising the flap is very important to the preservation of a good blood supply to its elongated apex, which has a relatively narrow base. Many arteries and veins are taken with the flap, as described by Buck-Gramcko [38]. The distal, rectangular part of the flap is fully released from its bed, but the more proximal dissection is carried out at the epifascial level, with careful preservation of the perforating vessels and the branches of the dorsal carpal arch and the radial artery (the first and second dorsal metacarpal arteries). Some of the terminal branches of these vessels may be ligated at the edge of the flap to allow greater arc of rotation. The tourniquet should be released intra-operatively to check good perfusion of the apex of the flap. All fibrous bands and contracted fascia between the first and second metacarpal bones are released in the conventional manner to allow full thumb abduction. The released web is maintained by two K-wires crossing between the first and second metacarpal bones. The flap is then advanced along the radial incision and rotated along the ulnar incision to occupy the first web space. It can then be sutured to the horizontal limb of the palmar inverted T incision well beyond the edge of the first.

The donor site is closed with direct sutures. Sometimes, it is necessary to excise a small Burrow's triangle on the larger wound margin on the ulnar side.

Dorsal Index-Combined Flap Technique (Fig. 18.11) [17]

The first incision starts at the radial aspect of the index proximal interphalangeal (PIP) joint at point A, extending proximally in the plane between the dorsal and palmar skin to the level of the thumb MCP joint (point B) (see Fig. 18.11a). The second incision passes proximally and dorsally from point A to point C to create an isosceles triangle with the apex not less than 20°. This creates the proximally based index flap (flap 1) (see Fig. 18.11a). Point B is the pivot point of this flap located on the dorsal aspect of the thumb index web commissure. A more proximal starting point is recommended for tight index finger digital skin. Ezaki and Oishi [37] recommended a ratio of 3:1 to keep the viability of this flap. This index flap (see Fig. 18.11a, b) encloses the excess radial skin at the index base, and continues over the dorsal aspect of the first web space. The third incision starts from point C at a 30–45° angle, directing distally half the length of the index flap to point D resulting in a dorsal triangle that comprise the dorsal triangular rotational flap (flap 2) (see Fig. 18.11a). The palmar rectangular flap (flap 3) is enclosed between two incisions, the first starts at point E (midway between points A and B) to point F at an angle of 60° and equal in length to line CD (see Fig. 18.11a). This incision releases the thumb web space and provides bed for the dorsal triangular rotational flap (see Fig. 18.11b). The release of the palmar skin contracture starts from point B as a curved incision across the palmar aspect of the thumb MCP joint crease, reaching the radial mid axial aspect of the thumb MCP joint at point G. This second incision completes the palmar rectangular flap and provides a bed that receives the dorsal index flap (see Fig. 18.11b, h). The index flap is rotated into the palmar aspect, curving around the base of the thumb at the level of the MCP joint (point A to point G) and the palmar rectangular flap dorsally to suture its proximal border to the distal border of the index flap and its advancing border BE to the line CD. The web width increases by the breadth of the two triangular flaps collectively. The palmer rectangular flap increases the web depth by suturing it proximally (see Fig. 18.11b, h).

Stabilization of MCP Joint

In the presence of ulnar collateral ligament instability, stability of the MCP joint is achieved by tightening the ulnar capsule of the MCP joint in a "double breasted" manner. If global instability or severe palmar contracture necessitates excessive capsular release, we prefer doing chondrodesis of the MCP joint. Chondrodesis usually alleviates the need for palmar release of the thumb. One or two Kirschner wires are used to stabilize the MCP joint in 10–20° of flexion. On doing chondrodesis, the articular surfaces of the joint are excised with a sharp knife until reaching the ossific nucleus. Care should be taken to avoid injury of the growth plate of the proximal phalynx.

Lengthening of the FPL

It should be released after release of the palmar contracture of the thumb. Chondrodesis usually alleviates the need for lengthening of the FPL. Lengthening is done at the level of distal forearm by Z-lengthening or intramuscular tenotomy [17].

Rehabilitation after Surgery

The operative splint and K wires are removed after 6 weeks of surgery. Skin care and gentle massage and stretching are done at home. Children start to move the thumb spontaneously. We do not ask for professional physiotherapy. The position is maintained in a night splint with the thumb extended for at least 6 months postoperatively, and daytime active use of the thumb is encouraged.

Evaluation of Results of Treatment

There are no universal criteria for the evaluation of the results of management of clasped thumb, due to the difficulty in assessing the thumb function at that young age, and different systems used by authors for evaluation of their results. Some authors used the degree of active extension of first MCP joint as the reference for evaluation [11, 18]. Tsuyuguchi et al. [12] added the degree of active radial abduction of the CMC joint to their system of evaluation. Lipskeir and Weizenbluth [32] added the width of the first web space to their scoring system, and they mentioned that active extension of first MCP joint is the most important factor for the prehension of large objects.

Because it is of no value to achieve active thumb extension without having stable MCP joint or without widening of the web, it is very important to consider these parameters in evaluation. Using the active extension as the sole criteria for assessment is possible in type I cases where this is the only deficient function.

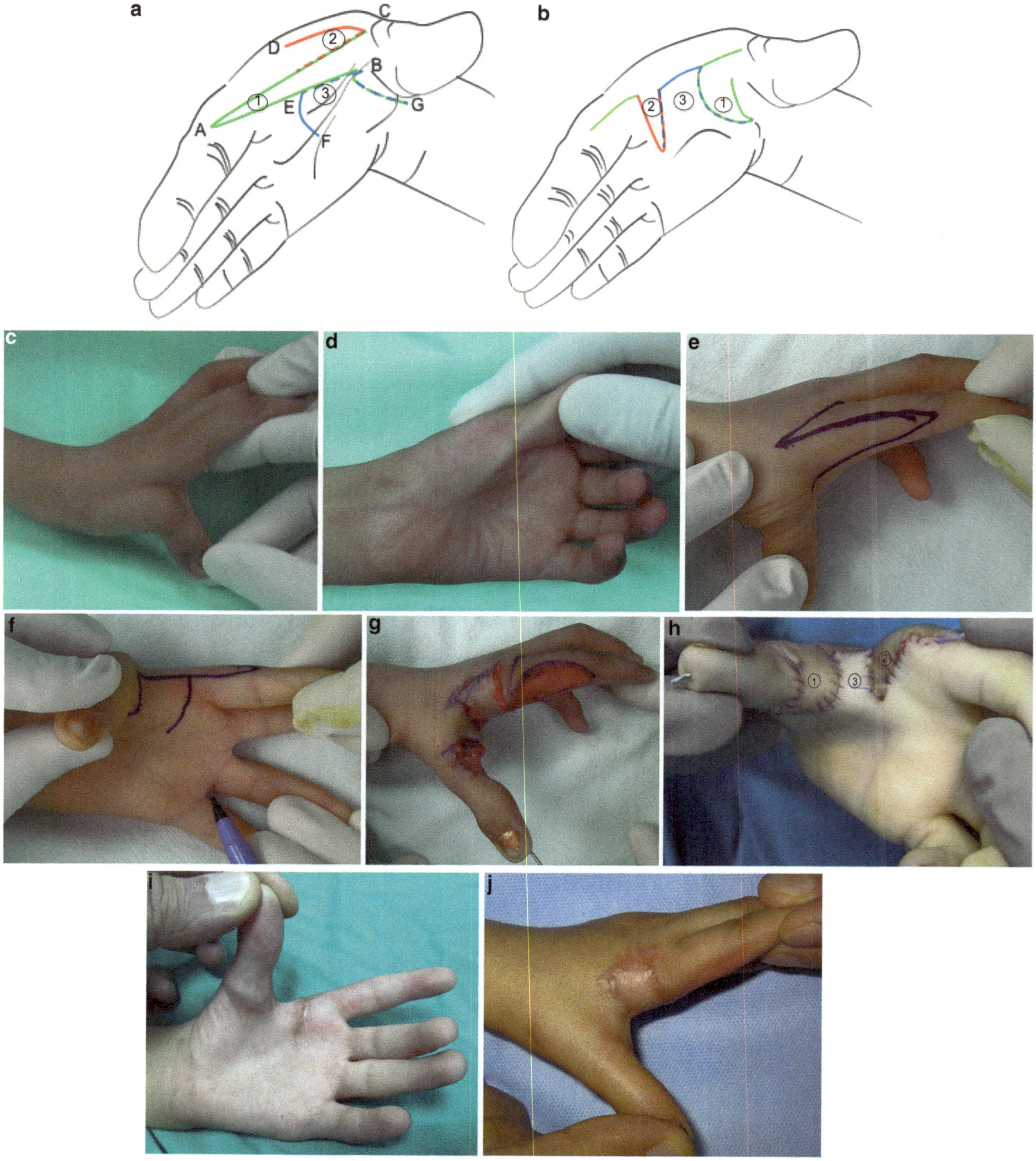

Fig. 18.11 (**a**) Diagram of the dorsal index combined flap. The green bordered angle joining the points C–A–B represent the dorsal index flap (no. 1). The red bordered angle created by line C–D represents the dorsal triangular rotation flap (no. 2). The palmar flap is bordered by lines joining points F–E–B–G (no. 3). (**b**) Drawing of the flap after transposition. (**c**) A case of congenital clasped thumb with unstable MCP joint and severe narrowing of the web space. (**d**) Very evident palmar thumb contracture. (**e, f**) Drawing of the dorsal index-combined flap. (**g, h**) Transposition of the flaps. (**i, j**) Clinical appearance after healing of the flap with widening of the web and release of palmar thumb contracture

Table 18.1 Gilbert's method of assessment of thumb function (personal communication)

Abduction (°)	Rotation (°)	Stability	Opposition	Results
40–45	110–120	Very stable (normal stability in all planes)	With little	Excellent
30–40	90–100	Stable (stable at the ulnar side)	With ring	Good
10–30	80–90	Mild instability (no problem at pinch)	With middle	Fair
0–10	<80	Unstable	None	Poor

We used a combination of criteria to evaluate results of surgery and thumb function [9]:

I. Parents' satisfaction: regarding cosmetic appearance and function
II. Thumb position and appearance: degree of abduction and rotation
III. Stability of MCP joint
IV. Thumb function: degree of opposition and the ability to grasp different objects

The degree of abduction, rotation, stability, and opposition were graded into four grades according to Gilbert (personal communication) (Table 18.1).

Using this system of evaluation, Abdel-Ghani et al. assessed postoperative results in 28 hands [9]. Parents of all the patients were satisfied with the results. Cosmetic appearance was not satisfactory with simple Z-plasty. The appearance of the first web space was better with the other techniques. The modified dorsal rotational advancement flap allowed a maximum degree of widening more than the other techniques used. In the case of ulnar collateral ligament instability of the MCP joint, ligamentous stabilization is a prerequisite for tendon transfer. Although the ligament reconstruction did not give excellent stability, the residual instability did not interfere with thumb function. In the case of global instability of the MCP joint, chondrodesis is the best way to achieve stability, and usually obviates the need for tendon transfer [9]. Our results of chondrodesis [9] are better than that reported by Tsuyuguchi et al. [12] and Lipskeir and Weizenbluth [32]. There was improvement of the grasp pattern in all the operated thumbs.

Properly planned treatment according to the type of the deformity improves the cosmetic appearance and functional capabilities of the hand (see Fig. 18.9).

References

1. Weckesser EC. Congenital flexion-adduction deformity at the thumb (congenital clasped thumb). J Bone Joint Surg. 1955;37A:977–84.
2. Miller JM, Varus P. A report of two cases. Univ Hosp Bull, Ann Arbor. 1944;10:10–1.
3. White JW, Jensen WE. The infant's persistent thumb-clutched hand. J Bone Joint Surg. 1952;34A:680–8.
4. Matev I. Surgical treatment of spastic 'thumb in palm' deformity. J Bone Joint Surg Br. 1963;45B:703–8.
5. Broadbent TR, Woolf RM. Flexion-adduction deformity of the thumb–congenital-clasped thumb. Plast Reconstr Surg. 1964;34:612–6.
6. Anderson TE, Breed AL. Congenital clasped thumb and the Moro reflex. (Letter). J Pediatr. 1981;99:664–5.
7. Manske PR. Longitudinal failure of upper limb formation. An Instructional Course Lecture, The American Academy of Orthopaedic Surgeons. J Bone Joint Surg Am. 1996;78A:1600–23.
8. Wood VE. Another look at the causes of the windblown hand. J Hand Surg Br. 1994;19:679–82.
9. Abdel-Ghani H, El-Naggar A, Hegazy M, Hanna A, Tarraf Y, Temtamy S. Characteristics of patients with congenital clasped thumb: a prospective study of 40 patients with the results of treatment. J Child Orthop. 2007;1:313–22.
10. McCarroll Jr HR. Congenital flexion deformities of the thumb. Hand Clin. 1985;1:567–75.
11. Weckesser EC, Reed JR, Heiple KG. Congenital clasped thumb (congenital flexion-adduction deformity of the thumb). J Bone Joint Surg. 1968;50-A:1417–28.
12. Tsuyuguchi Y, Masda K, Kawabata H, Kawai H, Keiro O. Congenital clasped thumb: a review of forty-three cases. J Hand Surg Am. 1985;10-A:613–18.
13. Bamshad M, Van Heest AE, Pleasure D. Arthrogryposis: a review and update. J Bone Joint Surg Am. 2009;91 Suppl 4:40–6.
14. Hall JG. Arthrogryposis (multiple congenital contractures). In: Rimoin RL, Conner JM, Pyeritz RE, et al., editors. Emery and Rimoin's principles and practice of medical genetics, vol. 168. 5th ed. Philadelphia: Churchill Livingston; 2007. p. 3785–856.
15. Crawford HH, Horton CA, Adamson JE. Congenital aplasia or hypoplasia of thumb and fingers extensor tendons. J Bone Joint Surg. 1966;48-A:82–91.
16. Flatt AE. The care of congenital hand anomalies. 2nd ed. St. Louis: Quality Medical Publishing; 1994.
17. Mahmoud M, Abdel-Ghani H, Elfar JC. New flap for widening of the web space and correction of palmar contracture in complex clasped thumb. J Hand Surg Am. 2013;38(11):2251–6.
18. Lin SC, Hung TH, Hsu HY, Lin CG, Chiu HY. A simple splinting method for correction of supple congenital clasped thumbs in infants. J Hand Surg Br. 1999;24:612–4.
19. Temtamy S, McKusick V. The genetics of hand malformation. New York: Alan R. Liss; 1987.
20. McCarroll HR, Manske PR. The windswept hand. In: Buck-Gramcko D, editor. Congenital malformations of the hand and forearm. London: Churchill Livingstone; 1998. p. 313–25.
21. Beals RK. The distal arthrogryposes: a new classification of peripheral contractures. Clin Orthop Relat Res. 2005;435:203–10.
22. Hall JG. Arthrogryposis multiplex congenita: etiology, genetics, classification, diagnostic approach, and general aspects. J Pediatr Orthop. 1997;6(3):159–66.
23. Rink BD. Arthrogryposis: a review and approach to prenatal diagnosis. Obstet Gynecol Surv. 2011;66(6):369–77.
24. Mitrovic D. Development of the articular cavity in paralyzed chick embryos and in chick embryo limb buds cultured on chorioallantoic membranes. Acta Anat (Basel). 1982;113:313–24.
25. Hall JG, Reed SD, Driscoll EP. Part 1. Amyoplasia: a common sporadic condition with congenital contractures. Am J Med Genet. 1983;15:571–90.
26. Sung SS, Brassington AM, Krakowiak PA, Carey JC, Jorde LB, Bamshad M. Mutations in TNNT3 cause multiple congenital contractures: a second locus for distal arthrogryposis type 2B. Am J Hum Genet. 2003;73:212–14.

27. Toydemir RM, Chen H, Proud VK, Martin R, van Bokhoven H, Hamel BC, et al. Trismus-pseudocamptodactyly syndrome caused by recurrent mutations of MYH8. Am J Med Genet A. 2006;140:2387–93.
28. Toydemir RM, Rutherford A, Whitby FG, Jorde LB, Carey JC, Bamshad MJ. Mutations in embryonic myosin heavy chain (MYH3) cause freeman Sheldon syndrome and Sheldon-Hall syndrome. Nat Genet. 2006;38:561–5.
29. Alvarado DM, Buchan JG, Gurnett CA, Dobbs MB. Exome sequencing identifies an MYH3 mutation in a family with distal arthrogryposis type 1. J Bone Joint Surg Am. 2011;93:1045–50.
30. Kimber E, Tajsharghi H, Kroksmark K, Oldfors A, Tulinius M. A mutation in the fast skeletal muscle troponin I gene causes myopathy and distal arthrogryposis. Neurology. 2006;67:597–601.
31. Tajsharghi H, Kimber E, Kroksmark AK, Jerre R, Tulinius M, Oldfors A. Embryonic myosin heavy-chain mutations cause distal arthrogryposis and developmental myosin myopathy that persists postnatally. Arch Neurol. 2008;65(8):1083–90.
32. Lipskeir E, Weizenbluth M. Surgical treatment of clasped thumb. J Hand Surg Br. 1989;14:72–9.
33. Kozin S. Clasped thumb (Chapter 41). In: Green DP, Hotchkiss RN, Pederson WC, Wolfe SW, editors. Green's operative hand surgery. 6th ed. Philadelphia: Churchill Livingston; 2011. p. 1399–401.
34. Senrui H. Congenital contractures. In: Buck-Gramcko D, editor. Congenital malformations of the hand and forearm. Philadelphia: Churchill Livingstone; 1998. p. 295–309.
35. Zadek I. Congenital absence of extensor pollicis longus of both thumbs. Operation and cure. J Bone Joint Surg. 1934;16:432–4.
36. Mih AD. Congenital clasped thumb. Hand Clin. 1998;14:77–84.
37. Ezaki M, Oishi SN. Index rotation flap for palmar thumb release in arthrogryposis. Tech Hand Up Extrem Surg. 2010;14:38–40.
38. Buck-Gramcko D. Syndactyly between the thumb and index finger. In: Buck-Gramcko D, editor. Congenital malformation of the hand and forearm. New York: Churchill Livingstone; 1998. p. 141–7.
39. Abdel-Ghani H, Amro S. Characteristic of patients with hypoplastic thumb: a prospective study of 51 patients with the results of surgical treatment. J Pediatr Orthop. 2004;13(2 pt B):127–38.
40. Hirshowiz BAK, Rousso M. Combined double Z-plasty and Y-V advancement for thumb web contracture. Hand. 1975;7:291–2.
41. Ghani HA. Modified dorsal rotation advancement flap for release of the thumb web space. J Hand Surg Br. 2006;31(2):226–9.

Part IV

Duplication

Radial Polydactyly

19

Goo Hyun Baek

Radial polydactyly is sometimes called polydactyly of the thumb, preaxial polydactyly, thumb duplication, bifid thumb, or split thumb. It can be classified as a part of "duplication" [1], or a failure of formation and/or differentiation affecting the radial-ulnar axis of the hand plate [2].

Epidemiology and Genetics

Radial polydactyly is a common congenital difference of the upper extremity in all races, and about 20 % of them occur bilaterally. Its incidence had been reported at 0.08–1.4 per 1,000 live births [3, 4]. Syndactyly was more common than polydactyly in the study from University of Iowa [5]. However, in Asian countries such as Japan, Korea, and Hong Kong, polydactyly is more common than syndactyly [6, 7]. Most radial polydactyly occur sporadically. However, when associated with triphalangeal thumb, higher hereditary predisposition has been identified. Among 21 patients of radial polydactyly with triphalangeal thumb, ten patients had a family history of the same abnormality in close relatives [8]. Radial polydactyly can occur in rare syndromic diseases such as Fanconi's anemia, Holt–Oram syndrome, and Rubinstein–Taybi syndrome.

Sonic hedgehog (SHH) within the posteriorly located zone of polarizing activity is considered as the main controller of the anteroposterior axis of limb development. The zone of polarizing activity regulatory sequence (ZRS) is a long-range limb-specific SHH enhancer. Several point mutations in the ZRS have been described in humans, and caused variable phenotype of radial polydactyly and triphalangeal thumb [9]. Bone morphogenetic protein 7 (BMP-7) is expressed strongly in the interdigital mesenchyme of the vertebrate limb, which normally undergoes programmed cell death. Loss of BMP-7 likely allows for survival of programmed cell death, and can give rise to an extra digit [10]. GLI3 gene is crucial since all GLI3-associated human congenital diseases comprise limb malformations [11]. Mutations in this gene have been associated with several diseases including preaxial polydactyly and postaxial polydactyly.

Classification

The Wassel classification for polydactyly of the thumb, published in 1969 [5], has been most widely used. This classification system is simple in application and communication (Table 19.1). Wassel type 4 is the most common type, representing 29–43 % of all polydactyly of the thumb, while type 1 is the least common [5, 12].

The Wassel classification is based on an assessment of the skeleton. In young children whose skeleton is immature, the true nature of the thumbs may not be apparent. For instance, Wassel type 1 polydactyly can be classified as a type 2 until ossification of the distal phalangeal epiphysis becomes apparent [13]. Wassel type 7 polydactyly which has a triphalangeal component shows diverse manifestations, and is further subclassified into six types [8].

There are some types of radial polydactyly unclassifiable by the Wassel system. Pedunculated type, triplicated thumb, and extra-thumb, which do not have bony connection with the main thumb, cannot be classified.

Temtamy and McKusick classified radial polydactyly into four types—thumb polydactyly (type I), polydactyly of a triphalangeal thumb or opposable triphalangeal thumb (type II), polydactyly of an index finger or nonopposable triphalangeal thumb (type III), and polysyndactyly (type IV) [4].

Chung et al. proposed a new classification system based on the anatomic morphology at the origin of the extra digit [14]. Type I was defined as the joint type, where the extra digit has its own joint at its origin. In type II, the single epiphyseal type, the extra digit originates from the epiphysis directly. Type III, or osteochondroma-like

G.H. Baek, M.D., Ph.D. (✉)
Department of Orthopedic Surgery, Seoul National University Hospital, 101 Daehak-ro, Jongno-gu, Seoul 110-744, South Korea
e-mail: ghbaek@snu.ac.kr

D.R. Laub Jr. (ed.), *Congenital Anomalies of the Upper Extremity: Etiology and Management*,
DOI 10.1007/978-1-4899-7504-1_19, © Springer Science+Business Media New York 2015

Table 19.1 Wassel classification for polydactyly of the thumb [5]

Type 1:	A bifid distal phalanx with a common epiphysis that articulates with a normal proximal phalanx
	There may be one common nail, but usually there are two distinct nails with a groove between them
Type 2:	A completely duplicated distal phalanx
	Each distal phalanx usually has its own epiphysis that articulates with the normal proximal phalanx
Type 3:	A duplicated distal phalanx with a bifurcated proximal phalanx
	The distal phalanges usually diverge from the longitudinal axis, or they may be parallel
Type 4:	A complete duplication of the proximal phalanx
	Each proximal phalanx has its own epiphysis or a common epiphysis that articulates with a normal metacarpal or a metacarpal slightly widened to accommodate both proximal phalanges
Type 5:	A bifurcated first metacarpal
	Each head of the bifurcation articulates with a duplicated proximal phalanx which has its own epiphysis
Type 6:	Complete duplication of the entire first digit
	One side may be more rudimentary than the other
Type 7:	A triphalangeal thumb or elements of a triphalangeal thumb accompanied by a normal thumb

type, originates from the metacarpal or phalangeal shaft of the main digit. Type IV is a hypoplastic type in which there is no bony connection between two thumbs. This classification system is practical and closely related to the surgical strategies.

Preoperative Evaluation

Sufficient discussion and explanation to the parents who have a baby with radial polydactyly on its clinical features and surgical outcome is necessary to maintain good rapport after the surgery. It is very important to inspect both hands of the patient, when a baby with radial polydactyly and his/her parents visit the outpatient department (OPD). Most of the babies with unilateral involvement show smaller sizes of affected thumbs than those of contralateral normal thumbs. Thus, the parents should understand that even if the more dominant one is preserved in the affected thumb, it will be smaller in length and girth when compared to the unaffected side.

In babies with bilateral involvement, the nail size of index finger can be a reference to judge the size of the affected thumbs. The width of the index fingernail is about two-thirds of that of the thumb in normal babies.

Active motion of each joint is hard to observe because the babies usually clench their hands. Passive motion and varus and valgus stress tests of the joints, palpation of tendons (especially flexor tendons), and observation of skin crease may be helpful to evaluate the polydactylic thumbs. Little or absent passive motion at bifurcation site of minor thumb (usually the radial one) may suggest odd-numbered Wassel type 1, 3, or 5. It is much easier to reconstruct a thumb that has stable joints in radioulnar plane. If the flexor tendon is palpable while moving the joint passively, good active motion can be expected postoperatively. When the skin crease is faint or absent, there is a strong possibility that the affected joint does not have effective motor power or the joint is fused, as in symphalangism.

Simple radiographs are very helpful for Wassel typing and surgical planning. Although it is not easy to obtain a true PA and lateral view of the affected thumbs, it is absolutely necessary for surgical planning. Radiographs of normal side in unilateral cases are also very important in assessing the size and shape of bones and joints of the affected thumbs comparatively. Medical photos are also needed for documentation and later evaluation of surgical outcome.

Before surgery, the parents should be informed that even if the thumb is reconstructed successfully, it will not be the same as the contralateral normal thumb in terms of function and cosmesis. The patients and their parents sometimes complain of applying a long arm cast postoperatively. However, a short arm cast can be easily removed spontaneously especially in young children.

In a study of 66 years of experiences for surgery of the duplicated thumb [15], there were 27.94 % of patients with serious complications, 7.35 % of them unsalvageable by secondary surgery, and 20.59 % salvageable by secondary surgery. Recently, the complication rates are declining. When initial surgery was planned to restore all anatomic elements, the need for secondary surgery was quite unusual [16]. The primary issues affecting appearance after surgery for radial polydactyly were reduced nail width and angulation at interphalangeal joint. Reconstructed Wassel type 7 thumbs had lower satisfaction score than other types [17].

Timing of Surgery

There has been no general agreement on proper timing of operation for radial polydactyly. Kozin recommended performing surgery at about 1 year of age, before the development of thumb-index finger pinch [18]. Jobe recommended performing surgical reconstruction when the child is about 18 months old, but no later than 5 years old, if possible [19]. Indebted to recent advancement in pediatric anesthesia, most surgeries can be performed safely if the patient does not have serious associated problems such as severe cardiac anomaly or pancytopenia. In certain cases, Wassel type 7, for example, bony shape of the delta bone is sometimes very important for surgical planning in which the surgical timing is better to be postponed until it is clearly visible in radiographs. Thus, timing of surgery depends on general condition of the patient, priority of surgery in patients with multiple associated anomalies, types of radial polydactyly, and most importantly surgeon's judgement. There is no gold standard for surgical timing of radial polydactyly. However, earlier surgery is recommended when surgical planning is completed and the structures of the thumb are large enough to manipulate surgically.

Surgical Technique

The surgical goal for reconstruction of the radial polydactyly is to make a straight, mobile, and stable thumb of good appearance in size and shape. However, even after a successful reconstruction, the reconstructed thumb is not perfect in terms of function and cosmesis. We are trying to make a better thumb in a given situation, not the best or perfect thumb.

The patients with radial polydactyly show very diverse manifestations, from a rudimentary floating type to a complex one. Ligation or simple excision may be enough for floating types of radial polydactyly. However, simple ablation of one digit has not produced satisfactory outcomes in most cases of radial polydactyly and it has resulted in retained deviation, stiffness, and/or ligamentous instability of the thumb. Although surgical concepts and techniques are still evolving, there are several reconstructive strategies to achieve a functionally and cosmetically acceptable thumb.

Surgical techniques to reconstruct radial polydactyly can be classified into five types—ligation, simple excision, excision and reconstruction, combination procedures (Bilhaut-Cloquet operation), and on-top plasty.

The surgical wound is usually closed with absorbable 4-0 or 5-0 sutures. If the wound is closed with nonabsorbable sutures, sedation of the patients may be needed for removal of sutures. A long arm thumb spica cast with more than 90° of elbow flexion is recommended postoperatively, because a short arm thumb spica cast or a long arm cast in a position of a less flexed elbow can be easily taken off. Patients undergoing corrective osteotomy and/or reconstruction of collateral ligament should be immobilized for 4–6 weeks, depending on age. Postoperative physical therapy is not necessary in most patients.

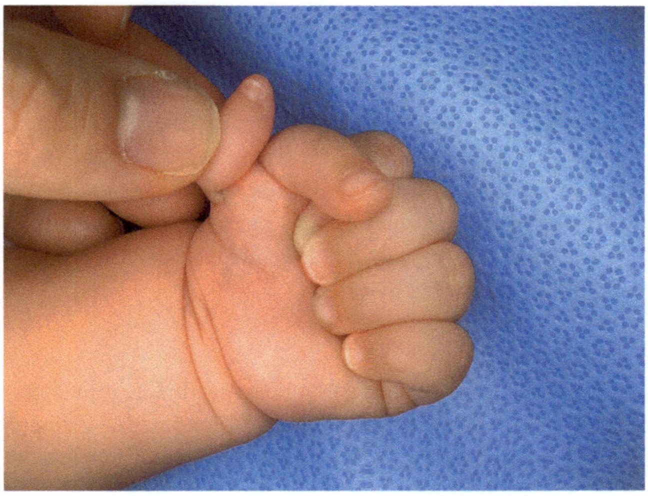

Fig. 19.1 A pedunculated type of radial polydactyly

Ligation

In a pedunculated type of radial polydactyly (Fig. 19.1), ligation at the base as close as possible to its root with 5-0 or 6-0 nylon with or without local anesthesia can be performed at OPD or nursery. Ligated hypoplastic thumb is mummified and usually falls off within 2 weeks. A nubbin usually remains after fall off. When the skin bridge measures more than 4 mm, excision under general anesthesia is recommended [13]. Even in the pedunculated type of polydactyly, painful neuroma may develop after the ligation, which is an indication for surgical exploration [20].

Simple Excision

Simple excision under general anesthesia is indicated, when there is no bony connection between two polydactyly thumbs, and a dominant thumb shows good stability, motion, and alignment (Fig. 19.2).

Technique: An elliptical incision is made around the minor thumb. The soft tissue pedicle usually contains neurovascular structures. To avoid bleeding, the vessels should be ligated or cauterized. To prevent painful neuroma, the nerve should be identified, sharply transected, and imbedded in the soft tissue.

Excision and Reconstruction

More than half of the patients with radial polydactyly can be successfully treated by the "excision and reconstruction" technique (Fig. 19.3). Main components of this technique are arthroplasty, corrective osteotomy, and tendon realignment.

When one of the two polydactylic thumbs is well developed, and the other one less developed, this technique is indicated. However, when both polydactylic thumbs are hypoplastic, this technique results in a small thumb, which is sometimes smaller than the index finger. Surgical technique for Wassel types 1 and 2 is similar. Also, similar surgical technique can be applied to Wassel types 3, 4, 5, and 6. For the diversity of clinical features, surgical technique for Wassel type 7 should be individualized case by case.

Arthroplasty

Arthroplasty consists of two components, that is, joint stabilization by ligamentoperiosteal flap [21] and partial excision of excessive portion of phalangeal or metacarpal head on which two thumbs sit.

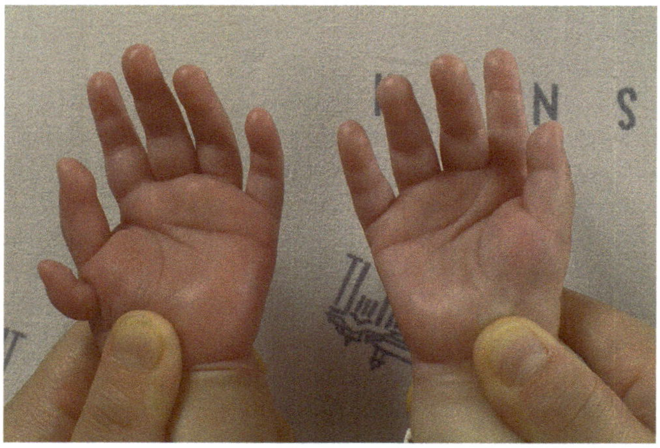

Fig. 19.2 When there is no bony connection between two thumbs, simple excision is indicated

Two thumbs sit on a single proximal phalangeal head in Wassel type 1 or 2 radial polydactyly, and on a single metacarpal in type 3 or 4. During dissection of minor thumb, distal insertion of collateral ligament should be preserved with adjacent periosteal tissue for later reconstruction. This ligamentoperiosteal flap will be reattached to the base of the phalangeal bone of the remaining main thumb after removal of the minor thumb. The phalangeal or metacarpal head, when the minor thumb is removed, is relatively large for the remaining dominant thumb. This size mismatching between two bones may cause angular deformity and/or bony prominence if it is not corrected. Thus, excessive portion of the head needs to be shaved or removed. Sometimes, a separate facet that articulates with the radial thumb to be deleted is observed. This facet can be used as a guideline to cut the excessive portion. An oscillating saw or osteotome cannot be used for very small phalangeal bones of young children. Their phalangeal bones are soft enough that shaving of articular cartilage and partial ostectomy can be performed by a small rongeur or a surgical blade. Excessive tension of the reconstructed collateral ligament to correct angular deformity at the joint level is not recommended because the deformity is likely to recur and stiffness of the joint may occur. However, angular deformity of less than 10° at the joint level can be corrected by this arthroplasty procedure. A longitudinal Kirschner wire (K-wire) is inserted to protect the reconstructed collateral ligament.

Corrective Osteotomy

Angulation at interphalangeal joint and reduced nail width are primary issues affecting appearance after the surgery [17]. More than 20° of angular deformity is not acceptable to

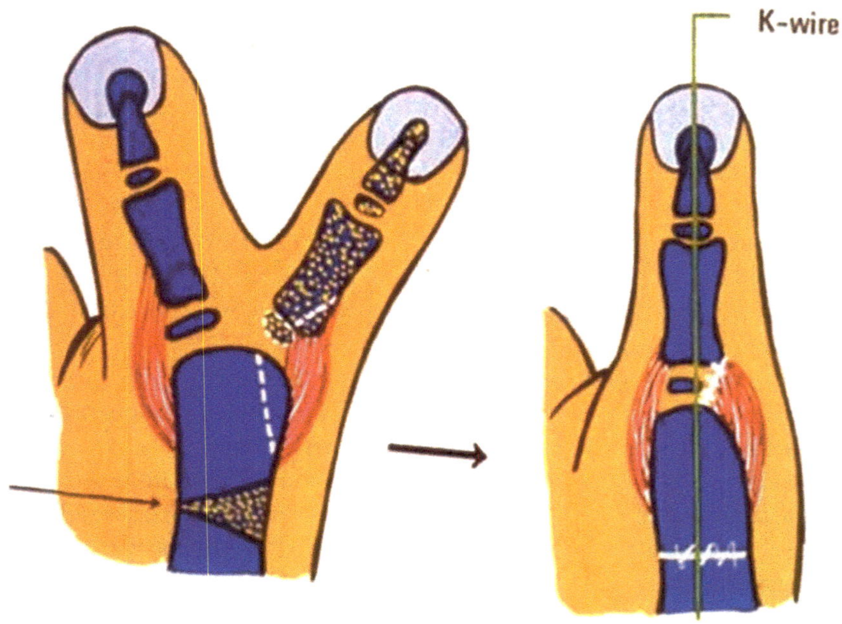

Fig. 19.3 A ligamentoperiosteal flap is raised to reconstruct the radial collateral ligament of the MP joint. The metacarpal head is excised partially to fit the base of the dominant proximal phalanx. If necessary, corrective osteotomy was added to make a straight thumb

most patients and parents. This can be corrected by closing wedge osteotomy. Double level osteotomy at proximal phalangeal and metacarpal levels can be indicated to align a severe divergent-convergent Wassel type 4.

Tendon Realignment

Abnormal insertions of flexor pollicis longus (FPL) and/or extensor pollicis longus (EPL) are not uncommon in radial polydactyly, especially in Wassel type 4. The FPL tendon attaches not only at its customary insertion, but also into the extensor by a tendon that passes around the radial aspect of the thumb. This anomalous muscle abducts the thumb instead of flexion, and is called as "pollex abductus" [22, 23]. The abnormal insertion of FPL and/or EPL may cause gradual angular deformity even after successful bony alignment has been achieved by corrective osteotomy. If there are abnormal insertions of FPL and/or EPL tendons, the insertion sites should be realigned to achieve good flexion-extension arc. The abnormal insertion can be completely detached and reattached into the correct position. The tendon can be sutured into the distal phalanx of young children using 4-0 or 5-0 nylon. When the phalangeal bone is too hard to be sutured by nylon suture, a pull-out suture technique can be used. When the distal portion of the tendon is bifid and inserted into both polydactylic thumbs, it usually inserts at ulnar side of the radial thumb, and radial side of the ulnar thumb. If the radial thumb is to be removed, the tendon is detached from the insertion of radial thumb and reattached into the ulnar side of dominant ulnar thumb in a "Y" shape to balance the vector forces (Figs. 19.4 and 19.5). During this procedure, the portion of tendinous insertion into the radial side of the remaining radial thumb needs to be detached to avoid abnormal abduction force.

In Wassel type 4, 5, 6, or 7 polydactyly of the thumb, some of thenar muscles insert into the radial side thumb. In most cases, the radial thumb is removed and the ulnar thumb is reconstructed. The insertion site of thenar muscles on radial thumb should be identified and dissected carefully for later reattachment to the main ulnar thumb.

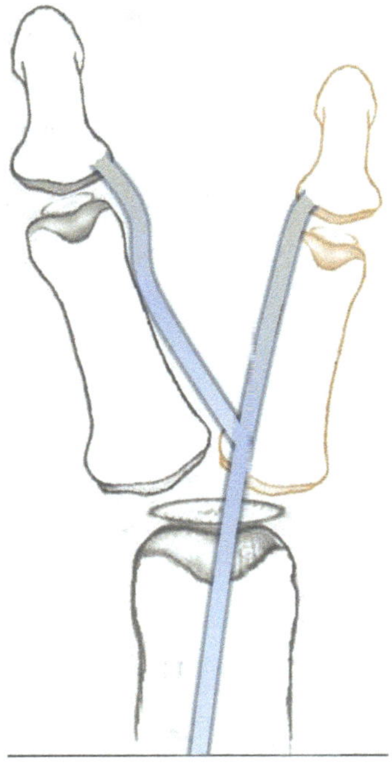

Fig. 19.4 The tendons frequently bifurcated distal to the MP joint, and insert to the side of each distal phalanx

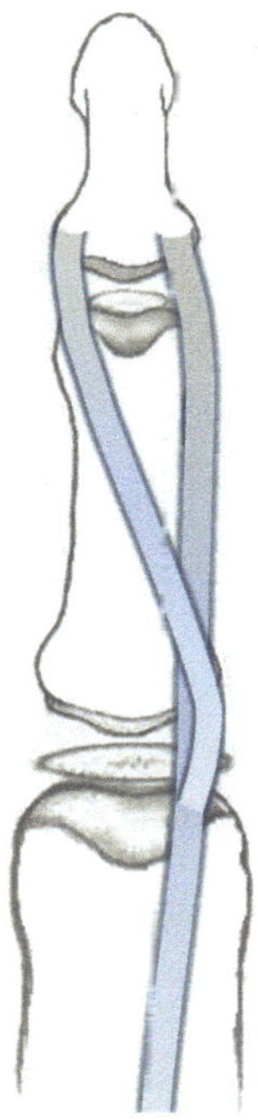

Fig. 19.5 The tendon insertion of minor thumb is detached and reattached to the main thumb in a Y shape to balance the vector force

Surgical Technique (Wassel Type 1)

A 7-month-old girl showed radial polydactyly on right thumb (Fig. 19.6). The nail size, length, and girth of ulnar side thumb of left hand were good enough to perform the "excision of radial thumb and reconstruction" procedure. As the epiphyses of phalanges and metacarpal were not observed in simple radiograph (Fig. 19.7), it was hard to assess the exact Wassel type but easy to decide the surgical plan as "arthroplasty" with or without "tendon realignment." Corrective osteotomy was not necessary because angular deformity at the IP joint is minimal. A racquet-shaped incision was designed. A zigzag incision has an advantage to prevent possible scar contracture, but this technique is not easy to apply to an infant with a thumb less than an inch in length. During dissection, it was confirmed that base of two distal phalanges was fused to be Wassel type 1. The dissection was deepened to expose distal phalangeal bone of the radial thumb, and a ligamentoperiosteal flap was raised. Distal phalanx of the radial thumb was cut to be removed, and the articular surface of this radial thumb was seen. Articular surface for the radial

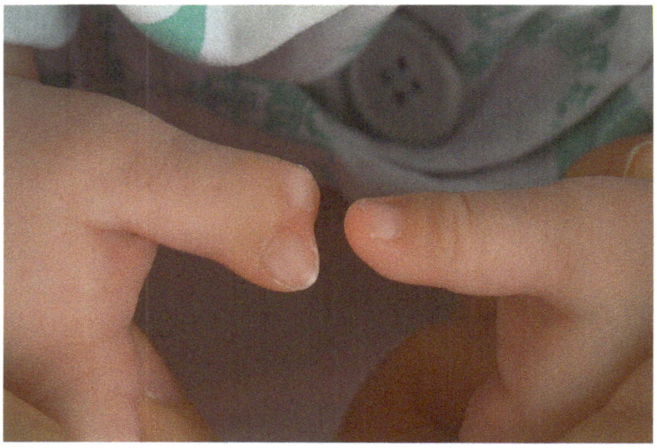

Fig. 19.6 Wassel type 1 polydactyly of right thumb. Ulnar thumb showed better configuration

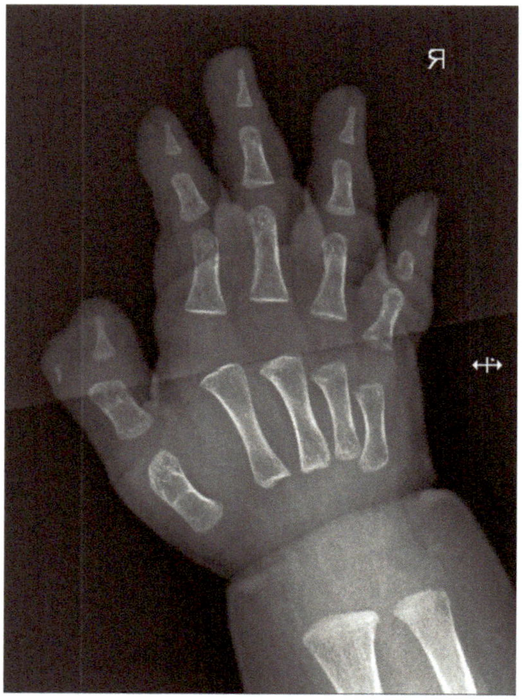

Fig. 19.7 Two thumbs sit on the proximal phalangeal head, and the head showed enlargement

thumb was cut using a number-15 blade scalpel (Fig. 19.8). The consistency of phalangeal bone in an infant is soft enough to be cut by surgical blade. There was no misalignment of tendons. After the arthroplasty procedure, the articular surface of the proximal phalanx fits that of the ulnar thumb. Before reconstruction of the collateral ligament, a 0.7-mm K-wire was inserted longitudinally to protect it. The ligamentoperiosteal flap was attached to the new insertion site by 5-0 absorbable suture, reconstructing the collateral ligament (Fig. 19.9). The reconstructed thumb looked straight (Fig. 19.10).

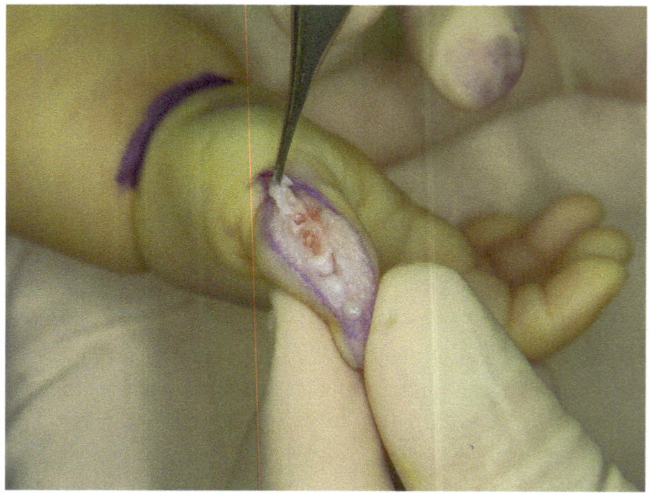

Fig. 19.8 A ligamentoperiosteal flap was raised (forcep), and the excessive portion of the proximal phalangeal head was removed

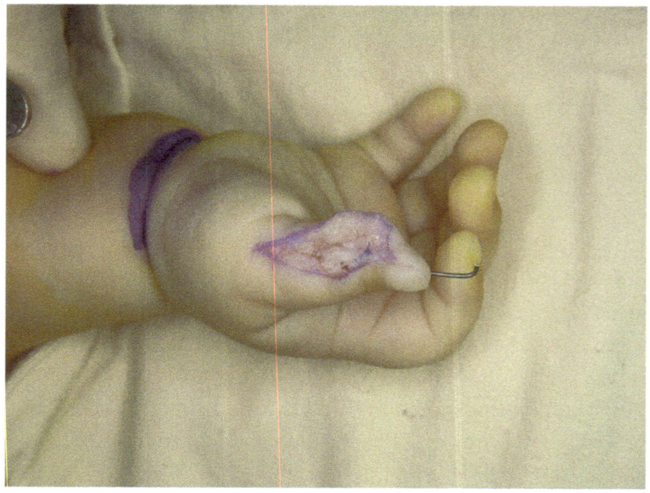

Fig. 19.9 A K-wire was inserted longitudinally, and the flap was reattached to the new insertion site

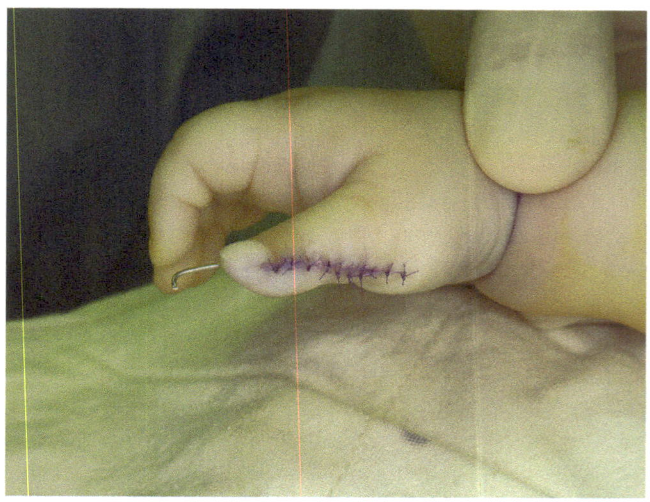

Fig. 19.10 Immediate postoperative finding

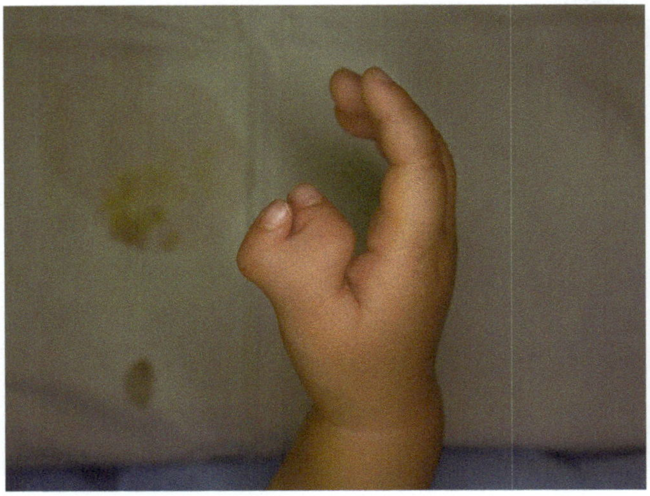

Fig. 19.11 A divergent-convergent Wassel type 4 radial polydactyly of a 14-month-old boy

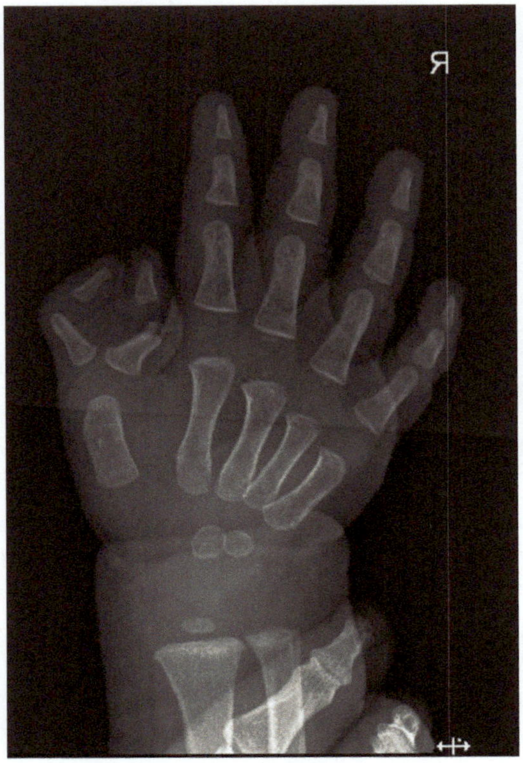

Fig. 19.12 The ulnar side thumb showed better bony development, although there was 35° of angular deformity at the IP joint

Surgical Technique (Wassel Type 4)

A 14-month-old boy showed a divergent-convergent Wassel type 4 radial polydactyly on the right side. The radial thumb was hypoplastic, but the ulnar thumb showed good size and shape (Fig. 19.11). There was 35° of angular deformity at the IP joint of ulnar thumb that needed corrective osteotomy at the proximal phalangeal neck level (Fig. 19.12). Medical photos and simple radiographs suggested strong possibility

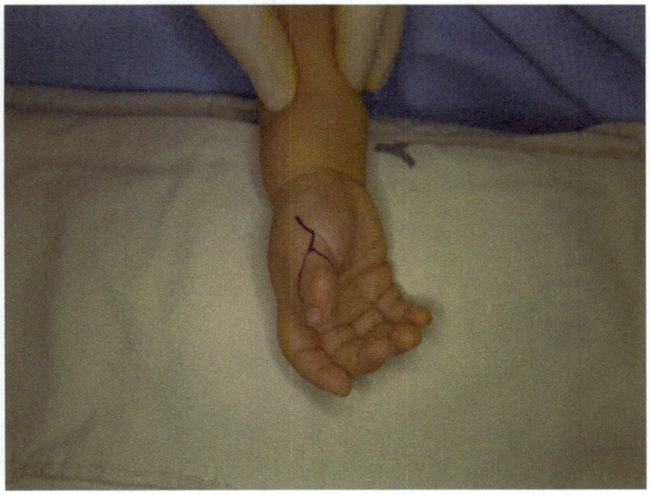

Fig. 19.13 Skin incision

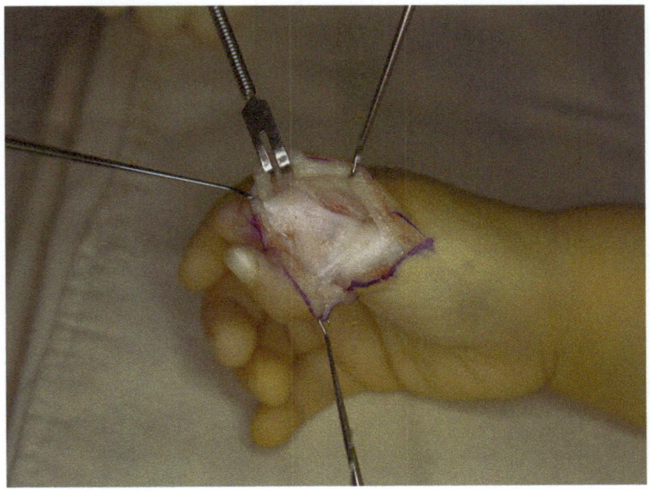

Fig. 19.14 The EPL tendon showed bifurcation at the MP joint level

that arthroplasty of MP joint and tendon realignment of EPL, FPL, and thenar muscles were necessary for proper reconstruction. The proximal phalangeal head of the ulnar thumb was underdeveloped, suggesting a potential recurrence of angular deformity postoperatively. A racquet-shaped incision was designed (Fig. 19.13) The EPL tendon was bifurcated at MP joint level, and inserted into both thumbs (Fig. 19.14). The insertion site of radial EPL slip was detached and sutured to the ulnar side of dominant thumb to balance the extension force. The FPL tendon showed the same pattern (Fig. 19.15). The insertion of the radial FPL slip was detached and tagged with suture for later reattachment into the ulnar side of dominant thumb (Fig. 19.16). The abductor pollicis brevis muscle insertion into the radial thumb was detached from the proximal phalangeal base for later reattachment into the reconstructed thumb. The radial thumb was removed, leaving ligamentoperiosteal flap for

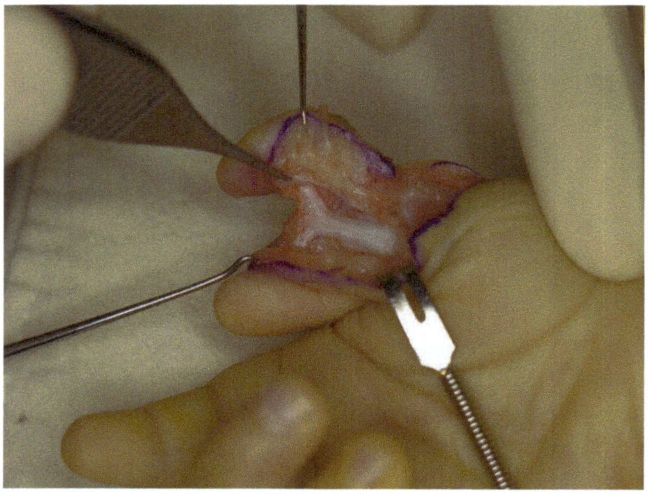

Fig. 19.15 The FPL tendon was bifurcated at the IP joint level

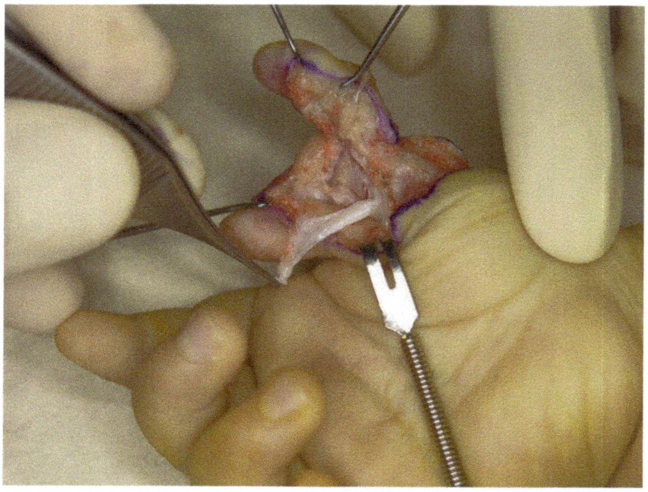

Fig. 19.16 The FPL insertion to the radial thumb was identified and preserved for later reattachment

later reconstruction of the MP joint. The portion of metacarpal head to be resected was lined (Fig. 19.17), and a ligamento-periosteal flap was raised and preserved. Excessive articular cartilage and bone was resected by number 15 blade and small osteotomes. The author finds that it is very difficult to do a fine osteotomy with power instruments like an oscillating saw. The ligamentoperiosteal flap and detached abductor pollicis brevis tendon were preserved for later reattachment (Fig. 19.18). The proximal phalanx was dissected subperiosteally for ulnarly based closing wedge osteotomy to correct angular deformity at the IP joint (Fig. 19.19). It is convenient to perform ulnarly based closing wedge osteotomy from a separate ulnar side incision. However, simultaneous medial and lateral incision on the same thumb may jeopardize blood circulation. The MP joint was fixed in a reduced position with a K-wire, and also osteotomy site of proximal phalanx was fixed with an additional K-wire (Fig. 19.20). Finally, the FPL tendon detached from the

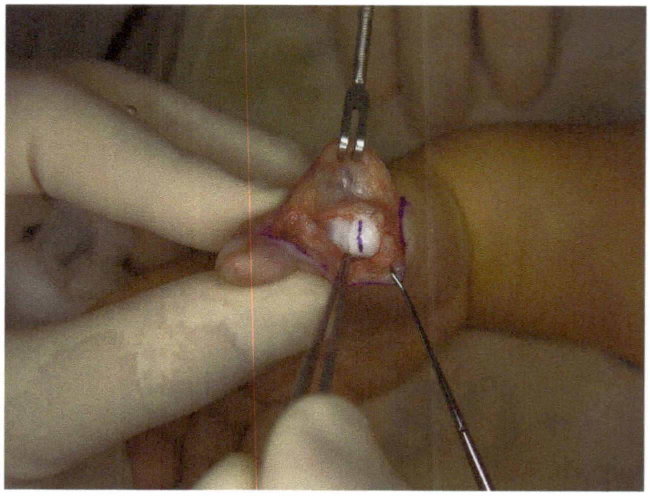

Fig. 19.17 Excessive portion of metacarpal head on which the removed radial thumb had sat was marked

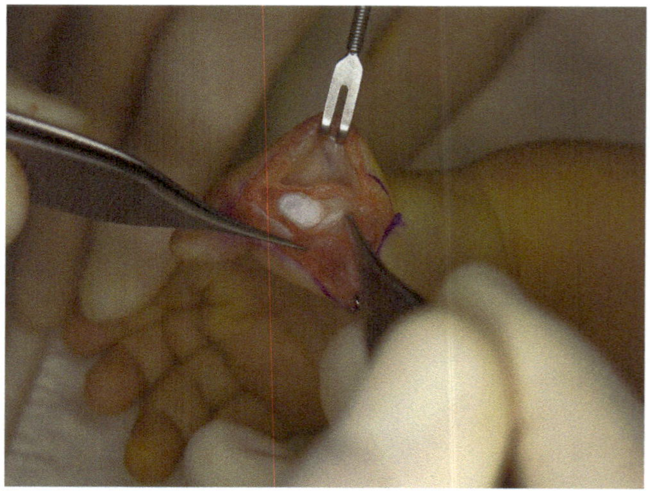

Fig. 19.18 After excision of the excessive portion of the metacarpal head, the detached tendon of APB (left forcep) and a ligamentoperiosteal flap (right forcep) were preserved

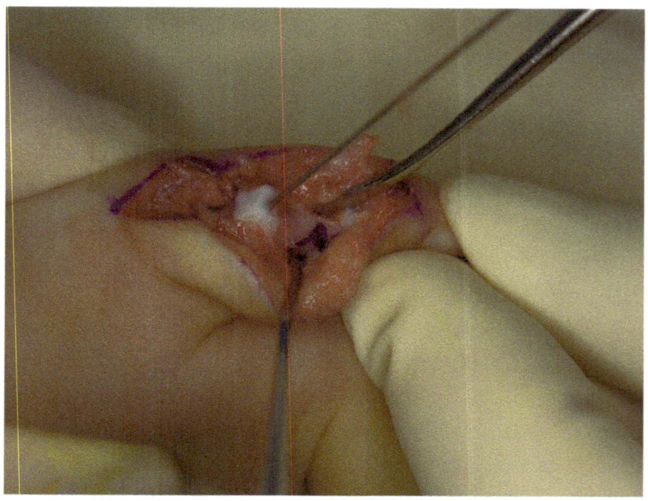

Fig. 19.19 The MP joint was fixed with a K-wire. Proximal phalanx was exposed subperiosteally for corrective osteotomy

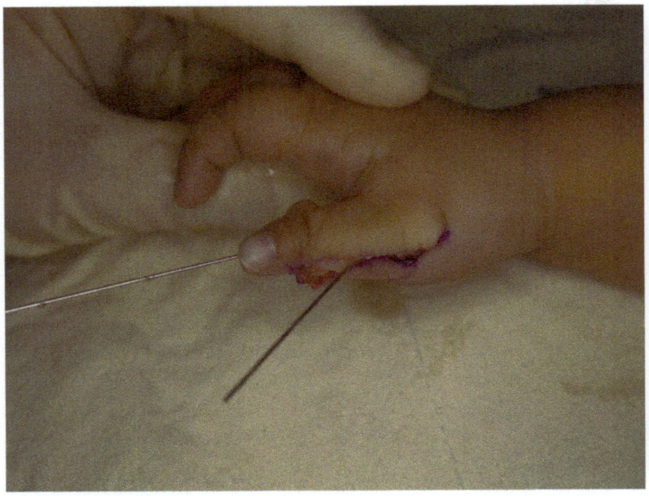

Fig. 19.20 The osteotomy site was fixed with a K-wire

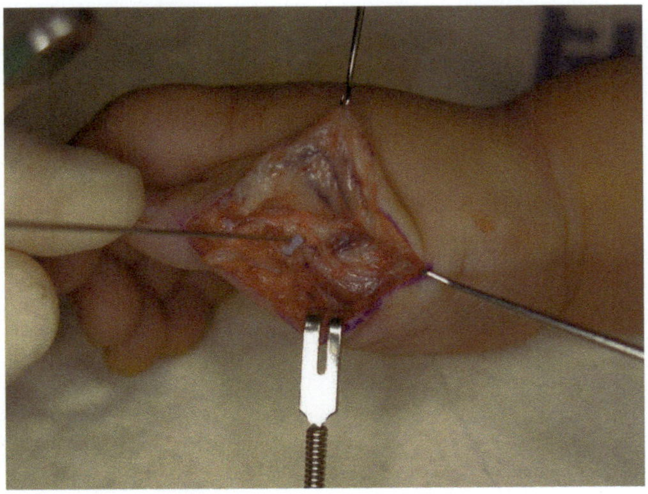

Fig. 19.21 The abductor pollicis brevis tendon detached from radial thumb as well as the previously raised ligamentoperiosteal flap were reinserted into the base of proximal phalanx

radial thumb was reattached into the ulnar side of reconstructed distal phalanx. The abductor pollicis brevis tendon detached from radial thumb as well as the previously raised ligamentoperiosteal flap for collateral ligament reconstruction was also reinserted into the base of proximal phalanx (Fig. 19.21). Alignment and appearance of the reconstructed thumb (Fig. 19.22) and the immediate postoperative radiograph (Fig. 19.23) showed good result.

Surgical Technique (Wassel Type 7)

Clinical features of Wassel type 7 radial polydactyly are so diverse that there is no standard surgical technique. In certain cases, simple excision is enough to correct deformity (Fig. 19.24). On the other hand, very complex reconstruction procedures are needed in certain cases (Fig. 19.25).

A 12-month-old girl showed a radial polydactyly, bifid at metacarpal shaft level. The ulnar thumb had delta middle phalanx with angular deformity (Figs. 19.26 and 19.27). A racquet-shaped incision was made along the radial thumb, and it was excised by dividing the bony connection at metacarpal shaft level. Another straight incision was made along the radial side of the ulnar thumb to excise the delta middle phalanx. After excision of the delta bone, the radial collateral ligament was sutured in proper tension. When the patient's age is less than 6 years, simple excision of the delta bone yields a good result [24]. The younger the patients, the better the surgical outcome. A longitudinal K-wire was inserted to protect reconstructed radial collateral ligament of IP joint (Fig. 19.28). Three years after the operation, alignment and range of motion were good (Figs. 19.29 and 19.30).

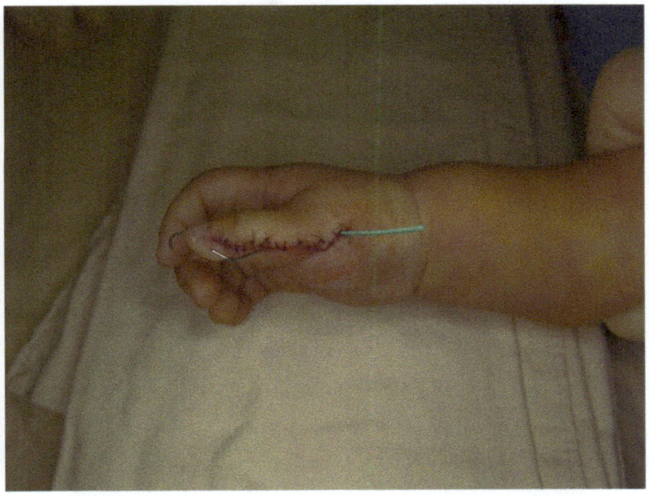

Fig. 19.22 A postoperative photo

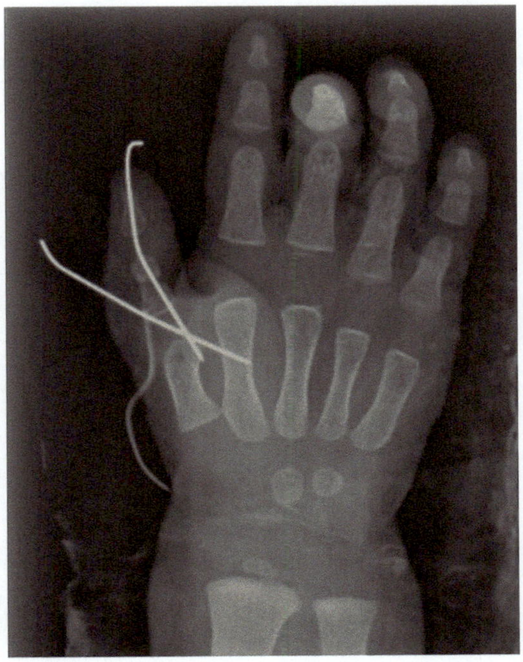

Fig. 19.23 Immediate postoperative radiograph

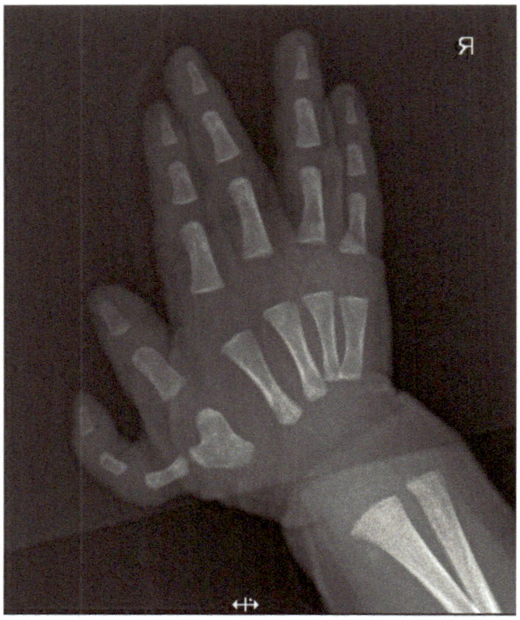

Fig. 19.24 A simple Wassel type 7 polydactyly. Radial triphalangeal thumb was hypoplastic, and ulnar thumb showed good IP and MP joints with straight alignment

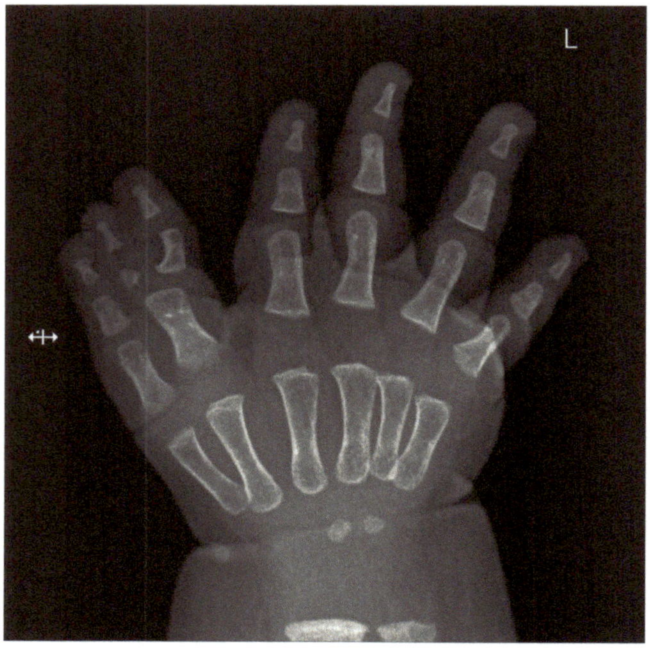

Fig. 19.25 A complex Wassel type 7 polydactyly

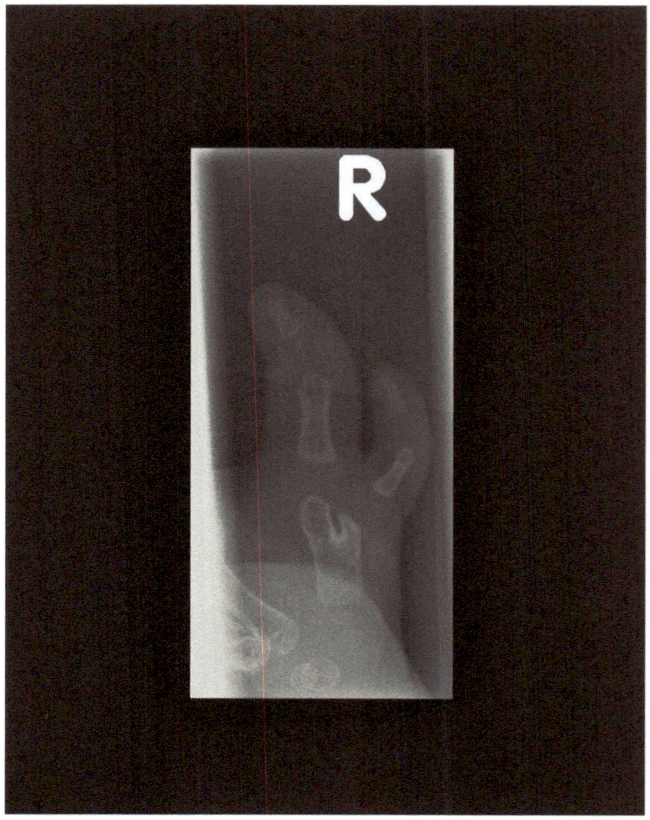

Fig. 19.26 A 12-month-old girl with Wassel type 7 polydactyly. The ulnar triphalangeal thumb had delta middle phalanx causing angular deformity

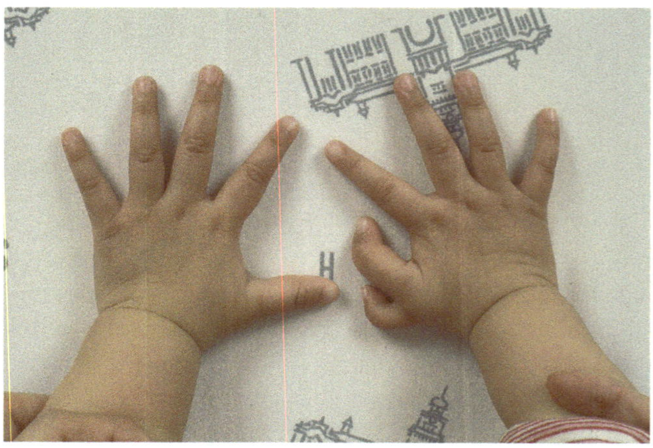

Fig. 19.27 Preoperative medical photo

Combination Procedure (Modified Bilhaut-Cloquet Procedure)

The original Bilhaut-Cloquet procedure (BC procedure) consists of resection of the central portion of duplicated segment and the coaptation of outer parts of bone, soft tissue, and nail tissue for the treatment of radial polydactyly [25]. This procedure has an advantage in obtaining a good-sized thumb with good IP joint stability. However, postoperative complications such as joint stiffness, physeal growth disturbance, and nail-plate deformity are common [15, 26, 27].

This original technique was modified to overcome these complications [28, 29]. There is no absolute indication for modified BC procedure. However, when both thumbs are hypoplastic and show almost symmetric appearance, this

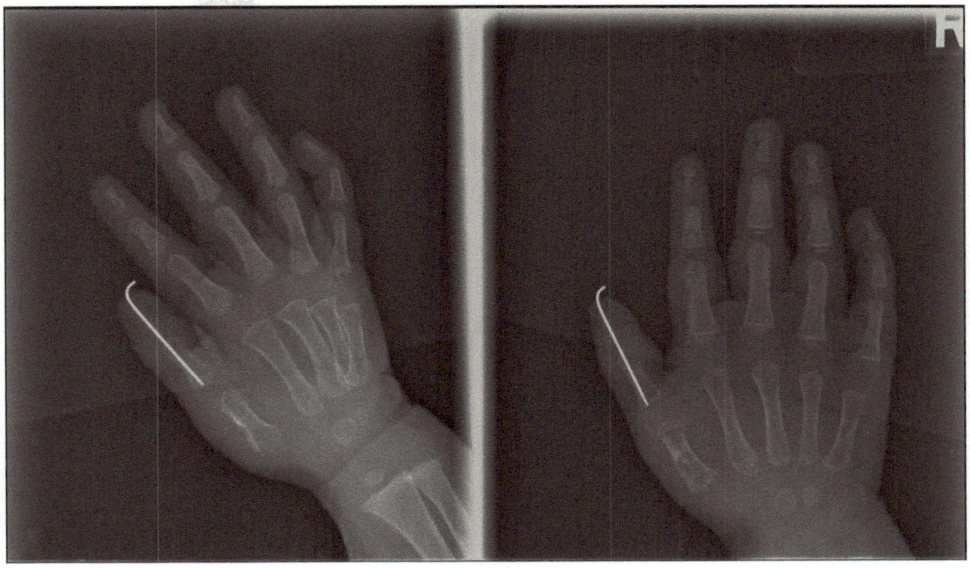

Fig. 19.28 Radial thumb was excised. The middle delta bone of the ulnar thumb was excised, and the collateral ligament was sutured in proper tension

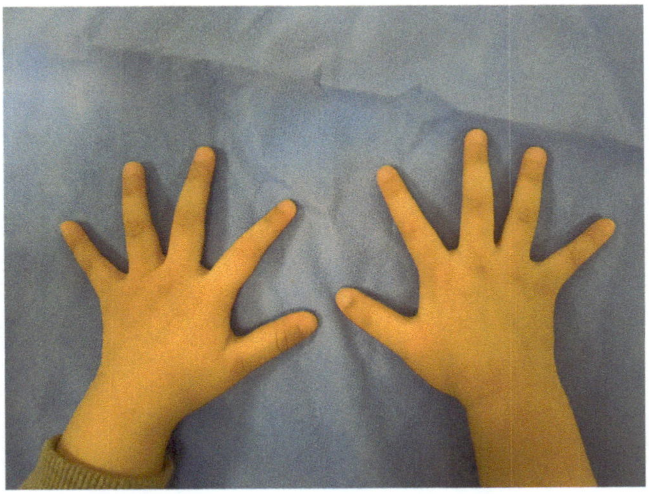

Fig. 19.29 Three years after the operation, alignment of the reconstructed thumb was straight

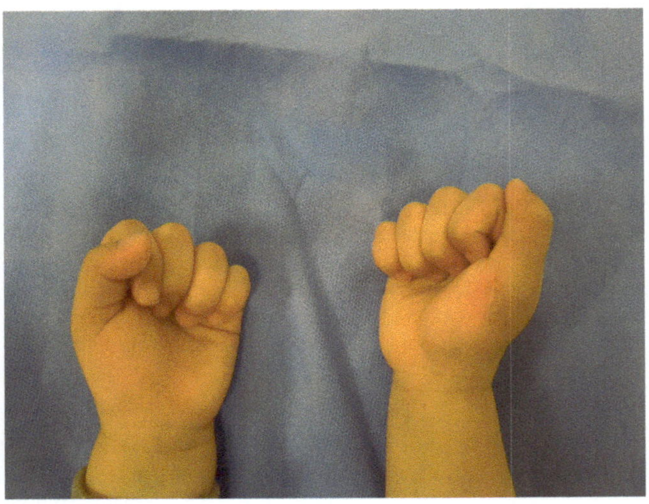

Fig. 19.30 Range of motion was good

procedure is indicated. Especially when the nail width is less than two-thirds of the contralateral normal side in unilateral cases, and when the nail width is less than that of index finger in bilateral cases, this modified technique is recommended. This modified procedure is different from the originally described method because it is an extra-articular procedure; the IP joint is reconstructed with one thumb and the other thumb contributes to only part of the distal phalanx for stability (Figs. 19.31 and 19.32). Both dorsal and volar incisions are necessary for this procedure. To prevent the so-called seagull deformity of the reconstructed nail, the contour of the nail bed can be manipulated. For example, a more rounded contour of the nail bed can be achieved by bending two parts more volarly. To make one smooth semicircular nail bed in the transverse plane, slight volar axial rotation is required (Fig. 19.33). Bony union between two distal phalangeal parts usually occurred within several months and rarely within a year.

For Wassel type 4 polydactyly, the original technique had been tried [30–32] and the authors reported good alignment and good joint stability. The medial portions of two distal phalanges as well as those of the two proximal phalanges should be resected for classic BC operation in Wassel type 4. However, it is almost impossible for phalangeal bones of bifid thumbs to be mirror images, especially in terms of height. A step-off between fused two proximal phalangeal bones at the IP joint is inevitable when the MP joint was coapted congruously. Otherwise, shaving of distal articular cartilage or shortening of one proximal phalangeal bone at shaft level is necessary.

When two bisected proximal phalanges are coapted, articular surface of proximal portion should be congruous because the MP joint is more important than IP joint functionally. There should be length mismatch between two portions at the IP joint level if two bones are not exactly the same height.

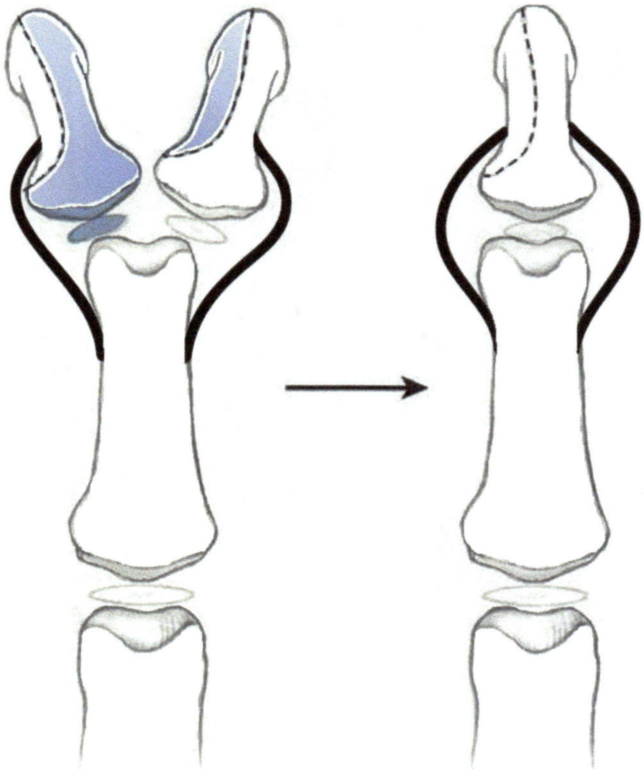

Fig. 19.31 Modified BC procedure for Wassel type 2. The shaded area is resected, and the two distal phalangeal bones are combined extra-articularly to preserve IP joint motion and to prevent epiphyseal plate injury

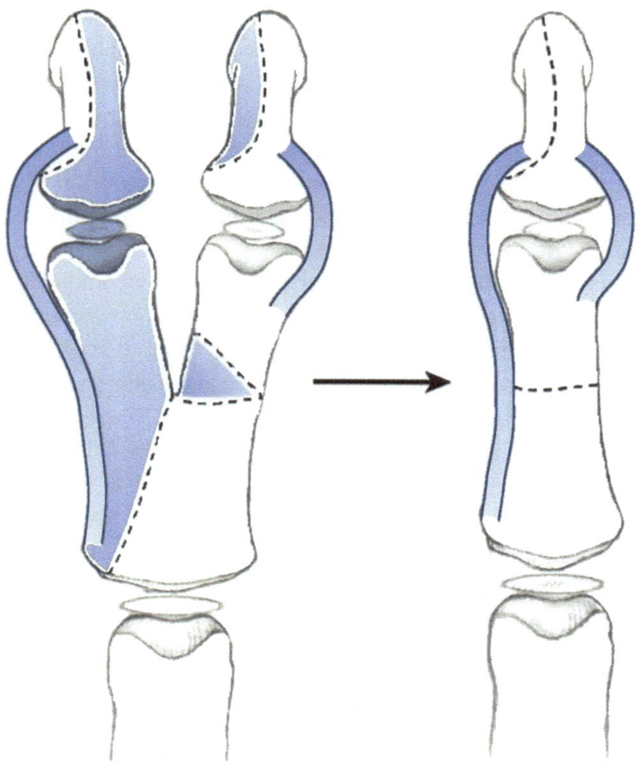

Fig. 19.32 Modified BC procedure for Wassel type 3. The corrective osteotomy of the proximal phalanx is performed when there is more than 20° of angular deformity

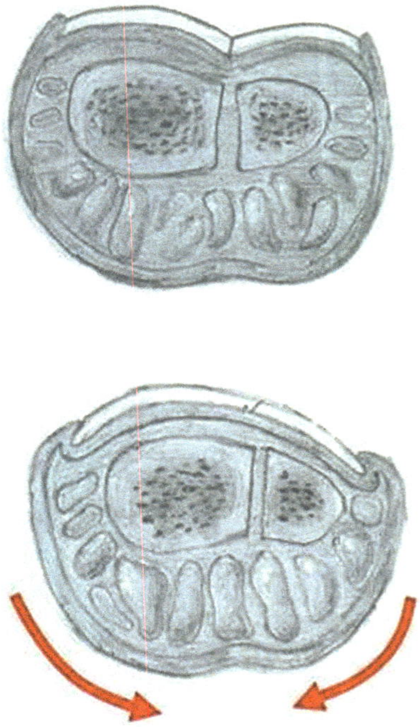

Fig. 19.33 Slight volar axial rotation is required to make smooth semi-circular nail bed

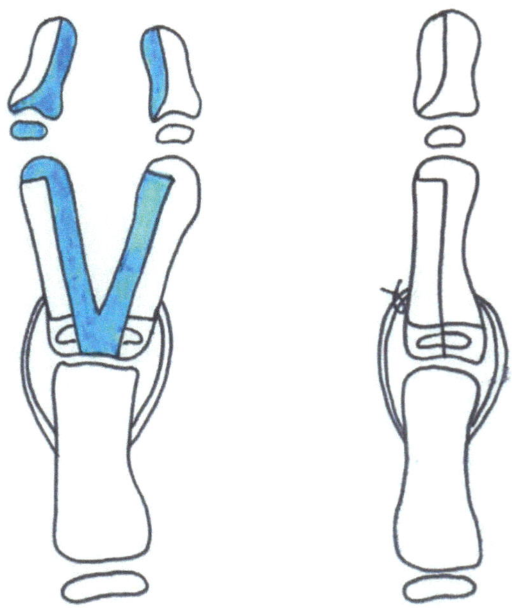

Fig. 19.34 Modified BC procedure for Wassel type 4. The articular surface of the MP joint is adjusted first after removal of central portions of two proximal phalanges. There is length discrepancy between two portions at the IP joint level if two bones are not exactly the same height. If the distal articular portion of proximal phalanx of dominant thumb is preserved, the remaining procedure is the same with that of type 2

If distal articular portion of proximal phalanx of dominant thumb is preserved and the same part of proximal phalanx of shorter minor thumb is removed, the reconstructed thumb will have a stable MP joint and mobile IP joint (Fig. 19.34). Previously mentioned modified BC technique is applied to at the IP joint and classic BC technique at the MP joint.

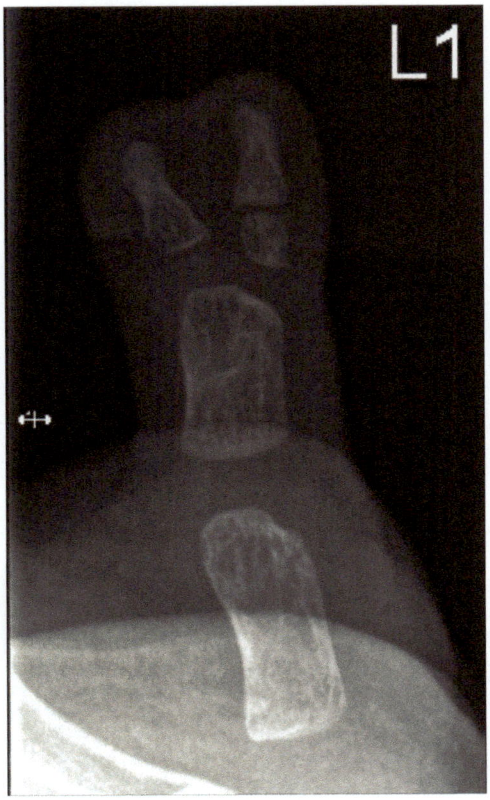

Fig. 19.35 The distal phalangeal epiphysis of the radial thumb showed abnormal triangular-shaped in this Wassel type 2 polydactyly

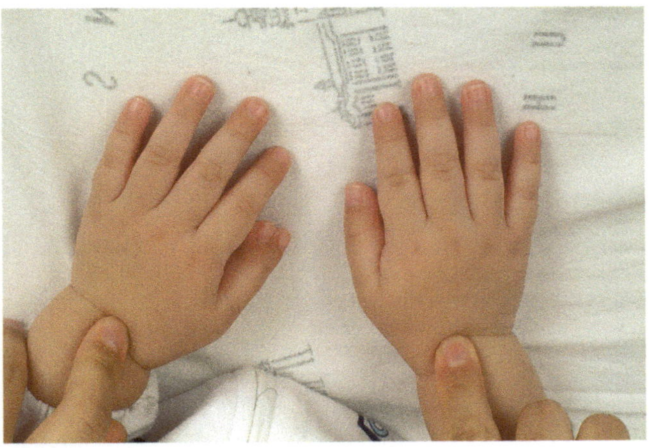

Fig. 19.36 The nail size of the polydactylic thumbs was smaller than those of the index fingers

Surgical Technique (Wassel Types 2, 3) [28, 29]

A 2-year, 1-month-old boy showed Wassel type 2 thumb polydactyly on the left hand. The distal phalangeal epiphysis of the radial thumb showed an abnormal triangular shape [33], while that of the ulnar thumb looked normal (Fig. 19.35). Thus, the ulnar thumb was chosen to be the main thumb of which most of the parts including IP joint would be preserved. The size of the nail of polydactylic thumbs was smaller than those of index fingers (Fig. 19.36).

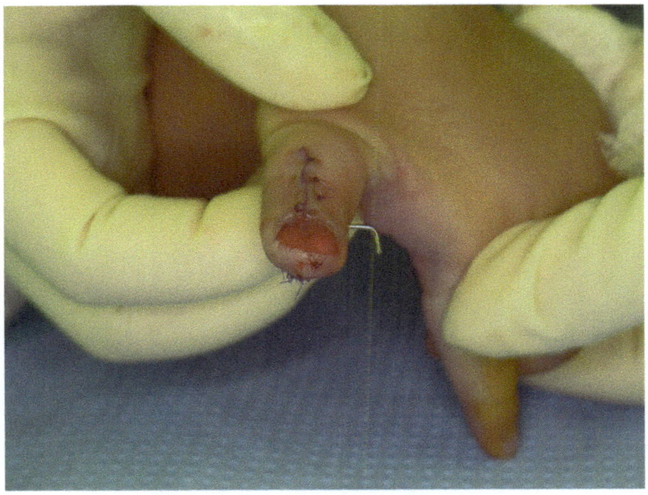

Fig. 19.37 A transverse K-wire was inserted for stability. The nail bed was repaired with 8-0 nylon sutures

Under tourniquet control, the nail plates were removed. Then soft tissues including skin and nail bed were removed along with the incision line. The base of the two distal phalanges was separated carefully. The main articulating digit, the ulnar side in this case, contained a major part of the distal phalangeal bone with the overlying nail bed. The radial minor thumb was made into a fillet flap containing only a small extra-articular part of the distal phalangeal bone supporting the incised nail bed and the collateral ligament attached to the proximal phalanx. Articular facet of proximal phalanx for minor radial thumb was shaved. The radial side of the main ulnar digit tuft was also trimmed with a small rongeur to make a better approximation with remaining portion of minor thumb.

The two distal phalangeal bones can be approximated and maintained by 5-0 nylon suture, one or two transverse K-wires, or a spinal needle in a very small thumb. The nail fold as well as nail bed was repaired with 8-0 nylon sutures (Fig. 19.37). The removed nail was trimmed and reinserted into the reconstructed nail fold for an internal splint. Two months after the operation, bony union was observed between the two portions of distal phalanges and the alignment was good (Fig. 19.38). Three months after the operation, the new nail grew well without deformity and IP joint motion was good (Figs. 19.39 and 19.40).

In a Wassel type 3 polydactyly, all the procedures are same as those of Wassel type 2 except the minor thumb is osteotomized at its bifurcation level. When there is more than 20° of angular deformity at the IP joint, a closed wedge osteotomy is performed at the proximal phalanx of the retained thumb. One or two K-wires are inserted to stabilize the osteotomy site.

All the K-wires are removed 4–6 weeks after the operation, even if the bony bridge is not observed between coapted distal phalanges, because bony union eventually be achieved.

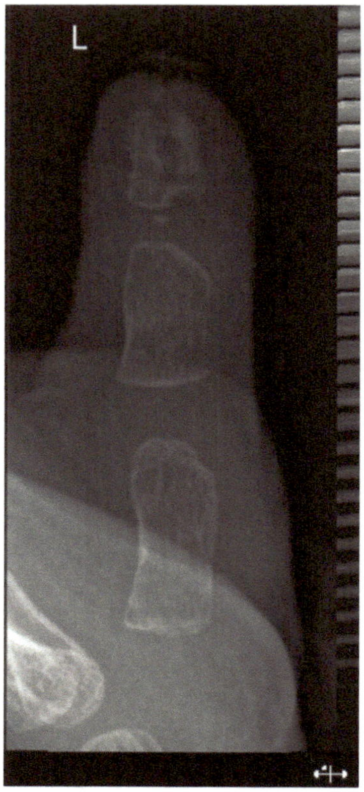

Fig. 19.38 Two months after the operation, bony union was achieved

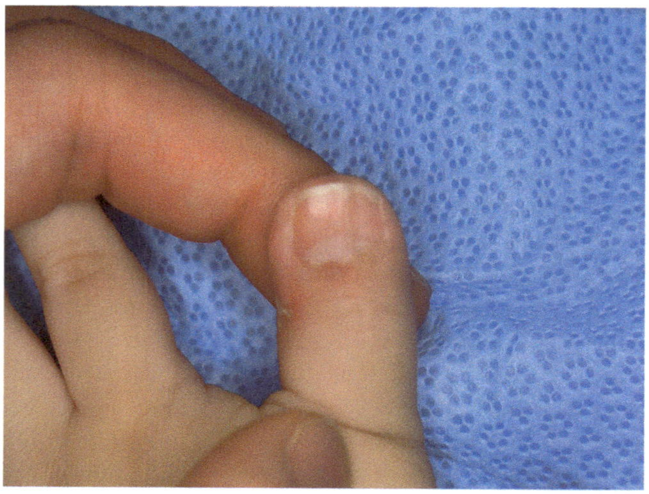

Fig. 19.39 Three months after the operation, the new nail grew well

Surgical Technique (Wassel Type 4)

A 15-month-old boy showed Wassel type 4 thumb polydactyly on right hand (Figs. 19.41 and 19.42). Dorsal and volar skin incisions were designed. Soft tissues were removed, and central portion of bifid proximal phalanges was resected. Two parts of proximal phalanges were coapted using 4-0 nylon to make the MP joint congruously. The EPL and FPL were realigned as previously described. For the IP joint, the same modified technique as in Wassel type 2 was applied.

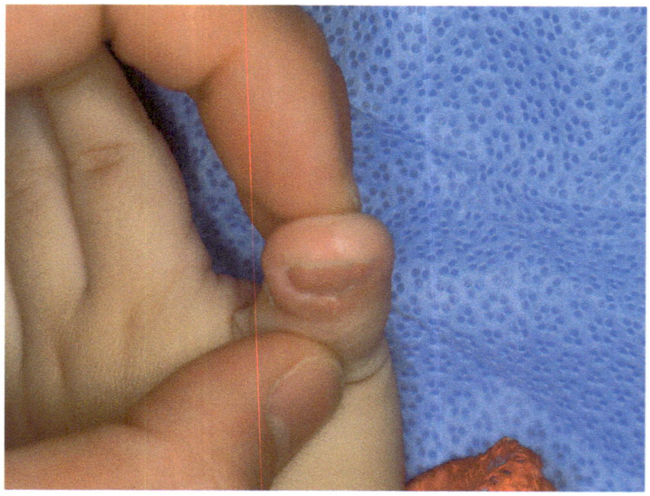

Fig. 19.40 The contour of the nail was smooth

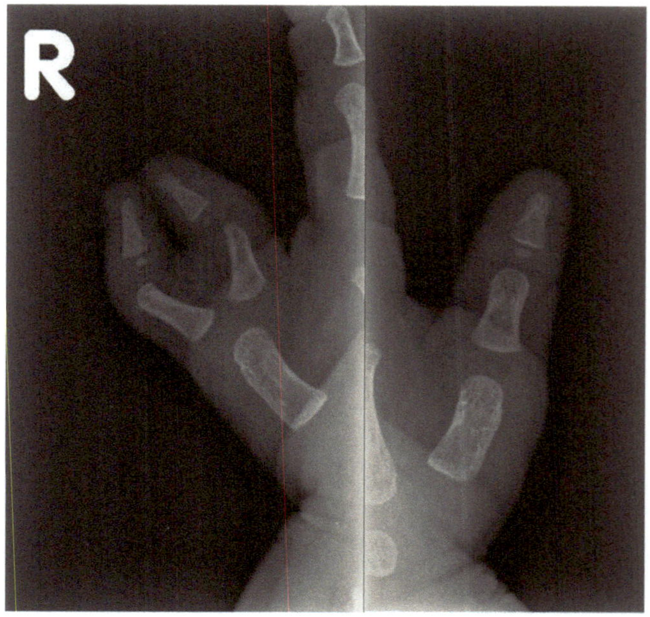

Fig. 19.41 Wassel type 4 polydactyly of right thumb. Bony hypoplasia of polydactylic thumbs was observed

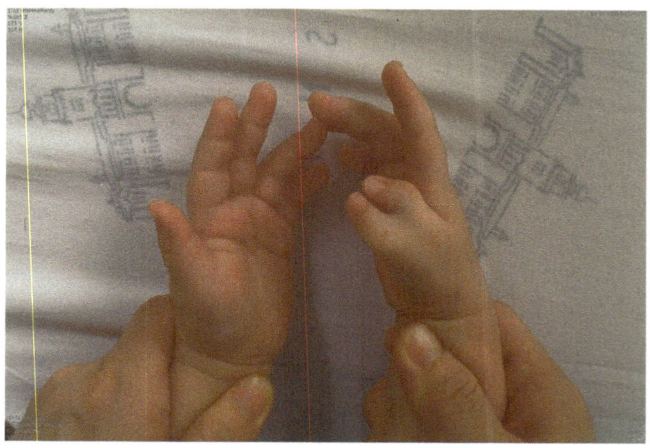

Fig. 19.42 The size of the nails of the polydactylic thumbs was smaller than those of index fingers

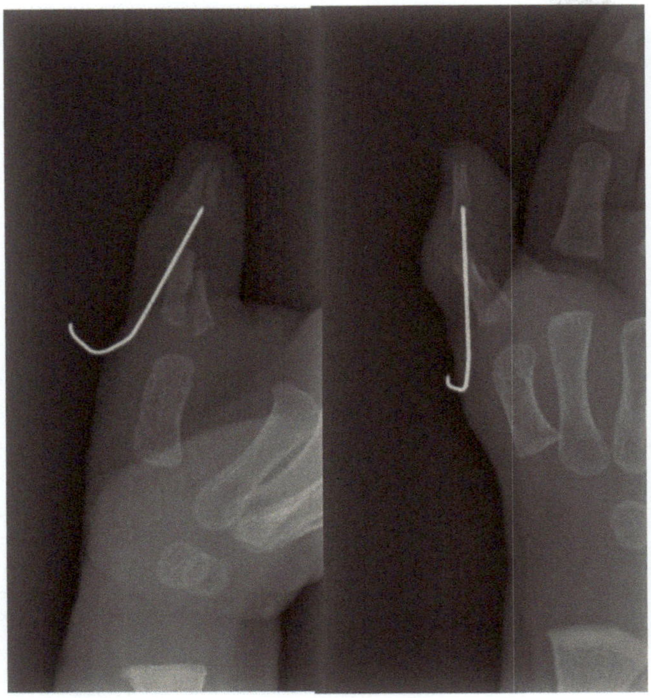

Fig. 19.43 Immediate postoperative radiographs after modified BC procedure

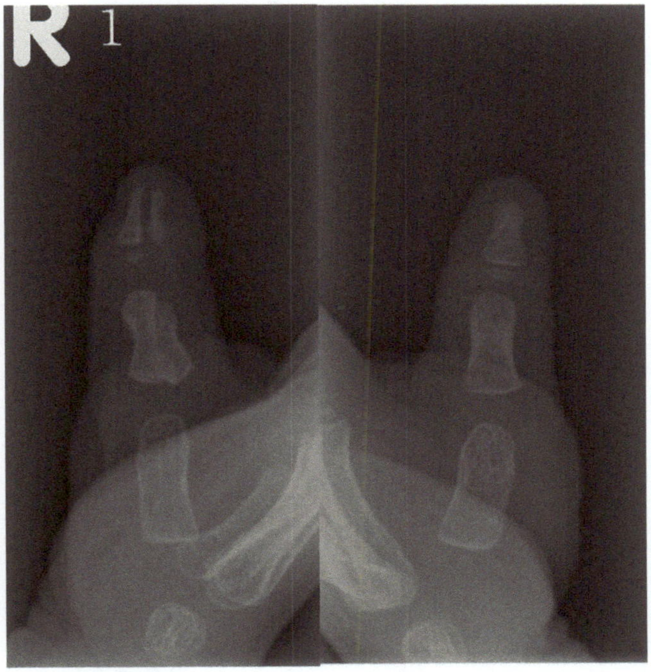

Fig. 19.44 At 4 months postoperatively, the MP joint became more congruous

After skin closure, removed nail was trimmed and reinserted. Although immediate postoperative radiographs showed an incongruous MP joint, the cartilaginous portions of coapted proximal phalanges were adjusted congruously (Fig. 19.43).

Four months after the operation, both IP and MP joints looked more congruous radiographically (Fig. 19.44). Three and half years after the operation, both IP and MP joints were becoming more congruous (Figs. 19.45 and 19.46). The epiphysis of the distal phalanx grew well without angular deformity. Two epiphyseal centers were noted at proximal portion of proximal phalanx. The flexion arcs of both MP and IP joints were almost equal to that of the normal side (Figs. 19.47 and 19.48).

On-Top Plasty

In certain patients with radial polydactyly, one thumb has a well-developed proximal part and a poorly developed distal part with an absent or hypoplastic nail, and the other thumb has a poorly developed proximal part but better distal parts, including nail and pulp. In this situation, better distal part of one thumb is transposed to the better proximal part of the other thumb. The transposed distal portion should have its own neurovascular bundle to feed itself, like a local neurovascular flap. The location of feeding artery to the transposed distal part can be traced by ultrasonography. At least one artery is usually identifiable.

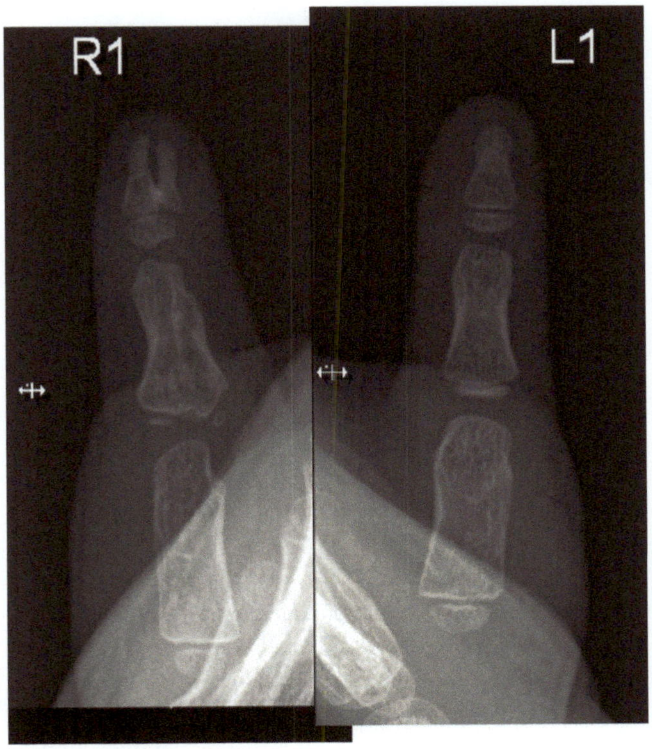

Fig. 19.45 Bony growth and alignment were good in AP view 3.5 years after the operation

Surgical Technique

An 11-month-old girl showed bilateral Wassel type 7 thumb polydactyly. The right side was operated on by the "excision and reconstruction" method. On the left hand, the radial-sided

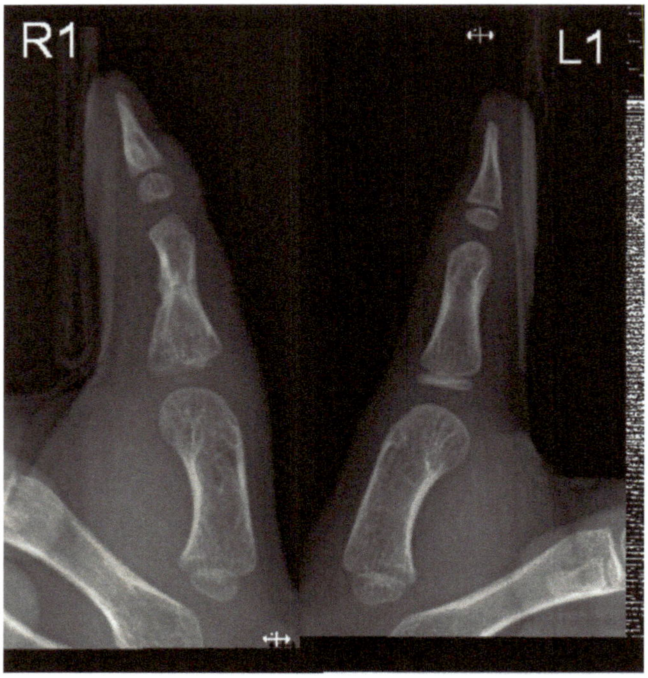

Fig. 19.46 Lateral views

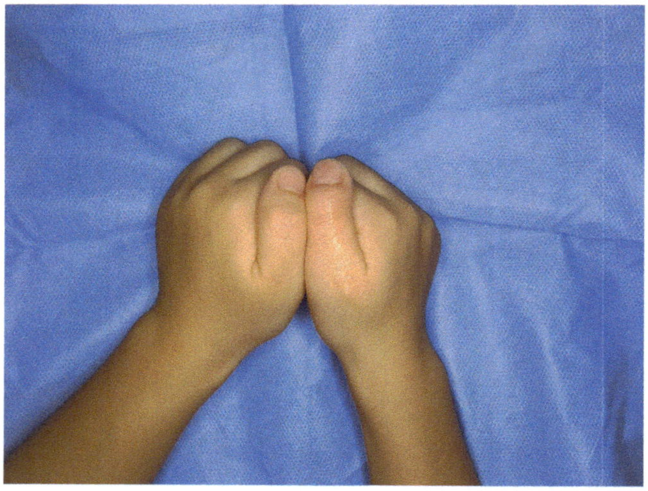

Fig. 19.47 Medical photos taken 3.5 years after the reconstruction

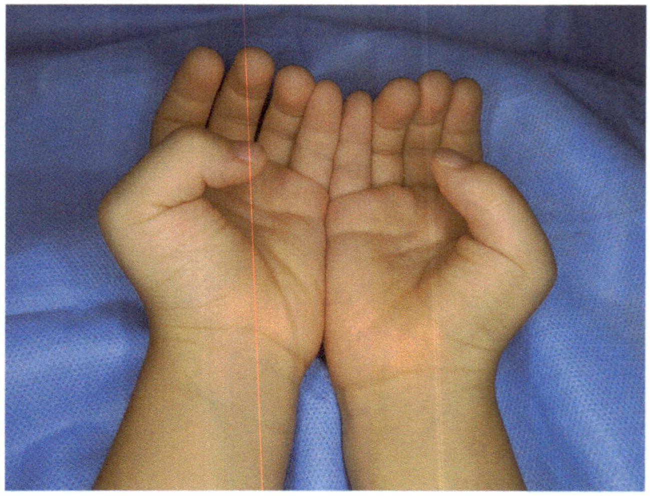

Fig. 19.48 Active range of motion was good at both IP and MP joints

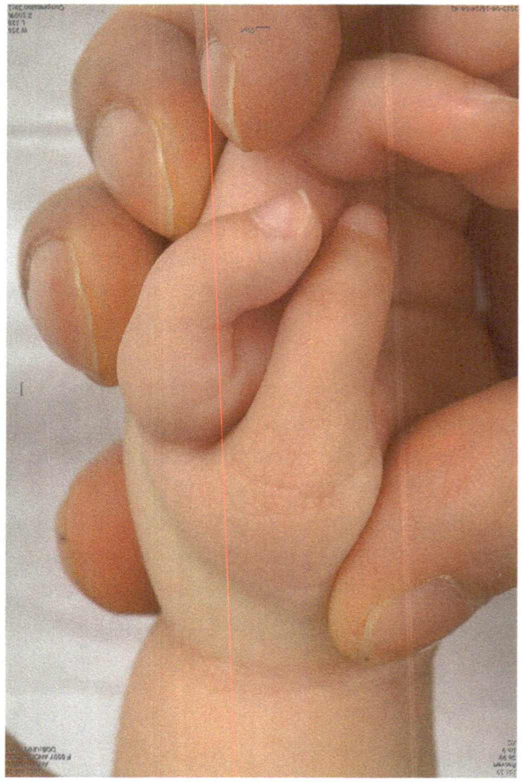

Fig. 19.49 Radial thumb showed good proximal part, and the ulnar thumb good distal part

thumb had a good proximal phalanx and MP joint, however, the distal phalangeal bone and nail were hypoplastic. The ulnar thumb had good nail, pulp, and distal phalangeal bone, but there was no bony connection with the radial thumb proximally (Figs. 19.49 and 19.50). Preoperative ultrasonography was performed to trace vascular supply to the ulnar thumb. Two vessels were identified dorsoradially and voloradially (Fig. 19.51). Skin incision was designed (Figs. 19.52 and 19.53). On the ulnar floating thumb, only the distal portion, including the nail and distal phalangeal bone, except the epiphysis, was isolated with vascular pedicle, and vascular perfusion was confirmed after tourniquet release (Fig. 19.54). On the radial main thumb, the distal portion, including the nail and distal phalangeal bone except epiphysis, was removed. Then a vascular pedicled portion of ulnar thumb tip was transposed to the top of radial thumb. The vascular bundle was buried into the soft tissue of ulnar

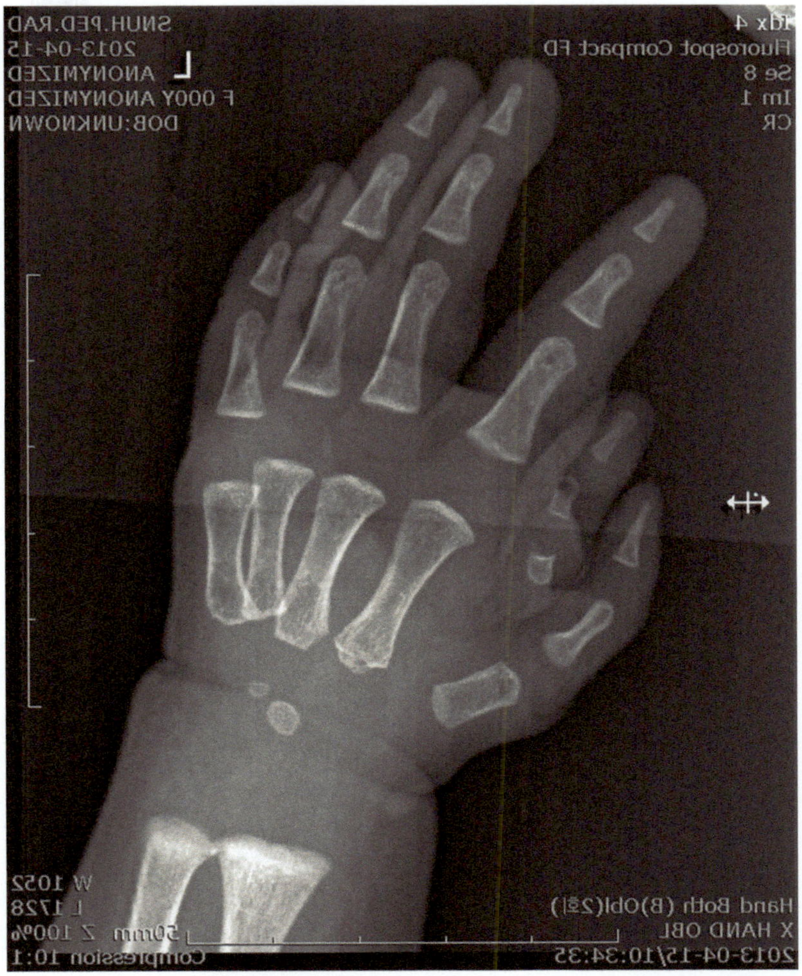

Fig. 19.50 The base of the ulnar thumb was not connected with the radial thumb

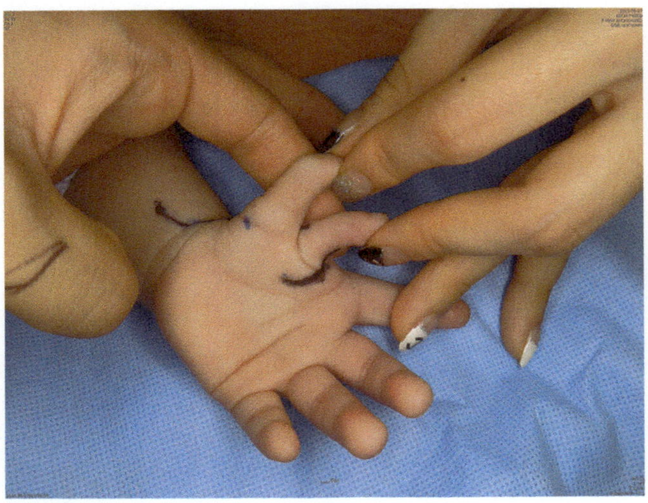

Fig. 19.51 Location of the vessels was identified by ultrasonography and marked

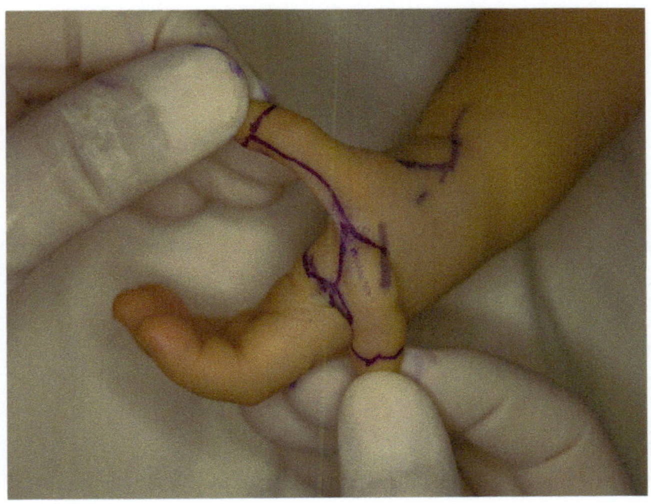

Fig. 19.52 Drawing of skin incision

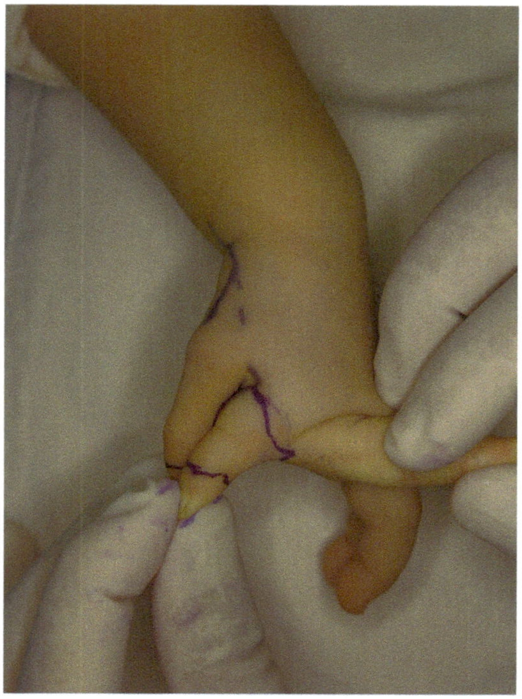

Fig. 19.53 Dorsal view of skin incision

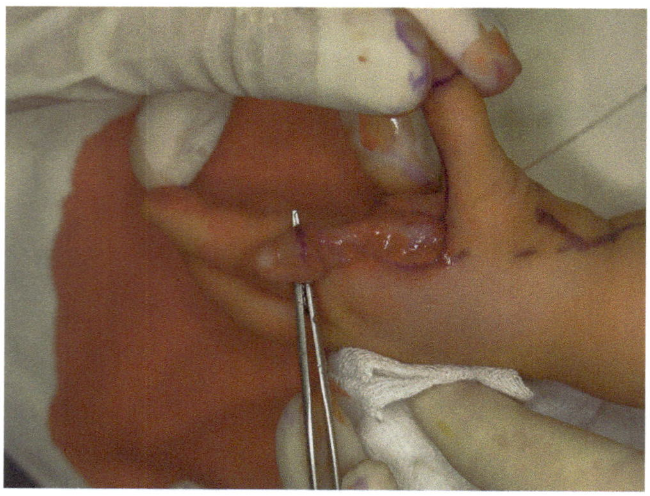

Fig. 19.54 Only the distal portion of ulnar thumb remained with vascular pedicles. Active bleeding and good circulation were noted after tourniquet release

side of the radial thumb. A longitudinal K-wire was inserted to fix the transposed part (Fig. 19.55). Immediate postoperative findings after the tourniquet release showed good alignment and circulation (Figs. 19.56, 19.57, and 19.58). Two months after the operation, the circulation of her left thumb maintained well and the thumb functioned nicely (Fig. 19.59).

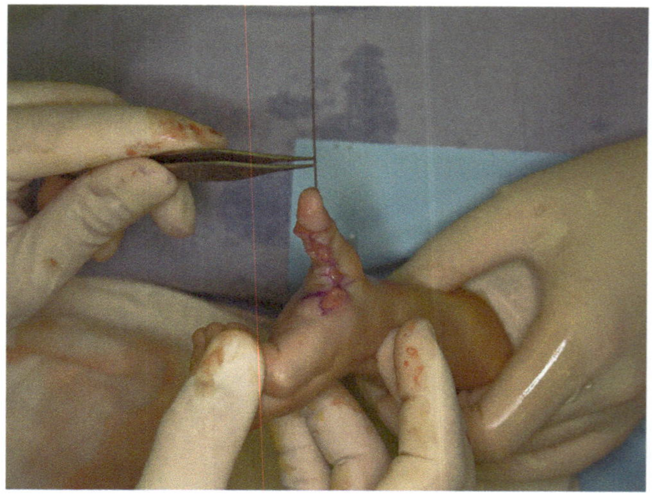

Fig. 19.55 The vascular pedicles were embedded on the ulnar side of the thumb. A K-wire was inserted for stability

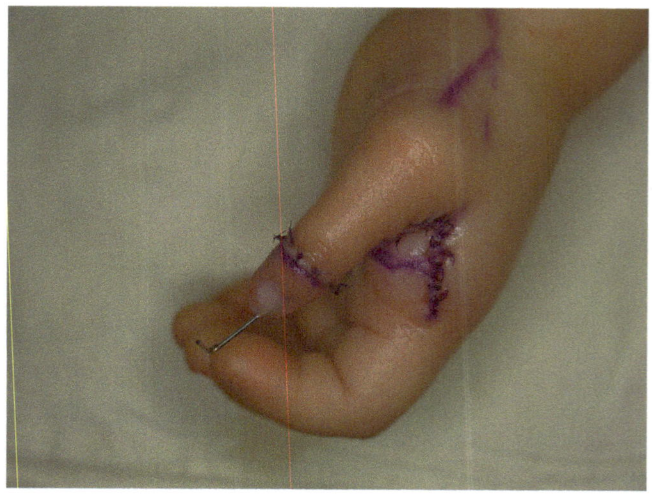

Fig. 19.56 Dorsal view of the reconstructed thumb

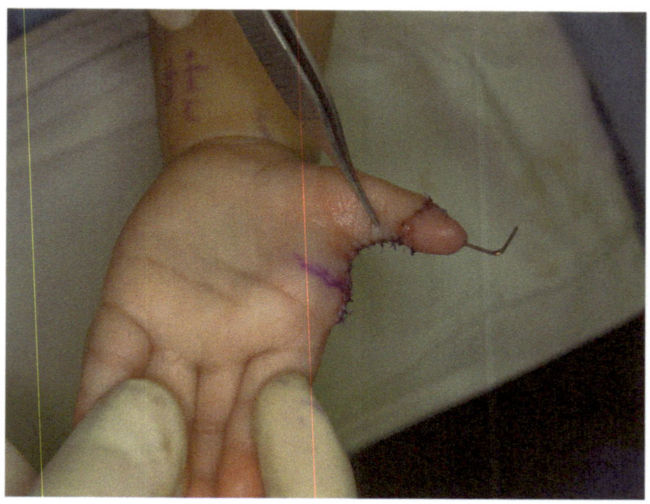

Fig. 19.57 First web space was well preserved

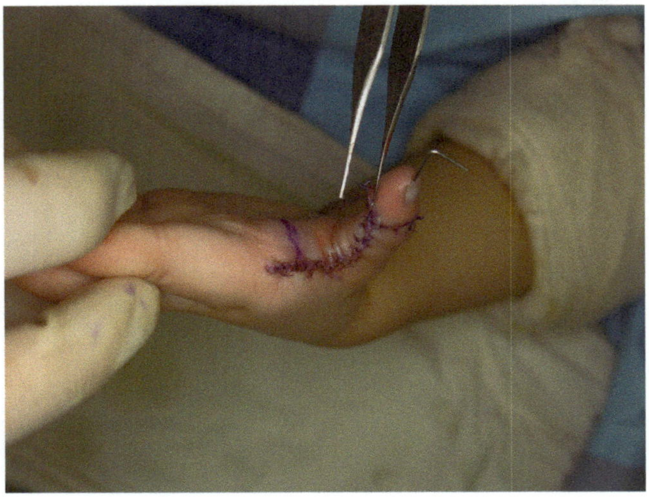

Fig. 19.58 After skin closure, the circulation of the transposed portion was well maintained

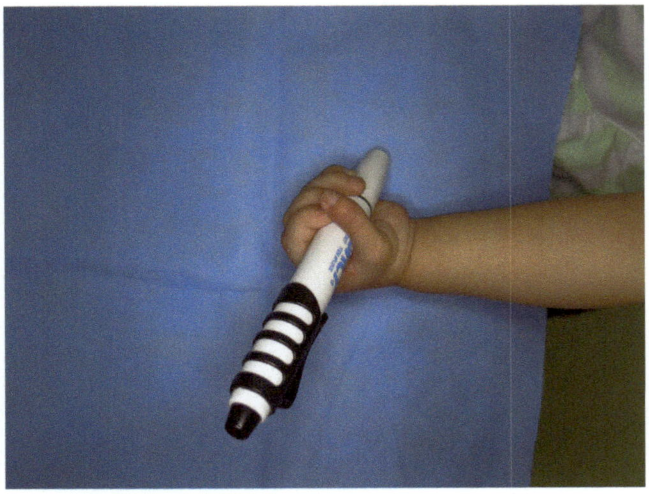

Fig. 19.59 Function and appearance were good 2 months after the operation

References

1. Upton J. Congenital anomalies of the hand and forearm. In: McCarthy JG, editor. Plastic surgery. Philadelphia: WB Saunders; 1980. p. 5240–398.
2. Oberg KC, Feenstra JM, Manske PR, Tonkin MA. Developmental biology and classification of congenital anomalies of the hand and upper extremity. J Hand Surg Am. 2010;35(12):2066–76. doi:10.1016/j.jhsa.2010.09.031.
3. Sesgin MZ, Stark RB. The incidence of congenital defects. Plast Reconstr Surg Transplant Bull. 1961;27:261–7.
4. Temtamy SA, McKusick VA. The genetics of hand malformations. Birth Defects (Original Article Series V). 1978;14:i–xviii, 1–619.
5. Wassel HD. The results of surgery for polydactyly of the thumb. A review. Clin Orthop Relat Res. 1969;64:175–93.
6. Ogino T, Minami A, Fukuda K, Kato H. Congenital anomalies of the upper limb among the Japanese in Sapporo. J Hand Surg Br. 1986;11(3):364–71.
7. Baek GH, Chung MS, Park YB, Yoo KH. The relative incidence of congenital anomalies of the hand. J Korean Orthop Assoc. 1997;32(4):796–801.
8. Wood VE. Polydactyly and the triphalangeal thumb. J Hand Surg Am. 1978;3(5):436–44.
9. Al-Qattan MM, Al Abdulkareem I, Al Haidan Y, Al Balwi M. A novel mutation in the SHH long-range regulator (ZRS) is associated with preaxial polydactyly, triphalangeal thumb, and severe radial ray deficiency. Am J Med Genet A. 2012;158A(10):2610–5. doi:10.1002/ajmg.a.35584.
10. Daluiski A, Yi SE, Lyons KM. The molecular control of upper extremity development: implications for congenital hand anomalies. J Hand Surg Am. 2001;26(1):8–22.
11. Hill P, Götz K, Rüther U. A SHH-independent regulation of Gli3 is a significant determinant of anteroposterior patterning of the limb bud. Dev Biol. 2009;328(2):506–16. doi:10.1016/j.ydbio.2009.02.017.
12. Al-Qattan MM. The distribution of the types of thumb polydactyly in a Middle Eastern population: a study of 228 hands. J Hand Surg Eur Vol. 2010;35(3):182–7. doi:10.1177/1753193409352417.
13. Tonkin MA. Thumb duplication: concepts and techniques. Clin Orthop Surg. 2012;4(1):1–17. doi:10.4055/cios.2012.4.1.1.
14. Chung MS, Baek GH, Gong HS, Lee HJ, Kim J, Rhee SH. Radial polydactyly: proposal for a new classification system based on the 159 duplicated thumbs. J Pediatr Orthop. 2013;33(2):190–6.
15. Townsend DJ, Lipp Jr EB, Chun K, Reinker K, Tuch B. Thumb duplication, 66 years' experience—a review of surgical complications. J Hand Surg Am. 1994;19(6):973–6.
16. Waters PM, Bae DS. Pediatric hand and upper extremity surgery. A practical guide. 1st ed. Philadelphia: Lippincott Williams & Wilkins; 2012. p. 41.
17. Goldfarb CA, Patterson JM, Maender A, Manske PR. Thumb size and appearance following reconstruction of radial polydactyly. J Hand Surg Am. 2008;33(8):1348–53. doi:10.1016/j.jhsa.2008.03.011.
18. Kozin SH. Deformities of the thumb. In: Wolfe SW, Hotchikiss RN, Pederson WC, Kozin SH, editors. Green's operative hand surgery. 6th ed. Philadelphia: Elsevier Churchill Livingstone; 2011. p. 1383.
19. Jobe MT. Congenital anomalies of the hand. In: Canale ST, Beaty JH, editors. Campbell's operative orthopaedics. 12th ed. St. Louis: Elsevier Mosby; 2013. p. 3755.
20. Leber GE, Gosain AK. Surgical excision of pedunculated supernumerary digits prevents traumatic amputation neuromas. Pediatr Dermatol. 2003;20(2):108–12.
21. Manske PR. Treatment of duplicated thumb using a ligamentous/periosteal flap. J Hand Surg Am. 1989;14(4):728–33.
22. Tupper JW. Pollex abductus due to congenital malposition of the flexor pollicis longus. J Bone Joint Surg Am. 1969;51(7):1285–90.
23. Lister G. Pollex abductus in hypoplasia and duplication of the thumb. J Hand Surg Am. 1991;16(4):626–33.
24. Hovius SE, Zuidam JM, de Wit T. Treatment of the triphalangeal thumb. Tech Hand Up Extrem Surg. 2004;8(4):247–56.
25. Bilhaut M. Guerison d'un poucebifide par un nouveau procedeoperatoire. Congr Fr Chirg. 1889;4:576–80.
26. Miura T. Duplicated thumb. Plast Reconstr Surg. 1982;69:470–81.
27. Tada K, Yonenobu K, Tsuyuguchi Y, Kawai H, Egawa T. Duplication of the thumb. A retrospective review of two hundred and thirty-seven cases. J Bone Joint Surg Am. 1983;65:584–98.

28. Baek GH, Gong HS, Chung MS, Oh JH, Lee YH, Lee SK. Modified Bilhaut-Cloquet procedure for Wassel type-II and III polydactyly of the thumb. J Bone Joint Surg Am. 2007;89(3):534–41.
29. Baek GH, Gong HS, Chung MS, Oh JH, Lee YH, Lee SK. Modified Bilhaut-Cloquet procedure for Wassel type-II and III polydactyly of the thumb. Surgical technique. J Bone Joint Surg Am. 2008;90(Suppl 2 Pt 1):74–86.
30. Hartrampf CR, Vasconez LO, Mathes S. Construction of one good thumb from both parts of a congenitally bifid thumb. Plast Reconstr Surg. 1974;54(2):148–52.
31. Samson P, Salazard B, Magalon G. The "Bilhaut-Cloquet" technique for treatment of thumb duplication. Handchir Mikrochir Plast Chir. 2004;36(2–3):141–5.
32. Tonkin MA, Bulstrode NW. The Bilhaut-Cloquet procedure for Wassel types III, IV and VII thumb duplication. J Hand Surg Eur Vol. 2007;32(6):684–93.
33. Baek GH, Chung MS, Gong HS, Lee S, Lee YH, Kim HH. Abnormal triangular epiphysis causing angular deformity of the thumb. J Hand Surg Am. 2006;31(4):544–8.

Ulnar Polydactyly and Ulnar Dimelia

20

Matthew E. Hiro, Hilton Phillip Gottschalk, and Terry R. Light

Overview

Ulnar polydactyly represents one of the most frequent hand congenital anomalies while ulnar dimelia is one of the most unusual congenital abnormalities. Ulnar polydactyly is common in many families particularly in families of African ancestry. Both conditions demonstrate variable pathologic anatomy due to failure of differentiation of the anterior–posterior axis of the upper limb. Other congenital abnormalities are commonly associated with each of these conditions. Ulnar polydactyly and ulnar dimelia may be diagnosed prenatally. Both diagnoses are apparent upon physical examination at birth. Appropriate diagnostic work-up should consider associated conditions. Surgical reconstruction of the affected extremity should improve the aesthetic appearance of the hand while preserving or improving upper extremity function.

Ulnar Polydactyly

Ulnar polydactyly, also known as postaxial polydactyly, represents a spectrum of disorders involving duplication of digits or parts of digits along the ulnar side of the hand. In contrast, radial, or preaxial polydactyly, involves the thumb and central polydactyly involves the index, middle, or ring fingers. Ulnar polydactyly arises due to failure of differentiation of the anterior–posterior axis of the hand plate during embryologic formation of the upper limb [1]. The epidemiology, genetics, and treatment of ulnar polydactyly are entirely unique [2, 3] and in many ways dissimilar from either radial or central polydactyly. Ulnar polydactyly is classified as *Class III/Duplication* using the International Federation of Societies for Surgery of the Hand (IFSSH) Classification [4]. The condition is categorized as *Class 1B2 Malformations/Failure of Axis of Formation of Hand Plate Anterioposterior Axis* according to the modified Oberg, Manske, Tonkin (OMT) Classification [5].

M.E. Hiro, M.D. (✉) • T.R. Light, M.D.
Department of Orthopaedic Surgery and Rehabilitation, Stritch School of Medicine, Loyola University Chicago, 2160 South First Avenue, Maywood, IL 60153, USA
e-mail: mhiro@lumc.edu; tlight@lumc.edu

H.P. Gottschalk, M.D.
Department of Pediatric Orthopaedics, Dell Children's Medical Center, 1301 Barbara Jordan Blvd., Ste 300, Austin, TX 78723, USA
e-mail: hpgottschalk@gmail.com

Classification

Supernumerary digits in ulnar polydactyly usually present as one of two forms described by Temtamy and McKusiak as Type A and Type B [6]. Type A ulnar polydactyly digits are well-developed digits located on the ulnar border of the small finger, whereas Type B describes a hypoplastic, pedunculated, or small finger nubbin. Several other classification schemes are described in Table 20.1 [2, 6–10].

Epidemiology

Ulnar polydactyly, the most frequent congenital hand difference in African American children occurs in approximately 1 in 150 newborns [3]. Although this condition is far less common in Caucasian (1:1,400), Mexican (1:700), and Middle Eastern patients (1:1,000), it is, nonetheless, one of the most frequently encountered congenital abnormalities of the upper limb. There are several differences in associations of ulnar polydactyly in children of different racial backgrounds [10, 11].

In African American children, the condition is usually inherited in an autosomal dominant pattern and is rarely associated with other hand anomalies, congenital syndromes, or non-syndrome systemic abnormalities. The ulnar polydactyly occurring in most African American children is usually classified as Type B ulnar polydactyly.

D.R. Laub Jr. (ed.), *Congenital Anomalies of the Upper Extremity: Etiology and Management*, DOI 10.1007/978-1-4899-7504-1_20, © Springer Science+Business Media New York 2015

Table 20.1 Classification schemes utilized in ulnar polydactyly

Temtamy classification [6]	Type A: well-formed and functioning digit on ulnar side of small finger
	Type B: small nonfunctioning digit that may be pedunculated or a nubbin
Stelling classification [7]	Type 1: digit with soft tissue only
	Type 2: digit with phalangeal elements
	Type 3: digit with phalangeal and metacarpal elements
Buck-Gramko classification [9]	Type V rud: digit with soft tissue only
	Type V distal phalanx: digit with bifid distal phalanx
"Universal" classification	Type V distal interphalangeal (DIP) joint: digit with two distal phalanges articulating at DIP joint
	Type V middle phalanx: digit with bifid middle phalanx
	Type V proximal interphalangeal (PIP) joint: digit with two middle phalanges articulating at PIP joint
	Type V proximal phalanx: digit with bifid proximal phalanx
	Type V metacarpal phalangeal (MCP) joint: digit with two proximal phalanges articulating at MCP joint
	Type V metacarpal: digit with bifid metacarpal
	Type V carpometacarpal (CMC) joint: digit with two metacarpals articulating with the CMC joint
Rayan classification [2]	Type I: small "wart-like" skin nubbin without a nail or bone
	Type II: digit with small nail and bone with or without a joint that has no tendons and no function
	Type III: digit that is more developed than type II with hypoplastic or absent PIP joint and articulation with MCP joint or bifid fifth metacarpal
	Type IV: fully developed sixth digit with a sixth metacarpal
	Type V: others; including ulnar polydactyly with syndactyly and other bony abnormalities
Al-Qattan classification [10]	Type I: small nubbin without bone or nail
"Modified Rayan"	Type IIA: Pedunculated non-functioning digit with narrow pedicle (<3 mm)
	Type IIB: Pedunculated non-functioning digit with wider pedicle (>3 mm)
	Type IIIA: Well-formed functioning digit articulating with bifid metacarpal or partially duplicated fifth metacarpal
	Type IIIB: Well-formed functioning digit with proximal phalanx fused to fifth metacarpal
	Type IV: digit with separate sixth metacarpal
	Type V: others; including polysyndactyly and triplication of small finger
Pritsch classification [8] for Type A only	Type I: fully developed sixth metacarpal that articulates at CMC joint "metacarpal type"
	Type II: digit on lateral side of fifth digit with intercalated distal metacarpal remnant "metacarpal phalangeal type"
	Type III: digit from hypoplastic sixth metacarpal or fused to fifth metacarpal "phalangeal type"
	Type IV: digit from metacarpal phalangeal joint "intercalated type"
	Type V: digit from bifid proximal phalanx "fully developed type"

Cases are usually bilateral (70 %). The left hand is more commonly affected in unilateral cases [2, 11]. There is equal sex distribution [10, 11].

In patients of non-African decent, ulnar polydactyly is usually sporadic. Only 5 % of patients of non-African decent demonstrate a recognizable pattern of inheritance. Non-African descent patients demonstrate both Type A and Type B ulnar polydactyly. Twenty percent of cases are bilateral and males are more commonly affected than females [11]. Non-African patients also demonstrate a higher incidence of associated hand conditions including polysyndactyly, mixed polydactyly, and isolated syndactyly than do African American children. Foot involvement (i.e., lateral toe polydactyly) may also be present in some children. Cases may also be associated with other congenital syndromes [12–15]. Associated syndromes and their inheritance patterns are listed in Table 20.2. Other congenital abnormalities not associated with one of the listed syndromes are uncommon [16].

Isolated, non-syndrome ulnar polydactyly is also strongly associated with genetic inheritance patterns. Both autosomal dominant and autosomal recessive patterns have been described. Genetic analysis has linked ulnar polydactyly to chromosomes 7, 13, and 19 [13, 17–21]. However, the exact pattern of inheritance of ulnar polydactyly is uncertain and most likely more complex than simple Mendelian genetics [11, 22]. Environmental exposure has been suggested as posing a risk for the development of ulnar polydactyly [23].

Pathogenesis

Although ulnar polydactyly is linked to failure of differentiation of the anterior–posterior axis of the developing limb bud,

Table 20.2 Syndromes associated with ulnar polydactyly [12–15]

Name	Associated anomalies	Inheritance
Ellis–van Crevald syndrome	Dwarfism, short limbs, small chest, dental abnormalities, cardiac defects	Autosomal recessive
Smith–Lemli–Opitz syndrome	Abnormal facies, microcephaly, intellectual disability, cardiac, renal, gastrointestinal and genital malformations, hypotonia,	Autosomal recessive
McKusick–Kaufman syndrome	Genital malformations (hydrometrocolpos), cardiac defects	Autosomal recessive
Trisomy 13/Patau syndrome	Intellectual disability, cardiac defects, brain/spinal cord abnormalities, microophthalmia, cleft lip/palate, hypotonia	Sporadic
Short rib-polydactyly I–III	Small chest, short limbs, cardiac defects, polycystic kidney disease, cardiac, gastrointestinal and genital abnormalities	Autosomal recessive
Orofaciodigital syndrome	Abnormal facies, oral and dental abnormalities, cleft lip/palate, polycystic kidney disease (type I only)	Type I: X-linked dominant Others: autosomal recessive
Bardet–Biedel syndrome	Visual loss, obesity, intellectual disability, hypogonadism, abnormal facies, cardiac, hepatic and gastrointestinal abnormalities	Autosomal recessive
Meckel syndrome	Occipital encephalocele, other neural tube defects, polycystic kidney disease, cirrhosis	Autosomal recessive
Greig cephalopolysyndactyly syndrome	Abnormal facies, macrocephaly, intellectual disability, large hallux/thumb	Autosomal dominant
Pallister–Hall syndrome	Brain abnormalities (hypothalamus hamartoma), bifid epiglottis, imperforate anus, renal abnormalities	Autosomal dominant
Weyers acrofacial dysostosis	Dental abnormalities, malformed nails, shortened limbs	Autosomal dominant
Joubert syndrome	Brain abnormalities (molar tooth sign), hypotonia, ataxia, intellectual disability, abnormal facies, retinal dystrophy, renal, hepatic and endocrine abnormalities	Autosomal recessive, rare X-linked recessive
Simpson-Galabi-Behmel syndrome	Abnormal facies, polythelia, diaphragmatic hernia, umbilical hernia, renal abnormalities, hepatosplenomegaly, intellectual disability, solid organ malignancy	X-linked dominant
Hydrolethalus syndrome	Abnormal facies, cleft lip/palate, hydrocephalus, brain abnormalities, cardiac defects, airway stenosis, omphalocele	Autosomal recessive
Acrocallosal syndrome	Macrocephaly, corpus callosum agenesis, abnormal facies, cleft lip/palate, cardiac abnormalities	Autosomal recessive
Asphyxiating thoracic dystrophy/Jeune syndrome	Small chest, short ribs, short limbs, pelvic abnormalities, respiratory failure	Autosomal recessive
Focal dermal hypoplasia/ Goltz-Gorlin syndrome	Multiple skin abnormalities, cutaneous papillomas, ocular abnormalities, dental abnormalities, cleft lip/palate	X-linked dominant

the exact mechanism is unknown. Embryologic limb development occurs in a coordinated fashion along the three spatial axes in a complex series of steps that begin with limb bud formation [1]. The embryologic formation of the upper limb is detailed in elsewhere in this book (Chap. 1). As the limb bud develops and lengthens along the proximal–distal axis, the zone of polarizing activity (ZPA) is established in the posterior mesoderm. Sonic hedgehog (SHH), elaborated by the ZPA, influences digital development and identity along the anterior–posterior axis. SHH contributes to the unique formation of the ulnar-sided structures of the forearm, wrist and hand including the ulna, the two ulnar columns of the carpal bones, and the small finger, ring finger, and the ulnar half of the middle finger. Deficiency of SHH leads to ulnar ray deficiency and overexpression of SHH leads to radial polydactyly [14]. Ulnar polydactyly has been linked to the Gli-3 transcription factor, an important protein in the signaling pathway of SHH located on chromosome 7 [24]. The Gli-3 protein exists in an active form (Gli-3A) and a repressor form (Gli-3R). Gli-3A exists primarily in the posterior mesoderm and displays the same gradient as SHH with decreasing concentrations anteriorly. Gli-3R has the opposite gradient with higher concentrations in the anterior mesoderm and decreasing concentrations posteriorly. Syndromes associated with ulnar polydactyly have been associated with defects in the Gli-3 gene as well as with defective processing of the Gli-3 protein into its active form [14, 25]. The normal balance of Gli-3 is disturbed when there is a relative increase in Gli-3R compared to Gli-3A. It has been proposed that this imbalance contributes to the formation of ulnar polydactyly [14].

Anatomy

Type B ulnar polydactyly includes rudimentary supernumerary digits that arise from the ulnar border of the small finger (Fig. 20.1). Because these digits lack bony elements and tendons, they are nonfunctional. The digits may be as small

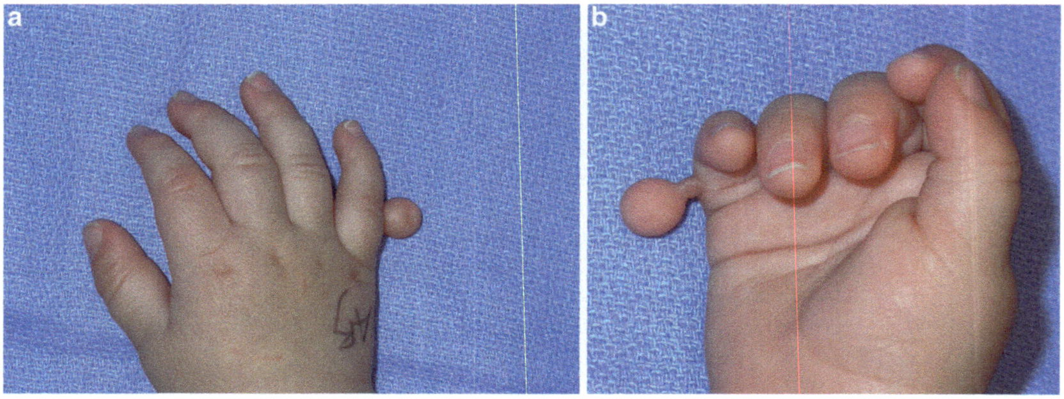

Fig. 20.1 (a) Dorsal and (b) volar views of a child with Type B ulnar polydactyly demonstrating a large pedunculated mass with a long stalk. There is a rudimentary nail present on dorsal aspect

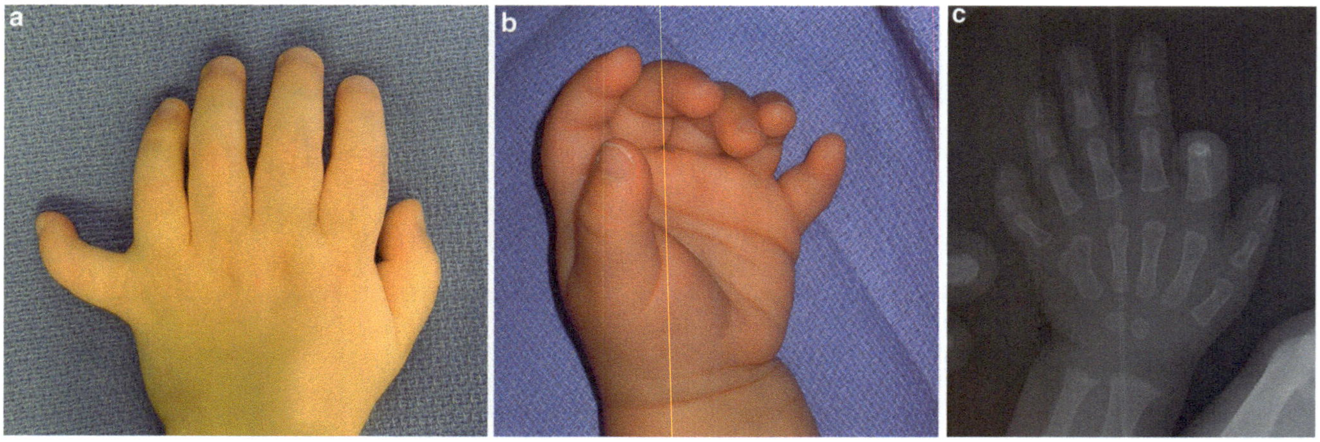

Fig. 20.2 (a) Dorsal and (b) volar views of a child with Type A ulnar polydactyly. The extra digit is fully formed with bony elements. There is some ulnar angulation of the digit compared to the adjacent small finger. (c) Hand radiographs demonstrate the proximal phalanx of the polydactylous digit is articulating with an abnormally broad metacarpophalangeal joint along the ulnar side of the joint. The joint surface is sloped ulnarly, which explains the angulation of the extra digit

as a wart-like bump on the ulnar side of the small finger proximal phalanx or may take the form of a somewhat more developed digit with a fibro-cartilaginous ossicle and a hypoplastic nail [3, 26]. The small, wart-like bumps, or rudimentary polydactyly, are considered to be remnant stumps from digits that were auto-amputated in utero [27, 28]. "Pacifier polydactyly" refers to a specific Type B polydactyly demonstrated by a very large and edematous soft tissue nubbin that is consistently sucked by the patient [29]. All Type B supernumerary digits, including rudimentary polydactyly, contain a neurovascular pedicle.

Type A ulnar polydactyly includes more developed digits with variable anatomy (Fig. 20.2). Type A digits always contain bony elements and may contain anomalous flexor and extensor tendons including the insertion for the abductor digiti minimi (ADM) and flexor digiti minimi brevis (FDMB) muscles. The interphalangeal joints are often hypoplastic and stiff. Digits that extend to or beyond the metacarpophalangeal (MCP) joint, either with a bifid metacarpal or a duplicated proximal phalanx articulating with a common metacarpal phalangeal joint, will include the insertion for the ulnar collateral ligament of the metacarpal phalangeal joint. A sixth metacarpal may include the insertions of the opponens digiti minimi (ODM) and be surrounded by the muscle bellies of the ADM and FDMB muscles. Type A digits contain digital nerves and arteries.

Diagnosis

Ulnar polydactyly, particularly Type A, may be diagnosed prenatally during routine second trimester ultrasound [15]. Remaining cases of ulnar polydactyly usually should be diagnosed during routine postnatal physical exams. Most cases of rudimentary ulnar polydactyly may be diagnosed by careful examination of the skin on the ulnar border of the

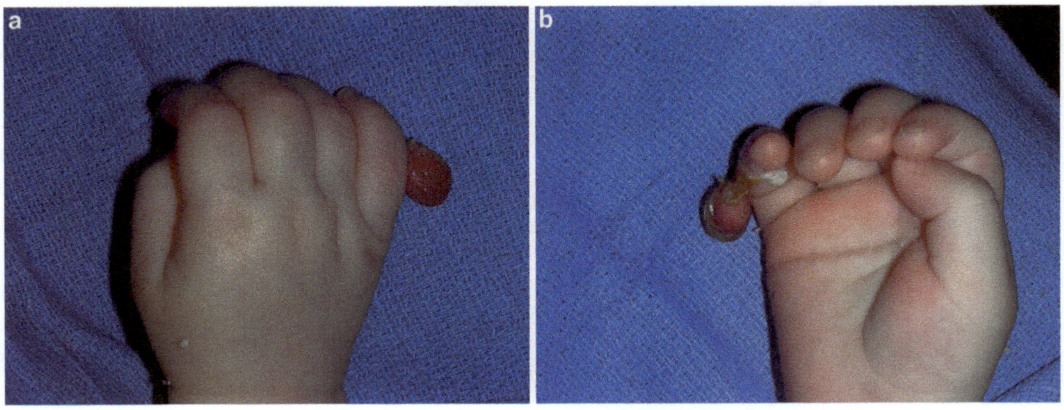

Fig. 20.3 (**a**) Dorsal and (**b**) volar views of a child treated with suture ligation of Type B ulnar polydactyly. One week after the suture was placed, the digit demonstrates significant edema and necrosis. The stalk can be seen to be separating from the ulnar aspect of the small finger. The digit subsequently fell off and the area went on to heal without complication

hand. The physical examination should focus on elements associated with syndromes that include ulnar polydactyly (see Table 20.2). In children with Type A ulnar polydactyly, anterior–posterior radiographs will help clarify the bony anatomy of the supernumerary digit. Family history should be obtained to determine a potential genetic causation. Referral to a geneticist should be considered in patients with evidence of congenital syndromes or isolated familial ulnar polydactyly. Referral to other pediatric specialists should precede surgical treatment of the ulnar polydactyly.

Treatment

The families of patients with Type A ulnar polydactyly are often surprised and distressed by their child's hand difference. The treatment of ulnar polydactyly is not an emergency. Type A ulnar polydactyly with a fully formed sixth ray may be functional. The family may still opt for surgery to give the hand a more "normal" appearance. In some cultures ulnar polydactyly is seen as a supernatural trait and individuals with extra digits were often given deferential treatment [30].

Many newborns with Type B ulnar polydactyly are treated by ligation without hand surgery consultation. Small, pedunculated digits are commonly treated by suture ligation by the nursery staff, pediatricians, obstetricians, and neonatal intensivists. With time the digit becomes ischemic and falls off days to weeks after the suture is applied [3] (Fig. 20.3). Vascular clips have also been used to cause ischemia by clamping across the pedicle of the digit. It has been reported that in untreated patients, the digit may auto-amputate and fall off without intervention [2]. Newborns with more completely developed ulnar polydactyly are usually referred to a hand surgeon [31].

Open excision of Type B digits in the nursery or office is an alternative to ligation that avoids the creation of a necrotic digit. The patient is soothed with a pacifier and the hand anesthetized with local anesthesia. The area is prepped and the supernumerary digit is excised in a fusiform pattern. The base of the wound is coagulated using a battery cautery, electrocautery, or topical silver nitrate and closed using simple absorbable suture. Topical antibiotic ointment or steristrips may be applied to the area as a dressing. The area typically heals with a small scar that is rarely problematic.

Because Type A polydactyly generally requires treatment under general anesthesia, surgery is delayed until the child is 6 months old. The goal of surgery is to excise abnormal bony and soft tissue elements while preserving function of the small finger. The incision should be designed using a racquet shape around the supernumerary digit preserving as much skin as possible. The incision can be extended proximally in the mid-lateral line of the finger and hand along the junction of the glabrous and non-glabrous skin. The skin is incised and sharp and blunt dissection is used to expose the bony elements of the digit. The bony elements are isolated from the surrounding subcutaneous tissue. Anomalous flexor and extensor tendons are sharply dissected, incised, and allowed to retract into the hand. The neurovascular bundles to the extra digit are identified. Traction neurectomies are performed on the digital nerves and the arteries are cauterized using bipolar cautery. The skin flaps are trimmed to allow for a linear closure that should lie in the midlateral line. Standing cutaneous deformities "dog-ears" should be corrected extending the incision longitudinally or along flexor creases.

Ulnar polydactyly that extends to or is proximal to the fifth metacarpal phalangeal joint deserves special attention. The hypothenar muscles, including the insertion of the ODM and muscle bellies of the ADM and FDMB, should be preserved and dissected from the extra metacarpal in the subperiosteal plane. In cases where the polydactyly extends proximal to the metacarpal phalangeal joint, the ADM insertion on the extra proximal phalanx is preserved with a

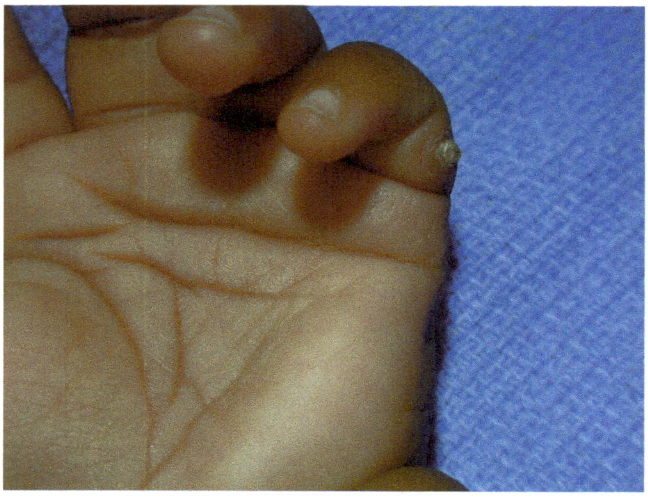

Fig. 20.4 A scar remained on the ulnar aspect of the small finger after suture ligation of Type B ulnar polydactyly. This area may be painful and contain a neuroma. Surgical correction including re-excision and traction neurectomies should be considered in patients who have problematic scars after suture ligation

periosteal sleeve. The ADM insertion is transferred to the base of the radial proximal phalanx to assure small finger abduction. If the polydactyly includes two proximal phalanges articulating with the small metacarpal at the MCP joint, the insertion of the ulnar collateral ligament on the base of the extra proximal phalanx should also be preserved with a periosteal sleeve. After excision of the ulnar digit, the ulnar collateral ligament should be transferred to the base of the retained proximal phalanx. When the metacarpal is bifid, osteotomy of the metacarpal creates a more normal contour of the residual small finger metacarpal. Angulation of the metacarpal should be corrected with closing wedge osteotomies and Kirschner wire fixation. The ulnar collateral stability of the reconstructed metacarpal phalangeal joint of the small finger should be tested. If additional stability is necessary, suture capsulorrhaphy with pin fixation of the MCP joint should be considered. The extrinsic flexor and extensor tendons should be centralized if eccentric.

Complications

Treatment-related complications are surprisingly more frequent in suture ligation than in surgical excision [2]. First, unless the suture is tied exactly at the base of the pedunculated digit, where it originates from the skin of the small finger, the skin that remains that is proximal to the suture may persist as a visible and palpable bump (Fig. 20.4); this occurs in up to 40 % of patients who undergo suture ligation [2, 3]. A painful neuroma may form at the amputation site. Improvement after excision of the remainder of the bump and traction neurectomies of the nerves has been demonstrated by several studies [32–34]. This occurrence of this complication may be minimized by surgical excision of pedunculated Type B ulnar polydactyly with traction neurectomy [35]. Other complications associated with suture ligation include bleeding, infection, and necrosis without amputation [2, 33].

Complications from treatment of Type A ulnar polydactyly are uncommon. Infection, bleeding, and wound healing difficulties have been reported but may be minimized with a well-planned and executed operation [2, 36]. Reconstruction of ulnar polydactyly tends to result in less symptomatic joint instability or stiffness compared to radial polydactyly. Nonetheless, cases with postoperative prominence of small finger metacarpal head, instability of the metacarpal phalangeal joint and intrinsic tightness have been reported [37].

Ulnar Dimelia

Ulnar dimelia is a rare form of duplication in which the ulnar side of the forearm, wrist, and hand is represented on both the preaxial as well as postaxial side of the limb. As with ulnar polydactyly, the condition is a result of abnormal differentiation along the anterior–posterior axis of the developing limb bud. Ulnar dimelia is included in the IFSSH *Class III/Duplication* category [4]. The condition is classified as Class 1A2 *Malformations/Failure of Axis of Formation of Entire Upper Limb Anterioposterior Axis* using the modified OMT Classification [5].

Classification

Most commonly, ulnar dimelia is characterized by duplication of the ulna, absence of the radius, absence of the thumb, and seven or eight digits symmetric about the midline. Because each patient demonstrates unique anatomic structural variations, a spectrum of mirror hand-multiple hand anomalies has been suggested [38]. A classification system of ulnar dimelia limbs is shown in Table 20.3. Type 1A is the most common form while the others (Type 1B–Type 5) are exceedingly rare [38].

Epidemiology

Ulnar dimelia is one of the most rare forms of upper extremity congenital difference. Most cases have been detailed as isolated reports or series with just over 60 cases reported in the literature [39]. Although ulnar dimelia is usually sporadic and unilateral [40, 41], it is a component of autosomal dominant syndromes including Laurin–Sandrow and Martin syndromes [38, 42–44].

Table 20.3 Classification for mirror hand-multiple hand spectrum[a]

Type	Name	Description
1A	Ulnar dimelia	Multiple fingers with two well-formed ulnae
1B	Ulnar dimelia	Multiple fingers with well-formed medial ulna, lateral ulna is hypoplastic
2	Intermediate type	Multiple fingers with two ulnae and a radius. Central ulna is vestigial [49]
3A	Intermediate type	Multiple fingers with one ulna and well-formed radius
3B	Intermediate type	Multiple fingers with one ulna and a hypoplastic radius
4A	Laurin–Sandrow syndrome	Bilateral multiple fingers, with two ulnae, complex syndactyly, multiple toes, nasal deformities
4B	Martin syndrome	Bilateral multiple fingers with a radius and an ulna, complex syndactyly, multiple toes, nasal deformities
5	Multiple hand	Complete hand duplication including thumb with normal forearm anatomy

[a]Adapted from J Hand Surg (Edinburgh, Scotland), 23/4, Al-Qattan MM, Al-Thunayan A, De Cordier M, Nandagopal N, Pitkanen J, Classification of the mirror hand-multiple hand spectrum, 534-6, Copyright 1998, with permission from Elsevier

Pathogenesis

The exact mechanism leading to ulnar dimelia has yet to be discovered. It is recognized that the ZPA is critical to defining the anterior–posterior axis of the developing limb bud; errors in differentiation of the ZPA are likely important to the etiology of ulnar dimelia. Several genes have been identified that result in atypical mirror hand (Type 3A/B) in animals including TWIST1, ALX4, and GLI-3 [45]. These genes can be associated with an abnormal increase in SHH activity on the anterior aspect of the limb bone leading to hypoplasia of the radius. Classic Type 1A ulnar dimelia may be a result of an error in the pre-patterning stage of limb development and may involve abnormal expression of the genes HOXB8, GLI-3, and HAND2 [45]. Type 4 is most likely related to gene mutations in SHH, while Type 5 may represent to be a true duplication of the ZPA [38].

Anatomy

The anatomy of ulnar dimelia is highly variable. The abnormal condition involves the entire upper extremity. Because the radius is absent, typical descriptions of anatomic structures should not be based on their location on the "radial" or "ulnar" sides of the forearm or hand. Instead, structures may be designated by their position on the medial (postaxial) or lateral (preaxial) side of the extremity.

Proximal elements of the arm may be abnormal including the scapula, clavicle, humerus, and glenohumeral joint [46–48]. The distal humerus articulates with both ulnas. The lateral aspect of the distal humerus exhibits a hypoplastic capitellum, which often resembles a poorly formed trochlea. The biceps and triceps may be underdeveloped or replaced with fibrous bands [48, 49]. The biceps may abnormally be inserted onto the distal humerus [50].

The forearm contains two parallel ulnae-like bones that are rotated from 70° to 180° to each other [41, 51]. The proximal portion of the lateral ulna often contains a broad articulation, not unlike an olecranon. However, since it is malrotated in the plane of the lateral hypoplastic trochlea, elbow motion is limited. The elbow is typically extended with a variable arc of passive and active flexion. Distally, the articular surfaces of the lateral or both ulnae are broad and often appear similar to the articular surface of the distal radius [41, 52]. The absence of a proximal or distal radioulnar joint results in little to no pronation or supination between the two forearm bones.

In the forearm, the flexor muscles tend to originate from both proximal ulnae. The medial musculature tends to be more developed with a normal appearing flexor carpi ulnaris. The lateral wrist flexor may be absent or abnormally inserted into the wrist capsule [49]. The wrist is typically flexed and deviated to either the medial or the lateral side. The presence of pronator teres and pronator quadratus has been described [49]. The flexor digitorum superficialis (FDS) and flexor digitorum profundus (FDP) may have common muscle bellies and have variable origins on the forearm bones. The FDS and FDP tendons are often present in each digit, though adjacent digits may share a common, bifurcated tendon. Function of the digital flexors can be highly variable and the proximal interphalangeal (PIP) and distal interphalangeal (DIP) joints are often stiff [46]. The extensor tendons are thin and may be duplicated to the central digit. Often the wrist and finger extensor muscles are absent with tendons that do not extend proximal to the wrist [49].

The carpus is symmetric with duplication of the ulnar elements including two pisiforms, two triquetrums, and two hamates. The central lunate or capitate may be fused or separated [46, 52]. The scaphoid and trapezium are absent. A hypoplastic trapezoid may be present at the distal aspect of the carpus articulating with the distal capitate and central metacarpals [46, 49]. The ulnocarpal joint is narrow and incongruent. The carpus may form a fibrous pseudoarthrosis in a volarly subluxed and flexed position [49].

The hand is broad and flat with absent thenar and hypothenar contours. Seven or eight digits may be arranged in separate clusters on the medial and lateral aspect of the hand.

Each digit may have an individual metacarpal or two adjacent digits may share a metacarpal. The metacarpals lack the normal cascade and are aligned in a single plane from medial to lateral. Digits are usually triphalangeal though biphalangeal digits have been seen [50, 53]. Syndactyly and clinodactyly may be present [46–48, 53]. Finger flexion is usually limited due to stiffness of the PIP and DIP joints and intrinsic function may be poor.

A large medial ulnar nerve innervates the more medial one and a half digits, like a normal ulnar nerve. An additional lateral ulnar nerve with an accompanying artery supplies the more lateral digits, or the sensory branch of the radial nerve may innervate them. The median nerve supplies the central digits although it may bifurcate in the forearm [49]. Electromyography demonstrates substantial cross innervation of the intrinsic muscles from both medial and lateral nerves to the median nerve [51].

The arterial anatomy of the ulnar dimelia hand is variable. The arterial anatomy may be asymmetric within the hand with a dominant medial ulnar artery supplying the majority of the digits. A smaller lateral artery perfused only the lateral two and a half of the seven digits in one studied hand. Another description demonstrated a large medial ulnar artery and a central median artery without a lateral vessel [49]. This asymmetry is interesting given the relative symmetry of bone and other soft tissue elements in ulnar dimelia. The arteries do not seem to communicate in a superficial arch, though a deep communication may be present [49, 52]. Anomalies in the common digital arteries have also been described [54].

Diagnosis

Due to the significant hand differences associated with ulnar dimelia, the clinical diagnosis is relatively straightforward and can often be detected on prenatal ultrasound.

Treatment

Ulnar dimelia is so uncommon that most hand surgeons will not encounter a single case in their practices. Hand and upper extremity surgeons should recognize the characteristic anatomic features of ulnar dimelia. Treatment begins with appropriate family counseling. They should be educated on the sporadic nature of ulnar dimelia though a brief family history should be included to ensure a syndromic form is not present.

A full physical exam including a comprehensive assessment of the upper extremity needs to be performed. Shoulder abnormalities are frequent in children with ulnar dimelia. All joints from the shoulder to the fingertip should be assessed for passive and active range of motion. Treatment should be designed to facilitate positioning of the hand in space, to normalize the appearance of the hand, and to maximize hand function. Thus, close observation of the child in clinic is important and can reveal significant information about the function of the upper extremity. Standard video assessments may also be of benefit. The parents often have insight into the child's successes and struggles with specific activities and should be encouraged to share their experiences. Repeat physical examinations may be necessary to accurately characterize the deficiencies present in a patient with ulnar dimelia [55].

Standard radiographs to include the hand, wrist, forearm, elbow, and shoulder will delineate the bony and joint anatomy of the involved extremity. Syndromic patients should have referral to appropriate pediatric subspecialists and genetic counselors as necessary.

Initial treatment should be designed to improve the wrist and elbow position and digital range of motion [52]. Passive range of motion with stretching and splinting should be initiated as early as possible to keep joints supple for future reconstruction if necessary. Once motion gain has plateaued with therapy, surgical reconstruction should be considered.

There are several reasons to consider operative treatment for ulnar dimelia. The elbow often lacks active or passive flexion making hand to mouth activities impossible. The flexed wrist often rests in flexion lacking active extension. The fingers, particularly the lateral digits, are usually stiff resulting in weak flexor function and poor positioning of the hand in space. Though the hand lacks traditional thumb opposition, the lateral cluster of digits is pronated in relation to the medial digits allowing some large object grasping activities. Finally, the unusual appearance of the mirror hand with its characteristic seven or eight digits and absent thumb attracts unwanted attention resulting in social challenges for the child.

Surgical treatment of the elbow aims to improve elbow flexion. The proximal portion of the lateral ulna abuts against the dysplastic distal humerus and blocks elbow and forearm motion. The biceps is often replaced with a fibrous cord. When passive motion is present, active motion depends upon the forearm flexor muscles. Several procedures have been described to improve elbow flexion. Subperiosteal resection of the proximal portion of the lateral ulna may permit the medial forearm to flex and extend at the lateral ulnotrochlear joint [50, 56] (Figs. 20.5 and 20.6). Other studies have shown modest improvement in supination and pronation with excision of the proximal lateral ulna [54]. The child should be monitored closely since regrowth of the proximal ulna may constitute a recurrent bony block [46]. Repeat resection should be undertaken and should include resection of the anterior distal humerus [50, 54]. Reconstruction of the lateral collateral ligament of the elbow may be necessary. Tendon transfer of the pectoralis major muscle for elbow flexion should be considered in patients with good passive but poor active elbow range of motion [51]. It is essential to preoperatively confirm function of the pectoralis prior to transfer since many patients with ulnar dimelia have hypoplasia of chest musculature. If an abnormal insertion of the biceps tendon onto the distal humerus is detected, transfer of the biceps insertion to the anterior forearm may also be of benefit [50]. If the forearm is positioned in an extreme of pronation or supination, rotational osteotomy of the one or both ulnae may bring the hand into neutral rotation or a slightly pronated position.

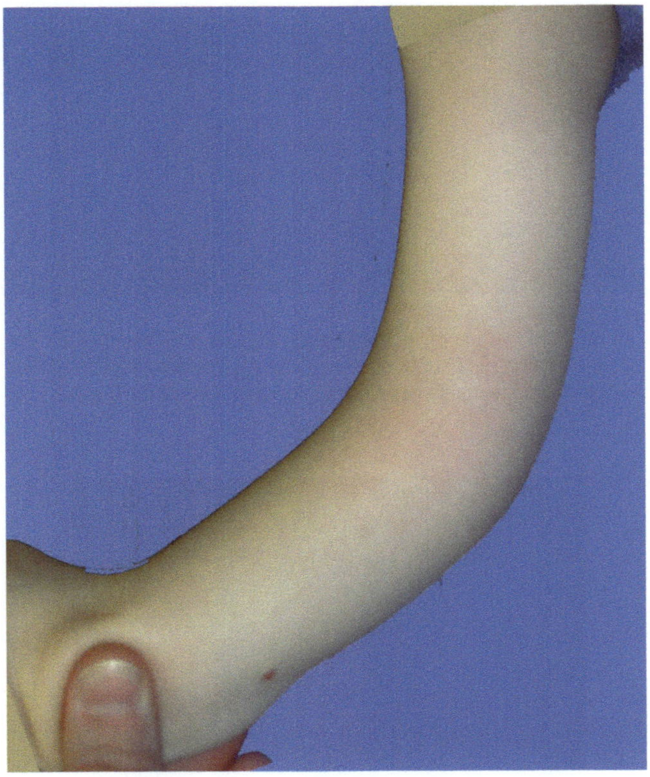

Fig. 20.5 Preoperative view of a child with ulnar dimelia with incomplete elbow flexion. The hand is to the left of the picture. Passive and active flexion of the elbow was limited to approximately 30°

Surgery of the wrist is designed to correct the flexed and deviated posture of the hand and establish active wrist extension. Procedures to release the flexion deformity and to augment wrist extension include palmar skin z-plasty, fractional lengthening of the flexor carpi ulnaris tendons, volar capsulotomy, dorsal capsule plication, extensor tendon shortening, or proximal carpectomy [50, 56]. Tendon transfer can confer active extension of the wrist. The transfer may be inserted into the extensor carpi radialis, if present, or directly into the second metacarpal. Donor motors include the flexor carpi ulnaris or residual flexor or extensor tendons from amputated fingers during digital reduction surgery [47, 50, 52, 53, 56]. Arthrodesis can help position the wrist and improve grip strength, but should be reserved for extreme cases not amenable to contracture release or tendon transfers [39].

The abnormal appearance of the seven or eight digit hand should be considered. The goals of hand reconstruction should include reduction in the number of digits to create a five-digit hand that includes a thumb for opposition.

The lateral cluster of digits should be reduced to a single digit while preserving the medial four digits. The medial cluster will serve as the index through small fingers. The lateral digits should be evaluated by physical exam findings and by observation of the child at play to determine which of these fingers is most readily reconstructed to function as a thumb. The other digits should be amputated.

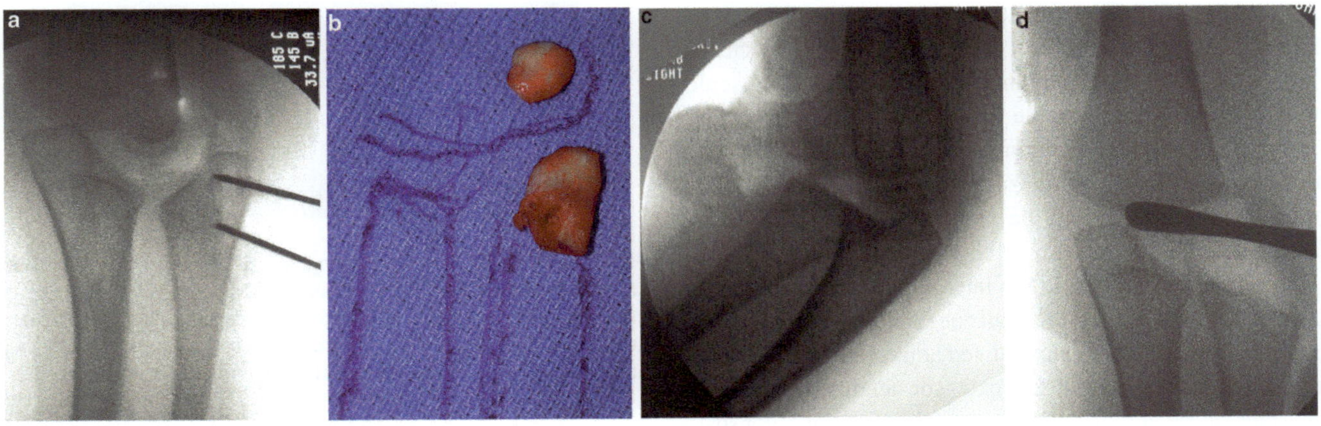

Fig. 20.6 Intraoperative views of the corrective surgery to improve elbow flexion. (**a**) Anterior fluoroscopic images of the abnormal elbow joint with two ulnae articulating with the humerus. The proximal aspect of the lateral ulna is blocking motion. Two Kirschner wires have been placed in the proximal lateral ulna designating the area to be resected. Subperiosteal dissection was used to expose this portion of the lateral ulna. After resection of this portion of the lateral ulna, full flexion was still restricted by an anterior projection from the articular surface of the hypoplastic capitellum. This was similarly excised. (**b**) The bony fragments removed demonstrating their relationship to the surrounding joint. (**c**) Anterior and (**d**) lateral fluoroscopic images of the elbow joint after excision of the proximal lateral ulna and portion of the capitellum. Full passive elbow flexion was achieved at the completion of the bony excision

Amputation of the redundant digits should be designed to preserve sufficient skin to resurface the reconstructed hand and first webspace. Tissues should be retained until the reconstruction is complete and it is certain that they could not be useful elsewhere [54]. Flexor and extensor tendons can be transferred for wrist extension or opponensplasty. Before completion amputation of the other digits, the blood supply of the digit that will become the new thumb should be confirmed. Aberrant arterial anatomy has been described and may make compromise the thumb reconstruction if it involves the selected digit [54].

Early techniques for thumb reconstruction involved merely amputating the redundant digits and leaving one to function as the thumb [46, 47, 55, 57]. Because the lateral cluster of digits is often pronated compared to the medial cluster, the retained digit was often adequately positioned to allow for opposition. Splinting the reconstructed thumb in abduction can improve the position [47]. Another technique involved creating a syndactyly between two of the lateral digits to make a broad and strong thumb [48, 58].

Others described a two-stage technique with the reconstruction beginning with reduction to a five-fingered hand and using redundant skin and subcutaneous tissue to resurface the first webspace [52]. The second stage involved rotational and shortening osteotomy of the metacarpal of the preserved lateral digit to a position that provides opposition with the medial cluster of digits. Some authors still recommend this technique with adequate long-term results [56]. The advantage of this technique is that it is simple and carries a low risk of vascular compromise. However, the reconstructed thumb will be triphalangeal and may appear too long compared to the contralateral thumb.

The amputation of two fingers in a seven-digit hand or of three digits in an eight-digit hand normalizes the number of digits (Figs. 20.7, 20.8, and 20.9). Pollicization of one of the lateral digits in the hand with ulnar dimelia is usually elected [50, 51, 53, 54, 59]. Though many digits and many musculotendinous units are available for this reconstruction, pollicization in these hands remains challenging. However, some differences between pollicization in ulnar dimelia and in thumb hypoplasia should be mentioned. The digital artery anatomy in ulnar dimelia may be abnormal and careful mapping of the arterial tree to the lateral cluster should be confirmed before selecting the digit for pollicization [54]. Since multiple digits are being amputated adjacent to the pollicized digit, redundant long flexor/extensor tendons or intrinsic muscles of the amputated digits may be used for reconstruction of the thumb intrinsic muscles. Opponensplasty at the time of pollicization should be considered, as the reconstructed intrinsic muscles are rarely adequate for opposition after surgery. Often, the lateral digits are short and the metacarpal shortening should be conservative to prevent the pollicized digit from being too small. An excellent review of pollicization in ulnar dimelia should be reviewed for additional technical details of this procedure [54].

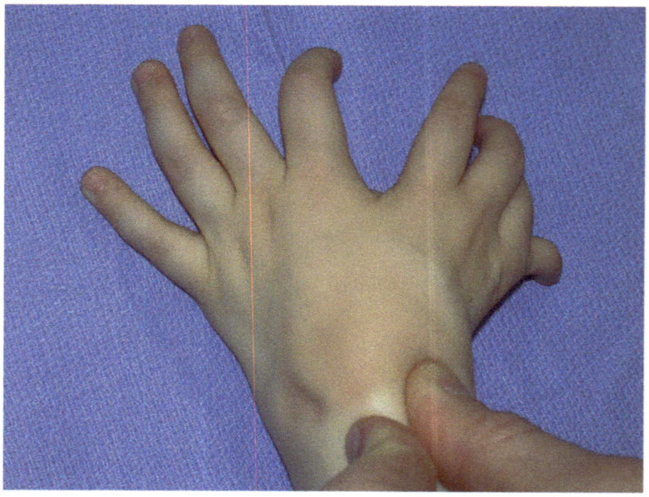

Fig. 20.7 Mirror hand with eight digits divided into two clusters. The lateral cluster is separated from the medial cluster by a central web and is slightly pronated in comparison to the remainder of the hand

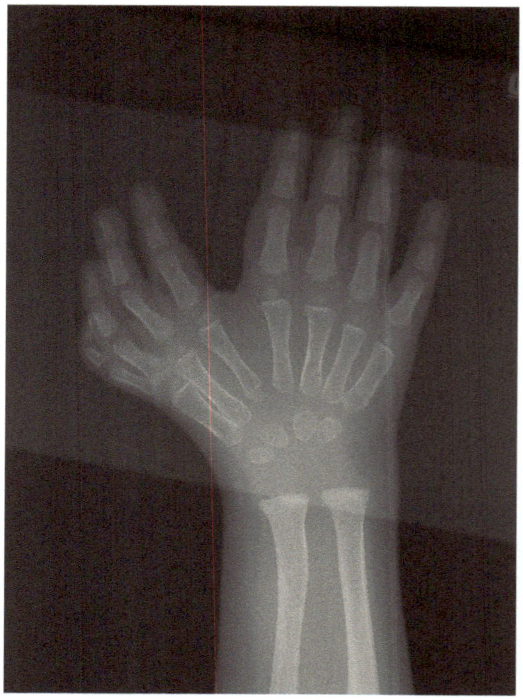

Fig. 20.8 Anterior–posterior radiograph of the hand demonstrating seven metacarpals and eight phalanges. The most lateral two digits articulate with a common metacarpal. Two capitates and two hamates are present at the carpal level. The distal articular surfaces of the medial and lateral ulna are broad like the articular surface of a normal radius

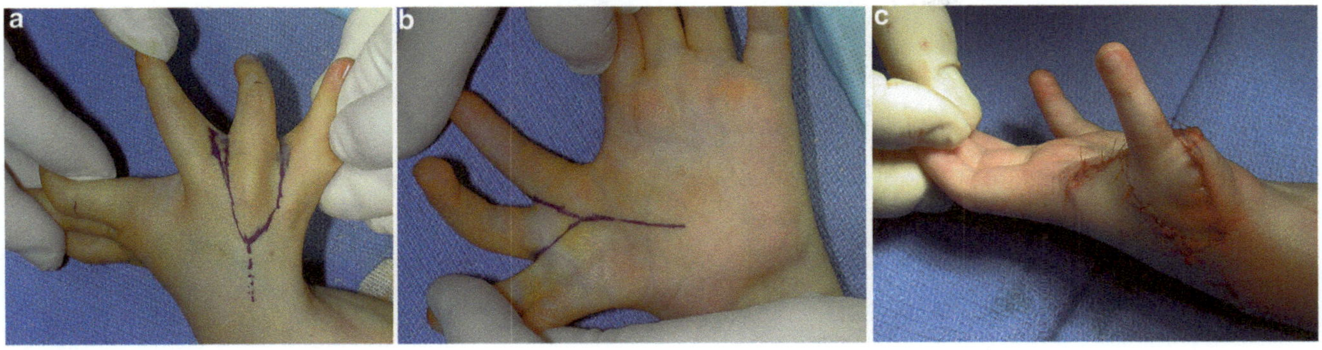

Fig. 20.9 After clinical evaluation of the child, the third most lateral digit was chosen for pollicization. (**a**) Dorsal and (**b**) volar views of the racquet incision used to isolate the pollicized digit. The remaining digits were amputated. (**c**) View of the completed pollicization. The digit is shorter and better positioned to function as a thumb. The remaining skin was used to create a first webspace and resurface the pollicized digit

Complications

Reconstruction of the upper extremity in patients with ulnar dimelia results in improved function. Procedures are challenging since tissues are often dysplastic and stiff. Complications may occur. Even with surgical release of the elbow with excision of the proximal lateral ulna, stiffness may occur with regrowth of the bone. Vascular compromise of a pollicized digit has been reported but may be avoided if arterial anomalies are recognized prior to transposing the digit [60]. The reconstructed thumb may be either too long or too short and opposition may be weak necessitating further tendon transfer.

References

1. Al-Qattan MM, Kozin SH. Update on embryology of the upper limb. J Hand Surg Am. 2013;38(9):1835–44.
2. Rayan GM, Frey B. Ulnar polydactyly. Plast Reconstr Surg. 2001;107(6):1449–54. discussion 55–7.
3. Watson BT, Hennrikus WL. Postaxial type-B polydactyly. Prevalence and treatment. J Bone Joint Surg Am. 1997;79(1):65–8.
4. Swanson AB, Swanson GD, Tada K. A classification for congenital limb malformation. J Hand Surg Am. 1983;8(5 Pt 2):693–702.
5. Tonkin MA, Tolerton SK, Quick TJ, Harvey I, Lawson RD, Smith NC, et al. Classification of congenital anomalies of the hand and upper limb: development and assessment of a new system. J Hand Surg Am. 2013;38(9):1845–53.
6. Temtamy SA, McKusick VA. Synopsis of hand malformations with particular emphasis on genetic factors. Birth Defects. 1969;3:125–84.
7. Stelling F. The upper extremity. Orthopedic surgery in infancy and childhood. Baltimore: WIlliams & Wilkins; 1963. p. 304–8.
8. Pritsch T, Ezaki M, Mills J, Oishi SN. Type A ulnar polydactyly of the hand: a classification system and clinical series. J Hand Surg Am. 2013;38(3):453–8.
9. Buck-Gramcko D, Behrens P. [Classification of polydactyly of the hand and foot]. Handchir Mikrochir Plast Chir. 1989;21(4):195–204.
10. Al-Qattan MM, Al-Shanawani B, Al-Thunayan A, Al-Namla A. The clinical features of ulnar polydactyly in a middle eastern population. J Hand Surg Eur Vol. 2008;33(1):47–52.
11. Castilla EE, da Graca Dutra M, Lugarinho da Fonseca R, Paz JE. Hand and foot postaxial polydactyly: two different traits. Am J Med Genet. 1997;73(1):48–54.
12. Simmons BP. Polydactyly. Hand Clin. 1985;1(3):545–65.
13. Umm e K, Basit S, Kamran-ul-Hassan Naqvi S, Ansar M, Ahmad W. Genetic mapping of an autosomal recessive postaxial polydactyly type A to chromosome 13q13.3-q21.2 and screening of the candidate genes. Hum Genet. 2012;131(3):415–22.
14. Al-Qattan MM, Al-Motairi MI. The pathogenesis of ulnar polydactyly in humans. J Hand Surg Eur Vol. 2013;38(9):934–9.
15. Bromley B, Shipp TD, Benacerraf B. Isolated polydactyly: prenatal diagnosis and perinatal outcome. Prenat Diagn. 2000;20(11):905–8.
16. Castilla EE, Lugarinho R, da Graca Dutra M, Salgado LJ. Associated anomalies in individuals with polydactyly. Am J Med Genet. 1998;80(5):459–65.
17. Galjaard RJ, Smits AP, Tuerlings JH, Bais AG, Bertoli Avella AM, Breedveld G, et al. A new locus for postaxial polydactyly type A/B on chromosome 7q21-q34. Eur J Hum Genet. 2003;11(5):409–15.
18. Galjaard RJ, van der Linde HC, Eussen BH, de Vries BB, Wouters CH, Oostra BA, et al. Isolated postaxial polydactyly type B with mosaicism of a submicroscopic unbalanced translocation leading to an extended phenotype in offspring. Am J Med Genet A. 2003;121a(2):168–73.
19. Radhakrishna U, Blouin JL, Mehenni H, Patel UC, Patel MN, Solanki JV, et al. Mapping one form of autosomal dominant postaxial polydactyly type A to chromosome 7p15-q11.23 by linkage analysis. Am J Hum Genet. 1997;60(3):597–604.
20. Radhakrishna U, Wild A, Grzeschik KH, Antonarakis SE. Mutation in GLI3 in postaxial polydactyly type A. Nat Genet. 1997;17(3):269–71.
21. Zhao H, Tian Y, Breedveld G, Huang S, Zou Y, Jue Y, et al. Postaxial polydactyly type A/B (PAP-A/B) is linked to chromosome 19p13.1-13.2 in a Chinese kindred. Eur J Hum Genet. 2002;10(3):162–6.
22. Zguricas J, Heutink P, Heredero L, Deurloo J, Oostra BA, Snijders PJ, et al. Genetic aspects of polydactyly. Handchir Mikrochir Plast Chir. 1996;28(4):171–5.
23. Man LX, Chang B. Maternal cigarette smoking during pregnancy increases the risk of having a child with a congenital digital anomaly. Plast Reconstr Surg. 2006;117(1):301–8.
24. Daluiski A, Yi SE, Lyons KM. The molecular control of upper extremity development: implications for congenital hand anomalies. J Hand Surg Am. 2001;26(1):8–22.

25. Al-Qattan MM. A novel frameshift mutation of the GLI3 gene in a family with broad thumbs with/without big toes, postaxial polydactyly and variable syndactyly of the hands/feet. Clin Genet. 2012;82(5):502–4.
26. Hare PJ. Rudimentary polydactyly. Br J Dermatol. 1954;66(11): 402–8.
27. Shapiro L, Juhlin EA, Brownstein MH. "Rudimentary polydactyly": an amputation neuroma. Arch Dermatol. 1973;108(2):223–5.
28. Kitayama Y, Tsukada S, Ishikura N, Ide Y, Kojima M. Rudimentary polydactyly: report of five cases. J Hand Surg Am. 1985;10(3): 382–5.
29. Kanter WR, Upton J. "Pacifier polydactyly": a transitional form between pedunculated polydactyly and rudimentary polydactyly. Plast Reconstr Surg. 1989;84(1):136–9.
30. Wrobel GD, Helmke C, Nash L, Awe JJ. Polydactyly and the Maya: a review and a case from the site of Peligroso, upper Macal River valley, Belize. Ancient Mesoamerica. 2012;23:131–42.
31. Dodd JK, Jones PM, Chinn DJ, Potokar T, Laing H. Neonatal accessory digits: a survey of practice amongst paediatricians and hand surgeons in the United Kingdom. Acta Paediatr. 2004; 93(2):200–4.
32. Heras L, Barco J, Cohen A. Unusual complication of ligation of rudimentary ulnar digit. J Hand Surg Br. 1999;24(6):750–1.
33. Patillo D, Rayan GM. Complications of suture ligation ablation for ulnar polydactyly: a report of two cases. Hand (N Y). 2011;6(1): 102–5.
34. Mullick S, Borschel GH. A selective approach to treatment of ulnar polydactyly: preventing painful neuroma and incomplete excision. Pediatr Dermatol. 2010;27(1):39–42.
35. Leber GE, Gosain AK. Surgical excision of pedunculated supernumerary digits prevents traumatic amputation neuromas. Pediatr Dermatol. 2003;20(2):108–12.
36. Taghinia AH, Upton J. Polydactyly. In: Weiss AC, editor. Textbook of hand and upper extremity surgery. Chicago: American Society for Surgery of the Hand; 2013. p. 1006–16.
37. Light TR, Buck-Gramcko D. Ulnar polydactyly. In: Buck-Gramcko D, editor. Congenital malformations of the hand and forearm. London: Churchill-Livingstone; 1998. p. 265–9.
38. Al-Qattan MM, Al-Thunayan A, De Cordier M, Nandagopal N, Pitkanen J. Classification of the mirror hand-multiple hand spectrum. J Hand Surg Br. 1998;23(4):534–6.
39. Chinegwundoh JO, Gupta M, Scott WA. Ulnar dimelia. Is it a true duplication of the ulna? J Hand Surg Br. 1997;22(1):77–9.
40. Burman M. An historical perspective of double hands and double feet. The survey of the cases reported in the 16th and 17th centuries. Bull Hosp Joint Dis. 1968;29(2):241–54.
41. Jameel J, Khan AQ, Ahmad S, Abbas M. Ulnar dimelia variant: a case report. J Orthop Traumatol. 2011;12(3):163–5.
42. Laurin CA, Favreau JC, Labelle P. Bilateral absence of the radius and tibia with bilateral reduplication of the ulna and fibula. A case report. J Bone Joint Surg Am. 1964;46:137–42.
43. Sandrow RE, Sullivan PD, Steel HH. Hereditary ulnar and fibular dimelia with peculiar facies. A case report. J Bone Joint Surg Am. 1970;52(2):367–70.
44. Martin RA, Jones MC, Jones KL. Mirror hands and feet with a distinct nasal defect, an autosomal dominant condition. Am J Med Genet. 1993;46(2):129–31.
45. Al-Qattan MM. Preaxial polydactyly of the upper limb viewed as a spectrum of severity of embryonic events. Ann Plast Surg. 2013;71(1):118–24.
46. Harrison RG, Pearson MA, Roaf R. Ulnar dimelia. J Bone Joint Surg Br. 1960;42-b:549–55.
47. Pintilie D, Hatmanu D, Olaru I, Panoza G. Double ulna with symmetrical polydactyly. Case report. J Bone Joint Surg Br. 1964;46: 89–93.
48. Davis RG, Farmer AW. Mirror hand anomaly; a case presentation. Plast Reconstr Surg Transplant Bull. 1958;21(1):80–3.
49. Barton NJ, Buck-Gramcko D, Evans DM. Soft-tissue anatomy of mirror hand. J Hand Surg Br. 1986;11(3):307–19.
50. Tsuyuguchi Y, Tada K, Yonenobu K. Mirror hand anomaly: reconstruction of the thumb, wrist, forearm, and elbow. Plast Reconstr Surg. 1982;70(3):384–7.
51. Harpf C, Hussl H. A case of mirror hand deformity with a 17-year postoperative follow up. Case report. Scand J Plast Reconstr Surg Hand Surg. 1999;33(3):329–33.
52. Gorriz G. Ulnar dimelia—a limb without anteroposterior differentiation. J Hand Surg. 1982;7(5):466–9.
53. Yang SS, Jackson L, Green DW, Weiland AJ. A rare variant of mirror hand: a case report. J Hand Surg Am. 1996;21(6):1048–51.
54. Barton NJ, Buck-Gramcko D, Evans DM, Kleinert H, Semple C, Ulson H. Mirror hand treated by true pollicization. J Hand Surg Br. 1986;11(3):320–36.
55. Kelley JW. Mirror hand. Plast Reconstr Surg Transplant Bull. 1962;30:374–7.
56. Al-Qattan MM, Al-Kahtani AR, Al-Sharif EM, Al-Otaibi NJ. Thumb reconstruction without formal pollicization in mirror hand deformity: a series of four cases. J Hand Surg Eur Vol. 2013;38(9):940–7.
57. Lichtblau PO. Mirror hand: one stage reconstruction. Orthopaedic Rev. 1981;10(12):77–80.
58. Bocca M, Ferraris E, Boccardo E. Polydactyly: the creation of a functional thumb in cases of mirror hand. Panminerva Med. 1968;10(4):164–70.
59. Gropper PT. Ulnar dimelia. J Hand Surg. 1983;8(4):487–91.
60. Pilkington S, Hearth M, Richards AM, Hobby JA. Laurin-Sandrow syndrome—a surgical challenge. Br J Plast Surg. 2000;53(1): 68–70.

Part V

Overgrowth, Amniotic Band, and Generalized Anomalies

Macrodactyly

21

Joseph Hardwicke and Ruth Lester

Definition

Macrodactyly (Greek *makros*, large, and *daktylos*, digit) is a descriptive term for a congenital malformation consisting of a significant increase in the length and girth of most or all of a digit compared to its contralateral digit (if unaffected), or compared to what would be expected for age/body build. The increased girth is accompanied by an increase in the dorso-ventral dimension and the lateral dimension of the digit [1]. The phalanges, tendons, nerves, vessels, subcutaneous fat, nails, and skin can all be enlarged [2].

The condition may present in an isolated digit, or multiple digits, and be unilateral or bilateral, symmetric or asymmetric, and simultaneously affect both hands and feet [3]. Previous terminologies that have been used to describe this condition include *megalodactyly*, *pachydactyly*, *gigantomegaly*, *dactylomegaly*, *digital gigantism*, *macrodactylia fibrolipomatosis*, *macrodystrophia lipomatosa*, and *local gigantism* [1, 4–6], with the last two terms usually referring to enlargement extending beyond the digit to involve more proximal structures. With even more proximal extension of overgrowth, macrodactyly can be seen as digital involvement in cases of hemihypertophy. Disappointingly, descriptors such as *banana fingers* [7] and *monstrous* [8] have been linked to this condition.

Other authors reserve the term *macrodactyly* for non-syndromic, congenital enlargement of a digit or digits that occurs in isolation without associated limb hemihypertrophy or vascular anomaly [4]. For the purposes of this chapter, *macrodactyly* will be used to describe subjective congenital digital enlargement of all causation, which may present at birth, or after, and in isolation, or in association with other signs or syndrome, sometimes referred to as *pseudomacrodactyly* [9]. It is our opinion that to limit this review to non-syndromic cases, or cases that do not extend beyond the digit or digits, will impact on the appreciation of the multidisciplinary management of the more complex cases. Although the majority of patients will present with isolated macrodactyly, a surgeon in a center treating such patients must be prepared to apply principles learned from these to all cases of enlarged digits.

J. Hardwicke, Ph.D., M.B.Ch.B., F.R.C.S. (Plast) (✉)
College of Medical and Dental Sciences, University of Birmingham, Edgbaston, Birmingham, West Midlands B15 2TT, UK
e-mail: J.Hardwicke@bham.ac.uk

R. Lester, M.B.Ch.B., D.Obst.R.C.O.G., D.C.H., F.R.C.S.
Department of Plastic Surgery, Birmingham Children's Hospital NHS Foundation Trust, Steelhouse Lane, Birmingham, West Midlands B4 6NH, UK
e-mail: ruth@Ruthlester.co.uk

History

The English philosopher and physician John Locke (1632–1704) may have been the first to describe a case of macrodactyly in his medical journals from 1675 to 1679 [10, 11]. Due to the rarity of macrodactyly of the hands and feet, it is usually reported on a case-by-case basis [2]. Between Polaillon (1884) and Humphry (1891), a total of 36 cases are presented from the literature between 1840 and 1891, although there is an overlap of citations [12, 13]. Sir George Murray Humphry describes six specimens from the Pathological Museum at the University of Cambridge, with a further 19 cases from the literature are also included in this review [13]. With the interpretation of the cases by today's standards, there appear to be examples of macrodactyly secondary to vascular anomaly, neurofibromatosis and Proteus syndrome, as well as progressive and static forms of the disease.

The next comprehensive review of macrodactyly was by Barsky in 1967 [2]. This review of 64 cases of upper limb macrodactyly consists of eight original descriptions and a review of the literature to that date, which relies heavily on the work of Polaillon. With the exclusion of cases prior to 1884, only 30 extra cases were published in intervening years. Macrodactyly of the upper and lower limb continues to be reported on a case-by-case basis and we estimate that fewer than 500 cases have been reported worldwide to date.

D.R. Laub Jr. (ed.), *Congenital Anomalies of the Upper Extremity: Etiology and Management*,
DOI 10.1007/978-1-4899-7504-1_21, © Springer Science+Business Media New York 2015

Classification

Macrodactyly is a congenital limb anomaly of overgrowth (IV) according to the modified Swanson/International Federation of Societies for Surgery of the Hand [14–16]. A recent reclassification has been proposed as dysplasia–hypertrophy–macrodactyly or dysplasia–hypertrophy–upper limb and macrodactyly, according to the Oberg–Manske–Tonkin (OMT) system, to reflect both the axis of formation/differentiation and the part of the limb predominantly affected [17].

In its own right, macrodactyly has been sub-classified in numerous ways. With no known unifying biological theory as to the causation, or progression, the only consistent feature is the subjective description of the enlarged digit. As such, there is overlap between classification systems, which must be considered as imperfect at the present time [4]. A brief review of the most commonly applied systems from the medical literature reveals three broad classes: relating to the tissues involved, rate of growth, and affiliation with different clinical signs or syndromes. Based upon these, we suggest a new inclusive classification system for macrodactyly.

To be classed as true macrodactyly, all elements of the digit must be enlarged [2, 18, 19]. This classification has been adapted to note that it is only tissues that respond late in development to neurogenic influence are enlarged, thus the tendon and blood vessels may be of normal size [20]. Digital enlargement may also occur secondarily to tumor or vascular anomalies and would be considered as pseudomacrodactyly [9], although the presentation and subsequent management may be similar in part (Fig. 21.1). There is no evidence that links outcomes with true or pseudomacrodactly.

The relative growth of the digit, compared to unaffected digits, may be considered as either (1) static or (2) progressive [2, 21], and may be symmetric or asymmetric [18, 22] (Fig. 21.2).

(a) In the static type, enlargement is present at birth and the affected limb grows in proportion to the child.

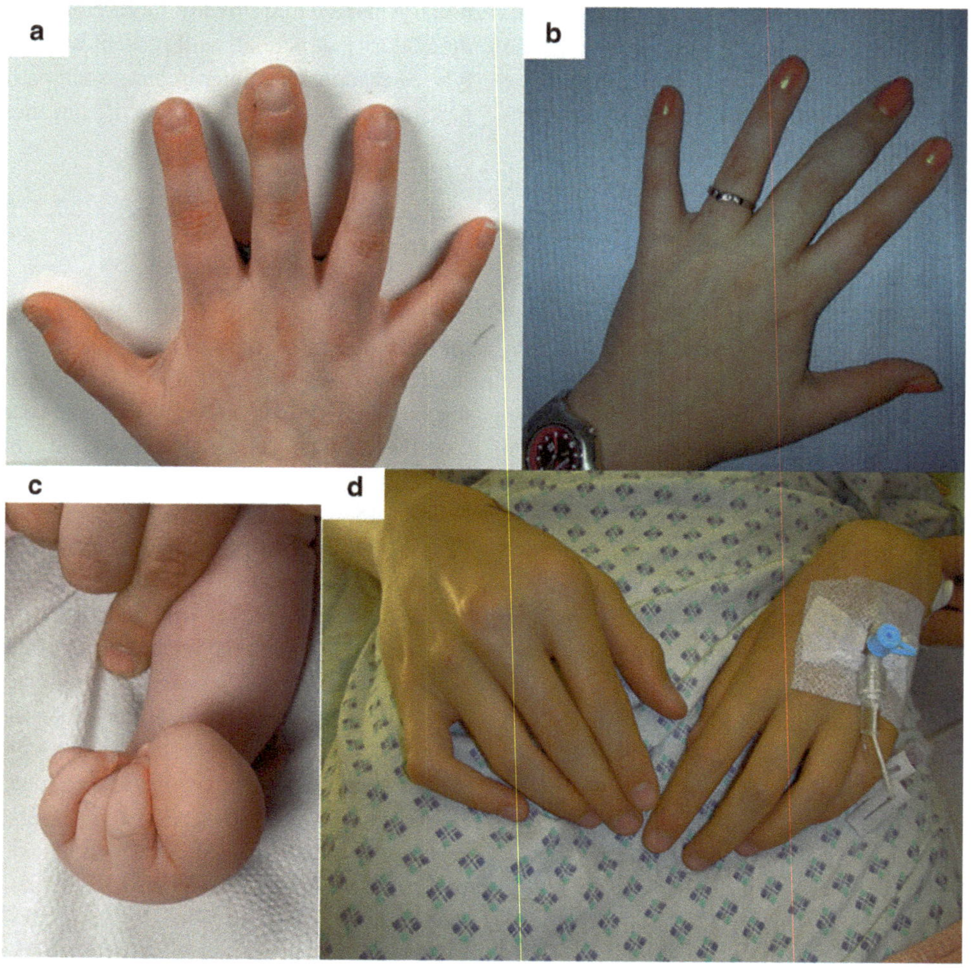

Fig. 21.1 Enlargement of the fingers or hand secondary to vascular malformations: (**a**) A lymphatic malformation of the tip of the middle finger. (**b**) An arteriovenous malformation of a finger leading to macrodactyly. (**c**) A venous malformation causing macrodactyly of the middle finger. (**d**) Muscle hypertrophy of the hand associated with a lymphatic malformation

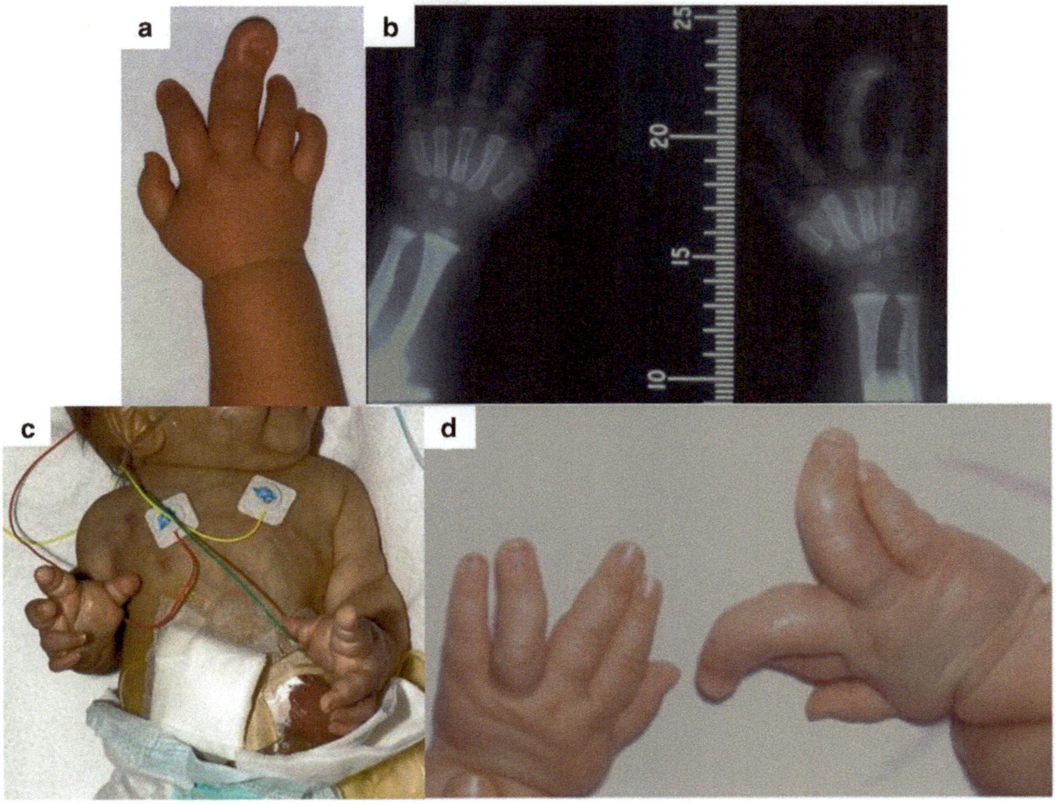

Fig. 21.2 The multiple variations of upper limb macrodactyly: (**a**) Progressive unilateral macrodactyly of the right middle finger. (**b**) Radiograph of the hands with the superimposition of a measure to allow for serial growth recording. (**c**) Bilateral, symmetrical macrodactyly in a child with an "unknown" syndrome which was fatal. (**d**) Bilateral, asymmetric macrodactyly

(b) In the progressive type, some overgrowth may be noted at birth, but at around 2 years of age there is evidence of slow, unrestricted, and disproportionate digital enlargement, which continues until closure of the epiphyses [23].

In our review of 32 patients with macrodactyly, approximately two-thirds had the static type, which is different from the findings of other authors [3, 4]. In our cohort of 20 patients, 6 required no surgical intervention. It has been observed that such patients usually present later with good function [21] but we did not note any significant difference in age at presentation between the static and progressive subtypes, although it was noted that those with static disease required fewer operations overall, which was significant. These findings are echoed by Cerrato et al. [4]. It is difficult to classify into static or progressive type before the age of two, as the only significant indicator of the prognosis in macrodactyly is by regular observation in the first few years of life.

The most comprehensive classifications to date are based upon the original work of Kelikian, and later modified by Dell, Flatt, and Upton [7, 23–26] (Table 21.1). Lipomatous macrodactyly is the most common form of overgrowth in the literature and is differentiated from NTOM by the absence of infiltration of the digital nerves upon microdissection and neurovascular structures are of normal caliber. NTOM was introduced by Kelikian [26] to differentiate the digital nerve involvement from that observed in neurofibromatosis-associated macrodactyly, and to emphasize the relationship between the enlargement of the nerve along with the bone and soft tissues. It is a common type of macrodactyly that is unilateral in 90 % of cases. As with lipomatous macrodactyly, it does not usually show a pattern of inheritance, nor association with other malformations [25–27]. The median nerve territory is more often affected, with 85 % of cases of macrodactyly affecting the thumb, index, or middle fingers [27]. Our recent review shows a similar distribution with involvement of these digits in 63 % of cases and out of the 32 cases presented, 27 were lipomatous or NTOM macrodactyly [3]. Cerrato et al. presented 21 cases of macrodactyly, of which 12 were NTOM and 9 lipomatous. No significant difference in patients, progression, number of operations, distribution, or associated anomalies was found [4].

Digital hyperostosis, or *hyperostotic digital gigantism*, also described by Kelikian, is a rare form of macrodactyly that is non-hereditary, and may present later [26, 28]. There is bilateral enlargement of the digits, which may be symmetric or asymmetric, without gross enlargement of the digital nerves or fat, but it can present in the median nerve distribution, with concurrent NTOM [7, 29]. Palpable periarticular

Table 21.1 Chronologic development of the different classification systems of macrodactyly

Author(s) (year of publication):	Holmes (1869)	Richardière (1891)	De Laurenzi (1962), Barsky (1967)	Kelikian (1974)	Upton (1990), Flatt (1994)	Upton (2006)
Classifications of macrodactyly	Symmetric	True	Static	Lipomatous macrodystrophy	Gigantism and (nerve oriented) lipofibromatosis	Nerve territory oriented macrodactyly
	Asymmetric	False	Progressive	Neurofibromatosis	Gigantism and neurofibromatosis	Lipomatous macrodactyly
				Nerve territory orientated macrodactyly	Gigantism and digital hyperostosis	Neurofibromatosis
				Hyperostotic variety	Gigantism and hemihypertrophy	Hyperostosis
						Hemihypertrophy
						Proteus syndrome
						Vascular malformations

Table 21.2 A proposed new system for the classification of macrodactyly

Characteristic	Classification			
1. Growth	Static		Progressive	
2. Associations	Isolated		Associated syndrome or anomalies	
3. Structure	Lipomatous	Nerve territory orientated	Hyperostotic	Vascular malformation

osteochondral masses arise from the volar plates of the metacarpals and phalanges, similar to the pattern seen in neurofibromatosis, and can lead to profound loss of motion [7, 23]. The joint involvement seen in hyperostosis and neurofibromatosis or Proteus syndrome will presumably lead to poorer functional outcomes, although this is not evidenced in the literature. The remaining subclasses associated with other anomalies or syndromes are discussed later.

The real value of a medical classification is to provide prognostic information, or to group patients for prospective analysis. With a confused variety of systems available for macrodactyly built upon phenotypic, intra-operative, histological, radiological, or genetic findings, the most effective classification should be based upon outcomes. It has been shown that patients with static disease need significantly fewer operations than those with progressive, although it must be acknowledged that the patient cohorts on which these assumptions are made were small and prone to variability [3, 4]. Macrodactyly associated with other anomalies or syndromes may also have poor functional outcomes due to joint involvement, flexion contracture, and other morbidity secondary to the syndrome involved.

With this established, we suggest a new three-layer classification based upon (1) growth progression, (2) associated anomalies, and (3) structures involved (Table 21.2). This encompasses all types of macrodactyly reported to date and can provide information about prognosis and allow grouping of similar patients for subsequent analysis. As such, a (1) *static*–(2) *isolated*–(3) lipomatous macrodactyly can be assumed to have a better prognosis in terms of function, fewer operations, and fewer surgical complications than a (1) *progressive*–(2) *syndrome-associated*–(3) hyperostotic macrodactyly.

Incidence

Macrodactyly is classed as a rare disease by the Office of Rare Disease Research, and thus affects less than 200,000 people in the USA [30]. With rare conditions, such as macrodactyly, a true population incidence is hard to calculate. The classic description by Flatt of an incidence of 0.9 % of all congenital hand anomalies is based upon the author's personal study of 2,758 patients, with 28 cases of macrodactyly in 26 patients [7]. This figure, although widely published, has no reference to the overall incidence in the general population. A similar number was found in Hong Kong in the 1980s, with two cases of macrodactyly from a cohort of 326 patients with congenital upper limb anomalies, equating to 0.5 % [31].

Congenital anomalies occur in 1–2 % of newborns, with 10 % of these affecting the upper limb [7]. National population studies from Sweden have also shown an incidence of upper limb anomalies to be approximately 1/500 [32–34] and one can therefore extrapolate the incidence of upper limb macrodactyly (~1 % of the total) to be around 1/50,000, but this is based upon many assumptions. Lower limb macrodactyly has been estimated to have an incidence of 1/18,000 [35]. In a large UK teaching hospital, one expects to see one to two new cases of upper limb macrodactyly per year, which echoes historic findings [36].

Associations

There are many reported associations of macrodactyly with other clinical signs or syndromes. In isolated non-syndromic macrodactyly, there can be concurrence of local anomalies such as syndactyly (occurring in 10 % of patients) [29] and clinodactyly or curvature of the enlarged digit. There is also a very rare entity of syndactyly associated with dorsal macrodactyly (Fig. 21.3)

Of the many reported syndromes that have presented with macrodactyly, none have it *per se* as a syndrome-defining feature. It is usually classified as part of an overgrowth component of the disease, which can be classified into (1) phakomatoses, (2) osteochondrodysplasias, (3) specific overgrowth syndromes, or (4) secondary to a vascular anomaly (Table 21.3).

1. The phakomatoses (or "neurocutaneous syndromes") include (a) neurofibromatosis type 1 and 2 (NF1 and NF2) and (b) the hamartoma syndromes.
   (a) NF1 and NF2 have both been associated with macrodactyly [7, 23, 25]. NF1 is the most commonly reported syndrome presenting with digital enlargement, as well as enlargement involving the upper and lower limbs, torso, and head and neck. It has an autosomal dominant inheritance pattern, with an incidence of 1/3,000 [37–39] and has specific diagnostic criteria [40]. Digital enlargement is frequently bilateral and presents in a similar manner to the previously described NTOM, or can be related to plexiform schwannomatosis [41]. It may also present with features of hyperostosis [25]. As has been shown in hyperostotic macrodactyly, bony

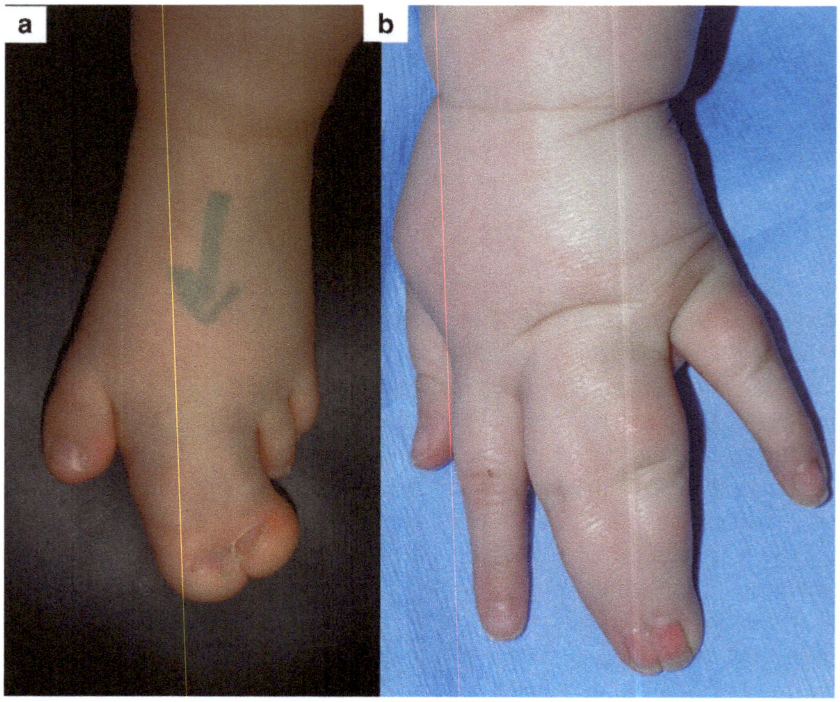

Fig. 21.3 Non-syndromic macrodactyly with associated malformations: (**a**) Macrosyndactyly of the second and third toes. (**b**) Subtle dorsal macrosyndactyly

Table 21.3 A classification for syndromes that have been associated with macrodactyly

Syndromes associated with macrodactyly			
1.	Phakomatoses	Neurofibromatosis type 1 and 2	
		Hamartoma syndromes	Proteus syndrome
			Tuberous sclerosis
2.	Osteochondrodysplasias	Enchondromatoses	Maffucci syndrome
			Ollier syndrome
		Monostotic fibrous dysplasia	
3.	Specific overgrowth syndromes	Beckwith–Wiedemann syndrome	
4.	Vascular anomalies	Vascular malformations	Klippel–Trénaunay syndrome
			Maffucci syndrome
			CLOVES syndrome

involvement can lead to limitation of movement and function. Growth is usually progressive and resection of the neurofibromas, or involved nerves, has been shown to limit advancement of the disease [42–44]. One must always consider the risk of malignant transformation and development of neurofibrosarcoma in the peripheral nerve [45, 46].

NF2 also has an autosomal dominant inheritance pattern but is 20 times less common than NF1. It manifests as bilateral vestibular schwannomas, spinal cord meningiomas or ependymomas and cataracts [47, 48]. Peripheral nerve involvement is rare, but macrodactyly secondary to a NF2 peripheral nerve schwannoma has been reported [49].

(b) Hamartomas are benign focal malformations that resemble a neoplasm in the tissue of its origin [50]. Multiple hamartomas are associated with syndromes such as Proteus syndrome and tuberous sclerosis (Fig. 21.4), both presenting with soft tissue and bone overgrowth [51, 52]. Proteus syndrome was described as a discrete clinical entity in 1979 [53] and assigned its name in 1983 [54] with reference to the Greek god who was gifted with the power to change his appearance at will. It is rare, and the first description is now attributed to Treves with his presentation of Joseph Merrick (the *Elephant Man*) to the Pathological Society of London in 1885 [55, 56]. It is not inherited, and displays genetic mosaicism [57–60]. After neurofibromatosis, it is the most widely reported syndrome associated with macrodactyly [61–65]. In this condition, macrodactyly can be highly variable, progressive, and asymmetric. Disproportionate growth throughout the body begins between the ages of 6–18 months and leads to severe overgrowth and flexion contractures and the hands, which, when combined with glabrous hyperplasia can preclude functional use of the hand [23, 66].

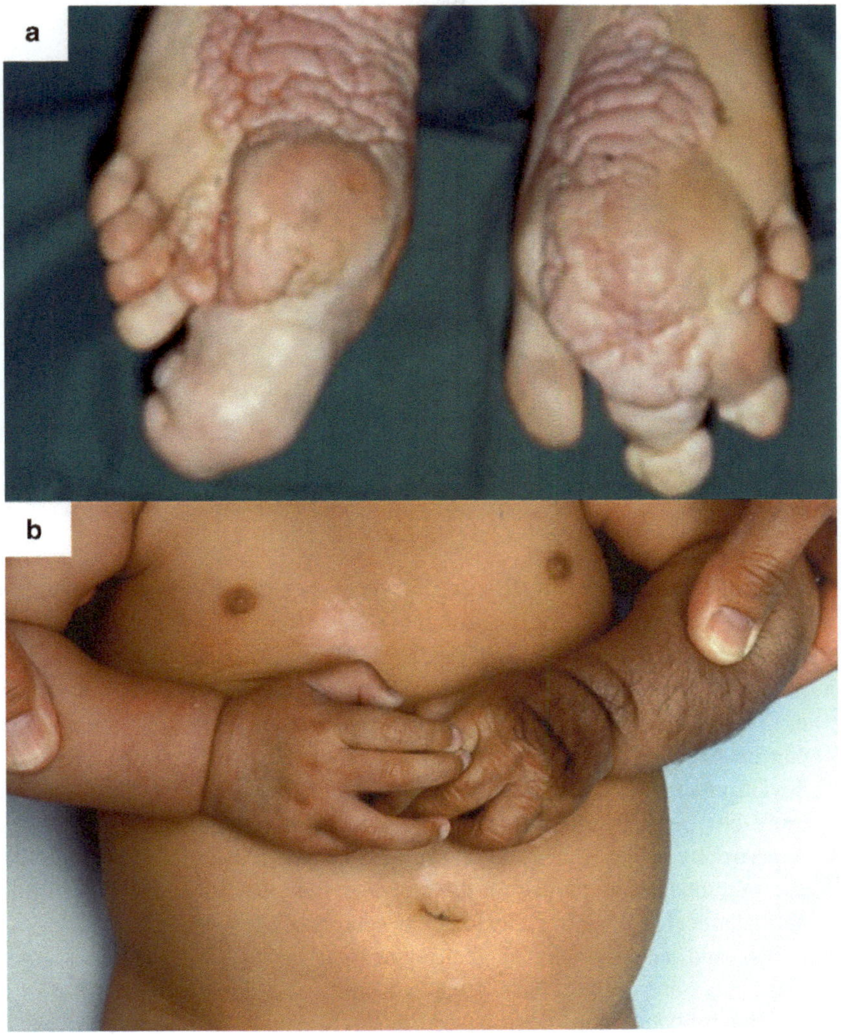

Fig. 21.4 Macrodactyly in association with hamartoma syndromes: (**a**) Bilateral macrodactyly of the toes and thickening of the plantar surfaces of the feet associated with Proteus syndrome. (**b**) Enlargement of the left hand associated with tuberous sclerosis

Tuberous sclerosis complex is an autosomal dominant disorder characterized by hamartomatous malformations in various organs such as brain, kidney, heart, and lung [67, 68]. Macrodactyly is rarely reported in association, with only ten cases identified up to 2000 [69]. There is a hyperostosis with cortical bone cysts, although the joints appear to be spared [70, 71]. The patients may have associated symptoms such as epilepsy or learning disability as a result of the primary diagnosis of tuberous sclerosis [72, 73].

2. The osteochondrodyplasias that may present in infancy include (a) the enchondromatoses and (b) fibrous dysplasia, which may present with digital enlargement secondary to bone overgrowth.
   (a) Muffuci syndrome and Ollier disease are both enchondromatoses, characterized by multiple enchondromas that are almost exclusively localized in the metaphysis of long bones and in the small bones of the hands and feet [74–77]. Enchondromas can result in severe growth abnormalities (more severe than those observed in multiple exostosis) and fingers often show irregular morphology and size, although are rarely reported in the literature [76, 78]. Radiological findings include ovoid, cystic, and highly radiolucent lesions, elongated parallel to the major axis of the bone, originating near the physis and migrating towards the diaphyses with growth [76, 79, 80]. Debulking of the enchondromas and hemangiomas forego amputation and can result in a hand that is improved in appearance and less prone to trauma [81].
   (b) Fibrous dysplasia may be monostotic or poylostotic in presentation, or have associated endocrinopathy in McCune–Albright syndrome. Rarely reported monostotic involvement in the digit [82] must be considered in the differential diagnosis of macrodactyly.
3. Overgrowth syndromes can be associated with hemihypertophy, of which macrodactyly can be a component. Beckwith–Wiedemann syndrome (BWS) is a rare and complex disorder of overgrowth with undetermined inheritance [83]. It was classically described as macrosomia, macroglossia, and an abdominal wall defect [84–86], but more recently has been noted to include hemihyperplasia

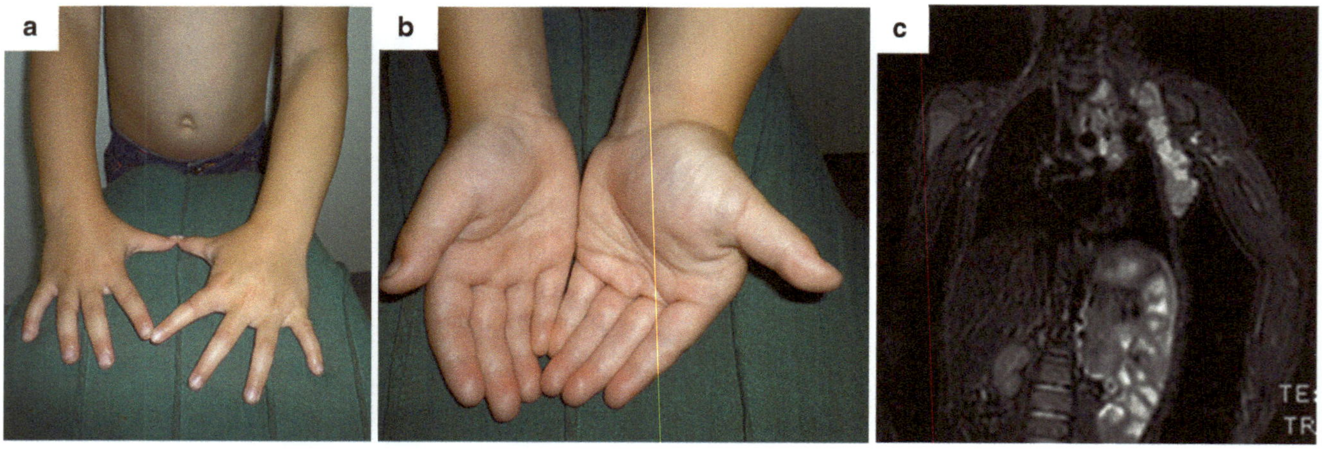

Fig. 21.5 Enlargement of the right hand musculature with sparing of the digits, in association with hemihypertrophy. (**a**) Dorsal view. (**b**) Anterior view. (**c**) Magnetic resonance imaging of the left upper limb showing generalized soft tissue hypertrophy

[87, 88]. Hemihypertrophy macrodactyly presents similarly to Proteus syndrome but with more uniform soft tissue overgrowth and muscular hypertrophy. The palm and hand are less enlarged in proportion to the ipsilateral forearm, due to increased muscle bulk, but in extreme cases can be fixed in flexion at the wrist with digits in ulnar deviation due to muscular imbalance, which becomes more obvious during adolescence [23]. Isolated muscle hypertrophy of the hand including muscular hyperplasia, aberrant muscles, ulnar drift of the fingers in the metacarpophalangeal (MP) joints, flexion contractures of the MP joints, and enlargement of the metacarpal spaces is extremely rare but we have seen two cases associated with a lymphatic malformation (see Fig. 21.1d) and localized gigantism of the upper limb (Fig. 21.5).

4. Vascular anomaly syndromes that are associated with digital enlargement include Klippel–Trénaunay syndrome (KTS) and CLOVES syndrome. The anomalies that are present are vascular malformations (VM) as per the International Society for the Study of Vascular Anomalies [89, 90]. Macrodactyly in such cases may be diagnosed and managed with a different strategy, focusing on destruction or disruption of the VM prior to surgical debulking. KTS was described in 1900 with three characteristic features: a vascular nevus; hypertrophy of all of the tissues, particularly the skeleton; and ipsilateral varicosities [91, 92]. McGrory reviewed 108 patients with KTS and found 26 had macrodactyly (79 digits) of the upper or lower limb, amongst other congenital hand and foot anomalies. There was predilection for the radial side of the hand and medial foot [93].

CLOVES syndrome consists of congenital lipomatous overgrowth, vascular malformations, epidermal nevi, and skeletal abnormalities [94]. It can span the classifications, being part of either the overgrowth or vascular anomaly subset. The presence of high flow lesions in these patients suggests that it may be clinically related to KTS, and as such we have classified it here. The presence of truncal lipomatous mass and a characteristic pattern of macrodactyly differentiates CLOVES from other syndromic forms of overgrowth [94, 95]. The macrodactyly consists of progressive soft tissue overgrowth in predominance to bone overgrowth, which may be nonprogressive and nondistorting in nature [96, 97], which is markedly different from that found in Proteus syndrome. Review of the historical literature reveals probable CLOVES syndrome that may previously have been described as gigantism [95] or Proteus syndrome [94].

Genetics

The majority of isolated, non-syndromic macrodactyly, whether it of the progressive or static subtype, is sporadic in nature with no known underlying genetic causation recorded on the Online Mendelian Inheritance in Man database [98]. At present, there is no modern molecular insight into macrodactyly and there are no cellular or animal models of macrodactyly [99]. Candidate genes have been proposed (Table 21.4) which include those coding for bone morphogenetic proteins 5 and 7 (BMP5 & 7), transforming growth factor beta 3 (TGF-B3), Wnt (wingless-type) signaling pathway proteins (Wnt-2, Wnt-5A), pleiotrophin (PTN) [99], natriuretic peptide receptor 2 (NPR2) [100], and phosphoinositide-3-kinase (PI3K) [101].

BMP5 and 7, TGF-B3, Wnt-2, and Wnt-5A are all overexpressed in macrodactyly, but PTN had the greatest fold-change when reported [99]. PTN is a promising candidate for the pathogenesis of macrodactyly because it promotes growth of nearly all the tissues affected by macrodactyly: PTN is necessary for neurite outgrowth and maturation in the central nervous system [102–104]. In the peripheral nervous system it promotes nerve regeneration following injury [105]. PTN is highly expressed in bone and cartilage, and is upregulated in response to mechanical loading [106–108], is an angiogenic factor, and supports endothelial cell proliferation [109].

Table 21.4 Genes associated with non-syndromic and syndromic macrodactyly

	Gene	Chromosome location	Encoded protein	Syndrome	Gene(s)	Chromosome location	Encoded protein(s)
Non-syndromic macrodactyly	*BMP5*	6p12.1	Bone morphogenetic protein 5	Neurofibromatosis type 1	*NF1*	17q11.2	Neurofibromin
	BMP7	20q13.31	Bone morphogenetic protein 7	Neurofibromatosis type 2	*NF2*	22q12.2	Merlin
	TGFB3	14q24.3	Transforming growth factor beta 3	Proteus syndrome	*AKT1*	14q32.33	RAC alpha serine/threonine-protein kinase
	WNT2	7q31.2	Protein Wnt-2	Proteus-like syndrome	*PTEN*	10q23.31	Phosphatase and tensin homolog
	WNT5a	3p14.3	Protein Wnt-5a	SOLAMEN syndrome	*PTEN*	10q23.31	Phosphatase and tensin homolog
	PTN	7q33	Pleiotrophin	Tuberous sclerosis	*TSC1*	9q34.13	Hamartin
					TSC2	16p13.3	Tuberin
	NPR2	9p13.3	Natriuretic peptide receptor 2	Beckwith–Wiedeman syndrome	*CDKN1C*, *H19*, *IGF2*, *KCNQ1OT1*	11p15.5	Cyclin-dependent kinase inhibitor 1C Insulin-like growth factor 2
	PIK3CA	3q26.32	Phosphoinositide-3-kinase	CLOVES syndrome	*PIK3CA*	3q26.32	Phosphoinositide-3-kinase

Overproduction of C-type natriuretic peptide (CNP) due to a chromosomal translocation was reported to cause skeletal dysplasia associated with tall stature [110, 111]. In addition, acromesomelic dysplasia, characterized by dwarfism and short limbs, is caused by loss of function mutations in the *NPR2* gene [112]. In a study by Miura et al., a three-generation family of tall stature and macrodactyly of the great toes had a gain of function mutation in the *NPR2* gene [100].

PI3K is an upstream regulator of the AKT-mTOR cell-signaling pathway, which has been implicated in non-syndromic macrodactyly and CLOVES syndrome [101, 113]. The PI3K/AKT/mTOR pathway is important in apoptosis and carcinogenesis [114, 115] and muscular hypertrophy [116].

In syndrome-associated macrodactyly, especially those with an autosomal dominant inheritance pattern, individual genes have been identified (see Table 21.4). A mutation in the *NF1* gene that encodes for neurofibromin leads to the development of NF1 [117, 118]. The *NF2* gene encodes for merlin (also known as schwannomin) and mutations lead to the development of NF2 [47, 48, 119]. Although its exact function is unknown, merlin is likely also involved in controlling cell movement, cell shape, and communication between cells [120–122], with mutations leading to the development of schwannomas, which may be associated with macrodactyly [49].

Proteus syndrome is caused by a mutation in the *AKT1* gene that encodes for RAC-alpha serine/threonine-protein kinase (AKT1), which regulates cell growth, proliferation, and apoptosis [123]. A mutation in *AKT1* leads to the abnormal growth characteristics of Proteus syndrome [66, 124]. Mutations in the *PTEN* gene, which encodes for phosphatase and tensin homolog (PTEN), have been associated with asymmetric overgrowth but do not meet the strict guidelines for a diagnosis of Proteus syndrome [125–127]. Instead, these individuals have Proteus-like syndrome, which is considered part of a larger group of disorders called PTEN hamartoma tumor syndromes. Segmental overgrowth, lipomatosis, arteriovenous malformation, and epidermal nevus (SOLAMEN) syndrome, another variant within this group with mosaic PTEN mutations, has presented with macrodactyly [128].

Tuberous sclerosis complex is caused by mutations in the *TSC1* or *TSC2* genes, which encode hamartin and tuberin, respectively [67]. The proteins act as tumor suppressors, and with loss of function mutations leads to the growth of tumors in many different organs and tissues [68, 72], which may lead to macrodactyly [69]. The genetic causes of BWS are complex [83, 129], and involve several genes that are intrinsic to normal growth, including the *CDKN1C*, *H19*, *IGF2*, and *KCNQ1OT1* genes [129–133]. The CLOVES syndrome is linked to *PIK3CA* gene mutations [113, 134] and is negative for *PTEN* gene mutations [94], which allows differentiation from similarly presenting PTEN hamartoma syndromes (e.g., SOLAMEN syndrome).

Imaging

Prenatal diagnosis of macrodactyly has been reported. Yuksel et al. present a case of macrodactyly of the second toe of the left foot, diagnosed at 24 weeks gestation on obstetric ultrasound scan (USS), with no other anomalies diagnosed [135]. Rypens et al. report a case of Proteus syndrome, diagnosed antenatally on USS, which presented with macrodactyly of the left middle finger and an associated massive axillary lymphangioma [136]. The evidence relating to the imaging of macrodactyly is not evident in the literature. In most cases, the diagnosis can be ascertained from the clinical history and examination after birth. If there is doubt as to the diagnosis, or if there is disproportionate growth of a previously *unaffected* digit, especially in adulthood, or after closure of the epiphyses, radiological investigation would be recommended.

Management

This section is inevitably anecdotal. Macrodactyly consists of a variety of conditions with many variations in presentation and growth patterns. It presents an almost unique situation whereby there is significant unpredictability of outcome with or without surgery. The management of macrodactyly demonstrates the need for very close observation of the child and detailed discussions with the parents and eventually the child throughout their growing years. It also requires considerable flexibility from a surgeon who has to consider the use of a wide variety of procedures and techniques. The aims of surgery are to allow a child to develop with minimum hindrance from their enlarged digit(s), e.g., by enabling them to be comfortable in shoes or to remove a digit, which is hindering their development of manipulative skills. This is done by attempting to reduce the disparity of the circumferential and longitudinal dimensions of the affected digit(s) when compared with the unaffected [25], with preservation of sensation, blood supply, and function, as far as is possible [23].

In terms of principles of surgery, the senior author currently uses a lateral approach to each individual digit tackling one side at a time with an interval of a few months between each operative procedure. With this approach, bone and soft tissues surgical reduction can be combined. Palmar or plantar soft tissue debulking can be carried out using a variety of incisions, including zigzag and longitudinal [7, 23, 26], as well as the use of skin grafts in the reconstruction [137]. The position of scars rarely causes a problem even when using a longitudinal plantar incision [3].

The need for repeated procedures must be highlighted in the cases of progressive macrodactyly. The eventual decision to carry out a ray amputation (Fig. 21.6) should not be considered a failure in management as it may take many years and several

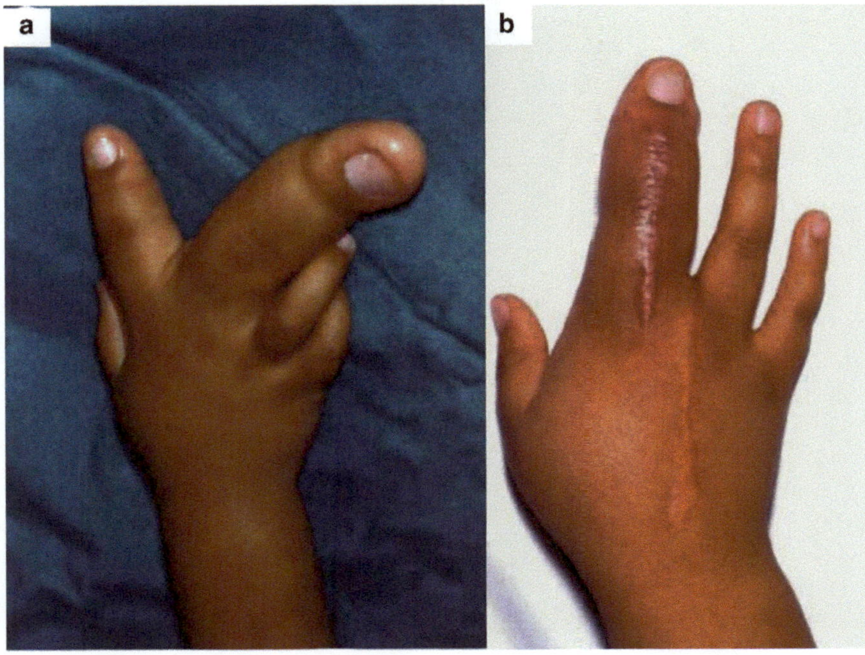

Fig. 21.6 Macrodactyly of the index and middle fingers: (**a**) Progressive macrodactyly of the right middle finger with the index finger affected to a lesser degree. (**b**) Postoperative image after ray amputation of the middle finger and soft tissue debulking of the index finger

operations to arrive jointly at this decision, which can transform the quality of life for these patients. In the vast majority of cases of surgically treated macrodactyly, the functional and cosmetic outcome will be acceptable to the patient [3].

The surgical management of macrodactyly can be classified by the treatment of the different tissues involved, i.e., soft tissue (skin and nerve) debulking, shortening of bone, correction of angulation of a digit, or attempting to arrest abnormal excessive growth by destruction of the growth plate. Macrodactyly associated with other anomalies, such as vascular anomalies, need to be treated individually according to problems reported by parents and/or child.

1. *Skin and soft tissue*: Excess fat can be radically reduced both dorsally and from around the nerve through a lateral incision. In isolated non-syndromic macrodactyly, there can be concurrent syndactyly (occurring in 10 % of patients) [29]. Syndactyly separation using either a volar or dorsal flap technique can be employed. If the fat is radically debulked at the same time, there is usually enough skin for direct closure without the need for skin grafts.
2. *Nerve*: McCarroll initially reported the cessation of abnormal growth after nerve excision in neurofibromatosis-associated macrodactyly [44]. Kelikian advocated excision of tortuous redundant digital nerve after neurolysis (defatting), and showed return of sensation by 3 months in six out of seven individuals, although no mention of continual growth is made [26]. Multiple authors have refuted nerve excision as a method of growth arrest this based on long-term outcomes, but this does include cases of partial nerve resection [42, 138–140]. The nerve can be radically debulked by a careful dissection and excision of infiltrated fat leaving only a small residual thickness of nerve tissue. Troublesome neuromata are rarely seen. Although the sensation of the digit may be reduced, this does not cause any functional problems, as the digit is unlikely to be used during fine manipulation.

   Nerve compression symptoms are reported in conjunction with enlargement of nerves in macrodactyly at both the cubital [141, 142] and carpal tunnel [143, 144]. Carpal tunnel syndrome is rare in children [145, 146] but has been reported in association with macrodactyly [147–151]. Release of the carpal tunnel and neurolysis has been shown to give symptomatic improvement [149]. The carpal tunnel decompression and neurolysis can be performed through an extended carpal tunnel incision, or in conjunction with other debulking procedures (Fig. 21.7).
3. *Bones, joints, and epiphyses*: Surgery to the bone including the joints can correct width, length, and angulation of a digit. If the epiphysis is included in the bony excisions, then ongoing growth of the length of the digit will be slowed down. Epiphyseal destruction will halt longitudinal growth if all centers involved in the enlargement of the digit are completely destroyed [23]. Early methods employed wiring or stapling of the growth plate [2] or the use of a motorized drill [152]. The use of a burr may not reliably destroy all growth centers and so some authors have moved to complete excision [7, 150]. Circumferential growth will continue and so will need addressing using osteotomy and bone trimming as described below. Epiphysodesis has been shown to be more reliable in longitudinal growth arrest from long-term follow-up than other methods, such as nerve excision [138].

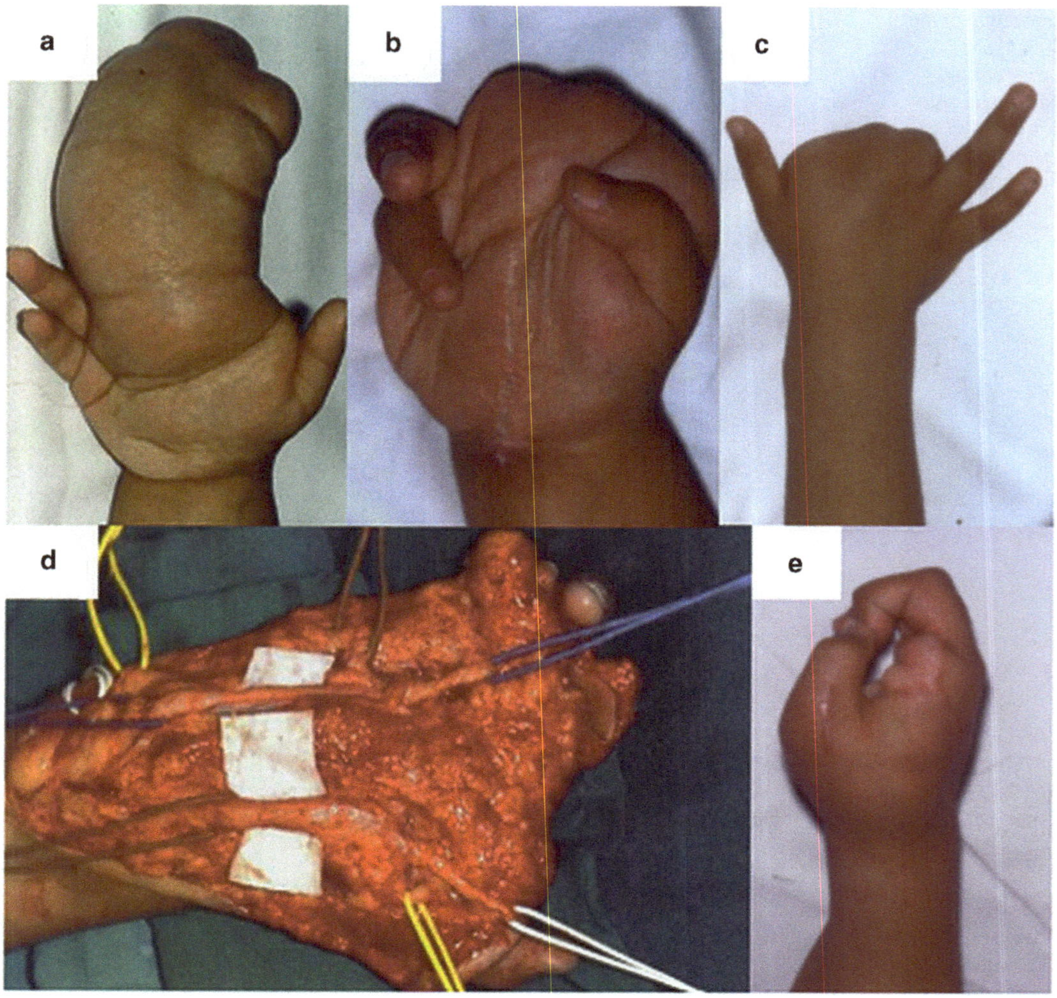

Fig. 21.7 Macrodactyly presenting with syndactyly of the index and middle fingers: (**a**) Gross macrosyndactyly with angulation leading to a nonfunctional hand. (**b**) The digits were initially amputated at MCP joint level but the hand remained encumbered. (**c**) Dorsal view. (**d**) A double ray amputation with debulking of the soft tissues of the palm was performed in conjunction with carpal tunnel decompression. (**e**) Lateral view showing a successful pinch grip

(a) *Width reduction*: Through the lateral incision used to debulk the soft tissue, enlarged phalangeal bones can be trimmed in the longitudinal direction. Joints are very often already stiff and therefore preservation of collateral ligaments becomes irrelevant. Bulky deposits of bone around the PIP joints can be trimmed and this can improve the range of movement of the joint without reducing the stability. In cases of hyperostotic macrodactyly, early diagnosis and resection of the osteochondral masses before significant impairment of joint function has occurred is advised [23, 25, 28].

(b) *Length reduction*: Length reduction should involve preservation of the nail bed, rather than just simple terminalization of the digit. The method attributed to Barksy shortens the middle phalanx with arthrodesis of the distal interphalangeal joint, transporting the distal phalanx and nail bed proximally, with plan for later soft tissue correction and narrowing of the nail bed if required [2] (Fig. 21.8). Tsuge described the "reverse" of this technique, with creation of a dorsal flap carrying the nail bed on one-third of the distal phalanx. The remainder of the distal phalanx is excised with the pulp and the nail bed transported proximally to the recipient middle phalanx, again with a plan for soft tissue correction at a later stage [153] (Fig. 21.9). However, simple excision of an already stiff distal interphalangeal joint will reduce the length of a digit, slow down the growth (by excision of the epiphysis), and improve the function and appearance of the digit. If this is carried out in association with a soft tissue debulking, any excess skin in the longitudinal direction will reduce spontaneously during the healing process. A single longitudinal/oblique K-wire can be used for fixation and removed in the outpatient department at around 6 weeks post-op.

(c) *Nail size and tip projection*: The nail width can be reduced at the same time as trimming of the bone and soft tissue debulking through a lateral incision.

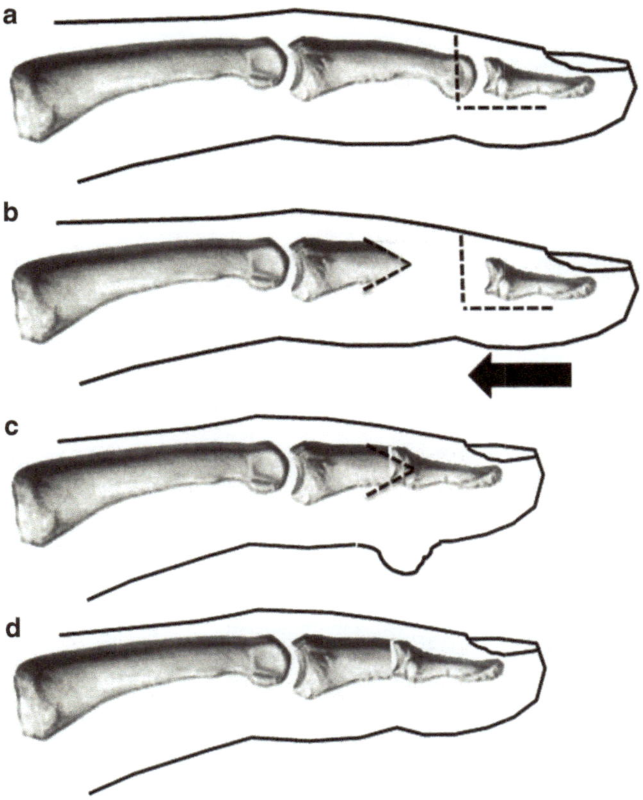

Fig. 21.8 Length reduction according to Barsky: (**a**) The enlarged digit with the skin incision as a *dashed line*. (**b**) The distal part of the middle phalanx is excised, proximal portion spiked and distal phalanx hollowed out. (**c**) The distal phalanx is transported proximally with a resulting volar hump. (**d**) The volar hump is excised at a later date. Adapted from [2]

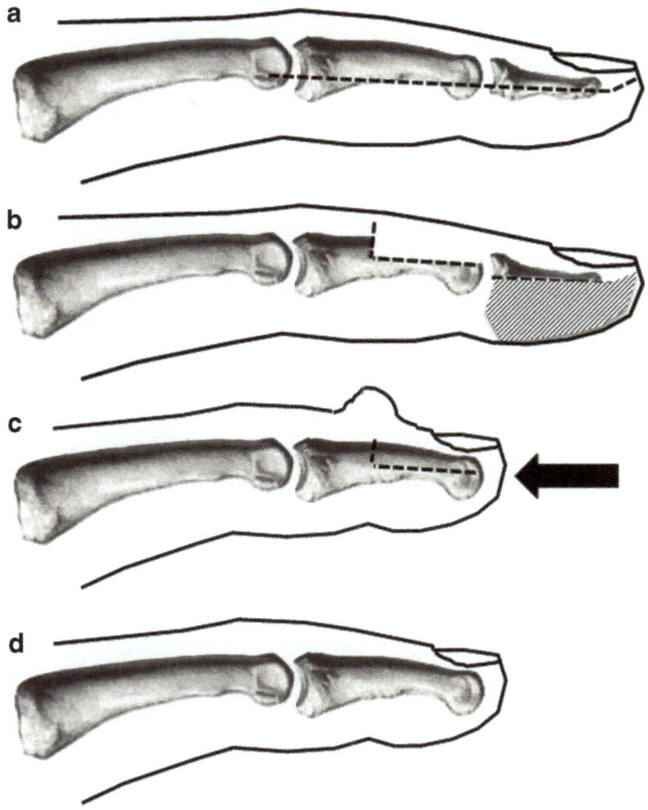

Fig. 21.9 Length reduction according to Tsuge: (**a**) Mid-lateral incisions to raise a dorsal flap to transport the nail. (**b**) The dorsal one-third of the distal phalanx is raised with the nail and redundant pulp and distal phalanx excised (*shaded*). (**c**) The distal phalanx and nail is transposed proximally, resulting in a dorsal hump. (**d**) The dorsal hump is excised at a later date. Adapted from [153]

This may need to be carried out on one side only. At the same time the excision of soft tissue around the tip of the digit can be performed close to the distal nail bed. The other side of the nail and further tip reduction can be performed 6 months later with debulking and narrowing of the digit through a lateral approach on the other side of the digit (Fig. 21.10).

(d) *Correction of angulation*: Closing wedge osteotomies at various sites in the phalanx will correct angulation and reduce the length of a digit or digits. A careful assessment of the X-ray and level of the angulation will determine where the osteotomy should take place. This can include the excision of the epiphysis. A whole stiff joint can be excised with minimal detriment to the function of the digit (i.e., an arthrodesis, Fig. 21.11). A single oblique K-wire is usually sufficient to encourage bone healing and can be simply removed in the clinic at around 6 weeks post-op.

(e) *Thumb*: The Millesi technique for thumb reduction is a combination of longitudinal and axial osteotomy of the distal phalanx with partial excision of the phalanx to provide shortening of the digit and narrowing nail bed in one stage (Fig. 21.12). This is further combined with oblique osteotomy of the proximal phalanx to allow shortening whilst maintaining the insertions of the extrinsic thumb flexor and extensor tendons [154]. It is also possible to consider a complete central resection of the bone and soft tissues.

4. *Ray Amputation*: In cases of progressive macrodactyly, the option for amputation should be raised early on in the treatment of the disease, especially if numerous operations and hospital admissions are anticipated. The parents and eventually the child need to be able to discuss this option freely but there is often a reluctance to consider this unless other attempts at surgical debulking have been tried in the first place. In the management of macrodactyly of the foot, it is often the best way to enable normal shoe fitting during the child's growing years. There should be no hesitation in carrying this operation out even in a young child, but significant soft tissue debulking both dorsally and on the plantar or volar side need to be carry-out at the same time. Longitudinal scars in this condition are not a problem on the sole of the foot. Historically, amputation of the thumb was strongly discouraged, with Kelikain favoring arthrectomy and fusion of the first

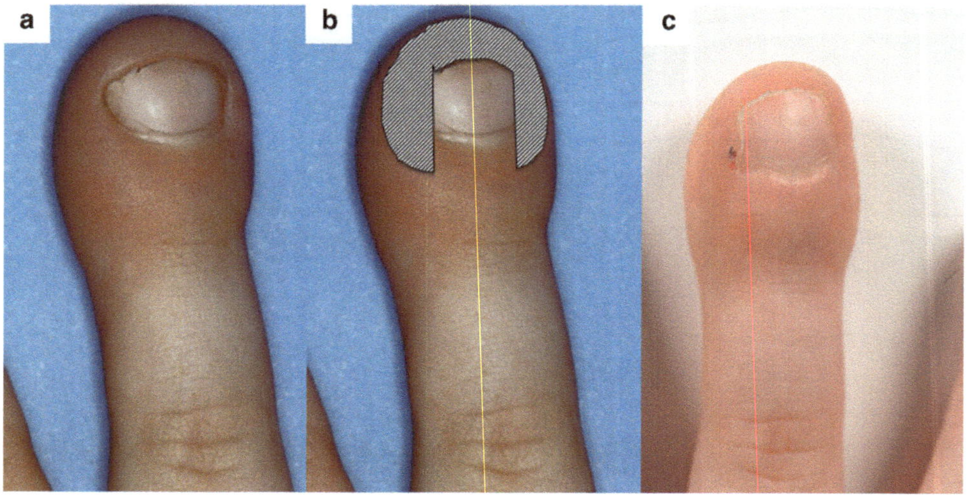

Fig. 21.10 Author's preferred method of reducing the nail: (**a**) Preoperative view. (**b**) Bilateral partial Zadeks procedure with bony and soft tissue reduction of the distal phalanx and finger tip. Excision area is *shaded*. (**c**) Postoperative view

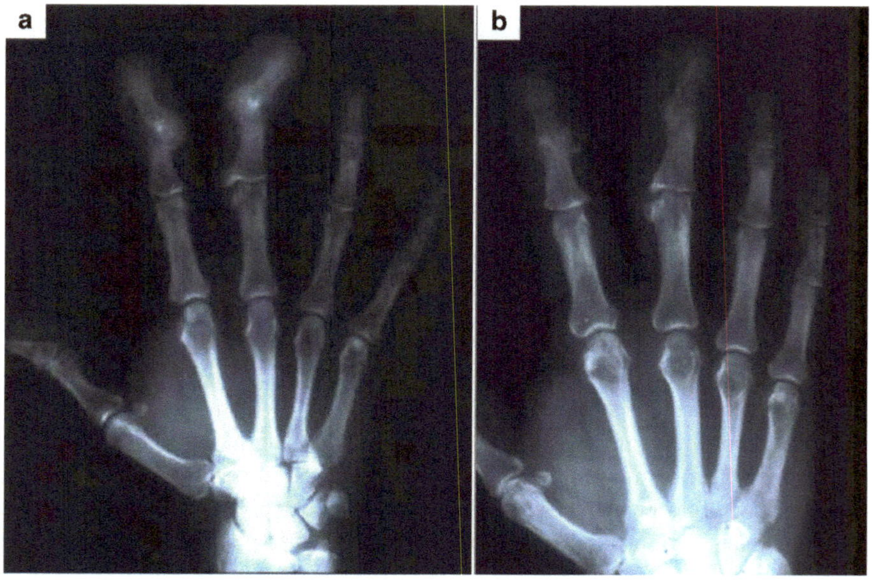

Fig. 21.11 (**a**) Pre- and (**b**) postoperative radiographs showing correction of angulation of the distal interphalangeal joint (DIPJ) of the middle finger, and hyperostosis of the DIPJ of the index finger, in conjunction with soft tissue debulking in an adult patient

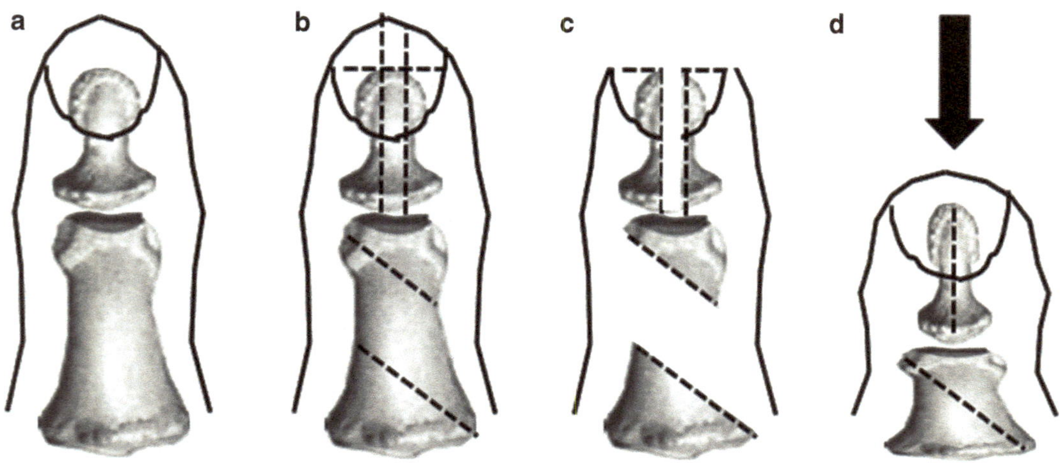

Fig. 21.12 Thumb reduction according to Millesi: (**a**) The enlarged thumb. (**b**) The central section of the distal phalanx and an oblique section of proximal phalanx is incised. (**c**) And removed. (**d**) The proximal and distal phalanges are reconstituted. Adapted from [154]

metacarpophalangeal joint [26]. More recently, digital transfer and free toe transfer have been used in the management of multi-digit macrodactyly affecting the thumb, middle, and index fingers [4].

Timing of Surgery

The surgeons' role in the management of this condition is to review and support the child through his growing years and alleviate some of the distress caused by this incurable condition. This requires the development of a close relationship, initially with the parents or guardians of the child, and gradual involvement of the child in the decision-making process with regards to the surgical technique and the timing of interventions. Surgery should be offered to correct problems with function and cosmesis as they arise. As repeated surgery may be necessary, consideration needs to be given to the child's general development and well-being.

Outcomes

In our analysis of macrodactyly affecting the upper and lower limbs, outcomes assessment was performed by postal questionnaire using validated tools, and the opinion of the surgeon [3]. The senior surgeon's outcome verdict was based on an overall combination of function, sensibility, growth arrest, and cosmesis, following discussion with the parents and child. It was interesting to note the difficulty in finding adequately fitting shoes in the cases of lower limb macrodactyly seemed disproportionate to the actual reported difference in shoe size. This is because the length of the toes is only a part of the overall increase in the size of the foot in that there is nearly always an associated increase in the depth and width of the foot due to the proximal enlargement of the bone and soft tissues of the forefoot (Fig. 21.13). There was a wide range in self-reported outcomes: The better outcomes were related to function and activity participation, which

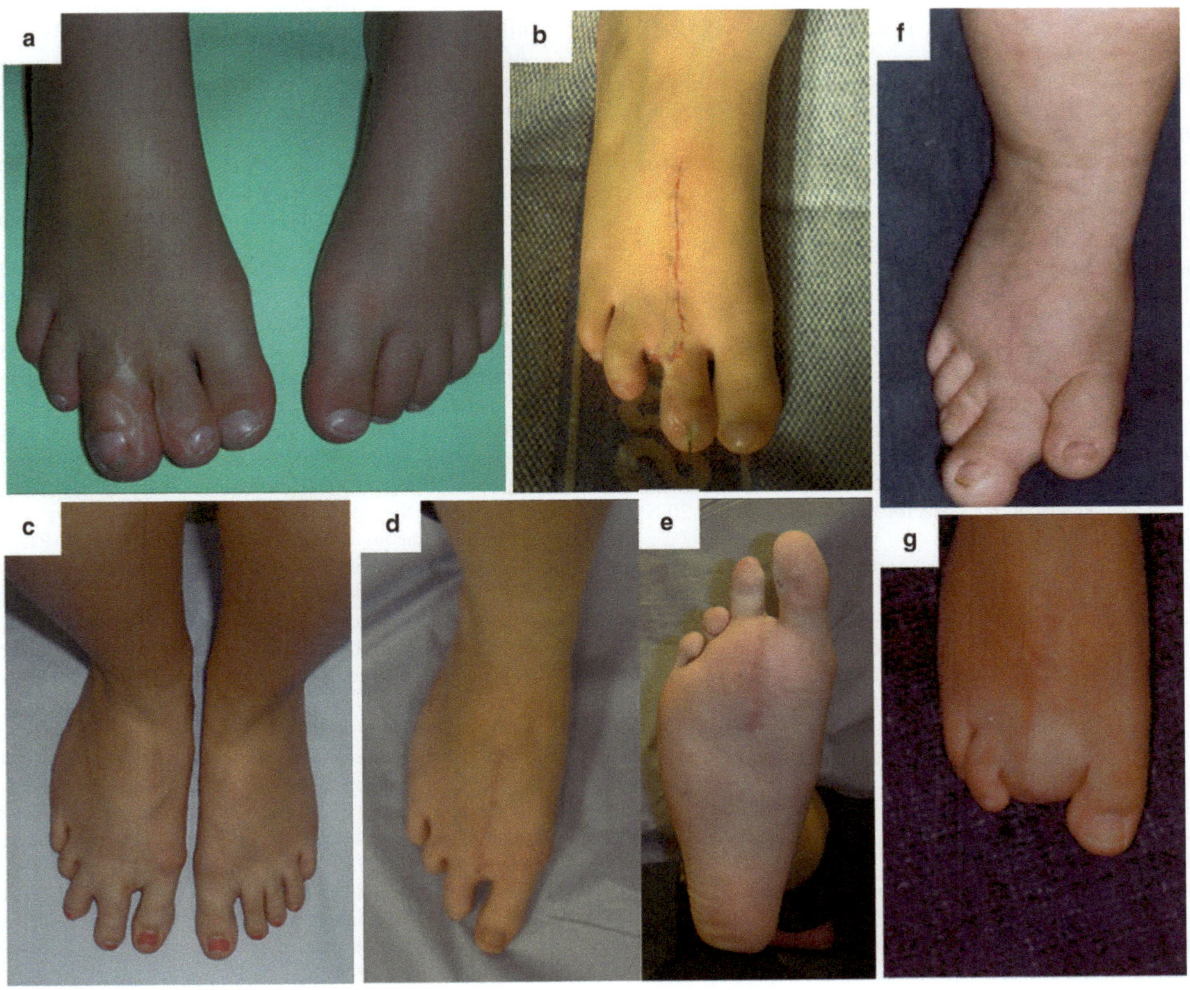

Fig. 21.13 Macrodactyly of the foot: (**a**) Macrodactyly of the right second and third toes. (**b**) Treated by third toe ray amputation and soft tissue debulking of the second toe enabling the reduction of shoe size discrepancy. (**c**) Macrodactyly of the right second toe leading to widening of the forefoot, which is not resolved by simple amputation of the toe—a full ray amputation is necessary. (**d**) Postoperative dorsal view. (**e**) The plantar scar is well tolerated. (**f**) Macrodactyly of the right second and third toes. (**g**) The forefoot width discrepancy is not resolved by digital amputation alone

could be assessed by the senior surgeon, whilst the poorer outcomes were related to happiness and satisfaction, which only were only revealed with self-reporting.

Summary

Macrodactyly represents a heterogeneous group of conditions. The parents and child deserve a detailed ongoing personalized assessment and review of their specific situation preferably with the same clinician for as long as possible. Many surgical techniques can be offered to alleviate functional and cosmetic problems. Surgeons managing this condition need to use all their craft skills to improve the quality of life of the child.

References

1. Biesecker LG, Aase JM, Clericuzio C, Gurrieri F, Temple IK, Toriello H. Elements of morphology: standard terminology for the hands and feet. Am J Med Genet A. 2009;149A:93–127.
2. Barsky AJ. Macrodactyly. J Bone Joint Surg Am. 1967;49:1255–66.
3. Hardwicke J, Khan MA, Richards H, Warner RM, Lester R. Macrodactyly—options and outcomes. J Hand Surg Eur Vol. 2013;38:297–303.
4. Cerrato F, Eberlin KR, Waters P, Upton J, Taghinia A, Labow BI. Presentation and treatment of macrodactyly in children. J Hand Surg Am. 2013;38:2112–23.
5. Yaghmai I, Mckowne F, Alizadeh A. Macrodactylia fibrolipomatosis. South Med J. 1976;1976(69):1565–8.
6. Thorne F, Posch J, Mladick R. Megalodactyly. Plast Reconstr Surg. 1968;41:232–9.
7. Flatt AE. The care of congenital hand anomalies. 2nd ed. St. Louis: Quality Medical; 1994. p. 47–62.
8. Lauschke H, Salminen S. Monstrous congenital macrodactyly with syndactyly of the foot—a case report. Acta Orthop Scand. 1998;69:201–2.
9. Fitoussi F, Ilharreborde B, Jehanno P, Frajman JM, Souchet P, Mazda K, Pennecot GF. Macrodactyly. Chir Main. 2009;28:129–37.
10. Price S, Williams AN. John Locke and a case of macrodactyly. Am J Med Genet A. 2009;149A:1364.
11. Dewhurst K. John Locke, 1632–1704, physician and philosopher; a medical biography with an edition of the medical notes in his journals. London: Wellcome Historical Medical Library; 1963.
12. Polaillon JFB. Chirurgie du doigt. Paris: G. Masson; 1884. p. 143–60.
13. Humphry SG. Macrodactyly, and some other forms of congenital overgrowth, and their relation to tumours. Med Chir Trans. 1891;74:165–80.
14. Swanson AB, Swanson GD, Tada K. A classification for congenital limb malformation. J Hand Surg Am. 1983;8:693–702.
15. Swanson AB. A classification for congenital limb malformations. J Hand Surg Am. 1976;1:8–22.
16. Swanson AB. A classification for congenital malformations of the hand. N J Bull Acad Med. 1964;10:166–9.
17. Tonkin MA, Tolerton SK, Quick TJ, Harvey I, Lawson RD, Smith NC, Oberg KC. Classification of congenital anomalies of the hand and upper limb: development and assessment of a new system. J Hand Surg Am. 2013;38:1845–53.
18. De Greef A, Pretorius LK. Macrodactyly. A review with a case report. S Afr Med J. 1983;63:939–41.
19. Richardière P. Hypertrophie congénitale de la main. Sem Méd. 1891;11:125.
20. Smith P. Lister's the hand, diagnosis and indications. 4th ed. London: Churchill Livingstone; 2002. p. 502.
21. De Laurenzi V. Macrodattilia del Medico. Gior Med Mil. 1962;12:401–5.
22. Holmes R. The surgical treatment of the diseases of infancy and childhood. Philadelphia: Lindsay and Blaketon; 1869. p. 207–21.
23. Upton J. Failure of differentiation and overgrowth. In: Mathes SJ, editor. Plastic surgery. 2nd ed. Philadelphia: Saunders Elsevier; 2006. p. 265–322.
24. Upton J. Overgrowth (gigantism) in congenital anomalies of the hand and forearm. In: May JW, Littler JW, editors. Plastic surgery. Philadelphia: WB Saunders; 1990.
25. Dell PC. Macrodactyly. Hand Clin. 1985;1:511–24.
26. Kelikian H. Congenital deformities of the hand and forearm. Philadelphia: WB Saunders; 1974. p. 939–75.
27. Wood V. Macrodactyly. J Iowa Med Soc. 1969;59:922–8.
28. Schuind F, Merle M, Dap F, Bour C, Michon J. Hyperostotic macrodactyly. J Hand Surg Am. 1988;13:544–8.
29. Kay SP, McCombe DB, Kozin SH. Deformities of the hands and fingers. In: Wolfe SW, Hotchkiss RN, Pederson WC, Kozin SH, editors. Green's operative hand surgery. 6th ed. Philadelphia: Elsevier; 2011. p. 1359–69.
30. ORDR. Office of Rare Disease Research. http://rarediseases.info.nih.gov/gard/8529/macrodactyly-of-thehand/resources/1. Accessed 11 Jan 2013.
31. Leung PC, Chan KM, Cheng JC. Congenital anomalies of the upper limb among the Chinese population in Hong Kong. J Hand Surg Am. 1982;7:563–5.
32. Ekblom AG, Laurell T, Arner M. Epidemiology of congenital upper limb anomalies in 562 children born in 1997 to 2007: a total population study from Stockholm, Sweden. J Hand Surg Am. 2010;35:1742–54.
33. Giele H, Giele C, Bower C, Allison M. The incidence and epidemiology of congenital upper limb anomalies: a total population study. J Hand Surg Am. 2001;26:628–34.
34. Lamb DW, Wynne-Davies R, Soto L. An estimate of the population frequency of congenital malformations of the upper limb. J Hand Surg Am. 1982;7:557–62.
35. Kowtharapu DN, Thawrani D, Kumar SJ. Macrodactyly. In: McCarthy JJ, editor. Drennen's the child's foot and ankle. 2nd ed. Baltimore: Lippincot Williams and Wilkins; 2009. p. 443–9.
36. Padgett EC, Stephenson KL. Reconstructive surgery of the skin and subcutaneous tissues of the extremities. In: Padgett EC, Stephenson KL, editors. Plastic and reconstructive surgery. Springfield: Charles C Thomas; 1948. p. 760.
37. Friedman JM, Riccardi VM. Clinical and epidemiological features. In: Neurofibromatosis: phenotype, natural history, and pathogenesis. 3rd ed. Baltimore: Johns Hopkins University Press; 1999. p. 29–86.
38. Gutmann DH, Aylsworth A, Carey JC, et al. The diagnostic evaluation and multidisciplinary management of neurofibromatosis 1 and neurofibromatosis 2. JAMA. 1997;278:51–7.
39. Huson SM, Harper PS, Compston DA. Von Recklinghausen neurofibromatosis: a clinical and population study in southeast Wales. Brain. 1988;111:1355–81.
40. NIH Consensus Statement. Neurofibromatosis. 1987;6:1–19.
41. Posner MA, McMahon MS, Desai P. Plexiform schwannoma (neurilemmoma) associated with macrodactyly: a case report. J Hand Surg Am. 1996;21:707–10.
42. Tsuge K. Treatment of macrodactyly. J Hand Surg Am. 1985;10:968–9.
43. Tsuge K, Ikuta Y. Macrodatyly and fibrofatty proliferation of the median nerve. Hiroshima J Med Sci. 1973;22:83–100.

44. McCarroll HR. Clinical manifestations of congenital neurofibromatosis. J Bone Joint Surg Am. 1950;32-A:601–17.
45. Riccardi VM. The genetic predisposition to and histogenesis of neurofibromas and neurofibrosarcoma in neurofibromatosis type 1. Neurosurg Focus. 2007;22:E3.
46. D'agostino AN, Soule EH, Miller RH. Sarcomas of the peripheral nerves and somatic soft tissues associated with multiple neurofibromatosis (von Recklinghausen's disease). Cancer. 1963;16: 1015–27.
47. Evans DG. Neurofibromatosis type 2 (NF2): a clinical and molecular review. Orphanet J Rare Dis. 2009;4:16.
48. Asthagiri AR, Parry DM, Butman JA, Kim HJ, Tsilou ET, Zhuang Z, Lonser RR. Neurofibromatosis type 2. Lancet. 2009;373:1974–86.
49. Bendon CL, Giele HP. Macrodactyly in the setting of a plexiform schwannoma in neurofibromatosis type 2: case report. J Hand Surg Am. 2013;38:740–4.
50. Albrecht (1904) Quoted by Anderson WAD. Pathology. 6th ed. St. Louis: CV Mosby; 1971. p. 980.
51. Hoey SE, Eastwood D, Monsell F, Kangesu L, Harper JI, Sebire NJ. Histopathological features of Proteus syndrome. Clin Exp Dermatol. 2008;33:234–8.
52. Norman-Taylor F, Mayou BJ. Macrodactyly in tuberous sclerosis. J R Soc Med. 1994;87:419–20.
53. Cohen Jr MM, Hayden PW. A newly recognized hamartomatous syndrome. Birth Defects Orig Artic Ser. 1979;15:291–6.
54. Wiedemann HR, Burgio GR, Aldenhoff P, Kunze J, Kaufmann HJ, Schirg E. The proteus syndrome. Partial gigantism of the hands and/or feet, nevi, hemihypertrophy, subcutaneous tumors, macrocephaly or other skull anomalies and possible accelerated growth and visceral affections. Eur J Pediatr. 1983;140:5–12.
55. Biesecker L. The challenges of Proteus syndrome: diagnosis and management. Eur J Hum Genet. 2006;14:1151–7.
56. Treves F. A case of congenital deformity. Proc Pathol Soc London. 1885;36:494–8.
57. Lublin M, Schwartzentruber DJ, Lukish J, Chester C, Biesecker LG, Newman KD. Principles for the surgical management of patients with Proteus syndrome and patients with overgrowth not meeting Proteus criteria. J Pediatr Surg. 2002;37:1013–20.
58. Biesecker LG, Happle R, Mulliken JB, Weksberg R, Graham Jr JM, Viljoen DL, et al. Proteus syndrome: diagnostic criteria, differential diagnosis, and patient evaluation. Am J Med Genet. 1999;84:389–95.
59. Biesecker LG, Peters KF, Darling TN, Choyke P, Hill S, Schimke N, et al. Clinical differentiation between Proteus syndrome and hemihyperplasia: description of a distinct form of hemihyperplasia. Am J Med Genet. 1998;79:311–8.
60. Clark RD, Donnai D, Rogers J, Cooper J, Baraitser M. Proteus syndrome: an expanded phenotype. Am J Med Genet. 1987;27: 99–117.
61. Angurana SK, Angurana RS, Panigrahi I, Marwaha RK. Proteus syndrome: clinical profile of six patients and review of literature. Indian J Hum Genet. 2013;19:202–6.
62. Morelli F, Feliciani C, Toto P, De Benedetto A, Tulli A. A minimal form of Proteus syndrome presenting with macrodactyly and hand hyperplasia. Eur J Dermatol. 2003;13:196–8.
63. Miura H, Uchida Y, Ihara K, Sugioka Y. Macrodactyly in Proteus syndrome. J Hand Surg Br. 1993;18:308–9.
64. Barmakian JT, Posner MA, Silver L, Lehman W, Vine DT. Proteus syndrome. J Hand Surg Am. 1992;17:32–4.
65. Desai P, Steiner GC. Pathology of macrodactyly. Bull Hosp Jt Dis Orthop Inst. 1990;50:116–25.
66. Biesecker LG, Sapp JC. Proteus syndrome. In: Pagon RA, Adam MP, Bird TD, Dolan CR, Fong CT, Stephens K, editors. GeneReviews™ [Internet]. Seattle: University of Washington; 1993–2013.
67. Orlova KA, Crino PB. The tuberous sclerosis complex. Ann N Y Acad Sci. 2010;1184:87–105.
68. Curatolo P, Bombardieri R, Jozwiak S. Tuberous sclerosis. Lancet. 2008;372:657–68.
69. Ghali FE. Macrodactyly in tuberous sclerosis. Pediatr Dermatol. 2001;18:364–5.
70. Tung HE, Shih SL. Tuberous sclerosis with rare presentation of macrodactyly. Pediatr Radiol. 2009;39:878.
71. Sahoo B, Handa S, Kumar B. Tuberous sclerosis with macrodactyly. Pediatr Dermatol. 2000;17:463–5.
72. Schwartz RA, Fernández G, Kotulska K, Jóźwiak S. Tuberous sclerosis complex: advances in diagnosis, genetics, and management. J Am Acad Dermatol. 2007;57:189–202.
73. Joinson C, O'Callaghan FJ, Osborne JP, Martyn C, Harris T, Bolton PF. Learning disability and epilepsy in an epidemiological sample of individuals with tuberous sclerosis complex. Psychol Med. 2003;33:335–44.
74. Superti-Furga A, Spranger J, Nishimura G. Enchondromatosis revisited: new classification with molecular basis. Am J Med Genet C Semin Med Genet. 2012;160C:154–64.
75. Pansuriya TC, Kroon HM, Bovée JV. Enchondromatosis: insights on the different subtypes. Int J Clin Exp Pathol. 2010;3:557–69.
76. Kaissi AA, Roetzer K, Klaushofer K, Grill F. Acroform type of enchondromatosis associated with severe vertebral involvement and facial dysmorphism in a boy with a new variant of enchondromatosis type I1 of Spranger: case report and a review of the literature. Cases J. 2008;1:324.
77. Spranger J, Kemperdieck H, Bakowski H, Opitz JM. Two peculiar types of enchondromatosis. Pediatr Radiol. 1978;7:215–9.
78. Al-Qattan MM, Javed K, Pant R. An unusual case of multiple hand enchondromas. J Hand Surg Eur Vol. 2010;35:321–2.
79. Casal D, Mavioso C, Mendes MM, Mouzinho MM. Hand involvement in Ollier Disease and Maffucci Syndrome: a case series. Acta Reumatol Port. 2010;35:375–8.
80. Silve C, Jüppner H. Ollier disease. Orphanet J Rare Dis. 2006;1:37.
81. Howard FM, Lee Jr RE. The hand in Maffucci syndrome. Arch Surg. 1971;103:752–6.
82. Vigorita V, D'Ambrosio F, Verde R, Kauderer C, Bryk E. Case report 784: fibrous dysplasia of the second pedal digit. Skeletal Radiol. 1993;22:441–3.
83. Weksberg R, Shuman C, Beckwith JB. Beckwith-Wiedemann syndrome. Eur J Hum Genet. 2010;18:8–14.
84. Best LG, Hoekstra RE. Wiedemann-Beckwith syndrome: autosomal-dominant inheritance in a family. Am J Med Genet. 1981;9:291–9.
85. Beckwith JB, Wang CI, Donnel GN, et al. Hyperplastic fetal visceromegaly with macroglossia, omphalocele, cytomegaly of adrenal fetal cortex, postnatal somatic gigantism and other abnormalties: newly recognized syndrome (Abst no 41). Proceedings of the American Pediatric Society, Seattle. 1964. p. 16–18.
86. Wiedemann HR. Familial malformation complex with umbilical hernia and macroglossia—a "new syndrome'? J Genet Hum. 1964;13:223–32.
87. Weksberg R, Shuman C, Smith AC. Beckwith-Wiedemann syndrome. Am J Med Genet C Semin Med Genet. 2005;137C:12–23.
88. Cytrynbaum CS, Smith AC, Rubin T, Weksberg R. Advances in overgrowth syndromes: clinical classification to molecular delineation in Sotos syndrome and Beckwith-Wiedemann syndrome. Curr Opin Pediatr. 2005;17:740–6.
89. ISSVA classification. In: Enjolras O, Wassef M, Chapot R, editors. Color atlas of vascular tumors and vascular malformations. New York: Cambridge University Press; 2007. p. 1–11.

90. Enjolras O. Classification and management of the various superficial vascular anomalies: hemangiomas and vascular malformations. J Dermatol. 1997;24:701–10.
91. Klippel M, Trénaunay P. Du naevus variqueux ostéohypertrophique. Archives générales de médecine. 1900;3:641–72.
92. Weber FP. Angioma formation in connexion with hypertrophy of limbs and hemihypertrophy. Br J Dermatol. 1907;19:231.
93. McGrory BJ, Amadio PC, Dobyns JH, Stickler GB, Unni KK. Anomalies of the fingers and toes associated with Klippel-Trenaunay syndrome. J Bone Joint Surg Am. 1991;73:1537–46.
94. Sapp JC, Turner JT, van de Kamp JM, van Dijk FS, Lowry RB, Biesecker LG. Newly delineated syndrome of congenital lipomatous overgrowth, vascular malformations, and epidermal nevi (CLOVE syndrome) in seven patients. Am J Med Genet A. 2007;143A:2944–58.
95. Alomari AI, Thiex R, Mulliken JB. Hermann Freiberg's case report: an early description of CLOVES syndrome. Clin Genet. 2010;78:342–7.
96. Bloom J, Upton J. CLOVES syndrome. J Hand Surg Am. 2013;38:2508–12. pii:S0363-5023(13)01188-X; doi:10.1016/j.jhsa.2013.08.120.
97. Gucev ZS, Tasic V, Jancevska A, Konstantinova MK, Pop-Jordanova N, Trajkovski Z, et al. CLOVE syndrome (congenital lipomatous overgrowth, vascular malformations, and epidermal nevi): CNS malformations and seizures may be a component of this disorder. Am J Med Genet A. 2008;146A(20):2688–90.
98. OMIM. www.omim.org. Accessed 11 Jan 2013.
99. Lau FH, Xia F, Kaplan A, Cerrato F, Greene AK, Taghinia A, et al. Expression analysis of macrodactyly identifies pleiotrophin upregulation. PLoS One. 2012;7:e40423.
100. Miura K, Namba N, Fujiwara M, Ohata Y, Ishida H, et al. An overgrowth disorder associated with excessive production of cGMP due to a gain-of-function mutation of the natriuretic peptide receptor 2 gene. PLoS One. 2012;7:e42180.
101. Rios JJ, Paria N, Burns DK, Israel BA, Cornelia R, Wise CA, et al. Somatic gain-of-function mutations in PIK3CA in patients with macrodactyly. Hum Mol Genet. 2013;22:444–51.
102. Kretschmer PJ, Fairhurst JL, Decker MM, Chan CP, Gluzman Y, Böhlen P, et al. Cloning, characterization and developmental regulation of two members of a novel human gene family of neurite outgrowth-promoting proteins. Growth Factors. 1991;5:99–114.
103. Merenmies J, Rauvala H. Molecular cloning of the 18-kDa growth-associated protein of developing brain. J Biol Chem. 1990;265:16721–4.
104. Rauvala H. An 18-kd heparin-binding protein of developing brain that is distinct from fibroblast growth factors. EMBO J. 1989;8:2933–41.
105. Blondet B, Carpentier G, Lafdil F, Courty J. Pleiotrophin cellular localization in nerve regeneration after peripheral nerve injury. J Histochem Cytochem. 2005;53:971–7.
106. Imai S, Heino TJ, Hienola A, Kurata K, Bu¨ki K, et al. Osteocyte-derived HB-GAM (pleiotrophin) is associated with bone formation and mechanical loading. Bone. 2009;44:785–94.
107. Tare RS, Oreffo ROC, Clarke NMP, Roach HI. Pleiotrophin/Osteoblast-stimulating factor 1: dissecting its diverse functions in bone formation. J Bone Miner Res. 2002;17:2009–20.
108. Azizan A, Gaw JU, Govindraj P, Tapp H, Neame PJ. Chondromodulin I and pleiotrophin gene expression in bovine cartilage and epiphysis. Matrix Biol. 2000;19:521–31.
109. Zhang N, Zhong R, Perez-Pinera P, Herradon G, Ezquerra L, Wang ZY, et al. Identification of the angiogenesis signaling domain in pleiotrophin defines a mechanism of the angiogenic switch. Biochem Biophys Res Commun. 2006;343:653–8.
110. Bocciardi R, Giorda R, Buttgereit J, Gimelli S, Divizia MT, Beri S, et al. Overexpression of the C-type natriuretic peptide (CNP) is associated with overgrowth and bone anomalies in an individual with balanced t(2;7) translocation. Hum Mutat. 2007;28:724–31.
111. Moncla A, Missirian C, Cacciagli P, Balzamo E, Legeai-Mallet L, Jouve JL, et al. A cluster of translocation breakpoints in 2q37 is associated with overexpression of NPPC in patients with a similar overgrowth phenotype. Hum Mutat. 2007;28:1183–8.
112. Bartels CF, Bükülmez H, Padayatti P, Rhee DK, van Ravenswaaij-Arts C, Pauli RM, et al. Mutations in the transmembrane natriuretic peptide receptor NPR-B impair skeletal growth and cause acromesomelic dysplasia, type Maroteaux. Am J Hum Genet. 2004;75:27–34.
113. Kurek KC, Luks VL, Ayturk UM, Alomari AI, Fishman SJ, Spencer SA, et al. Somatic mosaic activating mutations in PIK3CA cause CLOVES syndrome. Am J Hum Genet. 2012;90:1108–15.
114. Rodon J, Dienstmann R, Serra V, Tabernero J. Development of PI3K inhibitors: lessons learned from early clinical trials. Nat Rev Clin Oncol. 2013;10:143–53.
115. Miller TW, Rexer BN, Garrett JT, Arteaga CL. Mutations in the phosphatidylinositol 3-kinase pathway: role in tumor progression and therapeutic implications in breast cancer. Breast Cancer Res. 2011;13:224.
116. Bodine SC. mTOR signaling and the molecular adaptation to resistance exercise. Med Sci Sports Exerc. 2006;38:1950–7.
117. Williams VC, Lucas J, Babcock MA, Gutmann DH, Korf B, Maria BL. Neurofibromatosis type 1 revisited. Pediatrics. 2009;123:124–33.
118. Sabbagh A, Pasmant E, Imbard A, Luscan A, Soares M, Blanché H, et al. NF1 molecular characterization and neurofibromatosis type I genotype-phenotype correlation: the French experience. Hum Mutat. 2013;34:1510–8.
119. Trofatter JA, MacCollin MM, Rutter JL, Murrell JR, Duyao MP, Parry DM, et al. A novel moesin-, ezrin-, radixin-like gene is a candidate for the neurofibromatosis 2 tumor suppressor. Cell. 1993;72:791–800.
120. Zhou L, Ercolano E, Ammoun S, Schmid MC, Barczyk MA, Hanemann CO. Merlin-deficient human tumors show loss of contact inhibition and activation of Wnt/β-catenin signaling linked to the PDGFR/Src and Rac/PAK pathways. Neoplasia. 2011;13:1101–12.
121. Thaxton C, Bott M, Walker B, Sparrow NA, Lambert S, Fernandez-Valle C. Schwannomin/merlin promotes Schwann cell elongation and influences myelin segment length. Mol Cell Neurosci. 2011;47:1–9.
122. Stamenkovic I, Yu Q. Merlin, a "magic" linker between extracellular cues and intracellular signaling pathways that regulate cell motility, proliferation, and survival. Curr Protein Pept Sci. 2010;11:471–84.
123. Gonzalez E, McGraw TE. The Akt kinases: isoform specificity in metabolism and cancer. Cell Cycle. 2009;8:2502–8.
124. Cohen MM Jr. Proteus syndrome review: molecular, clinical, and pathologic features. Clin Genet. 2013. doi:10.1111/cge.12266 [Epub ahead of print].
125. Eng C. PTEN hamartoma tumor syndrome (PHTS). In: Pagon RA, Adam MP, Bird TD, Dolan CR, Fong CT, Stephens K, editors. GeneReviews™ [Internet]. Seattle: University of Washington; 1993–2013.
126. Hobert JA, Eng C. PTEN hamartoma tumor syndrome: an overview. Genet Med. 2009;11:687–94.
127. Eng C. PTEN: one gene, many syndromes. Hum Mutat. 2003;22:183–98.
128. Caux F, Plauchu H, Chibon F, Faivre L, Fain O, Vabres P, et al. Segmental overgrowth, lipomatosis, arteriovenous malformation and epidermal nevus (SOLAMEN) syndrome is related to mosaic PTEN nullizygosity. Eur J Hum Genet. 2007;15:767–73.

129. Choufani S, Shuman C, Weksberg R. Molecular findings in Beckwith–Wiedemann syndrome. Am J Med Genet C Semin Med Genet. 2013;163C:131–40.
130. Keniry A, Oxley D, Monnier P, Kyba M, Dandolo L, Smits G, Reik W. The H19 lincRNA is a developmental reservoir of miR-675 that suppresses growth and Igf1r. Nat Cell Biol. 2012;14: 659–65.
131. Maher ER, Reik W. Beckwith-Wiedemann syndrome: imprinting in clusters revisited. J Clin Invest. 2000;37:212–5.
132. Li M, Squire J, Shuman C, Fei YL, Atkin J, Pauli R, et al. Imprinting status of 11p15 genes in Beckwith–Wiedemann syndrome patients with CDKN1C mutations. Genomics. 2001;74:370–6.
133. Ramesar R, Babaya M, Viljoen D. Molecular investigation of familial Beckwith-Wiedemann syndrome: a model for paternal imprinting. Eur J Hum Genet. 1993;1:109–13.
134. Mirzaa G, Conway R, Graham Jr JM, Dobyns WB. PIK3CA-related segmental overgrowth. In: Pagon RA, Adam MP, Bird TD, Dolan CR, Fong CT, Stephens K, editors. GeneReviews™ [Internet]. Seattle: University of Washington; 1993–2013.
135. Yuksel A, Yagmur H, Kural BS. Prenatal diagnosis of isolated macrodactyly. Ultrasound Obstet Gynecol. 2009;33:360–2.
136. Rypens F, Dubois J, Garel L, Fournet JC, Michaud JL, Grignon A. Obstetric US: watch the fetal hands. Radiographics. 2006;26:811–29.
137. Edgerton MT, Tuerk DB. Macrodactyly (digital gigantism): its nature and treatment. In: Littler JW, Cramer LM, Smith JW, editors. Symposium on reconstructive hand surgery, vol. 9. St. Louis: CV Mosby; 1974.
138. Ishida O, Ikuta Y. Long-term results of surgical treatment for macrodactyly of the hand. Plast Reconstr Surg. 1998;102:1586–90.
139. Kalen V, Burwell DS, Omer GE. Macrodactyly of the hands and feet. J Pediatr Orthop. 1988;8:311–5.
140. Minguella J, Cusi V. Macrodactyly of the hands and feet. Int Orthop. 1992;16:245–9.
141. Meyer BU, Röricht S. Fibrolipomatous hamartoma of the proximal ulnar nerve associated with macrodactyly and macrodystrophia lipomatosa as an unusual case of cubital tunnel syndrome. J Neurol Neurosurg Psychiatry. 1997;63:808–10.
142. Silverman TA, Enzinger FM. Fibrolipomatous hamartoma of nerve. A clinicopathologic analysis of 26 cases. Am J Surg Pathol. 1985;9:7–14.
143. Tahiri Y, Xu L, Kanevsky J, Luc M. Lipofibromatous hamartoma of the median nerve: a comprehensive review and systematic approach to evaluation, diagnosis and treatment. J Hand Surg Am. 2013;38:2055–67.
144. Al-Jabri T, Garg S, Mani GV. Lipofibromatous hamartoma of the median nerve. J Orthop Surg Res. 2010;5:71.
145. Van Meir N, De Smet L. Carpal tunnel syndrome in children. J Pediatr Orthop B. 2005;14:42–5.
146. Lamberti PM, Light TR. Carpal tunnel syndrome in children. Hand Clin. 2002;18:331–7.
147. Nogueira A, Pena C, Martinez MJ, Sarasua JG, Madrigal B. Hyperostotic macrodactyly and lipofibromatous hamartoma of the median nerve associated with carpal tunnel syndrome. Chir Main. 1999;18:261–71.
148. Ulrich D, Ulrich F, Schroeder M, Pallua N. Lipofibromatous hamartoma of the median nerve in patients with macrodactyly: diagnosis and treatment of a rare disease causing carpal tunnel syndrome. Arch Orthop Trauma Surg. 2009;129:1219–24.
149. Salon A, Guero S, Glicenstein J. Fibrolipoma of the median nerve. Review of 10 surgically treated cases with a mean recall of 8 years. Ann Chir Main Memb Super. 1995;14:284–95.
150. Frykmann GK, Wood VE. Peripheral nerve hamartoma with macrodactyly in the hand: report of three cases and review of the literature. J Hand Surg Am. 1978;3:307–12.
151. Allende BT. Macrodactyly with enlarged median nerve associated with carpal tunnel syndrome. Plast Reconstr Surg. 1967;39: 578–82.
152. Clifford RH. The treatment of macrodactylism: a case report. Plast Reconstr Surg. 1959;23:245–8.
153. Tsuge K. Treatment of macrodactyly. Plast Reconstr Surg. 1967;39:590–9.
154. Millesi H. Macrodactyly: a case study. In: Littler JW, Cramer LM, Smith JW, editors. Symposium on reconstructive hand surgery, vol. 9. St. Louis: CV Mosby; 1974.

Amniotic Band Syndrome

22

Shady Abdel-Rehim and Kevin Chung

Amniotic band or constriction band syndrome (ABS) is a rare congenital disorder characterized by partial or complete constriction rings around limbs or digits that leads to deformation, malformation, and/or amputation of the extremities of the neonates [1]. Associated manifestations may include craniofacial, body-wall defects, and internal organ abnormalities. A prevalence rate of 1.16 per 10,000 live births has been reported in the USA, with defects occurring 1.76 times more often in African Americans than in Caucasians [2]. ABS occurs sporadically, and no autosomal inheritance or sex predilections have been recognized. The constellation of symptoms associated with ABS that often involves several body parts has led to various terms being used in the literature to describe this complex congenital anomaly. Traditionally, these terms included amnion rupture sequence, aberrant tissue band syndrome, constriction band syndrome, constriction ring syndrome, congenital annular constrictions, and Streeter dysplasia, among others. The presence of a large number of synonyms and acronyms may reflect the lack of consensus or perhaps the confusion among surgeons on the etiologies of this rare congenital disorder [3]. Rayan [4] more recently criticized the use of several terms to describe a single clinical entity in which he considered to be confusing to the reader. Instead he suggested the use of the terms "amniotic constriction bands" or "amniotic bands" that he believes to be the most accurate descriptions of the disease etiology. Despite the disease nomenclature, the resultant deformities and disability affecting newborns are usually alarming to the parents and their families and often pose a surgical challenge to the hand surgeon because of the unique presentation of each patient. Staged and multiple reconstructive procedures are often required, thus a good rapport and adequate family counseling is an integral part of the management of patients with ABS.

S. Abdel-Rehim, M.B.Ch.B., M.Sc., M.R.C.S. (Ed)
K. Chung, M.D., M.S. (✉)
Department of Plastic Surgery, University of Michigan Healthcare System, 2130 Taubman Center, SPC 5340, 1500 E. Medical Center Drive, Ann Arbor, MI 48109-5340, USA
e-mail: abdelreh@umich.edu; kecchung@umich.edu

Etiology of Amniotic Band Syndrome

Historically, the etiology of ABS has always been surrounded by controversies. The theories describing causes of congenital anomalies associated with ABS almost took a full circle from external compression to endogenous abnormalities of fetal development and back again. Hippocrates made the earliest recorded suggestion that antenatal malformation of the extremities may be caused by external compressive forces acting in utero (300 BC). Several theories regarding the etiology of ABS have been described since. Van Helmont (1652) reported a case of intrauterine amputation that he believed to be due to the sight of amputated soldiers by pregnant women. Chaussier (1812) later attributed limb amputations to a gangrenous process affecting the extremities in utero [5].

The first reported descriptions of "amniotic bands" as a cause of fetal limb amputations were made by Montgomery (1832), and then expanded upon by Simpson (1836). These authors suggested that intrauterine limb amputations result from the formation of constriction strings/bands that entangle fetal limbs and lead to their amputation [6, 7]. However, the idea of external mechanical compression by amniotic bands was rapidly dismissed when Streeter (1930) proposed his theory to suggest that constrictions rings were localized areas of imperfectly formed tissue due to defective areas of germ-line development [8]. Streeter's theory later became known as the "intrinsic theory" or "Streeter dysplasia" and was widely accepted by many. Similar to Streeter, Patterson (1961) also believed that an endogenous developmental error is most likely responsible for the congenital abnormalities associated with ABS [9]. In his thesis "Congenital ring-constrictions," Patterson performed histological studies suggesting that constriction rings occur primarily from failure of development of subcutaneous tissue that result in constriction bands resembling normal flexural creases. In its most severe form, these constriction bands would result in limb ischemia and amputation. Other authors, who support endogenous/intrinsic causes of ABS, have suggested a

D.R. Laub Jr. (ed.), *Congenital Anomalies of the Upper Extremity: Etiology and Management*,
DOI 10.1007/978-1-4899-7504-1_22, © Springer Science+Business Media New York 2015

multifactorial process in that a vascular compromise or tetratogenic insult of germ-line cells would result in the clinical manifestations associated with ABS [10–12]. However, there is little evidence to support these theories. Proponents of the intrinsic theory suggest that germ-line defects would explain most of developmental anomalies of ABS. Opponents argue that the clinical abnormalities resulting from germ-line defects should be more consistent and reproducible, which to a great extent is not the case in ABS as the clinical picture among patients is highly variable.

Tropin (1965) challenged Streeter's theory by proposing an alternative hypothesis in which he explained a sequence of events leading to fetal abnormalities that became known as the "extrinsic theory" [13]. Tropin's theory was simply a re-introduced of the intrauterine fibrous strand concept of deformity. He suggested that as the amnion ruptures during gestation, there is a tendency to form mesodermic fibrous strands that wrap around fetal extremities, as well as the neck and the umbilical cord of the fetus. Furthermore, the underlying layer of denuded chorion absorbs the amniotic fluid and causes a temporary oligohydramnios with compressive consequences of early constraint, such as scoliosis and clubfoot. In an experimental study involving rat models, Kino (1975) performed amniocentesis 15 days post conception thus inducing a state of oligohydramnios. He concluded that prenatal environmental factors such as intrauterine compression of the fetus during periods of decreased amniotic fluid could induce many of the various manifestations of ABS [14]. These findings reported by Kino supports Tropin's extrinsic theory. The timing of amniotic rupture is also believed to be a major factor determining the range and severity of ABS deformities. Higginbottom and colleagues (1979) reviewed 79 patients with deformities ranging from digital band constrictions to major craniofacial and visceral defects. The authors concluded that early amniotic rupture could lead to multiple fetal malformations, and visceral defects, whereas later ruptures predominantly affect the extremities [15]. Despite these findings, there is still an ongoing debate as to whether intrinsic or extrinsic or a combination of both causes is responsible for the clinical manifestations of ABS.

Diagnosis

The antenatal diagnosis of ABS can be established by ultrasonography. Visualization of amniotic bands is particularly difficult in the first trimester, especially if the bands are only limited to extremities. However, in the second and third trimesters it is relatively easier to detect amniotic bands abnormalities and restriction of motion associated with ABS [16]. When characteristic asymmetric fetal anomalies are observed by ultrasound, regardless of the presence or absence of fibrous membranes, ABS should be suspected. However, technological advancements of higher resolution (3D/4D) ultrasounds that are currently available can detect amniotic bands as early as 13 weeks of gestation [17–19]. An MRI can be useful to detect fetal structural abnormalities such as cranial defects associated with ABS [20]. MRI can also define the vascular anatomy, which may be anomalous, thus may help to prevent injury to the vessels during surgery. Serum markers such as elevated maternal serum alpha-fetoprotein and beta human chorionic gonadotropin have also been associated with cases of fetal ABS [21, 22]. Finally, at a few months of age, an X-ray is required to assess any associated bony abnormalities that may be present especially in syndactyly with amputated distal parts. The differential diagnosis for ABS includes symbrachydactyly and transverse deficiency. Symbrachydactyly is a term used to describe a group of deformities ranging from digital hypoplasia to aplasia or deficiency of the hand or forearm [23]. Unlike ABS where multiple extremities can be affected at different levels, symbrachydactyly is often unilateral and is characterized by the presence of distal ectodermal structures such as pulp, nail fold, and nail. Association with Poland syndrome has been recognized [24].

Transverse deficiency has an autosomal recessive inheritance pattern with variable expression. Transverse deficiency represents an arrest of formation of the limb linage and range from aphalangia to amelia. The stump is usually covered by soft-tissue and shows rudimentary digits at the end of the stump. The condition is classified by naming the level at which the remaining limb terminates with all structures distal to the level named being absent. The most common site of amputation is usually at the proximal third of the forearm [25, 26].

Clinical Presentation

The clinical manifestations of ABS typically involve various deformities that primarily affect the extremities as well as other parts of the body. The hand is the most commonly affected part with a tendency for involving the distal segments [3, 24]. Other associated abnormalities may include clubfoot, leg length discrepancies, scoliosis, craniofacial defects such as cleft lip and cleft palate, body-wall defects, and visceral abnormalities. However no two cases have the exact same findings [27, 28]. Risk factors such as fetal prematurity, low birth weight, and maternal co-morbidities (e.g., maternal illness during pregnancy and drug exposure) have been reported in 80 % of patients [29]. The presence of hand deformities should always alert the surgeon to the possibility of other occult existing anomalies. These abnormalities can be life or limb threatening and often require a thorough clinical evaluation by other specialists such as a pediatrician, a geneticist and/or a craniofacial surgeon, in addition to a hand surgeon.

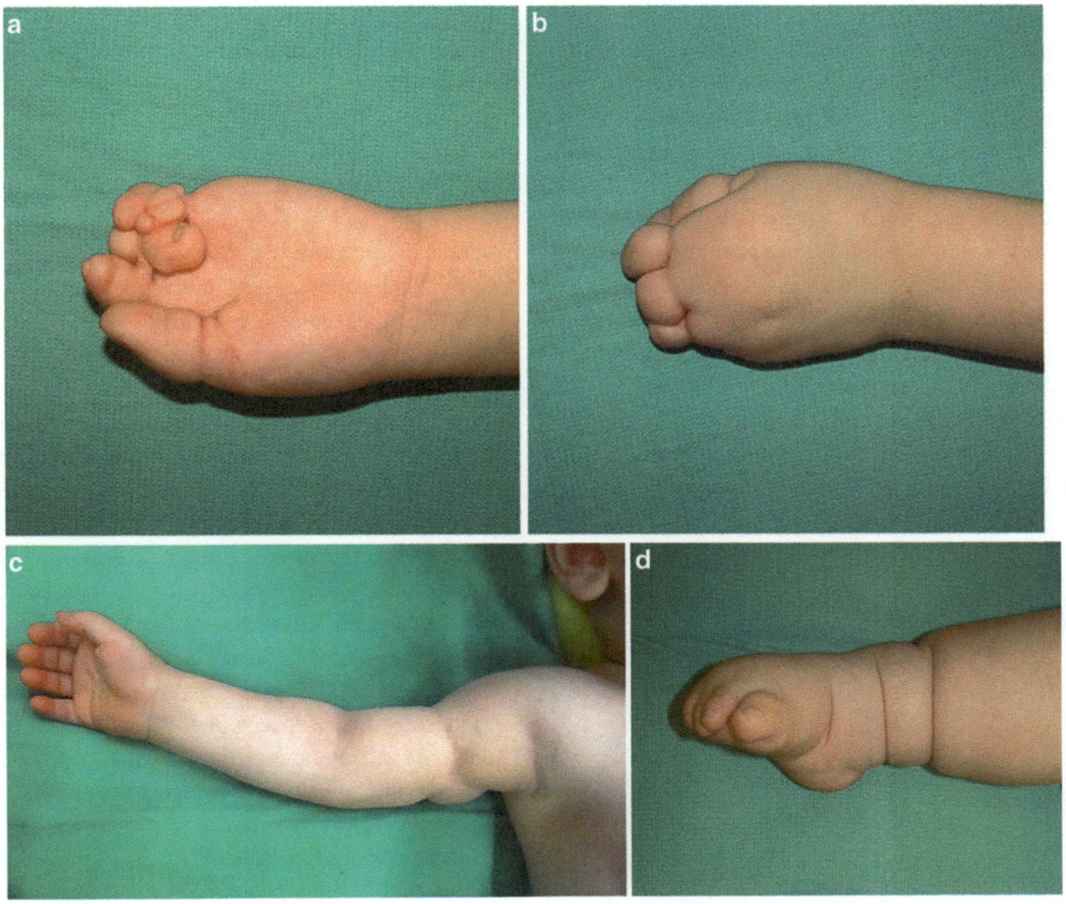

Fig. 22.1 Constriction bands involving the upper and lower extremities. The hand deformity shows constriction bands, lymphedema, acrosyndactyly, and digital amputations

In the hand, the spectrum of the clinical findings associated with ABS may vary from a simple indentation of the affected limb to a complete amputation of the limb or digit [27]. However, classic findings include constriction bands, lymphedema, acrosyndactyly, and/or distal amputations (Fig. 22.1). The histological specimens of mild constriction rings examined by Patterson [9] showed a defective subcutaneous dermal component covered by normal epidermis that resembles a normal flexural crease or skin fold. Scarring and dense fibrous tissue are commonly present in severe constriction rings that may lead to compression of nerves, vessels, and lymphatics [3]. The constriction bands are usually present at multiple levels and as the child grows, these bands may deepen and cause more compressive symptoms. This is believed to be due to a cycle of skin maceration, breakdown and healing by further scarring. The hand surgeon should therefore recognize the degree of severity in which the limb or digit is affected. Amputations often occur in utero that result from vascular insufficiency; however later in life this is rarely symptomatic. Temperature gradients and digital cyanosis have been reported across the constriction rings [30]. The amputated stumps may exhibit tapering skeletal elements with tight skin cover (Fig. 22.2). Neurological impairments such as nerve palsies are usually present since birth and are attributed to axonotmesis or neurotmesis. It is postulated that nerve compression or the development of compartment syndrome within the affected compartment distal to site of constriction are the main causes of nerve impairments associated with ABS. However, some authors believe that these neurological dysfunctions may be due to the absence of nerve fibers distal to the site of constriction [23].

Digital malformation is a classic clinical finding in ABS that is secondary to amputations and phalangeal hypoplasia. Acrosyndactyly is often associated with digital amputations. In acrosyndactyly there is a normal separation of the digits, however the digits are fused together distally. Proximal to the point of fusion, interdigital sinuses or tracts can be found and probed in between the digits (Fig. 22.3) that indicate normal separation of the fingers and remnants of webspaces, hence the synonyms pseudo-syndactyly or fenestrated syndactyly have been used to describe this condition. Contrary to true syndactyly, acrosyndactyly is almost always not associated with any underlying bony fusion. The frequency of digital involvement with ABS has been reported by Kino [14],

Flatt [30], and Foulkes and Reinker [29]. In those three reports central digits were the most affected whilst the thumb is the least affected digit with ABS. In the central digits the ring finger is most commonly involved followed by long then index and finally the small finger. Several reasons may explain why longer digits are more affected than the thumb. Kino stated that longer digits are more liable to external compression forces in the uterus, whereas in a clinched fist the other digits usually protect the thumb. A second reason could be the different embryonic stage of development of different digits. The development of the thumb precedes central digits and assuming that constriction bands occur after the period of major organogenesis as suggested by Foulker and Reinker, may explain the decreased tendency of thumb involvement in ABS. Finally, the time difference of fetal development of upper and lower limbs may also explain the different incidence of constriction band involvement of the hands and feet.

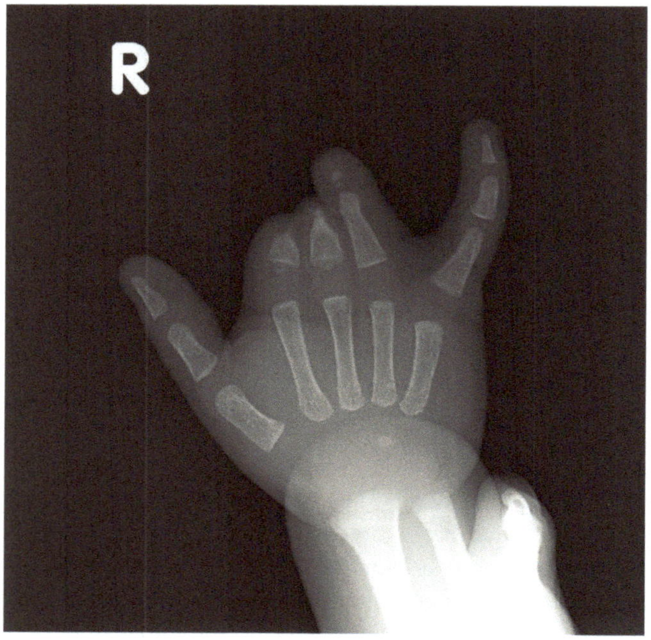

Fig. 22.2 An X-ray demonstrating transverse arrest of development and tapering of distal skeletal bones due to constriction bands

Classification

Several classifications have been devised for ABS based on the severity and location of the constriction bands [9, 31, 32]. Hall (1982) classified constriction rings into mild, moderate, and severe based on whether constriction rings are deep enough to cause lymphedema or amputations. He considered stage 1 as mild constrictions that do not result in lymphedema, stage 2 moderate constrictions resulting in lymphedema, and stage 3 as severe constrictions causing amputations. Weinzweig (1995) further subdivided Hall's classification by adding two intermediate stages that include a moderate constriction ring with distal deformity, syndactyly, or discontinuous neurovascular or musculotendinous structures without vascular compromise with or without lymphedema and severe constriction with progressive lymphaticovenous or arterial compromise with or without soft-tissue loss, and finally he added a fourth stage that include intrauterine amputation. Despite this, the most widely accepted and clinically relevant classification is the Patterson classification (1961), which has four categories:

1. Simple constriction rings
2. Constriction rings associated with deformity of the distal part with or without lymphedema
3. Constriction rings associated with acrosyndactyly
4. Intrauterine amputations

Additionally, cases that fall in the third category (constriction rings with acrosyndactyly) are further subdivided into three types:

- Type I: Conjoined fingertips with well-formed webs of the proper depth.
- Type II: The tips of the digits are joined, but web formation is not complete.
- Type III: Joined tips, sinus tracts between digits, and absent webs.

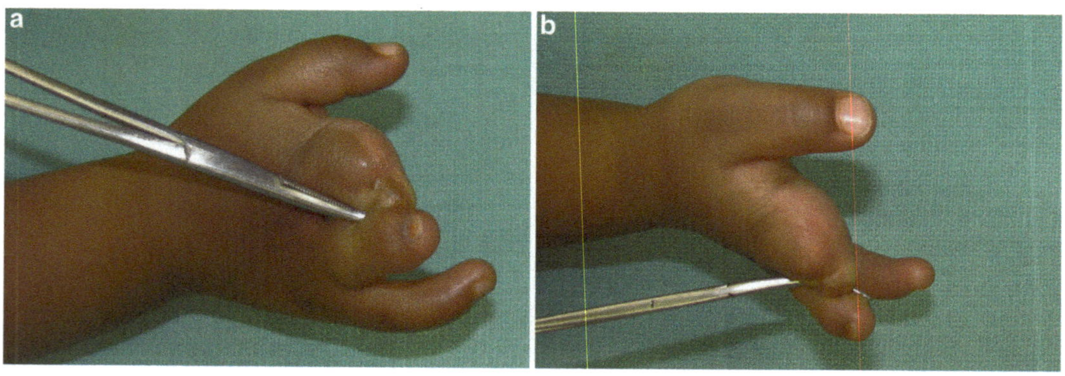

Fig. 22.3 Acrosyndactyly with a probe in the sinus tract

Treatment

The highly variable clinical picture among patients with ABS requires the treatment to be tailored to meet individual patient's requirements. A careful preoperative evaluation of underlying medical and surgical conditions must be considered to minimize the risk of anesthesia. The surgical treatment of ABS may range from an elective repair to an emergent limb-sparing or amputation procedures.

Superficial non-constrictive rings without distal swelling or neurovascular compromise may require no treatment or may be repaired electively to improve aesthetic appearance. For deep circumferential rings, the standard treatment includes Z-plasty and W-plasty in the presence of good distal function. In patients with acrosyndactyly, resurfacing of the webspace is required to separate digits and improve finger function. In cases of a constrictive band resulting in overt ischemia or osteomyelitis, distal amputation may be required [3, 23, 24]. Additionally, reconstructive procedures such as finger-to-toe transfers, bone-lengthening procedures, and pollicization procedures have been performed to restore function in cases of digital hypoplasia and amputation. Finally, fetoscopic band release for limb preservation in severe constriction rings has been used successfully [33, 34]. However, the rate of spontaneous abortion with these procedures has been reported between 6 and 10 %, a risk that should be carefully discussed beforehand with the parents together with all the pros and cons associated with this type of treatment.

Preoperative Considerations

Certain factors should be considered prior to surgery that include the appropriate timing for surgery, the amount of tissue to be excised or released, and the possibility for additional surgery of underlying structures such as tendons or nerves. The timing of surgery is mostly driven by the severity of the disease. Surgery should be considered in the first few days of life for constriction bands associated with severe distal edema and ischemia. In less severe cases, surgery should be performed electively, not "too early" to minimize the risk of anesthesia and not "too late" when hand function can be affected. In patients with acrosyndactyly, finger separation is usually recommended between 6 and 12 months to allow for longitudinal skeletal growth of the digits. Adhering to principles of congenital hand anomalies, the aim should be to complete all surgery before the child enters school, if possible. In the operating room, a two-team approach is recommended especially in cases of multiple limb involvement so that several procedures can be performed at the same setting, thus minimizing the total number of surgeries required.

The second preoperative consideration is the amount of tissue that needs to be released or excised. Most surgeons advocate the release of only 50 % of the constriction bands especially if the constrictions are located around the digits to preserve the vascular integrity. A second stage procedure can be scheduled 6–12 weeks following the first procedure to complete the repair. The third consideration is involvement of underlying structures. Underlying tendons and nerves can be affected by deep constriction bands and may require repair or reconstruction at the time of constriction band repair. The risk of additional procedures should therefore be discussed with the parents/family prior to surgery [3, 27].

Constriction Band Release

The standard treatment for constriction bands is excision of the constriction ring and the subcutaneous fibrous tissue followed by soft-tissue rearrangement by a Z-plasty or a W-plasty. A standard 60° Z-plasty with transposition of large skin flaps is recommended to preserve the viability of the skin flaps. The advantage of using a Z-plasty is twofold; first it breaks the tension line across the scar and second it adds length to the area of circumferential constriction (Fig. 22.4), whereas W-plasty only breaks the tension across the scar without incorporating further length. The two techniques alone do not address the resultant contour defect that arises after the excision of constriction rings and underlying subcutaneous tissue, an outcome that is considered not aesthetically pleasing. To prevent contour deformity, Upton [35] described a technique that involves excision of the constriction ring and underlying scarred tissue, then a portion of the adjacent healthy adipose tissue on both sides of the defect is separated from the dermis of overlying skin and mobilized to the center of the defect to fill the void. Subcutaneous veins should be preserved to facilitate venous drainage and prevent post-operative congestion. The skin flaps of the Z-plasty are then transposed separately over the adipose tissue. The skin suture line should be closed a few millimeters away from the underlying adipose suture line (Figs. 22.5 and 22.6). Repair of constriction rings around the fingers follows the same principles; however, skin incisions constituting the Z-plasty should be designed in a way that the final scar is placed along the midlateral lines to minimize skin contractures and visible scarring. At times the constriction ring is broad enough that an excision and closure by a Z-plasty is not possible. In these circumstances a local skin flap such as a cross finger flap can be executed to cover the resultant skin defect [27].

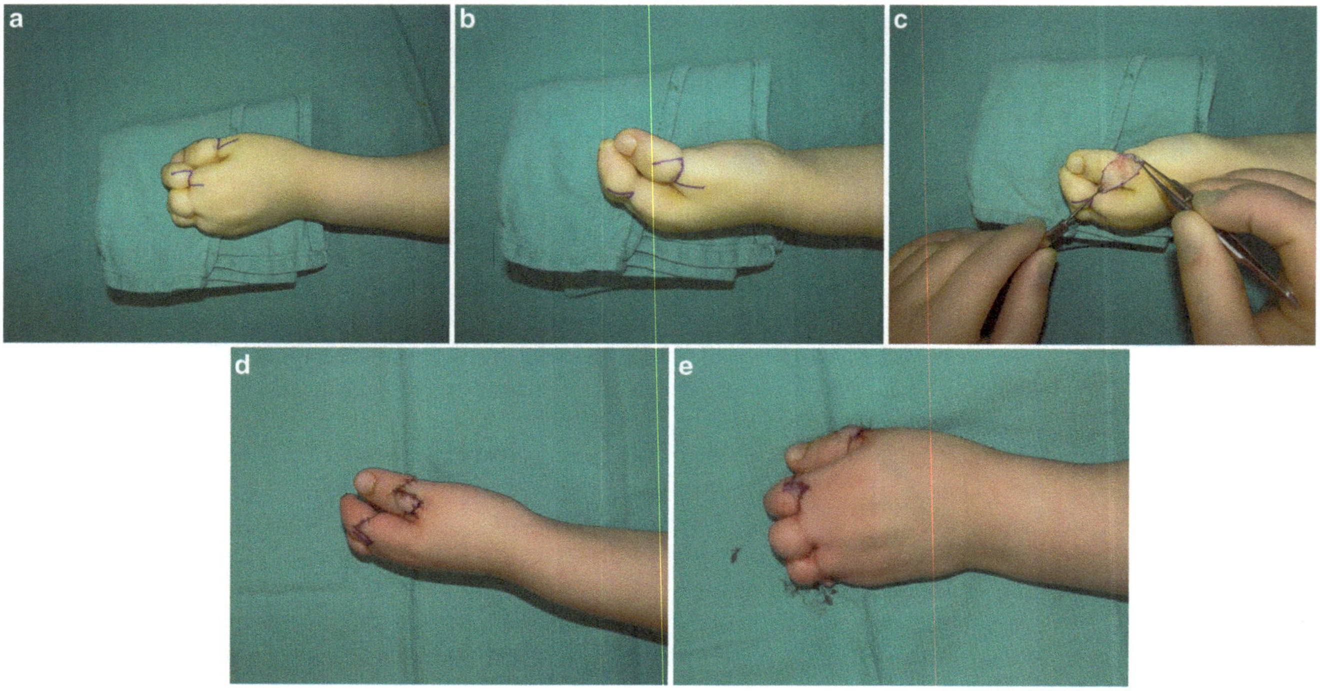

Fig. 22.4 Correction of constriction rings around digits using a Z-plasty

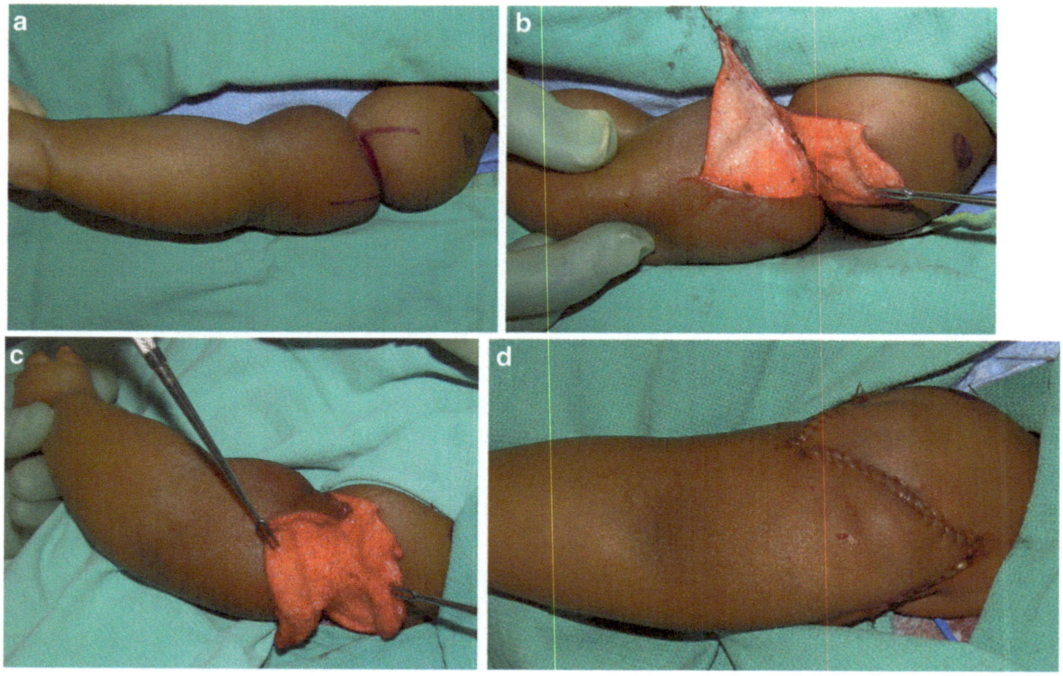

Fig. 22.5 Correction of a circumferential constriction band around the arm using a Z-plasty

Acrosyndactyly Repair

Acrosyndactyly is a condition in which two or more fingers are fused at their terminal portions with proximal epithelial lined clefts or sinuses between the fingers. Finger separation and resurfacing of the interdigital spaces and webspace is the final goal of surgery. Additional reconstructive procedures may be required to optimize functional and aesthetic results. In that respect several authors stated that the number of digits is not as important as their spacing, length, bulk, stability, and control [3, 24, 27]. Yet, acrosyndactyly often presents the surgeon with several challenges. First, the digits are usually merged together and are not clearly defined distal to the point

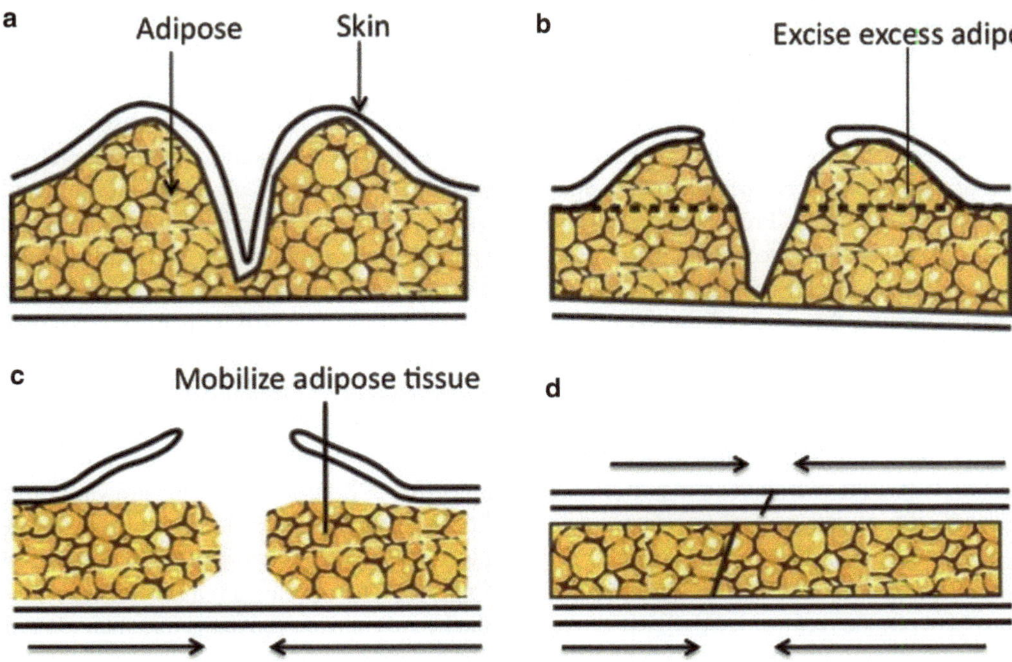

Fig. 22.6 Schematic drawings for releasing of the constriction band with Upton's technique. (**a**) Excision of all skin in the side walls. (**b**) Debulking of excess adipose tissue. (**c**) Subcutaneous adipose flaps are mobilized as needed to correct the contour deformity. (**d**) Skin and subcutaneous closures are preferably staggered

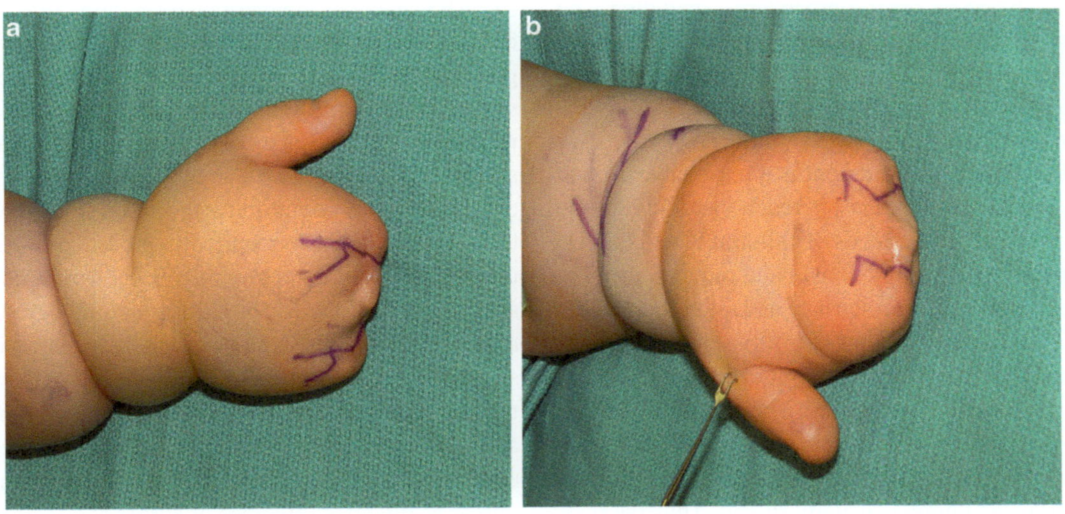

Fig. 22.7 Demonstrating surface marking of proximally based dorsal rectangular finger flap to resurface the webspace

of fusion, with several associated nail deformities. Therefore, it is often difficult to determine which fingertip belongs to which finger. A good reference point that has been noted is that the long finger is usually the most volar structure within the finger mass. In all cases the preservation of the fingertips is favored over amputations in order to preserve the finger length. Proximally, the webspaces are often absent especially in type III deformity (joined tips, sinus tracts between digits, and absent webs). In these cases the sinus is not sufficient to recreate the webspace, thus webspace resurfacing using a local flap is usually indicated. Finally, phalangeal hypoplasia and finger length discrepancies may require multiple secondary surgeries or digit lengthening procedures to deepen the commissures in patients with severe syndactyly.

The repair of acrosyndactyly requires a standard syndactyly technique for finger separation consisting of interdigitating Z-plasties and a rectangular, proximally based dorsal flap. The dorsal flap should be designed long enough to recreate the webspace. The surface marking of the proximally based dorsal rectangular flap extends from the level of the metacarpal joint proximally up to the level of middle of proximal phalanx (Fig. 22.7). Care must be taken when raising the skin flaps of the zigzag incisions of the Z-plasty as the neurovascular bundles may be displaced anteriorly. The dissection usually proceeds from proximal to distal. Distally, finger fusion at the fingertips should be carefully divided using sharp scissors. At all times the surgeon should preserve the viability and length of the fingertips, but occasionally amputation of necrotic parts is inevitable. Preserved yet imperfectly aligned digits can be reconstructed when the child is older. Blood vessels and nerves are preserved and the closure is performed by approximating the edges of the skin flaps. Tight closure of the skin due to skin shortage may jeopardize skin perfusion. In these instances, a full thickness skin graft can be harvested from the groin and used to resurface the defect on the sides of the finger. Before applying the skin grafts it is essential to deflate the tourniquet and perform an adequate hemostasis. By releasing the tourniquet the surgeon should be able to perform a final check of the adequacy of perfusion of the skin flaps. Finger dressings are then applied to prevent adhesions between the reconstructed digits.

Reconstruction of Digital Hypoplasia

Reconstruction of digital hypoplasia associated with ABS can be accomplished by several procedures, including webspace deepening, composite transfer of part of a finger (ontop plasty), pollicization procedures, toe-to-hand transfer, and bone lengthening procedures. The goal of surgery is to optimize hand performance. However, if the hand function is considered acceptable, no treatment is a reasonable alternative [27]. A thoughtful surgical approach can address both the functional and aesthetic needs of children with ABS. The minimal requirement of a functional hand requires the presence of two digits that are sensate and pain free. Other requirements are a movable digit to grasp objects and a stable digit against which the mobile digit can pinch. For optimal function, a third digit is required. The presence of a third digit allows the patient to have a chuck grip and perform powerful pinch and grasp movements [24]. In the majority of cases with ABS, the thumb is usually spared. Thus the treatment is usually directed at improving the function of the remaining four digits. From the reconstructive standpoint and in transverse absence of the digits such as in ABS, the proximal structures of the digits are normal which enables several reconstructive procedures to be performed.

Digital reconstruction depends on the number and length of the affected digits as well as the condition of surrounding soft-tissue. Local soft-tissue rearrangement such as a Z-plasty or a Jumping man flap (five flap plasty) can be performed to deepen the first webspace to increase the handgrip and thumb excursion. In cases where the thumb is short but present, a lengthening procedure such as on-top plasty can be preformed. On-top plasty involves the transposition of the distal end of the finger metacarpal and proximal phalanx on a neurovascular pedicle to lengthen the thumb or sometimes the long finger [36]. Other thumb augmenting procedures may include free phalangeal transfer, or distraction lengthening with or without bone grafts. In cases where there is complete absence of the thumb, a toe-to-finger transfer is the procedure of choice. If all digits are absent, toe-to-finger transfer with toes taken from both feet can be performed. One toe can be used to reconstruct the thumb and the other toe to create an ulnar digit to allow pinch movement. Bilateral toe-to-finger transfer can also be performed in cases where the thumb is present to create three digits to provide a chuck grip. Vilkki reported that the ability to pinch was restored in 14 of 17 congenitally defective extremities. [37]. A good range of motion of transferred toes has been reported by several authors [37–39]. Furthermore, the growth of transferred toes has been found to achieve comparable growth to normal toes in the foot [40]. Most importantly, children who receive a toe-to-finger transfer develop a remarkable functional adaptation of their newly transferred digits into their pattern of life.

Complications

Postoperative complications following surgical procedures for ABS includes hematoma formation, infection, wound dehiscence, neurovascular injury, skin flap necrosis, and skin graft failure. To minimize complications, a meticulous dissection under strict hemostasis facilitates identifying pertinent structures of the hand. Local skin flaps such as Z-plasties should be designed wide enough to transpose without undue tension that may compromise the blood supply. Additionally, tension free closure is required to prevent constriction of the underlying vessels and minimize local wound complications such as wound dehiscence. For optimal graft-take, nonadherent dressings should be applied together with adequate splinting of the mobile parts to decrease shearing forces at the skin-grafted areas. Finally, reviewing patients regularly at outpatients' clinic appointments together with parents' education regarding wound healing and scar management, improves the final outcomes of surgery.

Summary

Amniotic band syndrome is a rare congenital disorder that leads to several clinical manifestations predominantly affecting the extremities. The management of ABS is primarily focused on optimizing function and development whilst providing acceptable aesthetic results. Because of the variability of clinical presentation among patients, treatment strategy should be individualized to each specific condition. Finally, parents and children should be properly counseled and explained that several procedures may be required to achieve the desired outcomes.

References

1. Goldfarb CA, Sathienkijkanchai A, Robin NH. Amniotic constriction band: a multidisciplinary assessment of etiology and clinical presentation. J Bone Joint Surg Am. 2009;91 Suppl 4:68–75.
2. Garza A, Cordero JF, Mulinare J. Epidemiology of the early amnion rupture spectrum of defects. Am J Dis Child. 1988;142(5):541–4.
3. Kawamura K, Chung KC. Constriction band syndrome. Hand Clin. 2009;25(2):257–64.
4. Rayan GM. Amniotic constriction band. J Hand Surg Am. 2002;27(6):1111.
5. Baker CJ, Rudolph AJ. Congenital ring constrictions and intrauterine amputations. Am J Dis Child. 1971;121(5):393–400.
6. Montgomery W. Spontaneous amputation in utero. Dublin J Med Sci. 1832;2:49.
7. Simpson J. Essays on diseases of the placenta. Dublin J Med Sci. 1836;10:220.
8. Streeter G. Focal deficiencies in fetal tissues and their relation to intrauterine amputations. Contributions to embroyology. Vol. 22. No. 126. Washington: Carnegie Institute of Washington; 1930. p. 1–46.
9. Patterson TJ. Congenital ring-constrictions. Br J Plast Surg. 1961;14:1–31.
10. Van Allen MI. Fetal vascular disruptions: mechanisms and some resulting birth defects. Pediatr Ann. 1981;10:219–33.
11. Lockwood C, Ghidini A, Romero R, Hobbins JC. Amniotic band syndrome: reevaluation of its pathogenesis. Am J Obstet Gynecol. 1989;160(5 Pt 1):1030–3.
12. Bamforth JS. Amniotic band sequence: Streeter's hypothesis reexamined. Am J Med Genet. 1992;44:280–7.
13. Torpin R. Amniochorionic mesoblastic fibrous strings and amniotic bands: associated constricting fetal malformations or fetal death. Am J Obstet Gynecol. 1965;91:65–75.
14. Kino Y. Clinical and experimental studies of the congenital constriction band syndrome, with an emphasis on its etiology. J Bone Joint Surg Am. 1975;57(5):636–43.
15. Higginbottom MC, Jones KL, Hall BD, Smith DW. The amniotic band disruption complex: timing of amniotic rupture and variable spectra of consequent defects. J Pediatr. 1979;95(4):544–9.
16. Walter Jr JH, Goss LR, Lazzara AT. Amniotic band syndrome. J Foot Ankle Surg. 1998;37(4):325–33.
17. Paladini D, Foglia S, Sglavo G, Martinelli P. Congenital constriction band of the upper arm: the role of three-dimensional ultrasound in diagnosis, counseling and multidisciplinary consultation. Ultrasound Obstet Gynecol. 2004;23:520–2.
18. Hata T, Tanaka H, Noguchi J. 3D/4D sonographic evaluation of amniotic band syndrome in early pregnancy: a supplement to 2D ultrasound. J Obstet Gynaecol Res. 2011;37(6):656–60.
19. Inubashiri E, Hanaoka U, Kanenishi K, Yamashiro C, Tanaka H, Yanagihara T, Hata T. 3D and 4D sonographic imaging of amniotic band syndrome in early pregnancy. J Clin Ultrasound. 2008;36(9): 573–5.
20. Lee SH, Lee MJ, Kim MJ, Son GH, Namgung R. Fetal MR imaging of constriction band syndrome involving the skull and brain. J Comput Assist Tomogr. 2011;35(6):685–7.
21. Aitken DA, May HM, Ferguson-Smith MA, Howat R, Kohler HG. Amniotic band disruption syndrome associated with elevated amniotic AFP and normal acetylcholinesterase gel test. Prenat Diagn. 1984;4(6):443–6.
22. Sifakis S, Mantas N, Konstantinidou A, Koukoura O, Avgoustinakis E, Koumantakis E. A stillborn fetus with amniotic band syndrome and elevated levels of alpha-fetoprotein plus beta-human chorionic gonadotropin: a case report. Fetal Diagn Ther. 2008;24(2):111–4.
23. Kay SP, McCombe DB, Kozin SH. Deformities of the hand and fingers. In: Wolfe S, editor. Green's operative hand surgery. 6th ed. New York: Churchill Livingstone; 2011.
24. Moran SL, Jensen M, Bravo C. Amniotic band syndrome of the upper extremity: diagnosis and management. J Am Acad Orthop Surg. 2007;15(7):397–407.
25. Swanson AB, Swanson GD, Tada K. A classification for congenital limb malformation. J Hand Surg Am. 1983;8(5 Pt 2):693–702.
26. Ogino T, Saitou Y. Congenital constriction band syndrome and transverse deficiency. J Hand Surg Br. 1987;12(3):343–8.
27. Wiedrich TA. Congenital constriction band syndrome. Hand Clin. 1998;14(1):29–38.
28. Coady MS, Moore MH, Wallis K. Amniotic band syndrome: the association between rare facial clefts and limb ring constrictions. Plast Reconstr Surg. 1998;101(3):640–9.
29. Foulkes GD, Reinker K. Congenital constriction band syndrome: a seventy-year experience. J Pediatr Orthop. 1994;14(2):242–8.
30. Flatt AE. Constriction ring syndrome. In: Flatt AE, editor. The care of congenital hand anomalies. St. Louis: CV Mosby; 1977. p. 214.
31. Hall EJ, Johnson-Giebina R, Vasconez LO. Management of the ring constriction syndrome: a reappraisal. Plast Reconstr Surg. 1982;69(3):532–6.
32. Weinzweig N. Constriction band-induced vascular compromise of the foot: classification and management of the "intermediate" stage of constriction-ring syndrome. Plast Reconstr Surg. 1995;96(4):972–7.
33. Soldado F, Aguirre M, Peiró JL, Carreras E, et al. Fetoscopic release of extremity amniotic bands with risk of amputation. J Pediatr Orthop. 2009;29(3):290–3.
34. Richter J, Wergeland H, DeKoninck P, De Catte L, et al. Fetoscopic release of an amniotic band with risk of amputation: case report and review of the literature. Fetal Diagn Ther. 2012;31(2):134–7.
35. Upton J, Tan C. Correction of constriction rings. J Hand Surg Am. 1991;16(5):947–53.
36. Ogino T, Kato H, Ishii S, Usui M. Digital lengthening in congenital hand deformities. J Hand Surg. 1994;19(1):120–9.
37. Vilkki S. Advances in microsurgical reconstruction of the congenitally adactylous hand. Clin Orthop Relat Res. 1995;314:45–8.
38. Van Holder C, Giele H, Gilbert A. Double second toe transfer in congenital hand anomalies. J Hand Surg Br. 1999;24:471–5.
39. Foucher G, Medina J, Navarro R, Nagel D. Toe transfer in congenital hand malformations. J Reconstr Microsurg. 2001;17:1–7.
40. Kay SP, Wiberg M. Toe to hand transfer in children. Part 1. Technical aspects. J Hand Surg Br. 1996;21:723–34.

Arthrogryposis

23

Ann E. Van Heest

Introduction

Arthrogryposis is a descriptive term that describes an individual with congenital contractures of three or greater joints. Arthrogryposis is a congenital disorder of formation within the neuromuscular axis. Classification of arthrogryposis can include: classic, distal, and syndromic arthrogryposis. Classification helps us understand the extent of the disability.

By definition, arthrogryposis is congenital contractures of three or greater joints in multiple body areas. It is nonprogressive. Its incidence is 1 in 3,000–5,000 live births. Arthrogryposis is not a specific diagnosis, but rather a clinical finding. It is a characteristic that is seen in over 300 different disorders. An isolated congenital contracture affects only a single area of the body, such as seen in congenital club foot, which occurs in 1 of every 500 live births. This is distinctly different than arthrogryposis, which affects two or more different joints of the body. Treatment is based on functional disabilities and is aimed at improving functional abilities by improving limb position, strength, and mobility. The primary long-term goals of treatment are to improve use of adaptive patterns to allow for walking and independence with activities of daily living.

Classification

As shown in Fig. 23.1, congenital contractures can be divided into *isolated* congenital contractures, such as club foot, or *multiple* congenital contractures which are termed arthrogryposis [1]. Hall (1983 reference) has classified arthrogryposis as limb only, limb and viscera, or limb and CNS (Table 23.1).

A.E. Van Heest, M.D. (✉)
Department of Orthopaedic Surgery, University of Minnesota, 2450 Riverside Avenue South, Suite R 200, Minneapolis, MN 55454, USA
e-mail: vanhe003@umn.edu

Clinically, this presents as three distinct types: classic (amyoplasia), distal, and syndromic.

Classic arthrogryposis is also known as amyoplasia, or arthrogryposis multiplex congenital (AMC). This is a distinct form of arthrogryposis with characteristic clinical findings. Amyoplasia refers to *a* = no, *myo* = muscle, *plasia* = growth. In this condition, the shoulders are usually internally rotated and adducted, the elbows are extended, the wrists are flexed and ulnarly deviated, the fingers are stiff, and the thumbs are in the palm (Fig. 23.2). If there is lower extremity involvement, the hips may be dislocated, the knees are extended, and the feet often have severe equinovarus contractures. Many patients have a mid-facial hemangioma. Associated conditions can exist. In one series, 10 % of children had gastroschisis or bowel atresia [2]. In most clinical series, symmetrical involvement of the upper and lower extremities occurs. Other variations include upper extremity only, lower extremity only, or asymmetric involvement. In Hall's original description of 135 patients with amyoplasia, all cases were sporadic; however, there was an increased prevalence in twins and it occurred more commonly in conditions that would lead to decreased intrauterine limb movement, such as a bicornuate uterus, oligohydramnios, or intrauterine crowding [3].

Distal arthrogryposis includes ten distinct types as seen in Table 23.2. As described in the Online Mendelian Inheritance in Man® (OMIM®) [4], distal arthrogryposis includes what was previously called Freeman–Sheldon syndrome, Sheldon–Hall syndrome, Gordon syndrome, and multiple pterygium syndrome. Specific diagnostic criteria are necessary to make a diagnosis of a distal arthrogryposis. In the upper limb, major diagnostic criteria include camptodactyly, hypoplastic or absent flexion creases, overriding fingers, and ulnar deviation of the wrist (Fig. 23.3). This is commonly referred to as "the windblown hand." For the lower limb, major diagnostic criteria include talipes equinovarus, calcaneovalgus deformities, congenital vertical talus, and/or metatarsus adductus. To be affected, an individual must exhibit two or more major criteria; however, when a first

D.R. Laub Jr. (ed.), *Congenital Anomalies of the Upper Extremity: Etiology and Management*,
DOI 10.1007/978-1-4899-7504-1_23, © Springer Science+Business Media New York 2015

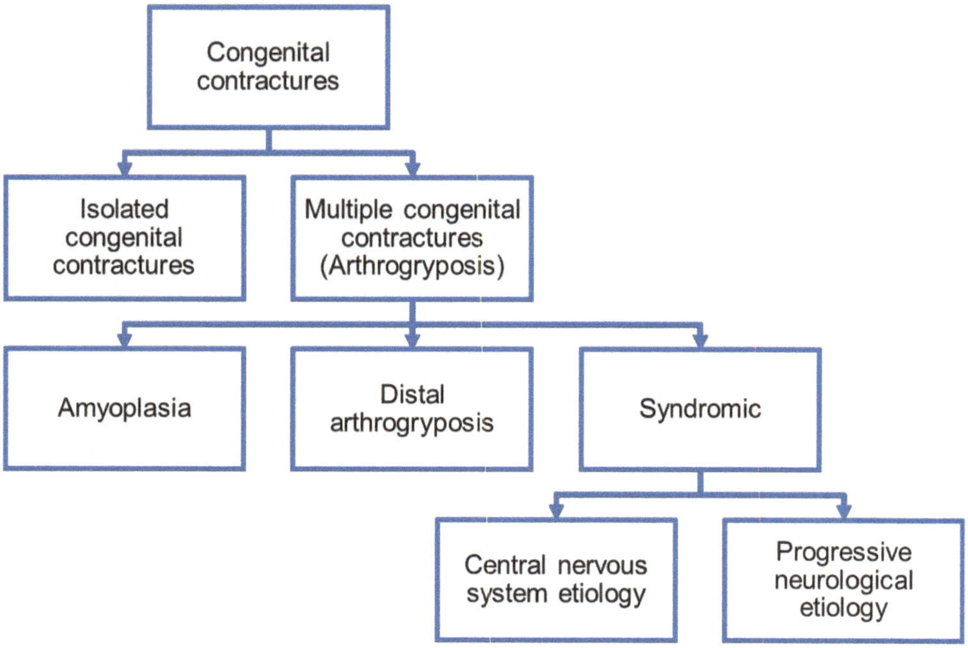

Fig. 23.1 Classification of types of arthrogryposis [1]

Table 23.1 Types of arthrogryposis as classified by Hall[a]

1. Limb only
(a) Classic arthrogryposis (Amyoplasia)
(b) Distal arthrogryposis (10 types)
2. Limb and viscera (syndromic)
3. Limb and CNS (lethal)

[a]Reprinted with permission from Hall JG, Reed SD, McGillivray BC, Herrmann J, Partington MW, Schinzell J, et al. Part II. Amyoplasia: Twinning in amyoplasia – a specific type of arthrogryposis with an apparent excess of discordantly affected identical twins. Am J Med Genet Part A 2005: 591–9. Copyright © 1983 Wiley-Liss, Inc., A Wiley Company

degree family member meets diagnostic criteria, other family members only need one major criterion to be affected.

Syndromic arthrogryposis includes multiple CNS disorders or neuromuscular diseases, which include multiple congenital contractures. Developmental abnormalities that affect the forebrain, such as microcephaly, are sometimes associated with arthrogryposis. Genetic peripheral neuropathies with an onset during fetal life are rare causes of arthrogryposis. Neuromuscular junction blockade in fetuses carried by mothers with myasthenia gravis or autoantibodies against fetal acetylcholine receptors can result in arthrogryposis [5].

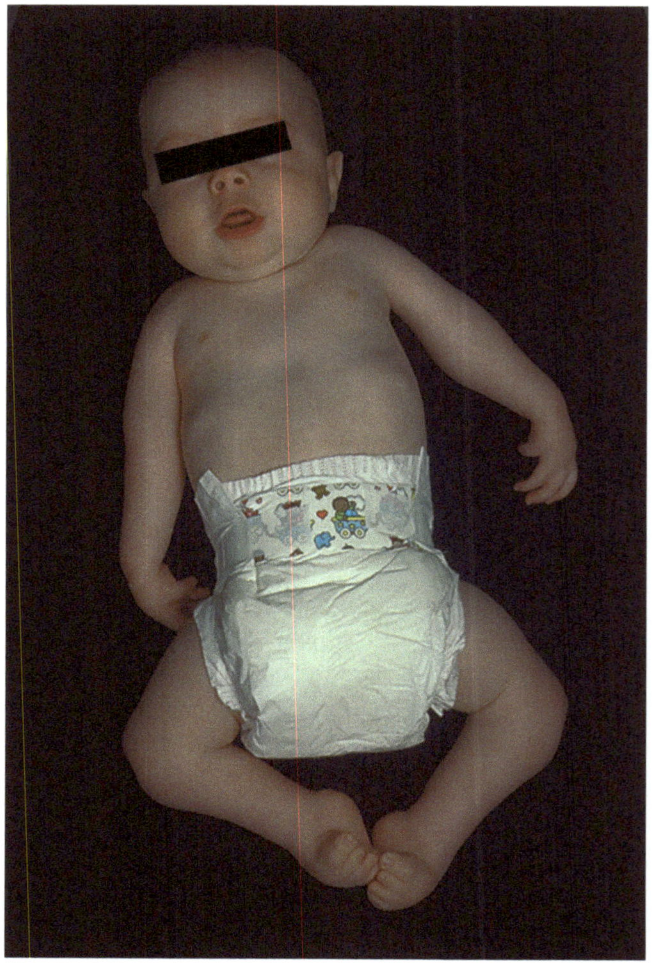

Fig. 23.2 A baby with classic arthrogryposis shows the typical features of internally rotated shoulders, extended elbows, flexed and ulnarly deviated wrists, stiff fingers, and the thumbs are in the palm. Additionally, her hips are dislocated, her knees are extended, and her feet have severe equinovarus contractures

Table 23.2 Distal arthrogryposis syndromes

Syndrome	New label	OMIM[a] number
Distal arthrogryposis type 1	DA1	108120
Distal arthrogryposis type 2A (Freeman–Sheldon syndrome)	DA2A	193700
Distal arthrogryposis type 2B (Sheldon–Hall syndrome)	DA2B	601680
Distal arthrogryposis type 3 (Gordon syndrome)	DA3	114300
Distal arthrogryposis type 4 (scoliosis)	DA4	609128
Distal arthrogryposis type 5 (opthalmoplegia, ptosis)	DA5	108145
Distal arthrogryposis type 6 (sensorineural hearing loss)	DA6	108200
Distal arthrogryposis type 7 (trismus pseudo-camptodactyly)	DA7	158300
Distal arthrogryposis type 8 (autosomal dominant multiple pterygium syndrome)	DA8	178110
Distal arthrogryposis type 9 (congenital contractural arachnodactyly)	DA9	121050
Distal arthrogryposis type 10 (congenital plantar contractures)	DA10	187370

[a]Online Mendelian Inheritance in Man® (OMIM®)

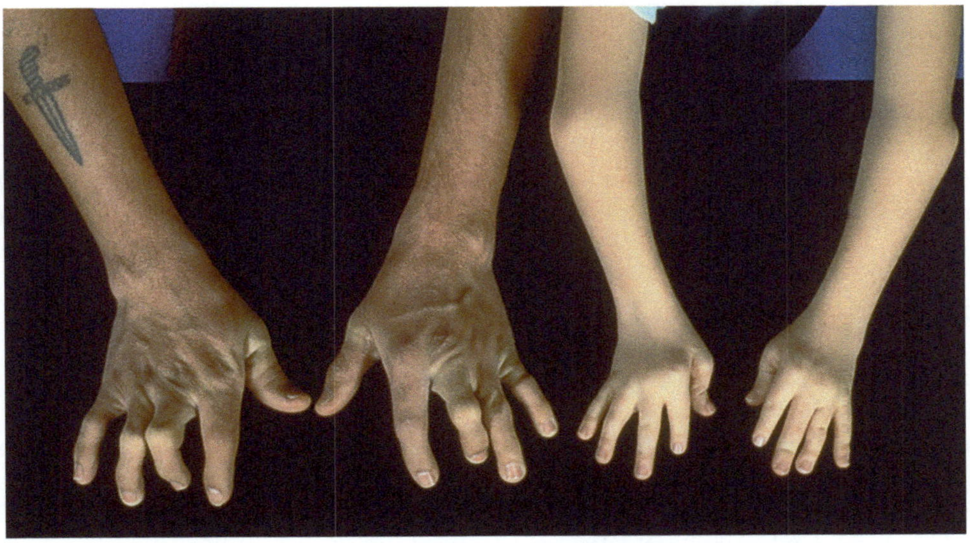

Fig. 23.3 Clinical features of distal arthrogryposis are seen in this father and son. The autosomal dominant disorder shows camptodactyly in the digits, with mild ulnar deviation of the wrists. Dislocated radial heads are noted by the prominence in the lateral elbow for the son

Etiology

Multiple congenital contractures appear to have a final common pathway. In the normal fetus, joint formation occurs by cavitation between 26 and 52 days post-fertilization. In order for normal joint development to occur, there must be adequate space, nerve supply, and muscle activity to promote normal joint formation. A disruption in any of these elements will lead to loss of normal joint movement, causing congenital contracture [1, 5]. Restricted movement can occur through fetal crowding with multiparous births, or uterine abnormalities such as a bicornuate uterus. Maternal illness can cause restricted movement, such as myasthenia gravis. Abnormal muscle or nerve development additionally leads to congenital contractures. Oligohydramnios has a known association with multiple congenital contractures. Classic arthrogryposis (amyplasia) is not known to have a specific genetic cause.

Distal arthrogryposes are a group of autosomal dominant disorders that mainly involve the distal aspects of the limbs, characterized by primary hand and foot involvement, limited involvement of proximal joints, and variable expressivity [6]. Mutations in at least five genes (TNN12, TNNT3, TPM2, MYH3, and MYH8) that encode components of the fast twitch contractile myofibers have been associated with distal arthrogryposis [7–9]. For example, in approximately 90 % of cases of distal arthrogryposis type 2, mutations are found in MYH3, a gene that encodes embryonic myosin. Mechanisms by which altered contractility leads to congenital contracture are not known.

Syndromic arthrogryposis is commonly most severe and includes many CNS and muscular diseases [1]. CNS malformations that are associated with diminished corticospinal activation of spinal cord motor neurons, such as hydranencephaly or microcephaly, most likely contribute to fetal hypomobility and development of congenital contractures [10]. Congenital neuropathies, myopathies, and muscular dystrophies may similarly lead to multiple congenital contractures due to lack of normal fetal movement.

Historical Perspective

Adolph Wilhelm Otto first described an infant with multiple congenital contractures noted at autopsy in 1841. He described this as "a monster with inwardly curved extremities." This has been credited as the first written description of arthrogryposis.

Clinical Manifestations of Arthrogryposis

The most common presentation to the hand surgeon includes classic arthrogryposis and distal arthrogryposis. Many children with syndromic arthrogryposis that includes limb and viscera are not surgical candidates. Patients with limb and CNS involvement have a lethal presentation as stillborn.

Classic Arthrogryposis (Amyoplasia)

Patients with classic arthrogryposis (amyoplasia) most commonly have lack of formation of normal musculature. The lack of normal muscles leads to multiple congenital joint contractures in the upper extremity. The most common pattern of deformity in the upper extremity is internal rotation of the shoulder with weak or absent shoulder girdle muscles; extension contracture of the elbow with weak or absent biceps and brachialis muscles; pronated, flexed, and ulnarly deviated wrists, with weak or absent wrist extension; and rigid digits with thumb and palm deformity. The degree of stiffness and weakness ranges from mild to severe and is not progressive.

The goal of treatment for children with arthrogryposis is to improve their quality of life by facilitating functional independence. At birth, nonoperative measures are initiated, with range of motion exercises, muscle and joint stretching, and splinting of specific joints to improve passive range of motion. Treatment to improve the function of the upper limb requires comprehensive planning with simultaneous assessment of shoulder, elbow, wrist, forearm, and hand function.

Nonoperative management is initiated at birth, and most commonly carried out for at least 12 months. Improvement of joint mobility is common, particularly at the elbow and wrist. The elbow is most critical in terms of achieving passive mobility to gain hand-to-mouth function. If after nonoperative treatment functional independence is still not possible, consideration for surgical treatment is explored [11]. Possible surgical treatment options are shown in Table 23.3.

Table 23.3 Surgical treatment options in amyoplasia

Shoulder	Derotational humeral osteotomy
Elbow	Elbow capsular release
	Elbow tendon transfers
	Radial head excision
Wrist	Dorsal carpal wedge osteotomy
	Tendon transfer
Digits	Syndactyly release
Thumb	Tendon transfer
	First web release
	Thumb adductor release

Clinical Features of Amyoplasia

The joints of the upper and lower extremities are stiff in varying degrees. The skin is smooth over the joints, with reduced or absent skin creases. Oftentimes at large joints, particularly the shoulders, skin dimples are seen. Reduced mass of the muscles is visualized, and palpation shows an increase of firm tissue with an increase in fibrous tissue. A similarity in facial appearance is notable; intellectual development is usually normal.

Treatment of the Shoulder

In most patients, shoulder internal rotation is an integral part of their ability to perform bi-manual skills as the shoulder internal rotation helps bring their hands to midline and cross over to assist with grasp, as shown in Fig. 23.4. However, in some children, if the internal rotation contracture is severe and actually interferes with function, an external rotational osteotomy of the proximal humerus can be performed to improve function.

Treatment of the Elbow

Nonoperative management is initiated at birth, and most commonly carried out for at least 12 months. Improvement of joint mobility is common, particularly at the elbow and wrist. The elbow is most critical in terms of achieving passive mobility to gain hand-to-mouth function. If after nonoperative treatment elbow flexion is insufficient to allow passive mobility of hand to mouth, surgical treatment would be indicated. Specifically, if less than 90° of flexion is achieved and the hand cannot be brought to the mouth passively, a posterior elbow capsulotomy with triceps lengthening would be indicated [11]. Indications for surgery are less than 90° of passive elbow flexion and an inability to reach the hand to the mouth.

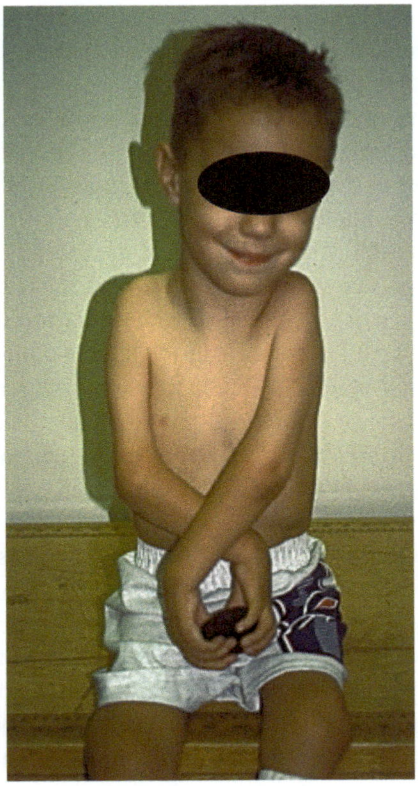

Fig. 23.4 De-rotation osteotomy of the shoulder can be indicated for severe internal rotation positioning of the limb causing significant dysfunction. Care must be taken with judicious use of this operation as most children with amyoplasia use the shoulder internal rotation to assist with bimanual hand use as shown in this figure

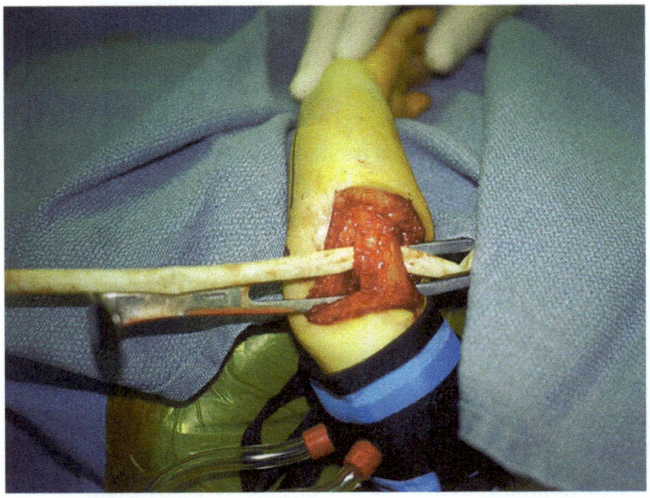

Fig. 23.5 Posterior elbow capsular release with triceps lengthening is performed through a posterior incision. The triceps is isolated, as shown here, and is subsequently lengthened using a Z-lengthening technique

Surgical Technique

Posterior elbow capsulotomy with triceps lengthening is performed with the patient in a lateral decubitus position. A sterile tourniquet is used, at least through initial dissect to allow identification and protection of the ulnar nerve. The posterior aspect of the elbow is identified by palpation. Caution should be taken that oftentimes the limb is so internally rotated that the medial epicondyle can be mistaken for the olecranon. A curvilinear incision is made down the posterior aspect of the elbow. In arthrogryposis, significance of cutaneous tissue with minimal tissue planes is a common pathological finding. The ulnar nerve is identified as it passes through the inner muscular septum and through the cubital tunnel. Osborne's fascia is released, and the ulnar nerve is protected with a vessel loop. The sterile tourniquet then can be removed to allow greater proximal dissection and triceps mobilization once the ulnar nerve has been identified and protected, particularly in the small child. The tricep is isolated on its insertion at the olecranon. Dissection is carried out medially and laterally, isolating the triceps tendon back to the level of the musculotendinous junction as shown in Fig. 23.5. A Z-lengthening or V-Y advancement is performed; at least doubling the length of the tendon will be necessary to provide appropriate elbow flexion.

The posterior aspect of the capsule is then incised, exposing the joint surface. The arthrotomy is extended medially and laterally to allow maximum elbow flexion with gentle passive stretch. It is important to be careful about increasing the joint mobility, as physeal fractures can occur if excessive force is used. Dissection most commonly needs to be carried out at least to the mid-axial line and may include the posterior aspects of the medial and lateral ligaments. Full flexion of the elbow is the goal of the posterior capsular release. The triceps is then repaired in an elongated position with use of a non-absorbable or reinforced suture. The skin is closed, and a light dressing applied. The limb is then placed in a hinged elbow brace or a long-arm cast in at least 90° of flexion. Passive range of motion to allow joint mobility is initiated as soon as tolerated by the patient. Therapy is advanced to include hand-to-mouth activities with passive flexion. During the first month, this is limited to 90° to protect the triceps lengthening, and advanced thereafter to full passive flexion. Use of a splint to maximize flexion during the day is possible with a hinged splint and use of rubber bands anteriorly as shown in Fig. 23.6. If an elbow flexion contracture ensues, alternative nighttime flexion splinting alternated with extension splinting can be initiated.

Surgical Outcomes

Several series examining results of posterior capsular release with triceps lengthening report excellent results. For example, Van Heest et al. [11] reported on a study group of 23 children treated between 7 months and 13 years of age with an average follow-up of 5.4 years. Prior to the surgery, the average arc of passive motion was 32°, with an average of 38° of flexion. An arc of at least 90° of passive flexion was achieved in all children intraoperatively. At an average follow-up of 5.4 years, 22 of the 23 children were able to feed themselves with the hand on the operated side. Twenty-one of the children with less than grade three elbow flexion strength required the use of passive assistance. No further muscle transfers were performed in these children, as adaptive mechanisms, as shown in Fig. 23.7, allowed independent activities of daily living.

Operative Outcomes with Muscle Transfer

Several options exist for muscle transfers. First, if passive range of motion has been achieved either operatively or non-operatively, passive adaptive maneuvers can be performed by the child for functional use of the elbow. Such is described by Van Heest et al. [11]. Nonoperative intervention for active elbow flexion requires the use of passive elbow flexion, and adaptive maneuvers such as tabletop push (see Fig. 23.7a), swinging of the arms (see Fig. 23.7b), or contralateral arm use (see Fig. 23.7c, d) to bring the hand to the mouth. Many children are quite creative in being able to passively achieve hand-to-mouth function.

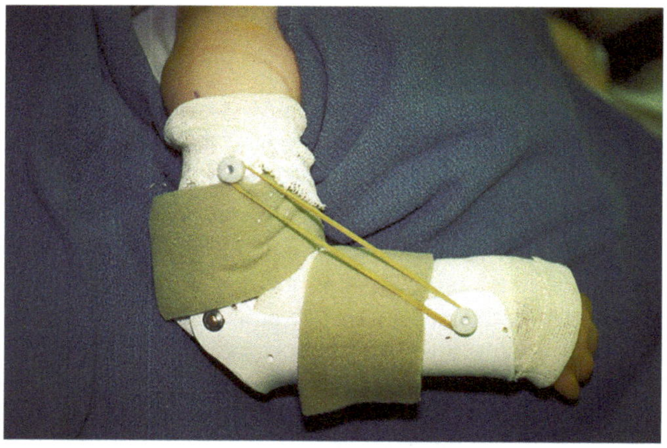

Fig. 23.6 Use of a splint to maximize flexion during the day is possible with a hinged splint and use of rubber bands anteriorly as shown. During the first month, this is limited to 90° to protect the triceps lengthening, and advanced thereafter to full passive flexion

Operative measures to improve active elbow flexion include transfer of the flexor pronator origin (Steindler) [12, 13]; transfer of the pectoralis muscle; transfer of the triceps muscle; free muscle transfer of the grascilis; or, most recently, transfer of a single head of the triceps on its separate neurovascular pedicle. One review of the results of surgical treatment of arthrogryposis with tendon transfer surgery examined 18 tendon transfers in 14 children with an average follow-up of 4 years [14]. Using functional outcome criteria, six of nine transfers provided good function, one provided fair, and two provided poor. The most common reason for downgrading was development of an elbow flexion contracture, which precluded active and passive elbow extension after triceps transfer. Subsequent studies have similarly shown severe elbow flexion contractures and, most commonly, triceps to biceps tendon transfer is no longer recommended [15]. The pectoralis transfer can be used as a unipolar [16], partial bipolar [17], or complete bipolar transfer [18]. The advantage of the pectoralis transfer is that additional muscle mass is added to the hypoplastic limb. The disadvantage is the extensive dissection necessary. It may also be contraindicated for use in females because of the chest wall deformity; lack of predictability of strength is common as well. The third available option for transfer is the latissimus dorsi muscle. Muscle mass is added from the chest wall to the hypoplastic limb without significant loss of function. However, in many children with arthrogryposis, the latissimus dorsi muscle is underdeveloped and insufficient for transfer. Several authors have recommended pre-operative evaluation by MRI scan or intraoperative assessment of muscle quality prior to transfer. Additionally, due to its shape as a long muscle, extension is difficult to assess. The Steindler

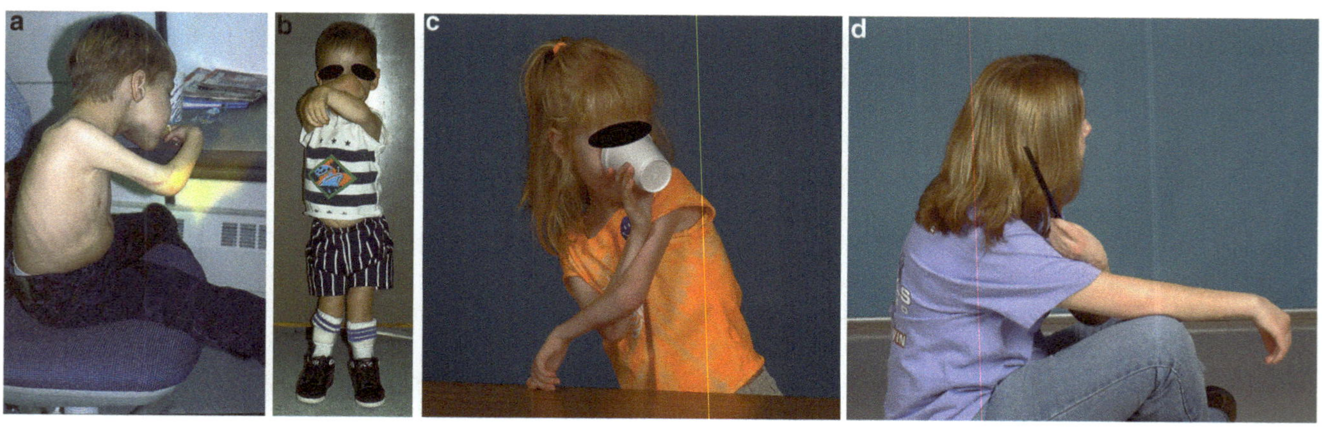

Fig. 23.7 Nonoperative intervention for active elbow flexion requires the use of passive elbow flexion, and adaptive maneuvers such as tabletop push (**a**), swinging of the arms (**b**), or contralateral arm use (**c, d**) to bring the hand to the mouth. Many children are quite creative in being able to passively achieve hand-to-mouth function, so that operative treatment with muscle transfer is not necessary

transfer, as described by Goldfarb et al. [12], is a less invasive elbow flexion transfer. The medial epicondyle origin of the flexor pronator muscle is divided and transferred to the anterior portion of the humerus. This transfer has been shown to improve initiation of elbow flexion, but has difficulty with achieving the full arc of elbow flexion for hand-to-mouth function. Additionally, critics have been concerned about enhancing the Steindler effect in requiring simultaneous wrist and elbow flexion in children who already have a wrist flexion contracture. Lastly, transfer of a single head of the triceps has recently been described by Ezaki [19]. Isolation of a single head of the triceps would allow transfer of one head while maintaining the other two heads as an antagonist elbow extensor. Theoretically, this would avoid the elbow flexion contractures seen after triceps to biceps transfer. The difficulty with the muscle transfers described above is that most children with amyoplasia have weak muscles, and transferring a weak muscle does not provide significant strength; thus, most of the outcomes of muscle transfer surgery are only good, not excellent.

Radial Head Dislocations

Some children with arthrogryposis will present with radial head dislocations. On physical examination, prominence of the radial head may be seen or palpated (Fig. 23.8); radiographs will reveal a radial head dislocation. If this occurs, assessment of the effect of loss of range of motion must be conducted. For example, an anteriorly dislocated radial head can block terminal flexion. Resection of the radial head can, in some cases, restore or improve function [20].

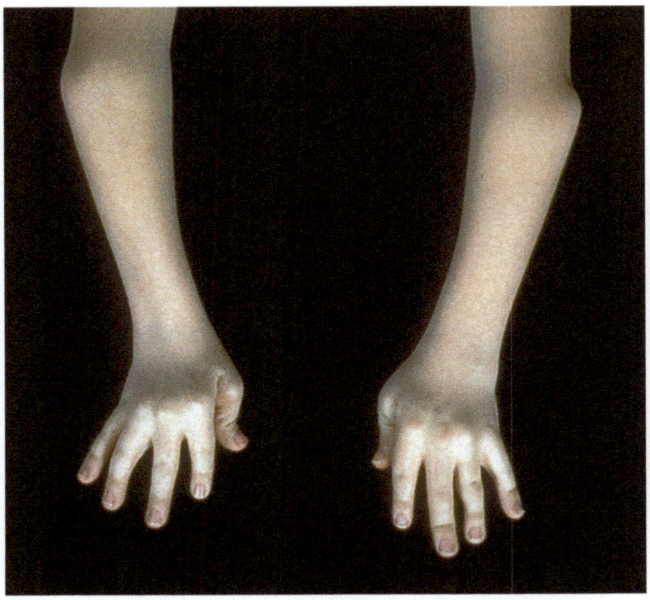

Fig. 23.8 A dislocated radial head can be diagnosed on physical examination by prominence of the radial head at the lateral head as seen here. Motion of the radial head can be palpated during pronation and supination

Treatment of the Wrist

Nonoperative management of the wrist includes passive range of motion and splinting. Most commonly, a wrist hand orthosis is worn at night to improve passive extension of the wrist and fingers (Fig. 23.9). During the day, wrist splints are avoided because movement of the wrist is already limited in these stiff joints, and further splinting most commonly does not enhance function.

The most common treatment of the wrist is dorsal carpal wedge osteotomy. Dorsal carpal wedge osteotomy was first described by Ezaki in 1993 [19]. Surgical indications for dorsal carpal wedge osteotomy include excessive wrist flexion contracture deformity which limits upper extremity function, having failed nonoperative treatment. Of particular note is that some children with severely stiff upper limbs do use their wrist flexion posturing in order to achieve hand-to-mouth function or to assist in crawling and standing up (Fig. 23.10). If this is the case for a child, straightening

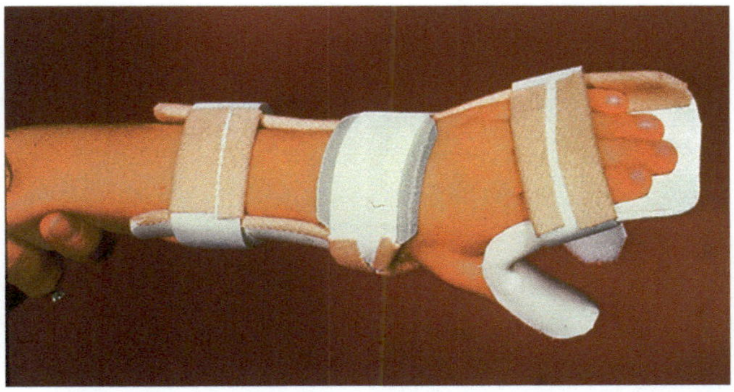

Fig. 23.9 Wrist hand orthosis worn at night to improve passive extension of the wrist and fingers. During the day, wrist splints are avoided because movement of the wrist is already limited in these stiff joints, and further splinting most commonly does not enhance function

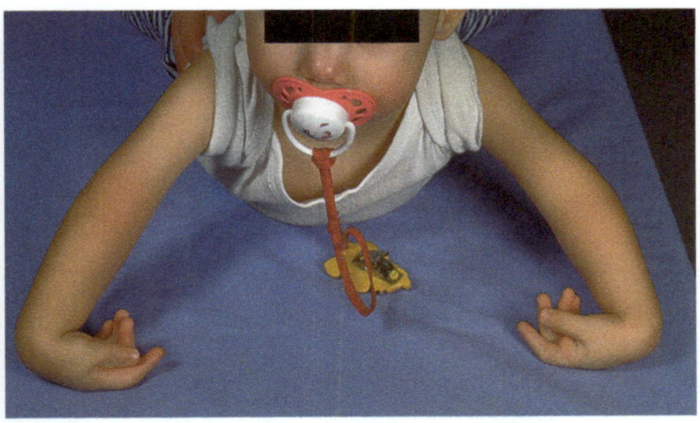

Fig. 23.10 Some children with arthrogryposis have severely stiff upper limbs and they use their wrist flexion posturing in order to achieve hand-to-mouth function or to assist in crawling and standing up, as shown here. If this is the case for a child, straightening the wrist would worsen their abilities. Only in children with adequate elbow flexion should wrist extension osteotomies be performed

the wrist would worsen their abilities. Only in children with adequate elbow flexion should wrist extension osteotomies be performed.

Surgical Technique

Dorsal carpal wedge osteotomy is performed using a dorsal approach to the wrist; the digital and wrist extensor tendons are isolated and protected. A dorsal capsulotomy is then performed. At the level of the midcarpus (Fig. 23.11), a dorsal wedge osteotomy is made sufficient to correct the wrist flexion deformity to at least a neutral position, taking care that noteworthy finger flexor tightness is not produced by tenodesis. If ulnar deviation correction is required as well, the dorsal carpal wedge can resect more bone on the radial side to provide biplanar deformity correction. This position is held in place with two cross K-wires. In addition, tendon transfer of the extensor carpi ulnaris (ECU) to the extensor carpi radialis brevis may be performed to correct the ulnar deviation deformity or wrist extension weakness, or both, if the ECU tendon is noted to have sufficient excursion intraoperatively. After the procedure, the patient is placed in a cast for 1 month. If radiographs show healing of the osteotomy, the cast is removed and the K-wires are pulled. The patient is given a wrist splint for protection and begins to participate in occupational therapy activities for wrist range of motion, particularly wrist extension, and hand function. Removable night splints are indicated on a case-by-case basis if needed for further improvement of wrist extension.

Surgical Outcomes

An evaluation of 20 wrists in 13 children with an average 4 years follow-up revealed a mean improvement of 43° of wrist extension with a loss of 35° of wrist flexion [21]. No significant change in the arc of motion was seen; however, extension was relocated into a more functional extended position. In one review [21] children older than 7 years of age at the time of surgery had significantly greater extension improvement than those less than 7 years of age. Additionally, patients who had a concomitant ECU tendon transfer at the

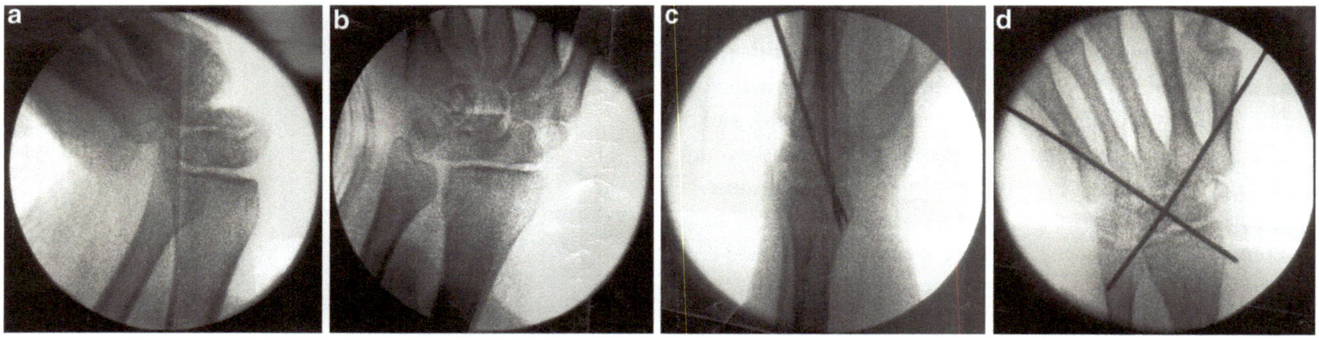

Fig. 23.11 Dorsal carpal wedge osteotomy is performed using a transverse dorsal incision and dorsal capsulotomy. A dorsal wedge of carpus is excised through the midcarpal joint (**a**, **b**), which is often synostostotic. Preservation of the radiocarpal joint is essential to maintain the limited arc of motion present. Pinning in a position of extension (**c**, **d**) with cast for 4–6 weeks to allow for bone healing is recommended. Concomitant centralization of the ECU tendon can improve long-term results for maintaining wrist extension

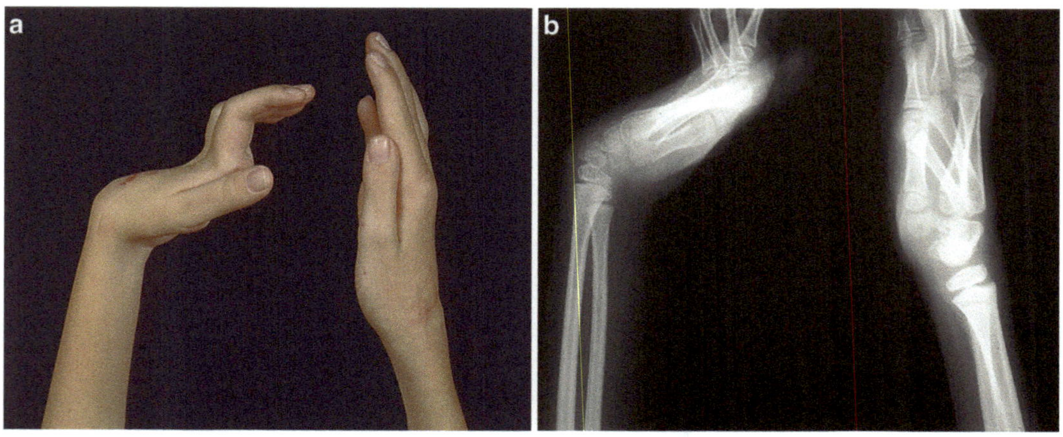

Fig. 23.12 This patient presents after a left wrist dorsal carpal wedge osteotomy (DCWO) requesting that the right wrist be treated. Part (**a**) shows a clinical picture of the post-op DCWO on the left wrist and a pre-op DCWO on the right wrist. Part (**b**) shows the lateral radiograph of the post-op DCWO on the left wrist and a pre-op DCWO on the right wrist. Prior to the surgery, the left wrist had similar deformity to the right wrist

time of dorsal carpal wedge osteotomy had a greater improvement in wrist extension. Dorsal carpal wedge osteotomy can significantly improve wrist extension while at the same time preserving the arc of motion (Fig. 23.12).

Treatment of the Hand

Syndactyly releases are most commonly a partial syndactyly and can be performed using local flaps with or without skin graft. The patterns in the hand with amyoplasia are similar to those with distal arthrogryposis and will be discussed together.

Distal Arthrogryposis

The second type of arthrogryposis commonly seen by hand surgeons is distal arthrogryposis. Features shared by all distal arthrogryposes include a consistent pattern of hand and foot involvement, limited proximal joint involvement, and variable expressivity. Ten different types of distal arthrogryposes have been described to date (see Table 23.2). Most commonly in these types of arthrogryposis the "windblown hand" is seen. The windblown hand includes ulnar deviation of the digits through the metacarpophalangeal (MCP) joint, stiff digits, and thumb-in-palm. The digits can be stiff in flexion, such as seen in camptodactyly, or stiff in extension, with side-to-side intrinsic grasp patterns. The thumb is typically flexed across the palm with adduction of the ray through the carpometacarpal joint, as well as flexion of the MCP joint. Simple incomplete syndactyly is common (Fig. 23.13).

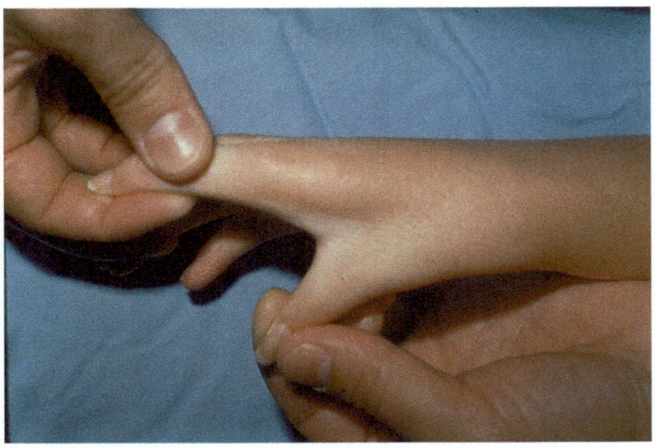

Fig. 23.13 Simple incomplete syndactyly is common in arthrogryposis and can be treated with local flaps or full thickness skin grafts if functionally limiting finger or thumb use

Treatment of the Hand

The mainstay of treatment for the windblown hand is nonoperative management with splints for improved positioning and passive range of motion of the joint, starting as an infant when the diagnosis is first made. In the early school-age child, if positioning has not improved then surgical management can be considered.

Surgical management in the windblown hand would include release of contractures. Release of camptodactyly has been disappointing, so that stiff digits are most commonly treated nonoperatively.

Treatment of the Thumb-in-Palm Deformity

Treatment of thumb-in-palm deformity involves repositioning of the thumb through osteotomies, fusions, or tendon transfers. Release of the first web can include a dorsal rotation flap, a Z-plasty, or volar skin grafting. Release of the thumb adductor is performed as described by Matev [22], with release of the origin of the thumb adductor from the third metacarpal, thus preserving its pinch power through preserving its nerve supply. This is important in children who are already weak when maximum thumb pinch strength needs to be preserved. If posturing across the palm is severe, consideration of an MCP fusion to position the thumb MCP joint in greater extension can be considered in the older child. In the younger child, release of the volar capsule and augmentation of the dorsal capsule with pinning for 4–6 weeks to allow healing can be considered. Augmentation of the extensor pollicus brevis tendon through transfer from the extensor indicis proprius has been used as shown in Fig. 23.14. Transfer of the extensor carpi radialis longus tendon, if present, to the first ray can improve abduction of the ray itself. Large series are not available for either of these surgical techniques. Adduction of the first metacarpal with contracture of the first web and volar skin is often accompanied by contracture of the thumb adductor and deficient thumb extension. Thus, a thumb reconstruction would include release of the first web, with possible skin grafting on its volar aspect.

In some cases, children with arthrogryposis will present with hyperextension deformity through the MCP joint as shown in Fig. 23.15. Most likely this will be due to adduction of the first metacarpal across the palm, with secondary stretching of the volar capsule in hyperextension, which can lead to dislocation of the MCP. Release of the first ray using the Matev procedure [15] with a volar capsulotomy as described by Tonkin et al. [23] has been conducted. Surgical operations for the windblown hand reviewed by Wood [24]

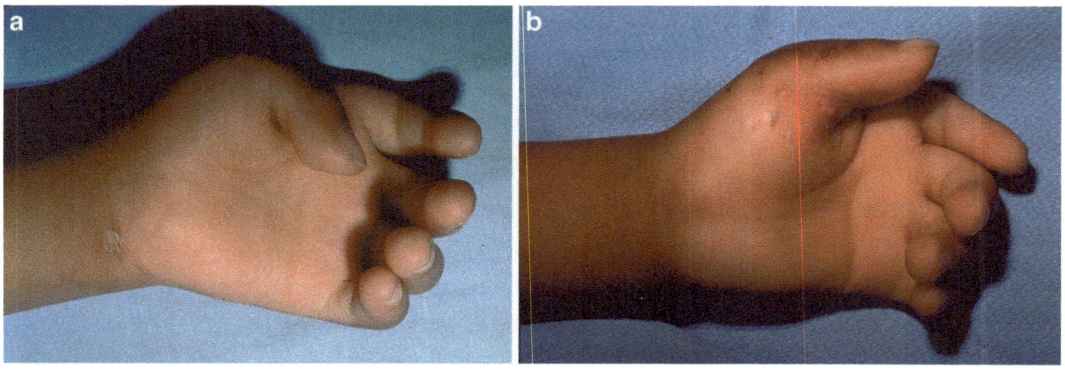

Fig. 23.14 Thumb-in-palm deformity is a common feature of both amyoplasia and many types of distal arthrogryposes (**a**). Surgical treatment with Z-plasty of the contracted volar skin, MP dorsal capsulodesis, and augmentation of thumb extension with transfer of the EIP tendon to EPB can improve thumb position and function (**b**)

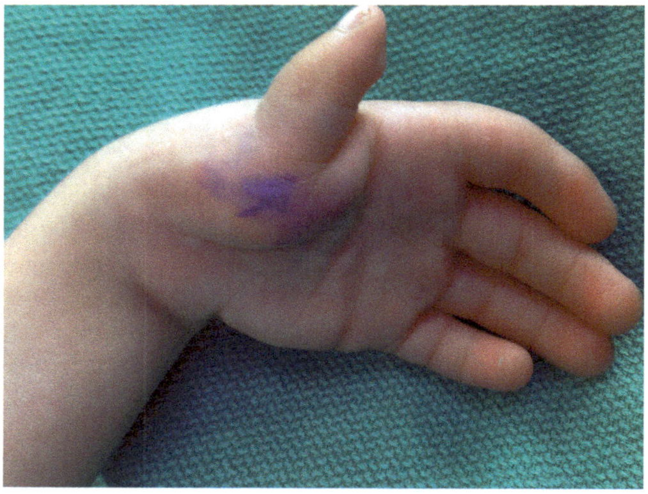

Fig. 23.15 Thumb-in-palm can on occasion cause adduction of the first ray with secondary hyperextension of the MCP joint. In cases such as these, volar capsulodesis would be necessary as part of surgical treatment. In the older child, MCP joint fusion may be an option

concluded that the most common procedure was Z-plasty of the thumb, followed by release of the thumb adductor, extensor indices proprius transfer to extensor pollicis longus or extensor pollicis brevis, with dorsal rotation flap or skin grafting. In three cases lengthening of the flexor pollicis longus tendon was necessary.

Summary

In summary, arthrogryposis is a disorder of joint formation of the neuromuscular axis leading to multiple congenital contractures. Classification as classic arthrogryposis (amyoplasia), distal arthrogryposis, and syndromic arthrogryposis helps us understand the extent of disability and its treatment. Amyoplasia is the most common arthrogryposis that is treated surgically. Elbow capsular release with triceps lengthening, dorsal carpal wedge osteotomies, and thumb-in-palm correction are the most common surgical procedures. Treatment is based on functional positioning and use of the limb. The goal of management of the child with arthrogryposis is to increase independence by improving joint position and mobility.

References

1. Bamshad M, Van Heest AE, Pleasure D. Arthrogryposis: a review and update. J Bone Joint Surg Am. 2009;91 Suppl 4:40–6. PubMed PMID: 19571066.
2. Hall JG, Reed SD, McGillivray BC, Herrmann J, Partington MW, Schinzel A, et al. Part II. Amyoplasia: twinning in amyoplasia—a specific type of arthrogryposis with an apparent excess of discordantly affected identical twins. Am J Med Genet. 1983;15(4):591–9.
3. Hall JG, Reed SD, Driscoll EP. Part I. Amyoplasia: a common, sporadic condition with congenital contractures. Am J Med Genet. 1983;15(4):571–90.
4. OMIM® Online Mendelian Inheritance in Man® [Database]. Johns Hopkins University; 1966 [updated 6 December 2013 8 December 2013]. An Online Catalog of Human Genes and Genetic Disorders]. http://omim.org/.
5. Polizzi A, Huson SM, Vincent A. Teratogen update: maternal myasthenia gravis as a cause of congenital arthrogryposis. Teratology. 2000;62(5):332–41. PubMed PMID: 11029151.
6. Bamshad M, Jorde LB, Carey JC. A revised and extended classification of the distal arthrogryposes. Am J Med Genet. 1996;65(4):277–81.
7. Sung SS, Brassington AM, Grannatt K, Rutherford A, Whitby FG, Krakowiak PA, et al. Mutations in genes encoding fast-twitch contractile proteins cause distal arthrogryposis syndromes. Am J Hum Genet. 2003;72(3):681–90. PubMed PMID: 12592607.
8. Sung SS, Brassington AM, Krakowiak PA, Carey JC, Jorde LB, Bamshad M. Mutations in TNNT3 cause multiple congenital contractures: a second locus for distal arthrogryposis type 2B. Am J Hum Genet. 2003;73(1):212–4. PubMed PMID: 12865991.
9. Toydemir RM, Rutherford A, Whitby FG, Jorde LB, Carey JC, Bamshad MJ. Mutations in embryonic myosin heavy chain (MYH3)

cause Freeman-Sheldon syndrome and Sheldon-Hall syndrome. Nat Genet. 2006;38(5):561–5. PubMed PMID: 16642020.
10. Pakkasjarvi N, Ritvanen A, Herva R, Peltonen L, Kestila M, Ignatius J. Lethal congenital contracture syndrome (LCCS) and other lethal arthrogryposes in Finland—an epidemiological study. Am J Med Genet A. 2006;140A(17):1834–9. PubMed PMID: 16892327.
11. Van Heest A, James MA, Lewica A, Anderson KA. Posterior elbow capsulotomy with triceps lengthening for treatment of elbow extension contracture in children with arthrogryposis. J Bone Joint Surg. 2008;90A(7):1517–23. PubMed PMID: 18594101.
12. Goldfarb CA, Burke MS, Strecker WB, Manske PR. The Steindler flexorplasty for the arthrogrypotic elbow. J Hand Surg Am. 2004;29(3):462–9.
13. Steindler A. Tendon transplantation in the upper extremity. Am J Surg. 1939;44(1):260–71.
14. Van Heest A, Waters PM, Simmons BP. Surgical treatment of arthrogryposis of the elbow. J Hand Surg Am. 1998;23(6): 1063–70.
15. Doyle JR, James PM, Larsen LJ, Ashley RK. Restoration of elbow flexion in arthrogryposis multiplex congenita. J Hand Surg Am. 1980;5(2):149–52.
16. Clark JM. Reconstruction of biceps brachii by pectoral muscle transplantation. Br J Surg. 1946;34(134):180. PubMed PMID: 20278126. Epub 1946/10/01. eng.
17. Schottstaedt ER, Larsen LJ, Bost FC. Complete muscle transposition. J Bone Joint Surg Am. 1955;37-A(5):897–918; discussion, 918–9. PubMed PMID: 13263337. Epub 1955/10/01.eng.
18. Atkins RM, Bell MJ, Sharrard WJ. Pectoralis major transfer for paralysis of elbow flexion in children. J Bone Joint Surg Br. 1985;67(4):640–4.
19. Ezaki M. Treatment of the upper limb in the child with arthrogryposis. Hand Clin. 2000;16(4):703–11.
20. Campbell CC, Waters PM, Emans JB. Excision of the radial head for congenital dislocation. J Bone Joint Surg Am. 1992;74(5): 726–33. PubMed PMID: 1624487.eng.
21. Van Heest AE, Rodriguez R. Dorsal carpal wedge osteotomy in the arthrogrypotic wrist. J Hand Surg Am. 2013;38(2):265–70. PubMed PMID: 23267756. Epub 2012/12/27. eng.
22. Matev I. Surgery of the spastic thumb-in-palm deformity. J Hand Surg Br. 1991;16(2):127–32. PubMed PMID: 2061648. Epub 1991/05/01. eng.
23. Tonkin MA, Beard AJ, Kemp SJ, Eakins DF. Sesamoid arthrodesis for hyperextension of the thumb metacarpophalangeal joint. J Hand Surg Am. 1995;20(2):334–8.
24. Wood VE. Another look at the causes of the windblown hand. J Hand Surg Br. 1994;19(6):679–82. PubMed PMID: 7706863. Epub 1994/12/01. eng.

Madelung Deformity

24

Sarah E. Sibbel, Andrea S. Bauer, and H. Relton McCarroll

History and Epidemiology

The first description of the Madelung deformity is attributed to a lecture given by Guillaume Dupuytren in 1834 [1]. However, it became Otto von Madelung's deformity namesake after he thoroughly characterized the findings that others had described, offering a potential cause and treatment options for the deformity. Madelung actually advocated the term *manus valga* for the deformity and did not credit himself with discovering the disease or for being the first to document it [2].

Madelung deformity observations precede the availability of X-rays and were based upon clinical observation. He described prominence of the distal ulna, volar subluxation of the wrist, and volar angulation of the distal radial epiphysis. He noted limitations in range of motion of the forearm and wrist. He also noticed that the deformity was twice as common in women and generally bilateral, with symptoms beginning at an average age of 13 years [3].

The exact etiology of Madelung deformity is unknown. Most cases occur sporadically, without any defined inheritance pattern or known genetic association. In 1929, Leri and Weill described a familial mesomelic dwarfism, characterized by short stature and the Madelung wrist deformity [4]. The Madelung deformity is a consistent characteristic of Leri–Weill dyschondrosteosis (LWD), which is also characterized by deformities of the proximal radius, tibia, and fibula. Leri–Weill dyschondrosteosis is inherited in a pseudo-autosomal dominant manner [5], while idiopathic Madelung deformity is sporadic. The short stature homeobox-containing gene (SHOX) was first described in 1997 and linked to idiopathic short stature and Turner syndrome [6]. Shortly thereafter, point mutations in the SHOX gene were found in families with Leri–Weill dyschondrosteosis [7, 8].

Madelung deformity and Leri–Weill dyschondrosteosis are rare. In 1977, Flatt reported on a series of over 1,400 patients with congenital upper limb differences, only 1.7 % of which represented Madelung deformity [9]. Subtle deformity is likely present for years before it is noticed clinically due to the fact that the magnitude of the deformity tends to worsen with skeletal growth.

Anatomy

Madelung deformity is characterized by a shortened radius that curves palmarly and ulnarly, a dorsally prominent ulnar head, and a triangular arrangement of the carpal bones [2, 10, 11]. The hand appears to be translated palmarly and ulnarly relative to the wrist. Since the ulna is unaffected, it continues to have normal longitudinal growth that gives it an elongated and prominent appearance (Fig. 24.1). In severe cases, the distal radioulnar joint (DRUJ) may become incongruent, and the carpus will migrate proximally and palmarly, causing decreased range of motion, pain, and for some, an undesired aesthetic appearance of the wrist [12]. This deformity is due to a growth disturbance at the ulnar and volar aspects of the distal radius physis. In 1992, Vickers and Nielsen described the Vickers ligament, an abnormal volar ligament that is thought to tether the lunate to the volar distal radius. The authors suggested that this ligament contributes to the radial deformity seen in Madelung deformity due to asymmetric reduced growth at the compressed area of the physis. This is hypothesized to lead to the characteristic appearance of lunate subsidence between the ulna and the radius [13]. Others believe that the Vickers ligament is hypertrophied wrist capsule that replaces the missing volar 40–60 % of the lunate fossa, and that it is secondary to the deformity, not the primary cause [15].

S.E. Sibbel, M.D. • A.S. Bauer, M.D. (✉) • H.R. McCarroll, M.D.
Department of Orthopaedic Surgery, Shriners Hospital for Children Northern California, 2425 Stockton Boulevard, Sacramento, CA 95817, USA
e-mail: sarah.sibbel@childrenscolorado.org; anbauer@shrinenet.org; hreltonm@comcast.net

D.R. Laub Jr. (ed.), *Congenital Anomalies of the Upper Extremity: Etiology and Management*, DOI 10.1007/978-1-4899-7504-1_24, © Springer Science+Business Media New York 2015

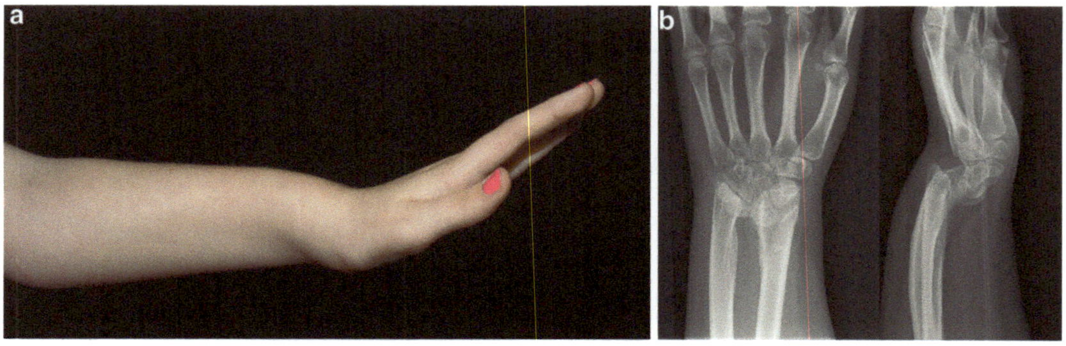

Fig. 24.1 (a) Clinical photograph and (b) AP and lateral wrist radiographs of patient with Madelung deformity. Reproduced with permission from Shriners Hospitals for Children—Northern California

On physical examination, the deformity is most noticeable observing the subluxation from the ulnar side. The forearm is of normal shape. The distal end of the ulna is distinct under the skin and the styloid process and articular surface can be recognized. The hand is normal, but has dropped palmarly. The diameter of the wrist is almost twice normal. The hand, viewed from the radial side, is less obviously displaced. The extensor tendons, which pass over the radius towards the dorsum of the hand, bridge and obscure the step that is so noticeable on the ulnar side. The anteroposterior diameter of the wrist appears almost double that of the contralateral side. When the distal end of the radius is palpated with the hand dorsiflexed, and the extensor tendons relaxed, a large portion of the articular surface of the radius may be palpated. At the same time it is noticeable that the posterior lip of the distal radius, which is normally rather sharp, is more obscure. If it is compared with the radius of the healthy side, it is noticed that the whole distal epiphysis of the radius is angulated palmarly [3].

Associated Conditions/Differential Diagnosis

Leri-Weill dyschondrosteosis is a dominantly inherited skeletal dysplasia that is frequently associated with Madelung deformity. Those affected present with normal intelligence, short stature, mesomelic limb shortening, and Madelung deformity. Mesomelia is defined as when the middle portion of a limb is shortened in relation to the proximal portion and is the most frequent clinical finding in LWD [16]. In 2001, Ross et al. [17] performed a study of 43 patients with LWD and found that 32 (74 %) had Madelung deformity. Both Madelung deformity and LWD are more common in females, possibly due to the role estrogen plays in the development of dyschondrosteosis and the effect of estrogen on the physis [17, 18].

The short stature homeobox (SHOX) gene is expressed by both sex chromosomes in males and females and is thought to play a role in bone growth and development. Haploinsufficiency of the SHOX gene, which is located in the pseudo-autosomal region of the chromosomes, results in the genetic defect that causes LWD [17]. Due to recombination between sex chromosomes during meiosis, the SHOX defect is passed to offspring in a pseudo-autosomal dominant inheritance pattern instead of in a sex-linked pattern. Therefore, the offspring of a person with a SHOX haploinsufficiency disorder have a 50 % chance of acquiring the genetic mutation. Langer mesomelic dysplasia (LMD) results from a homozygous deletion or compound heterozygous mutation of SHOX. LMD may occur in offspring where both parents have LWD. It is characterized by severe skeletal dysplasia and short stature, with shortening of the long tubular bones more marked in the proximal portion of the extremity. Madelung deformity is much rarer in those with LMD than those with LWD [16].

Turner syndrome (TS) is a genetic disorder (45, XO) that is also due to haploinsufficiency of the SHOX gene and includes short stature, primary amenorrhea, neck webbing, lymphedema, high-arched palate, short metacarpals, scoliosis, hearing difficulties, cardiac and renal anomalies, hypothyroidism, and glucose intolerance [16]. Madelung deformity may be seen in up to 7 % of affected individuals. The reason for the relatively low incidence in TS versus the high incidence in LWD is not clear, but may be due to the influence of estrogen exposure on the development of Madelung deformity. Those with TS may be protected from developing Madelung deformity by their sex steroid deficiency, whereas LWD females generally have normal ovarian function [17].

Cases of Madelung deformity have also been reported in those with psuedohypoparathyroidism types 1a and 1b, due to a mutation in the GNAS gene [19, 20]. It has also been reported in the setting of nail-patella syndrome, which is inherited in an autosomal dominant fashion with variable penetrance [21]. Both of these syndromes share no known relationship with SHOX gene mutations and illustrate the complexity of the genetic origins of the deformity. Idiopathic cases may represent de novo or as uncharacterized mutations [18]. Further research is needed to identify the genetic mutations associated with this deformity.

The theory that Madelung deformity is caused by wrist trauma has been debated for decades, with argument against this cause dating as far back as Anton et al. in 1938 [22]. It is disputed that since most cases present in young females with no history or exposure to trauma, it is unlikely that this could be the reason for the deformity. However, in a more recent study, a Madelung-like deformity has been described in female gymnasts that are believed to be the result of physeal trauma due to repetitive loading of the wrist joint.

So-called reverse Madelung deformity was recognized by Kirmisson as a similar yet separate deformity in 1902. Since that time, there have been only a handful of cases reported in the literature. In the reverse Madelung deformity, the radius is bowed dorsally, displacing the distal ulna palmarly. The articular surface of the radius is angulated dorsally, shifting the carpus dorsally as well. It is unknown whether this deformity is mediated by the same genetics as true Madelung deformity, or whether it represents a separate form of skeletal dysplasia.

Diagnosis

Most patients with Madelung deformity initially present to the physician somewhere between 8 and 14 years of age [12]. The primary complaint is often that of wrist pain and stiffness, but may include difficulty with school, sports, or other activities of daily living, as well as concern over the appearance of the wrist itself [18]. Physical examination will reveal the prominent distal ulna with volar subluxation of the carpus relative to the forearm. Supination and wrist extension may be limited and there may be instability of the DRUJ depending upon the severity of the deformity. Distal hand function and elbow motion are unaffected [12]. Spontaneous rupture of extensor tendons has been reported in the literature, associated with the dorsal prominence of the distal ulna, and may lead to a diagnosis in those with longstanding disease. A comprehensive history and physical examination of the patient is essential to evaluate for associated diagnoses, such as LWD, or other unrelated causes for the patient's complaints. In cases where LWD is suspected, younger siblings should be examined and radiographed as well, as it may be possible to intervene with less-invasive procedures prior to symptoms appearing.

Radiographs will confirm the diagnosis of Madelung deformity. Early reports on the radiographic appearance of the wrist in this disorder described features such as "pyramidalization" of the carpus as a result of the proximal subsidence of the lunate, the absence or narrowing of the ulnar aspect of the distal radial physis, anterior bowing of the radial shaft, and dorsal subluxation of the ulnar head [22]. Several radiographic parameters have been proposed to identify, quantify, and categorize Madelung deformity. Measurements were initially based on the radius [13], but this is unreliable due to the anatomic variability of the radius in this condition. More recent criteria have been based on the ulna, as it is thought to be normal. McCarroll et al. [23] identified five radiographic parameters for Madelung deformity, including ulnar tilt, lunate subsidence, lunate fossa angle, palmar tilt, and palmar carpal displacement. They found that ulnar tilt, lunate subsidence, and palmar carpal displacement are reliable and reproducible measurements for quantifying the severity of Madelung deformity on X-rays (Fig. 24.2). Measurement of palmar tilt is unreliable because of the superimposition of multiple structures on the lateral X-ray. In a later study performed by the same group, diagnostic threshold values for ulnar tilt, lunate subsidence, lunate fossa angle, and palmar carpal displacement were determined. The thresholds are defined as: an ulnar tilt of 33° or greater, lunate subsidence of 4 mm or more, lunate fossa angle of 40°

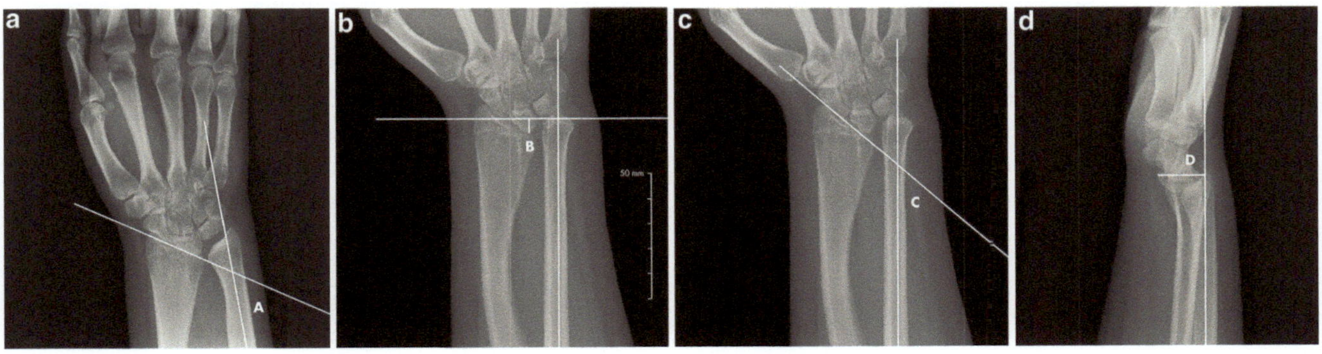

Fig. 24.2 Radiographic parameters of Madelung deformity. (**a**) (Ulnar tilt): Ulnar tilt is defined on the PA X-ray as the complement (90°-angle A) of the acute angle (angle A) between the longitudinal axis of the ulna and a line tangential to the proximal surfaces of the scaphoid and lunate. (**b**) (Lunate subsidence): Lunate subsidence on a PA X-ray is defined as the distance in millimeters (distance B) between the most proximal point of the lunate and a line perpendicular to the longitudinal axis of the ulna and through its distal articular surface. The measurement is positive if the ulna extends distal to the proximal surface of the lunate. (**c**) (Lunate fossa angle): Lunate fossa angle on a PA X-ray is defined as the complement (90°-angle C) of the acute angle (angle C) between the longitudinal axis of the ulna and a line across the lunate fossa of the radius. (**d**) (Palmar carpal displacement): Palmar carpal displacement on a lateral X-ray is defined as the distance in millimeters (distance D) between the longitudinal axis of the ulna and the most palmar point on the surface of the lunate or capitate. Reproduced with permission from Shriners Hospitals for Children—Northern California

or greater, and palmar carpal displacement of 20 mm or more. The lunate fossa angle was found to be especially useful in the early diagnosis of Madelung deformity [24].

There is little information written regarding the use of MRI in the diagnosis and evaluation of Madelung deformity. Vickers and Nielsen [13] advocate for the use of MRI in their 1992 study, suggesting that the early identification of the thickened volar radiolunate (Vickers) ligament may allow for prophylactic excision. Other studies [25, 26] have confirmed the presence of the Vickers ligament as well as an anomalous thickened volar radiotriquetral ligament. However, the clinical usefulness of MRI in Madelung deformity has not yet been evaluated critically and is not currently part of our institution's routine workup.

Treatment Methods

Appropriate treatment of Madelung deformity remains controversial. This is in part due to the fact that many patients are very concerned with the appearance of the wrist, making it difficult to tease out other functional concerns. Patients who present simply because they notice the bony deformity do not necessarily require treatment. In our experience, however, this scenario is quite rare, and most patients present with limitations in range of motion along with pain. Nonsurgical treatment is limited to symptom relief—splinting and activity modification may help those with mild, intermittent symptoms. However, since Madelung deformity is an anatomic problem, definitive treatment is generally surgical. Surgical treatment of the Madelung deformity can be divided into three categories: early prevention, late correction, and salvage procedures. First, early deformity in young patients with open physes can be treated in a preventative manner with physiolysis and release of Vickers ligament. Second, various osteotomies of the radius and ulna have been described to correct the bony deformity in patients with limited growth remaining. Lastly, some patients may not present for treatment until adulthood, generally with complaints related to ulnocarpal impaction. In these patients, an ulnar shortening osteotomy, with or without a concomitant osteotomy of the distal radius, may be appropriate. Partial or complete wrist arthrodesis may also be considered in the setting of an arthritic joint.

Physiolysis and Vickers Ligament Release

In their 1992 study, Vickers and Nielsen [13] identified two distinct lesions that are central to the pathogenesis of Madelung deformity. The principal lesion is growth arrest in the ulnar zone of the distal radial physis, which slows the growth in this area asymmetrically resulting in volar and ulnar bowing of the distal radius. They also identified the Vickers ligament, which, as discussed previously, is an abnormally thickened short radiolunate ligament that tethers the lunate to the distal radius, leading to the classic pyramidalization of the carpus. This ligament may also contribute to the partial growth arrest of the distal radial physis secondary to compression. Vickers and Nielsen [13] recommended addressing both of these lesions through a transverse volar approach, but modifications in this approach have been made more recently to utilize a standard longitudinal volar incision [27].

This procedure is reserved for young patients with open physes and is intended to prevent further deformation of the wrist. A traditional Henry approach to the volar distal radius is utilized. The thickened Vickers ligament is identified deep to the pronator quadratus and transected, releasing the soft-tissue tether. The bony bridge on the volar-ulnar aspect of the distal radial physis is identified via a combination of preoperative imaging, intraoperative fluoroscopy, and direct visualization. This area is then curetted, with care being taken to avoid injuring the adjacent healthy physeal cartilage. Pronator muscle or fat is then interposed to replace the resected segment and to prevent physeal bar formation (this is also known as the Langenskiöld procedure). Once the soft tissues are repaired, the wrist is placed into a short-arm cast for 2 weeks (Fig. 24.3). The patient's growth is followed closely with radiographs every 6 months. If the ulna appears to be overgrowing, epiphysiodesis should be considered [12]. The efficacy of this release is unknown. Vickers and Nielsen [13] treated 15 wrists in 11 skeletally immature patients and reported no progression of deformity.

There is a paucity of additional publications on physiolysis for Madelung deformity. There are "word of mouth" reports of serious complications following the procedure, possibly secondary to loss of the support of the Vickers ligament, which is the only support for the volar aspect of the lunate. Until the usefulness of the procedure is further defined, the authors advise caution and care in its use. Also, the procedure described by Vickers and Nielson does not correct preexisting deformity, nor does it provide a solution for the more typical Madelung deformity patient who presents with marked deformity and little growth potential remaining [10, 28]. This led to the development of techniques to correct the bony deformity through a radial osteotomy, which may be performed in isolation or in combination with release of Vickers ligament. All of the recent publications describing osteotomy of the radius in patients with Madelung deformity have a common goal in preserving the DRUJ.

Radial Dome Osteotomy

A standard Henry volar approach to the distal radius is performed. Release of the Vickers ligament may be performed, if desired. Circumferential periosteal elevation of the distal radius metaphysis and placement of small Homan or Bennett

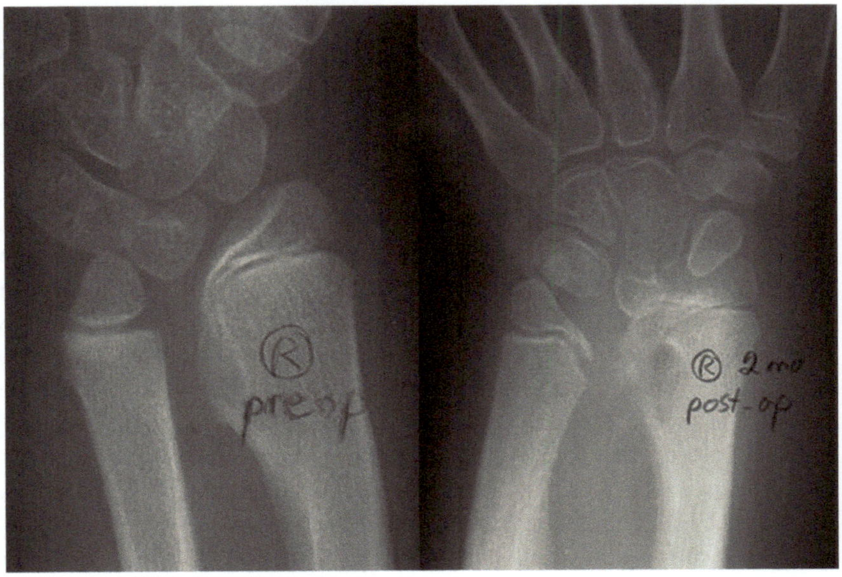

Fig. 24.3 AP wrist radiograph before and 2 months after Vicker ligament release and physiolysis. Reproduced with permission from Shriners Hospitals for Children—Northern California

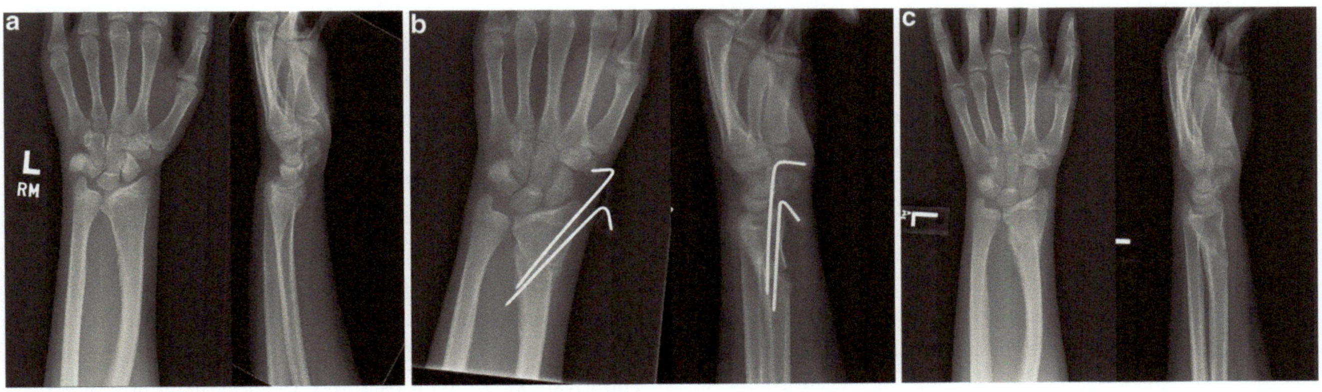

Fig. 24.4 Correction of Madelung deformity via distal radius dome osteotomy. (**a**) Preoperative radiographs. (**b**) Postoperative radiographic appearance, immediately before pin removal. (**c**) Final radiographic appearance at 3 months after surgery. Reproduced with permission from Shriners Hospitals for Children—Northern California

retractors is then performed. The osteotomy is planned under combined direct visualization and fluoroscopic guidance with great attention to avoid violation of the DRUJ and, if still open, the radial physis. It is of utmost importance to plan the osteotomy concave distal, allowing for appropriate correction to be made [28]. In contrast, a convex distal osteotomy will create a prominent metaphyseal spike on the distal fragment that will impede radial deviation and extension of the osteotomy. Waters and Bae [12] use the saying "If you make the osteotomy look like a smile, not a frown, you will end up happy." The path of the planned osteotomy is fenestrated using a K-wire or drill bits and completed using curved osteotomes. A DomeSaw® (Matrix Orthopaedics, Inc. Twin Falls, ID) may also be utilized. The curve of the osteotome blade or DomeSaw® creates an osteotomy plane that is concave distal in both the frontal and sagittal planes, allowing for multiplanar correction of the deformity. Longitudinal traction is used to reduce the hand to the ulna, as well as create radial deviation and extension of the distal fragment. Dorsal displacement of the distal fragment is also performed. The corrected position is held by two K-wires placed from the radial styloid, across the osteotomy site and into the proximal fragment [28]. These wires may be placed into the distal fragment prior to creation of the osteotomy and used as a joystick to facilitate reduction [12]. Often a spike of bone may need to be removed from the proximal volar cortex, and this can be used as local bone graft in the osteotomy site. Fluoroscopic images are obtained to confirm desired correction (Fig. 24.4).

Distal ulnar epiphysiodesis may be performed in conjunction with radial dome osteotomy in a young patient who is at risk for further deformity due to continued ulnar growth. The distal ulnar physis is located with fluoroscopy and a longitudinal incision is made centered over this area. The dorsal ulnar sensory nerve is identified and protected. A 25-gauge needle can be placed in the physis and to confirm its location using fluoroscopy. Subperiosteal dissection is performed and the physis is drilled or curetted under direct visualization, leaving the periosteum on the far side undisturbed. Once adequate physeal destruction is confirmed under fluoroscopic imaging, the periosteum of the ulna is repaired [12].

In patients who present late with little skeletal growth remaining, or in those who have advanced deformity with positive ulnar variance, an ulnar shortening osteotomy may be necessary in combination with a radial dome osteotomy. A longitudinal incision is carried out over the ulnar border of the distal forearm with care being taken to protect the dorsal ulnar sensory nerve. Subperiosteal dissection is performed and the plate of choice is applied to the ulna, making sure that the length of the plate will accommodate the osteotomy site. The distal holes are drilled with partial placement of screws and the osteotomy site marked. The plate and screws are removed. Two parallel oblique passes are made with a sagittal saw to correspond with the desired amount of shortening. The ring of bone is removed and the plate and screws are reapplied. The osteotomy is reduced and proximal fixation is achieved with screws applied in compression. Fluoroscopic imaging is utilized to assess plate placement and osteotomy alignment.

For all of the above procedures, prophylactic fasciotomy should be considered, as the amount of correction can be quite dramatic. Once the incisions have been closed and dressed, the extremity should be immobilized in a well-padded long arm splint or bivalved cast. The pins from the dome osteotomy are removed when radiographic healing is evident, anywhere between 4 and 8 weeks. Gentle ROM is started once the pins are removed, and a removable wrist splint is worn for activity and weaned over the next 2 weeks as comfort allows.

Very Distal Radius Osteotomy

In 2010, McCarroll and James [15] described a distal radius osteotomy technique that allows correction of the palmar tilt, ulnar tilt, and the radial bow present in Madelung deformity (Fig. 24.5). They begin by approaching the ulna and provisionally placing an ulnar plate to plan the ulnar shortening osteotomy. A transverse osteotomy is utilized and the cut ends of the ulna are allowed to move into bayonet apposition with one another. It is important that the ends of the ulna can overlap so the ulna does not limit mobility of the radial osteotomy. A dorsal approach is then taken to the distal radius and the extensor tendons are retraced out of the way. A small capsulotomy into the wrist joint is made and a K-wire placed across the articular surface in order to estimate palmar tilt. Another K-wire is placed into the radial styloid, just proximal and parallel to the articular surface. This wire is used as a guide to the radial tilt and as a joystick to facilitate reduction. A second joystick is placed into the distal radius from dorsal to volar, parallel to the previously placed joystick. A dorsal buttress T-plate is then tentatively selected. A marking pen is used to draw a guide line across the dorsal radius parallel to the radius articular surface. The line is drawn as distal as possible, but sufficient length of the distal fragment of the radius must be preserved to attach the T plate securely. A second guide line is drawn from the proximal margin of the DRUJ perpendicular to the axis of the radius. This will be the approximate site of the second osteotomy. A third line is drawn between the first two guidelines but at half the angle to the perpendicular line. This is the line of the distal osteotomy and will correct the ulnar tilt of the articular surface by 50 %. The ulnar extent of the osteotomy must be proximal to the DRUJ. A sagittal saw is then used to make the osteotomy cut following the central guide mark in a radial-ulnar direction and parallel to the vertical joystick and the K-wire across the articular surface of the radius in a dorsal to palmar direction. The joysticks are then used to move the distal articular fragment into a corrected position of palmar tilt and ulnar tilt.

If the distal osteotomy is acceptably aligned, only a transverse osteotomy of the proximal shaft of the radius is needed. If the visual assessment suggests additional correction is indicated the proximal osteotomy can be altered slightly to incorporate the needed correction. At this point in the procedure the proximal radius will have a very sharp dorsal point

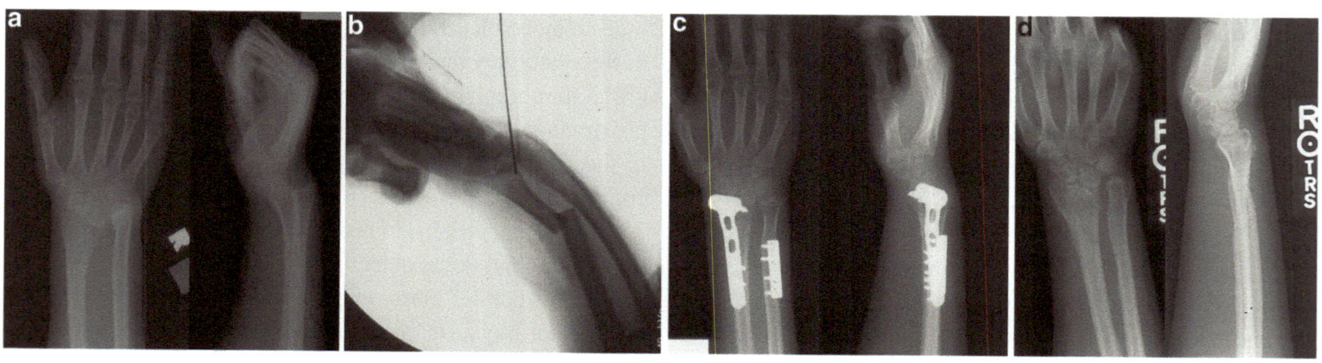

Fig. 24.5 Correction of Madelung deformity via very distal radius osteotomy. (**a**) Preoperative radiographs. (**b**) Intraoperative fluoroscopic image. The ulna has been cut and allowed to move into bayonet apposition. A K-wire has been inserted across the radiocarpal joint. (**c**) Postoperative radiographs at 6 months after surgery demonstrating healed osteotomies with hardware still in place. (**d**) Final postoperative radiographs 2 years after initial surgery, hardware has been removed. Reproduced with permission from Shriners Hospitals for Children—Northern California

that will provide very poor support to a properly aligned distal fragment. Sufficient bone must be removed from the proximal radius to provide a flat, stable surface to support the distal fragment. Enough shortening of the radius is needed to reduce the two radial fragments without excessive soft tissue tension. A choice must be made that represents a compromise between shortening of the radius and support for the distal fragment. When an acceptable position is selected, the osteotomy site is temporarily fixed with K-wires and X-ray imaging used to check the alignment.

A final choice of T-plate for fixation is made. Some contouring of the plate is always needed. Once a satisfactory contour is obtained, the plate is fixed to the radius with multiple screws taking care that the distal screws do not enter the radiocarpal or DRUJs. Once fixation is complete, the position of the osteotomy, plate, and screws can be assessed under fluoroscopy.

The previously selected ulnar plate is attached to the distal fragment of the ulna using the pre-drilled holes. Manual traction is applied to the distal ulna and the remaining overlap between the distal and proximal ulna is marked. An osteotomy is performed of the proximal fragment to the desired level. The fragments are aligned and fixation is completed.

The periosteum is closed over the plate and soft tissues repaired. The forearm and hand are immobilized in a short arm cast that is bivalved to allow for swelling. Six weeks after surgery the cast is removed and X-rays of the wrist and distal forearm obtained. A removable wrist splint is provided and ROM exercises initiated. X-rays are checked at 4–6 week intervals until solid union is documented. The patient is then allowed to slowly discontinue the splint and increase use and exercise as tolerated.

Multiple Osteotomies Using Three-Dimensional Modeling

Historically, osteotomies performed to correct Madelung deformity have been based upon surgical planning using plain radiographs [10, 12–15, 18, 28, 29]. However, evaluation of the deformity in two dimensions is difficult due to the complex three-dimensional nature of the anatomy. Recent technological advances in computed tomography (CT) imaging and computer programming have enabled us to evaluate the deformity in three dimensions and allowed for comparisons to the contralateral limb. This technology assists the surgeon in accurately planning and performing three-dimensional osteotomies using customized guides.

To plan a corrective osteotomy, three-dimensional imaging of the deformity is required. This is most easily achieved via CT with three-dimensional reconstruction. The specific protocol for the CT is dictated by the computer software that is used to model the osteotomies. In some instances, the use of the computer simulation may be facilitated by an engineer familiar with the particular program. Since bilateral involvement is typical of Madelung deformity, the use of the contralateral wrist as a model for comparison can be difficult. If the contralateral wrist is asymptomatic and not severely affected, it can be used as the comparison model. Other options for comparison models include generic bone models and those of prior patients. Generic bone models are typically based upon an "average adult male," which makes comparison to pediatric patients difficult. If models from a previous patient are used, the surgeon may be able to match for gender, age, and size.

The three-dimensional models of the affected bone can be superimposed onto the goal model and osteotomies planned. From this data, physical bone models can be fabricated, along with customized guides to assist with plate and screw placement and the pre-planned osteotomy sites.

Corrective osteotomies using this three-dimensional modeling technique are still in its early stages of development. To date, there is only one case report in the literature of using three-dimensional computer-simulated bone modeling in Madelung deformity [32]. Our experience with this technique is limited as well, but early results using the Materialise system (Plymouth, MI) have been promising (Fig. 24.6).

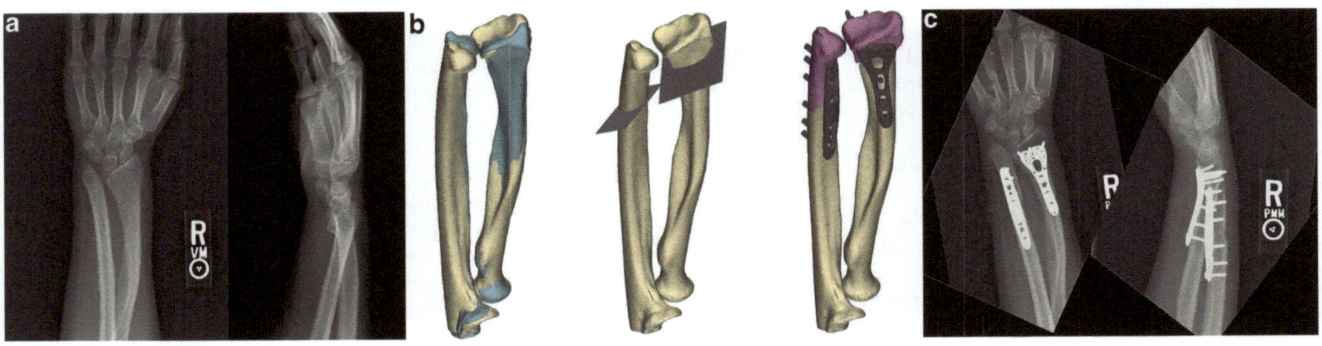

Fig. 24.6 Correction of Madelung deformity via multiple osteotomies using three-dimensional modeling. (**a**) Preoperative wrist radiographs. (**b**) Preoperative plan. The first image shows the preoperative state (in *white*) superimposed on a mirror image of the contralateral side (in *green*). Next, the planned osteotomy sites are indicated. Lastly, the planned outcome with hardware in place; corrected distal fragments in *purple*. (**c**) Final radiographic appearance at 4 months after surgery. Reproduced with permission from Shriners Hospitals for Children—Northern California

Summary

Madelung deformity is a complex entity that is not completely understood. It is a relatively rare condition, leading to a paucity of long-term follow-up of the natural history of the disease, as well as data on those that have had surgical intervention. It is difficult to determine whether or not surgery is beneficial in relieving pain or improving function over the long term, when the natural course is unknown. Vickers ligament release, physiolysis, radial osteotomies, and/or ulnar shortening procedures may effectively correct radiologic alignment and provide improvement in aesthetic appearance and pain. There is a risk of recurrent deformity however, particularly in the younger patient. The recent advent of a measurement system that is applicable to Madelung deformity will allow surgeons to intelligently discuss the advantages of various techniques by how they correct the deformity, not just whether they relieve pain or alter the range of motion. It is hoped that further insight into the natural history will be forthcoming. The osteotomy techniques described reliably improve the cosmetic appearance of the hand and wrist and, by relieving pain, improve function.

References

1. Lecon GD. Orale de Clinique Chirurgicale Faites a l'Hotel-Dieu de Paris. 1834;4:197.
2. Arora AS, Chung KC, Otto W. Madelung and the recognition of Madelung's deformity. J Hand Surg Am. 2006;31(2):177–82.
3. Madelung OW. Die spontane subluxation de hand nach vorne. Verh Dtsch Ges Chir. 1878;7:259–76.
4. Leri A, Weill J. Une affection congenitale et symetrique du developpement osseux: la dyschondrosteose. Bull Mem Soc Med Hosp Paris. 1929;53:1491–4.
5. Roubicek M, Arriazu MC, Isaac G. SHOX deficiency phenotypes. J Clin Endocrinol Metab. 2003;88(8):4004.
6. Rao E, Weiss B, Fukami M, Rump A, Niesler B, Mertz A, et al. Pseudoautosomal deletions encompassing a novel homeobox gene cause growth failure in isiopathic short stature and Turner syndrome. Nat Genet. 1997;16(1):54–63.
7. Belin V, Cusin V, Viot G, Girlich D, Toutain A, Moncla A, et al. SHOX mutations in dyschondrosteosis (Leri-Weill syndrome). Nat Genet. 1998;19(1):67–9.
8. Shears DJ, Vassal HJ, Goodman FR, Palmer RW, Reardon W, Superti-Furga A, et al. Mutation and deletion of the pseudoautosomal gene SHOX cause Leri-Weill dyschondrosteosis. Nat Genet. 1998;19(1):70–3.
9. Flatt AE. The congenital hand anomalies. St. Louis: CV Mosby; 1977. p. 50.
10. Harley BJ, Carter PR, Ezaki M. Volar surgical correction of Madelung's deformity. Tech Hand Upper Extremity Surg. 2002;6:30–5.
11. Canale ST. Madelung deformity. In: Campbell's operative orthopedics. 10th ed. St. Louis: Mosby; 2002. p. 76.
12. Waters PM, Bae DS. Pediatric hand and upper limb surgery: a practical guide. Philadelphia: Wolters Kluwer Health; 2012.
13. Vickers D, Nielsen G. Madelung deformity: Surgical prophylaxis (physiolysis) during the late growth period by resection of the dyschondrosteosis lesion. J Hand Surg Br. 1992;17(4):401–7.
14. McCarroll HR, James MA. Very distal radial osteotomy for Madelung's deformity. Tech Hand Up Extrem Surg. 2010;14(2): 85–93.
15. Munns C, Glass I. SHOX-related haploinsufficiency disorders. In: Pagon R, Bird T, Dolan C, editors. Gene reviews. Seattle: University of Washington; 2005. Updated 2008.
16. Ross JL, Scott Jr C, Marttila P, Kowal K, Nass A, Papenhausen P, et al. Phenotypes associated with SHOX deficiency. J Clin Endocrinol Metab. 2001;86(12):5674–80.
17. Ghatan AC, Hanel DP. Madelung deformity. J Am Acad Orthop Surg. 2013;21:372–82.
18. Sanchez J, Perera E, Jan de Beur S, Ding C, Dang A, Berkovitz GD, et al. Madelung-like deformity in pseudohypoparathyroidism type 1b. J Clin Endocrinol Metab. 2011;96(9):E1507–11.
19. Rump P, Jongbloed JD, Sikkema- Raddatz B, Mundlos S, Klopocki E, van der Luijt RB. Madelung deformity in a girl with a novel and de novo mutation in the GNAS gene. Am J Med Genet A. 2011; 155A(10):2566–70.
20. Ioan DM, Maximilian C, Fryns JP. Madelung deformity as a pathognomonic feature of the onycho-osteodysplasia syndrome. Genet Couns. 1992;3(1):25–9.
21. Anton JI, Reitz GB, Spiegel MB. Madelung's Deformity. Ann Surg. 1938;108(3):411–39.
22. De Smet L, Claessens A, Lefevre J, Beunen G. Gymnast wrist: An epidemiologic survey of ulnar variance and stress changes of the radial physis in elite female gymnasts. Am J Sports Med. 1994;22(6):846–50.
23. Fagg PS. Reverse Madelung's deformity with nerve compression. J Hand Surg Br. 1988;13(1):23–7.
24. Ducloyer P, Leclercq C, Lisfranc R, Saffar P. Spontaneous ruptures of the extensor tendons of the fingers in Madelung's deformity. J Hand Surg Br. 1991;16:329–33.
25. Jebson P, Blair WF. Bilateral spontaneous extensor tendon ruptures in Madelung's deformity. J Hand Surg Am. 1992;17:277–80.
26. McCarroll HR, James MA, Newmeyer III WL, Molitor F, Manske PR. Madelung's deformity: Qualitative assessment of x-ray deformity. J Hand Surg Am. 2005;30(6):1211–20.
27. McCarroll HR, James MA, Newmeyer III WL, Manske PR. Madelung's deformity: Diagnostic thresholds of radiographic measurements. J Hand Surg Am. 2010;35A:807–12.
28. Cook PA, Yu JS, Lubbers L, Coleman CR, Cook II AJ, Kean JR, et al. Madelung deformity in skeletally immature patients: morphologic assessment using radiography, CT, and MRI. J Comput Assist Tomogr. 1996;20(4):505–11.
29. Stehling C, Langer M, Nassenstein I, Bachmann R, Heindel W, Vieth V. High resolution 3.0 Tesla MR imaging findings in patients with bilateral Madelung's deformity. Surg Radiol Anat. 2009;31(7):551–7.
30. Green DP, Hotchkiss RN, Pederson WC, Wolfe SW, editors. Deformities of the wrist and forearm. In: Green's operative hand surgery, vol. 2, 5th ed. Philadelphia: Elsevier; 2005. p. 1484–91.
31. Harley BJ, Brown C, Cummings K, Carter PR, Ezaki M. Volar ligament release and distal radius dome osteotomy for correction of Madelung's deformity. J Hand Surg Am. 2006;31:1499–506.
32. Imai Y, Miyake J, Okada K, Murase T, Yoshikawa H, Moritomo H. Cylindrical corrective osteotomy for Madelung deformity using a computer simulation: Case report. J Hand Surg Am. 2013;38A: 1925–32.

25 Epidermolysis Bullosa

Roberto Diaz, Jennifer M. Chan, and Amy L. Ladd

Background

Epidermolysis bullosa (EB) is a rare hereditary connective tissue disorder of the skin that leads to blister formation following minimal mechanical trauma. Gene mutations result in the production of abnormal structural proteins whose primary function is anchoring of the epidermis to the dermis, making the skin vulnerable to injury with trivial mechanical trauma. In the United States, the prevalence of EB was estimated at approximately 8 cases per one million population in 1990 based on the National EB Registry [1]. The incidence was estimated as 19 cases per one million between 1986 and 1990 [1].

The severity of the disease can vary from mild to severe and appears to be related to the degree of protein abnormality and quantities present [2]. EB can manifest in many areas of the body including extra-cutaneous sites such as the eyes, gastrointestinal tract, and genitourinary tracts. Severity and location will vary based on subtype of EB. Currently, there is no cure for EB and treatment is aimed at minimizing blister formation, preventing infection, optimizing nutrition, and maintaining hand function. One of the most disabling aspects of EB is the formation of pseudosyndactyly of the hands (Fig. 25.1) leading to progressive loss of hand function [3]. Hand involvement is most frequently observed in the recessive dystrophic epidermolysis bullosa subtype. The hands are particularly vulnerable to blister formation as they frequently experience sheer forces during various activities of daily living. Surgical treatment of the hand is aimed at improving hand function by restoring independent finger mobility, pinch, and grasp function. This chapter will focus on the treatment of hand deformities caused by EB, specifically those in children with recessive dystrophic epidermolysis bullosa as seen at our institution.

R. Diaz, M.D. • A.L. Ladd, MD (✉)
Department of Orthopaedic Surgery, Stanford University Medical Center, 450 Broadway, Pavilion A, Redwood City, CA 94063, USA
e-mail: ridiaz@stanford.edu; alad@stanford.edu

J.M. Chan, O.T.R., C.H.T.
Rehabilitation Services, Lucile Packard Children's Hospital at Stanford, 321 Middlefield Road, Menlo Park, CA 94025, USA
e-mail: jmchan@lpch.org

History

EB was first described by Austrian dermatologist Von Hebra in 1870 [4]. In 1879, Tilbury Fox, a British dermatologist, described the inheritance of EB in two cases involving a 6-year-old girl who presented with hand blisters and her sister, a 2-year-old with blisters on multiple areas and ulcerations on the tongue [5]. In 1886, this condition was named epidermolysis bullosa by Heinrich Koebner.

EB Types

There are four major types of EB based on the Report of the Third International Consensus Meeting on Diagnosis and Classification of EB [6]. EB is classified according to the level at which cleavage occurs: (1) EB simplex (intraepidermal separation), (2) junctional EB (intra-lamina lucida separation), (3) dystrophic EB (sub-basal lamina separation), and (4) Kindler syndrome (mixed cleavage points).

EB simplex (EBS) is the most common type that follows an autosomal dominant inheritance pattern with several subtypes having an autosomal recessive pattern of inheritance. It is characterized by localized or widespread blisters depending on subtype and typically presents at birth or early infancy. Blister formation occurs within the epidermis and blisters heal without scar formation. Most patients with the localized subtype will have a normal life expectancy [2, 7]. Nail dystrophy, milia, and mucosal involvement are rare in all types of EBS compared to the other major types [1].

D.R. Laub Jr. (ed.), *Congenital Anomalies of the Upper Extremity: Etiology and Management*, DOI 10.1007/978-1-4899-7504-1_25, © Springer Science+Business Media New York 2015

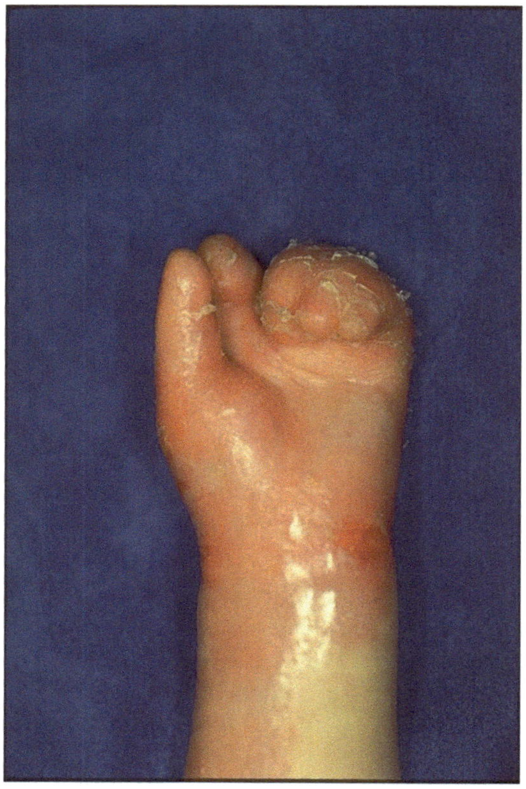

Fig. 25.1 Example of pseudosyndactyly

Junctional EB (JEB) is inherited in an autosomal recessive fashion and can vary from mild to severe disease. Cleavage occurs at the dermal–epidermal junction within the lamina lucida. The hallmark clinical feature of all forms of JEB is enamel hypoplasia that has an appearance of pitting on tooth surfaces [1]. There are two general subtypes of JEB, which include the JEB-Herlitz and the more common generalized atrophic benign EB [1, 2]. The junctional EB Herlitz variant is the most severe form that is present at birth and carries a high risk of death within the first 2 years of life. Blisters heal with atrophic scars. Manifestations can occur in the eyes, and gastrointestinal and genitourinary systems. Death is related to complications from malnutrition, infection, and respiratory failure [2, 7]. In the milder form, generalized atrophic benign EB, patients can have a normal lifespan. They may have scalp involvement, which can lead to hair loss.

Dystrophic EB is characterized by cleavage below the basal lamina and has both autosomal dominant and recessive inheritance patterns [1, 2, 7]. The autosomal dominate subtype (DDEB) has a milder presentation with blistering occurring primarily in the upper and lower extremities. In contrast, the recessive type (RDEB) manifests with widespread blistering with involvement of the eyes, gastrointestinal tract, genitourinary tract, kidney, and heart. Blisters heal with severe scar formation that can result in nail dystrophy, joint flexion contractures, and pseudosyndactyly of the fingers and toes. This ongoing process of blister and scar formation can result in significant hand dysfunction. There is also an increased risk of the development of squamous cell carcinoma in areas of chronic non-healing ulcers. Because there is mucosal involvement, scar formation and erosions can occur in the esophagus, cornea, and genitourinary and gastrointestinal tracts. Death typically ensues in early adult life secondary to malnutrition, infection, and cutaneous carcinomas.

Kindler syndrome is an autosomal recessive form of EB with cleavage occurring at multiple sites including intraepidermal, junctional, and sublamina densa [1, 2]. Blistering presents at birth and typically occurs in acral locations. Blister healing occurs with atrophic scar. Patients generally have a normal lifespan with blister formation decreasing with time. This form EB is associated with photosensitivity, skin atrophy, and dyspigmentation and can also have mucosal involvement [2].

Diagnosis

EB commonly presents at birth with skin blisters that must be distinguished from other skin lesions occurring during the neonatal period. The diagnosis of EB begins with a thorough history and physical examination including a family history to rule out inheritable causes of skin blisters and erosions [8]. The differential diagnosis of a newborn with skin blisters is quite extensive as described by Nischler et al. Some notable conditions include inheritable causes, traumatic blisters, infectious causes such as herpes simplex, staphylococcal scalded skin syndrome, bullous impetigo, and immunobullous disorders including bullous pemphigoid, and epidermolysis bullosa acquisita [8]. If there is a high suspicion for EB, a skin biopsy of a blister is required for a definitive diagnosis. Immunofluorescence mapping (IFM) of a skin biopsy is the primary diagnostic tool used in the diagnosis of EB and can identify the EB subtype in addition to the level of skin separation. If IFM is inconclusive, transmission electron microscopy and genetic testing can be performed to aid in the diagnosis [2, 6, 7].

Hand Contractures

Hand deformities can occur with all major types of EB; however, they more commonly occur with recessive dystrophic EB subtypes. Le Touze et al. described four characteristic lesions seen in EB affecting the hand: (1) complete loss of nails, (2) flexion contracture of fingers and palm, (3) thumb adduction contracture, and (4) pseudosyndactyly. Deformities develop from repeated blister healing that forms dense scar tissue causing partial fusion between digital web spaces. As this process continues, fusion of entire digits can result and scar tissue can eventually encase the entire hand, a condition referred to as a mitten hand (Fig. 25.2). This mitten hand restricts movement of fingers, causing finger contractures,

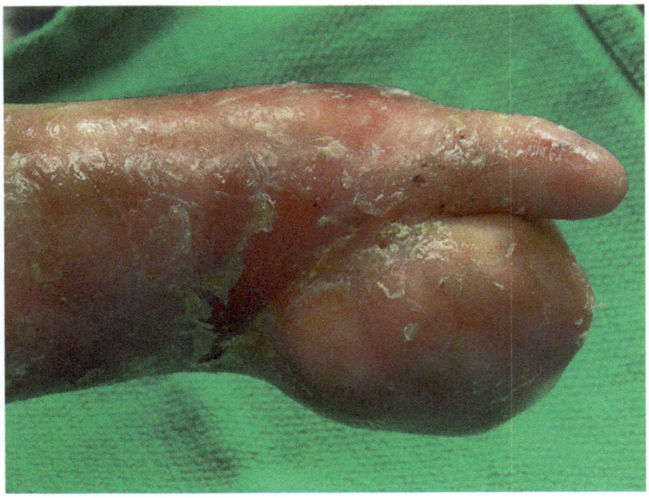

Fig. 25.2 Mitten hand

adduction contracture of the thumb and proximal muscle atrophy, and even joint destruction in cases with severe long-standing deformities [9]. This renders the hand non-functional, making it difficult for patients to carry out even simple tasks. Fine et al. reviewed the National Epidermolysis Bullosa Registry to determine the frequency and risk of developing hand and foot deformities in the major and subtypes of EB. This database contains information on 3,280 patients with EB that enrolled between the period of 1986 and 2002. There were 2,748 patients identified who had sufficient data to allow classification into 10 different subtypes of EB. The authors concluded that mitten hand deformities occur less commonly in EBS, JEB, and DDEB than in RDEB. The frequency of mitten hand deformities observed in EBS and JEB ranged from 0.0 to 4.39 % and 0.53 to 6.82 % depending on subtype. This is in comparison to 41.18 % and 51.13 % seen with non-Hallopeau-Siemens RDEB and RDEB-inversa, respectively. The highest frequency was observed in the Hallopeau-Siemens RDEB subtype at 95 %. The frequency of mitten hand deformities was only 2.35 % in the DDEB subtype.

Management

Nonoperative

Treatment of EB is best delivered in a multidisciplinary fashion with involvement of the patient's family, primary care physician, dermatologist, dentist, nutritionist, and physical and occupational therapists. Involvement of subspecialty services such as gastroenterology, urology, ophthalmology, pain management, plastic surgery, and hand surgery is determined based on need. Because there is currently no cure available for EB, nonoperative treatment is aimed at preventing blister formation by minimizing skin trauma, providing adequate nutrition, wound care, and preventing infection [2].

Operative Treatment Indications

The indications for operative treatment of the hand in patients with EB include progressive loss of hand function as demonstrated by decreased grasp or pinch, formation of pseudosyndactyly, loss of finger independence, flexion contractures, and formation of a mitten hand. The goals of surgery are to improve overall hand function by reestablishing pinch and grasp function, and to delay recurrence [2, 10, 11]. The timing of surgery will depend on surgeon preference. Although some patients will present with severe contractures and a mitten hand deformity, we prefer early surgical intervention when patients maintain some hand function with only mild to moderate contractures. Early surgical intervention is advocated in order to avoid interruptions in a developing child [3, 12]. Surgery is considered when parents and patients can cooperate with the postoperative regimen [3, 11].

Preoperative Considerations

It is important to recognize that EB can affect many areas of the body, and extreme care must be exercised when treating the patient. An air mattress should be utilized when possible. All bony prominences should be well-padded and sequential compression devices are preferentially not utilized as they can further damage fragile skin. No rubbing of skin should be allowed and the use of adhesive tape is contraindicated. A blood pressure cuff should only be applied to a well-padded extremity [12]. Electrocardiographic leads are placed over petroleum non-adhesive dressing as shown in Fig. 25.3 [1]. An intravenous line is placed after the patient has been adequately sedated and is sutured into place and secured with a cotton wrap and Coban (3 M Corp., St. Paul, MN) (Fig. 25.4). It is important that all members participating in the care of the patient are aware of these precautions.

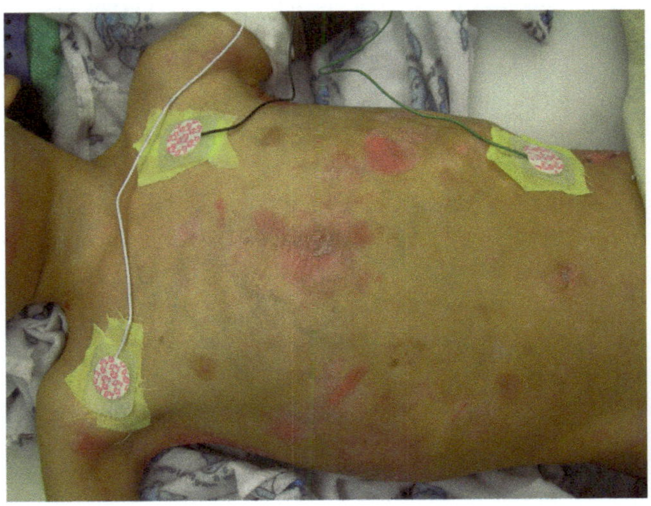

Fig. 25.3 Electrocardiographic leads placed over non-adhesive dressings

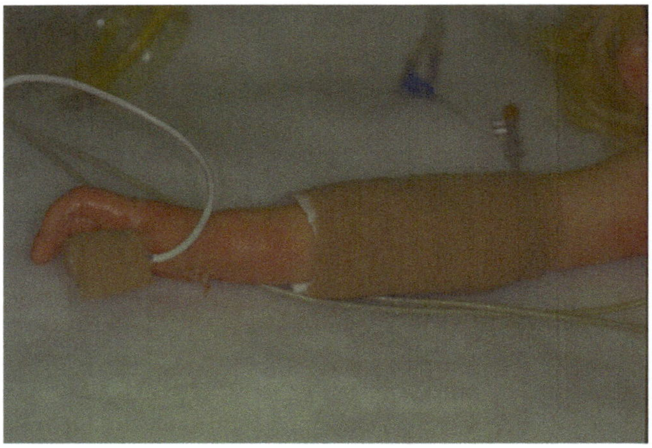

Fig. 25.4 Intravenous line secured with Coban

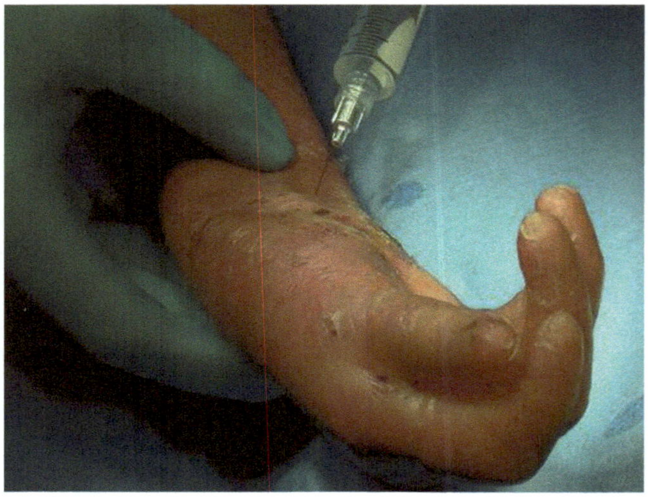

Fig. 25.5 Median nerve block

Surgical Technique

The operative technique performed by the senior author is similar to that described by several other surgeons [3, 12–15]. However, our technique differs such that no tourniquet is used, full thickness skin grafts are used instead of split thickness, and pinning of the thumb is not performed after release of its adduction contracture [11]. After carrying out the preoperative precautions described previously, the patient is placed on synthetic sheepskin overlying the operative table. Although some surgeons prefer the use of tourniquet [12–15], we elect not to use a tourniquet to avoid skin trauma at the site of tourniquet placement. The patient is given one dose of appropriately dosed cefazolin intraoperatively if there are no allergic contraindications. Bleeding generally consists of slow ooze that can be controlled with Hemostatic collagen (Avitene, Alcon Puerto Rico Inc., Humacao, Puerto Rico) or thrombin-soaked cellulose. There is also a constant serous ooze from the surgical sites that must be monitored carefully in order to adequately provide fluid resuscitation intraoperatively. A median nerve wrist block of dose appropriate 0.25 % bupivacaine with epinephrine 1:200,000 is administered. This block decreases anesthetic requirements and also helps with postoperative pain (Fig. 25.5). The abdomen and extremity are prepped without mechanical scrubbing, pouring dilute chlorhexidine soap over the proposed operative sites.

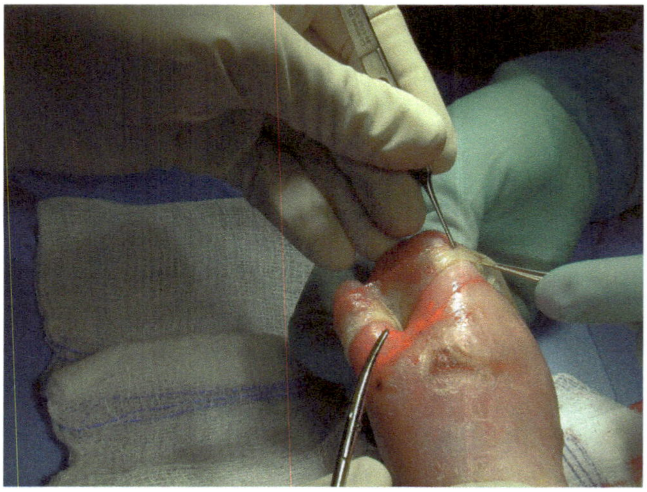

Fig. 25.6 Surgical "degloving" of hand

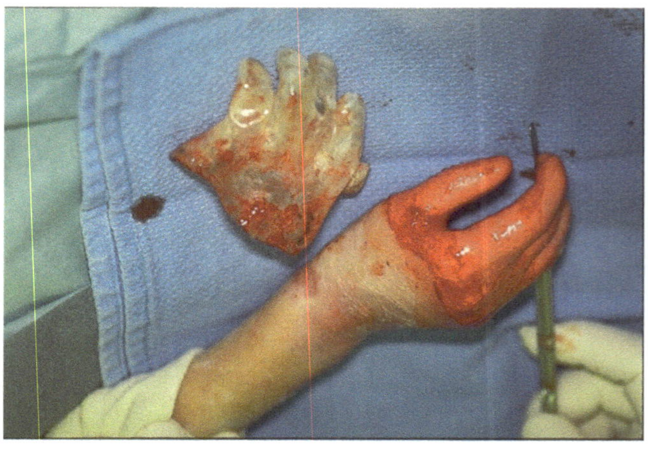

Fig. 25.7 Intraoperative image demonstrating the epidermal cocoon after degloving the hand

Surgery begins with epidermal degloving of the hand by scoring only the epidermis with a scalpel, then gently teasing away the epidermal cocoon using fine forceps, a Freer elevator, and selective separation with Littler scissors (Figs. 25.6 and 25.7). The pseudosyndactyly that forms between the fingers is released with the elevator, advanced with selective cuts, and gently separated with opposing traction on the digits. When applying traction, a single layer of gauze padding over each digit absorbs the ooze, which can create slippery

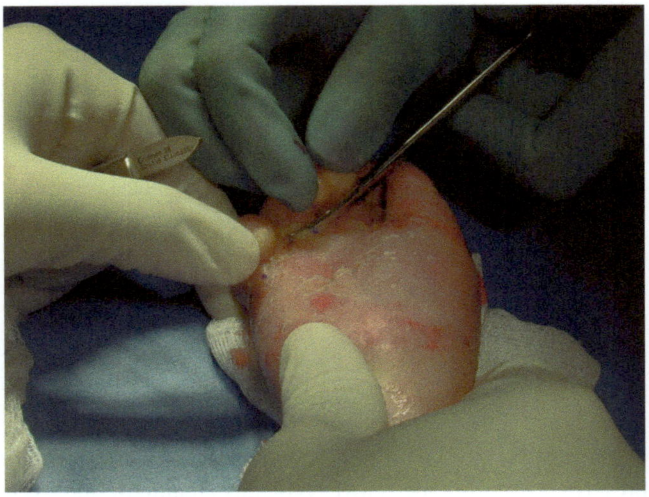

Fig. 25.8 Contracture release

surfaces. Degloving alone has proven to be ineffective and is associated with early recurrence [16]. The first web space contracture usually requires release of the adductor fascia, and only occasionally full thickness skin grafting. A four flap Z-plasty is not used to release the first web space contracture as the skin non-pliable.

Joint contractures are released by identifying areas of tension, using gentle passive extension forces. Sites of tension are released sharply along with gentle manipulation (Fig. 25.8). Care must be taken to prevent injury to the neurovascular structures. Complete contracture releases are often not possible; limitations to release include vulnerability of the neurovascular bundle and size of the subcutaneous defect. Fine K-wires are placed across the interphalangeal joints of the fingers to maintain the correction of the contractures achieved in surgery (Fig. 25.9). Full thickness skin grafts are applied to areas of skin deficits that are greater than 1 cm (see Fig. 25.9). Skin grafts are harvested from areas void of blisters, with the abdomen most preferred. It typically has areas free of blisters. Obtaining skin graft in patients with EB is more technically challenging than from harvesting from normal skin, especially since these children have little subcutaneous fat, have noncompliant skin, and variable location of clothing—underwear and waistband—can irritate the wound. Templates are recommended to plan precise areas of skin grafts, given the non-compliance of EB skin. We prefer to use full thickness skin grafts in contrast to other surgeons [10, 12–14, 16]. The epidermis readily sloughs off during the handling of the skin graft creating a dermal graft; however, we found that this does not affect graft acceptance or healing. The donor site is closed with absorbable subcuticular and interrupted epidermal sutures. Nonabsorbable sutures should be avoided as they can become buried in the healing scar. We prefer the use of 6-0 ophthalmic suture because the spatula needle and suture coating allows easy gliding through the sticky tissues. The graft incision is covered with nonadhesive dressings followed by gauze and flexible tubular fishnet bandage. The skin grafts are then sutured into the skin-deficient areas of the hand with running nonabsorbable sutures.

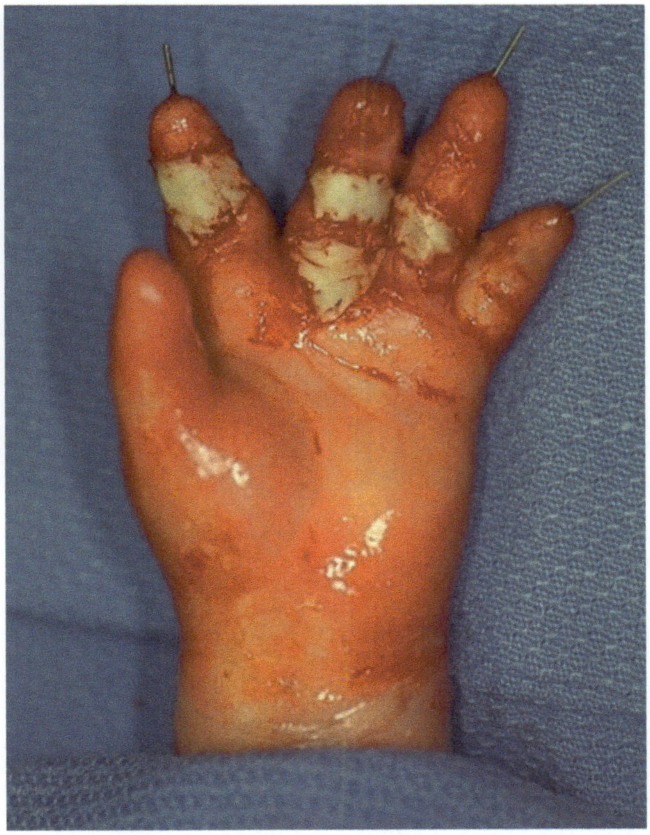

Fig. 25.9 Hand demonstrating finger pinning and full thickness skin grafts

In recent years we have moved away from obtaining skin graft when possible, given the rapid epithelialization in these patients and the associated donor site morbidity. Liberal use of antibiotic ointment is then applied to the hand wounds followed by petroleum gauze (Fig. 25.10). Mupirocin (Bactroban, GlaxoSmithKline) is preferred, providing coverage against the common contaminant, Pseudomonas. The web spaces are maintained open by placing bulky mineral oil-soaked cotton in between the digits over the non-adherent gauze. No K-wire is used for the thumb. Instead, the thumb is maintained in the abducted position by placing a 2″ roll bandage as a spacer. The extremity is then placed in a well-padded cast completely covering the hand; in young children we use a long arm cast (Fig. 25.11). Patients are typically discharged home on the day of surgery.

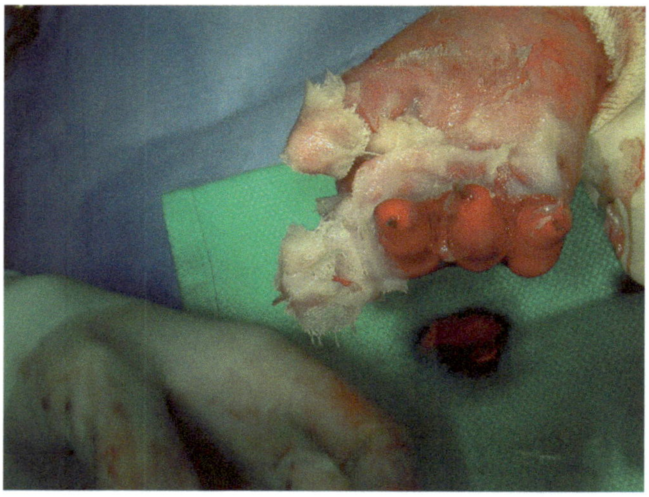

Fig. 25.10 Postoperative dressings demonstrating the use of antibiotic ointment and petrolatum gauze

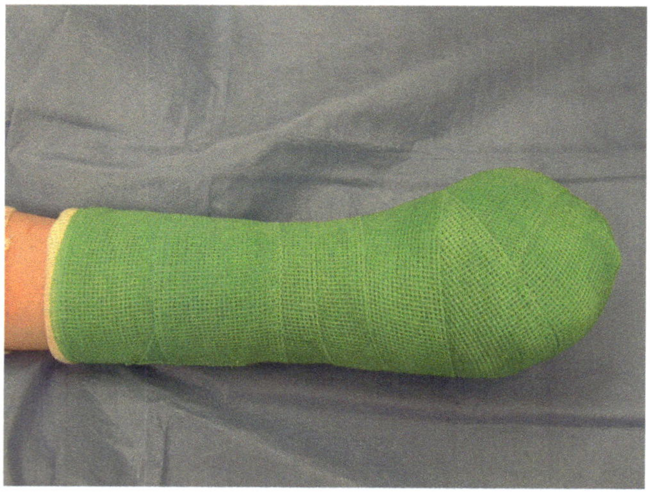

Fig. 25.11 Well-padded postoperative cast

Cast Removal

The second stage procedure is performed 10–14 days under anesthesia (IV sedation or brief intubation). This includes cast and pin removal, and splint fabrication with the therapists. One dose of prophylactic antibiotics is given. The cast is carefully removed with a cast saw and the dressings are soaked with normal saline and dilute peroxide to aid in careful dressing removal. The wounds are inspected and debrided; although the cast padding and dressings are typically replete with colored drainage and foul smell suggestive of pseudomonas, we have never encountered a deep infection. The wounds are then covered with dressings coated with a mixture of antibiotic ointment and an emollient cream (e.g., Aquaphor, Beiersdorf, Inc.) followed by non-adhesive petroleum gauze and dry gauze for drainage absorption. A splint is fabricated to maintain gains in range of motion; ideally the hand therapist prefabricates a thermoplastic splint using a hand tracing of similar size in the intraoperative setting. The splint will be modified as swelling subsides and may include the use of silicone putty partitions to maintain web spaces as shown in Fig. 25.12. Therapy and dressing changes begin typically 2–3 days after the cast removal. Adequate analgesics are required for dressing changes, which may be guided by the pain management service if available. The child is seen in hand therapy for assistance with dressing care, mobility and precision exercises, and swelling reduction. Therapy goals are focused on helping the patient improve hand function for daily living tasks. When wounds are sufficiently healed, either bandage wraps with downward pressure between the web spaces or elastic compressive custom-made glove typically maintain the web spaces. The splint is recommended to be worn at night indefinitely (Fig. 25.13). Therapy is continued as an outpatient.

Rehabilitation

Postoperative hand therapy serves a very important role in the management of EB. Following surgery, patients develop a close relationship with a therapist aimed at improving hand function and preventing recurrence of contractures as well as minimizing blister formation. At each visit, range of motion, fine motor movement, finger position, and any development of pseudosyndactyly are monitored to help guide the need for repeat surgical intervention [17]. Generally, gentle passive flexion and extension exercises are performed with care to limit skin trauma. Range of motion exercises are important during the early postoperative period as patients can develop stiffness from pin placement and immobilization. Thus, therapy consists of maintaining hand function by the use of thermoplastic splints, web space wrapping with gauze, or custom compressive gloves, and range of motion exercises. Several physicians believe that splinting and the use of compressive gloves can help delay recurrences [11, 12, 14]. Postoperatively, patients typically wear a thermoplastic splint fulltime for 2–4 weeks depending on the healing phase and remove it for dressing changes every 2–3 days. Gentle active range of motion exercises are performed 3–5 times per day with dressings on. Exercises should also be performed during dressing changes as patients can achieve greater ranges of motion with dressings removed. Therapy is performed on the wrist, fingers, and thumb. It is not uncommon for patients to experience significant pain during the early postoperative period and may only be able to perform limited therapeutic exercises initially. With progressive healing, range of motion, functional grasp, and pinch will also improve. Patients are then transitioned from full time splinting to a compressive glove or interdigital wrapping of the hands with gauze bandage to be worn during the day and continue with the splint at night indefinitely.

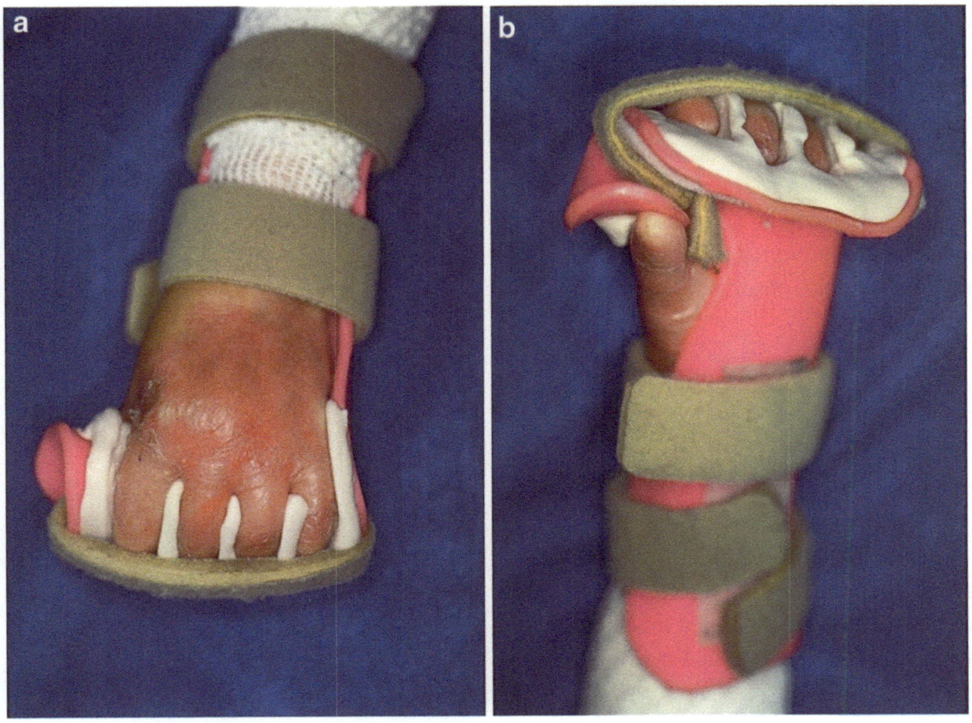

Fig. 25.12 (**a**, **b**) Thermoplast splint with silicone putty partitions

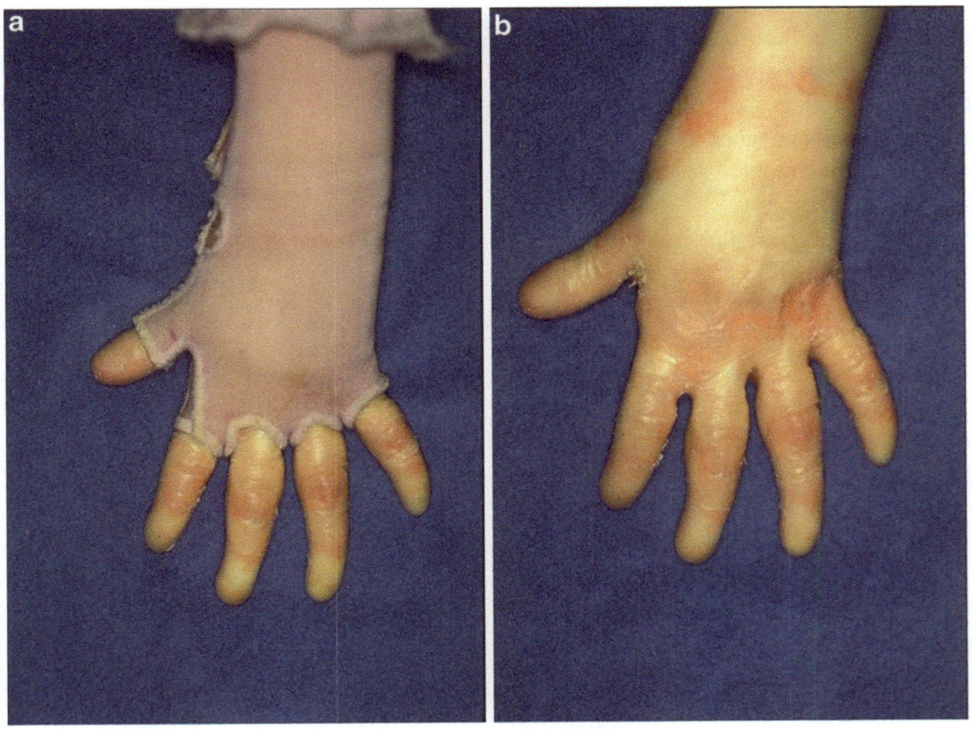

Fig. 25.13 (**a**) Elastic compressive custom-made glove worn at daytime. (**b**) Same hand with glove removed demonstrating maintenance of web spaces

Complications

Most complications occurring during the management of a patient with EB are related to skin fragility and mucosal involvement. Skin trauma resulting in blister formation can occur during the handling of the patient during any stage of treatment. Mask ventilation can result in skin blistering and intubation can result in mucosal injury. Poorly padded extremities during placement of blood pressure cuff cans cause severe blistering as can the use of adhesives such as placement of electrocardiographic leads directly on the skin.

Patients with EB have a higher incidence of gastroesophageal reflux and are at increased risk for aspiration [18]. Increased fluid losses can occur and should be monitored closely especially in patient with poor nutrition to prevent dehydration. Patients with EB are also at increased risk for thermal losses because of skin blisters and low body mass index [18]. EB patients are also at an increased risk of infection. However, we routinely only give prophylactic antibiotics intraoperatively and have not observed any postoperative infections using this protocol.

Outcomes

In 1982, Greider and Flatt published their results on the surgical treatment of nine hands in five patients with RDEB. Average patient age was 6 years at the time of surgery. There were no complications in this series. One patient had a marked recurrence on one hand and a moderate recurrence on the other hand. Two patients had a slow or slight recurrence at their 8- and 10-year follow-up, respectively. At a four year follow-up, a fourth patient had a recurrence of their thumb adduction contracture. One patient died within a year from surgery secondary to pneumonia and sepsis.

Le Touze et al. described their experience in four patients with hand deformities secondary to EB. They reported good immediate postoperative results with respect to finger independence, finger flexion and extension, and thumb opposition. They were to able maintain good hand function for 18–24 months with therapy, but report a recurrence between 4 and 6 years requiring repeat surgery.

Ladd et al. reported their results on nine hands in seven EB patients treated operatively with an average follow-up period of 17 months. There were no infections or wound complications. All patients had persistent or recurrent contractures measuring 15–30° at the interphalangeal joints and some form of metacarpal phalangeal joint extension contracture limiting flexion. Recurrence developed to a mild degree in two patients and moderate degree in three patients. Five patients who were compliant with the postoperative treatment regimen were observed to have good functional results demonstrated by grasp and pinch function (Fig. 25.14). Our experience over two decades suggests that recurrence is variable depending on severity of disease, compliance with splinting or wrapping, and medical attention. We have operated on some children several times. Most patients and families prefer the simple wrapping to maintain the webs compared to splinting, given its ease of use and freedom of the fingers. Although in our experience this provides excellent web maintenance, it leaves no check for the digital contracture in the anteroposterior plane.

Since there is no cure for EB, recurrence of hand deformities will likely occur despite surgical treatment [3, 14]. Surgery can provide significant improvement in hand function allowing patients to perform activities of daily living and continue psychomotor development. However, it is important to inform patients and parents that a second surgery will likely be needed as surgery does not change the underlying disease [3]. The following case illustrates hand deformities that may develop with long-standing recurrent blistering and scarring in patients with EB. The patient whose hand is shown in Fig. 25.15 has undergone multiple surgeries as a child beginning at age 4. At age 25, he presented to our clinic complaining of difficulty grasping objects and elected to undergo surgical treatment in an attempt to improve hand function. He underwent finger and thumb syndactyly and contracture releases in addition to release of his wrist contracture (Fig. 25.16). At his 4-month postoperative visit (Fig. 25.17), he was able to grasp an ace bandage and a pen (Fig. 25.18a,b). He is currently in college and is able to type by performing single key stokes with his thumb. He is scheduled to undergo a similar procedure of his left hand.

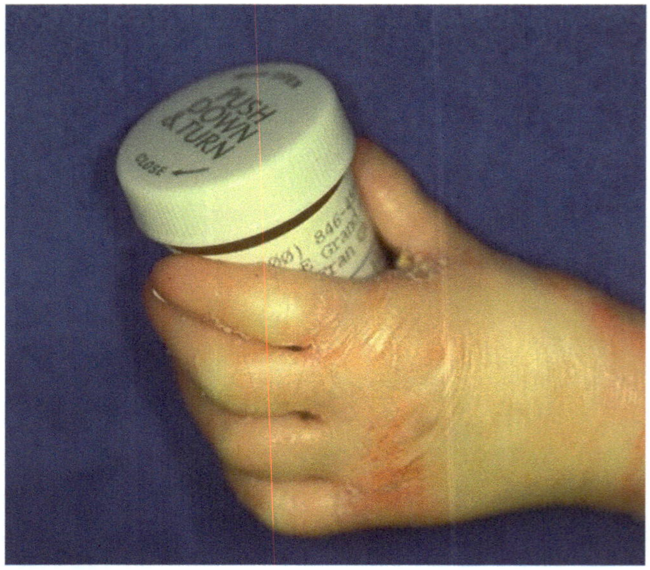

Fig. 25.14 Postoperative patient demonstrating ability to grasp objects

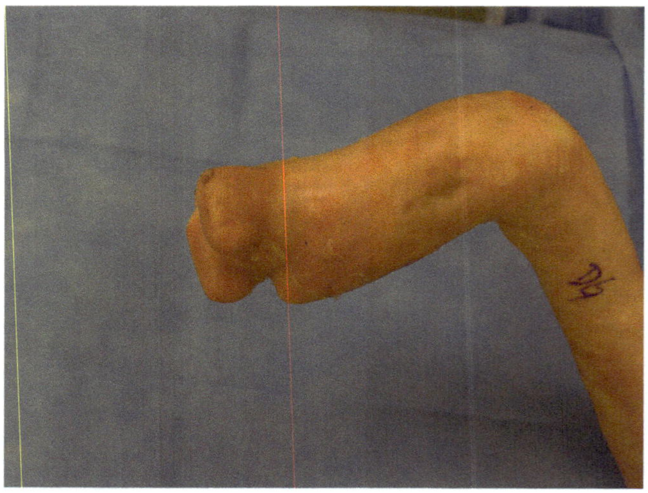

Fig. 25.15 Preoperative image of 25-year-old male who has undergone multiple surgeries for recurrence. He now reports difficulty with grasping objects

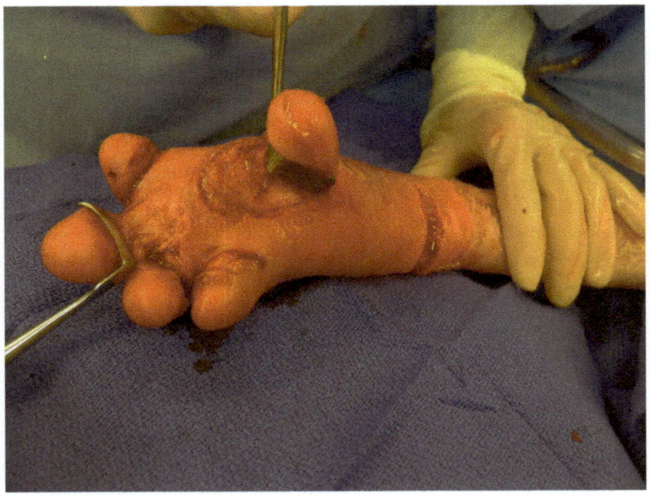

Fig. 25.16 Intraoperative image of patient in Fig. 25.15 after contracture release of wrist, thumb, and fingers

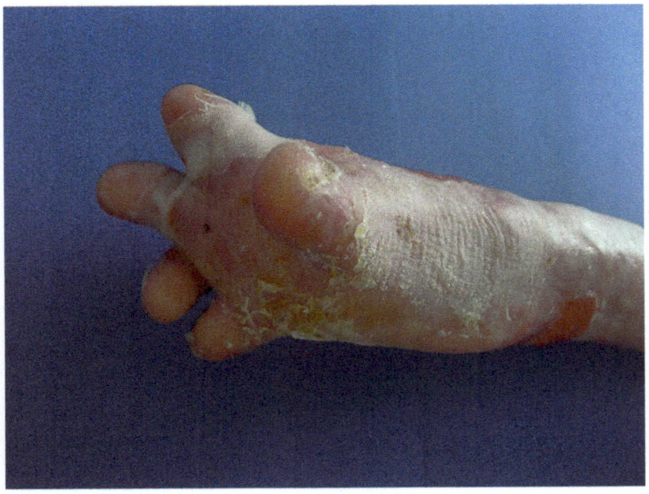

Fig. 25.17 Four-month postoperative image of patient in Fig. 25.15 following contracture releases

Conclusion

EB is a rare inherited disorder characterized by blister formation in the skin following minimal mechanical trauma. The severity of the disease will vary based on EB type. Hand deformities most commonly occur in patients with the RDEB subtype and can be a cause of significant disability in a child. The goal of surgical treatment is to improve hand function by restoring independent finger mobility, pinch, and grasp function. Patients and family members should be informed that recurrence is common and repeat surgery may be necessary to improve hand function.

References

1. Fine JD. Inherited epidermolysis bullosa. Orphanet J Rare Dis. 2010;5:12.
2. Gonzalez ME. Evaluation and treatment of the newborn with epidermolysis bullosa. Semin Perinatol. 2013;37(1):32–9.
3. Le Touze A, Viau D, Martin L, Depont R, Robert M. Recessive dystrophic epidermolysis bullosa: management of hand deformities. Eur J Pediatr Surg. 1993;3:352–5.
4. Von Hebra F. Pemphigus: Arzlicher Bericht des K.K. Allgemeinen Krankenhauses zu Wein vom Jahre 1870. Vienna, 1870;362–4.
5. Fox T. Notes on unusual or rare forms of skin disease. IV. Congenital ulceration of the skin (two cases) with pemphigus eruption and arrest of development generally. Lancet. 1879;I:766.
6. Fine JD, Eady RA, Bauer EA, Bauer JW, Bruckner-Tuderman L, Heagerty A, et al. The classification of inherited epidermolysis bullosa (EB): Report of the Third International Consensus Meeting on Diagnosis and Classification of EB. J Am Acad Dermatol. 2008;58:931.
7. Cooper TW, Bauer EA. Epidermolysis bullosa: a review. Pediatr Dermatol. 1984;1:181–8.
8. Nischler E, Lausegger A, Huttner C, et al. Diagnostic pitfalls in newborns and babies with blisters and erosions. Dermatol Res Pract. 2009;2009:320–403.
9. Fine J, Johnson L, Weiner M, Stein A, Cash S. Pseudosyndactyly and musculoskeletal contractures in inherited epidermolysis bullosa: experience of the national epidermolysis bullosa registry, 1986-2002. J Hand Surg Br. 2005;30(1):14–22.

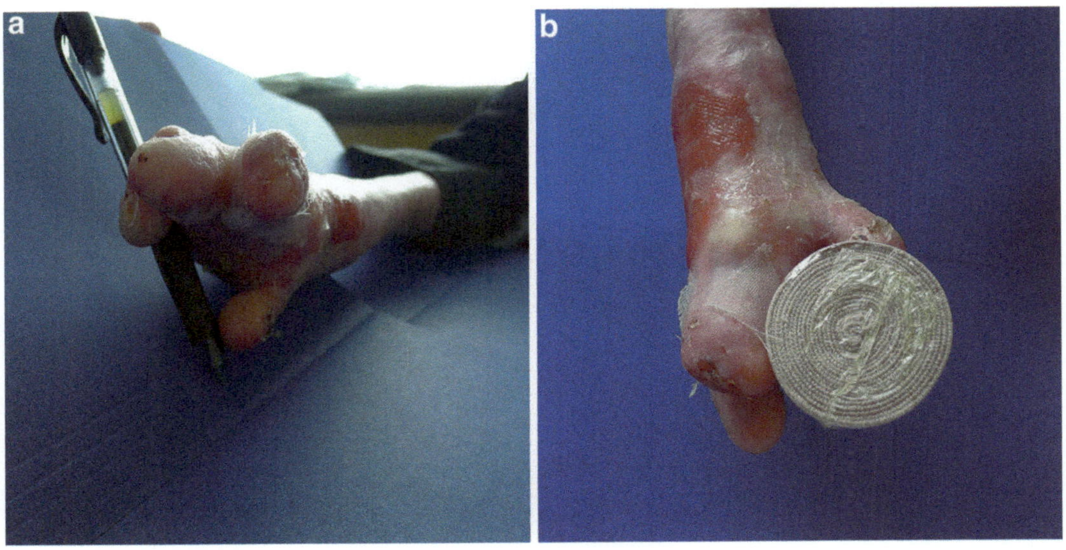

Fig. 25.18 (**a**, **b**) Four-month follow-up of patient in Fig. 25.15 demonstrating ability to grasp objects

10. Cuono C, Finseth F. Epidermolysis bullosa: current concepts and management of the advanced hand deformity. Plast Reconstr Surg. 1978;62:280–5.
11. Ladd AL, Kibele A, Gibbons S. Surgical treatment and postoperative splinting of recessive dystrophic epidermolysis bullosa. J Hand Surg Am. 1996;21A:888–97.
12. Greider J, Flatt AE. Care of the hand in recessive epidermolysis bullosa. Plast Reconstr Surg. 1983;72(2):222–8.
13. Greider JL, Flatt AE. Surgical restoration of the hand in epidermolysis bullosa. Arch Dermatol. 1988;124:765–7.
14. Terrill PJ, Mayou BJ, Pemberton J. Experience in the surgical management of the hand in dystrophic epidermolysis bullosa. Br J Plast Surg. 1992;45:435–42.
15. Zarem HA, Pearson RW, Leaf N. Surgical management of hand deformities in recessive dystrophic epidermolysis bullosa. Br J Plast Surg. 1974;27:176–81.
16. Horner RL, Wiedel JD, Bralliar F. Involvement of the hand in epidermolysis bullosa. J Bone Joint Surg. 1971;53A:1347–56.
17. Mullett F. A review of the management of the hand in dystrophic epidermolysis bullosa. J Hand Ther. 1998;11:261–5.
18. Goldschneider K, Lucky A, Mellerio J, Palisson F, Carmen Vinuela M, Azizkhan RG. Perioperative care of patients with epidermolysis bullosa: proceedings of the 5th international symposium on epidermolysis bullosa, Santiago, Chile, December 4–6, 2008. Paediatr Anaesth. 2010;20:797–804.

General Skeletal Disorders

26

Jennifer W. Lisle, Alex C. Lesiak, and Lauren E. Fonseca

Osteogenesis Imperfecta Background

Descriptions of osteogenesis imperfecta (OI) date back to Egypt from 1000 BC, when a mummy was characterized as having a wormian skull bone, amber-colored teeth, and bowed legs [1]. Olaus Jakob Ekman provided the first scientific description of OI in 1788; however, the first use of the phrase "osteogenesis imperfecta" to describe the condition was by Willem Vrolik in 1849 [1, 2]. Since then, numerous other names have been used to describe OI: mollities ossium, fragilitas ossium, osteopsathyrosis idiopathica, osteoporosis fetalis, osteomalacia congenital, Lobstein's disease, Vrolik's disease, Eddome syndrome, and van der Hoeve syndrome [1, 3].

Genetics

OI is characterized as a heterogeneous group of inherited disorders caused by mutations in genes that code for type I procollagen (COL1A1 and COL1A2) [1]. These genes are found on chromosomes 7 and 17, respectively [4], and 286 mutations of type I collagen have already been described [3]. The mutations of type I procollagen account for approximately 90 % of all cases of OI [2] with the majority of these cases inherited in an autosomal dominant fashion or caused by a sporadic mutation [4]. More recently, research has identified eight other genes associated with a portion of the remaining 10 % of OI cases. These are autosomal recessive in inheritance and all but two affect type I collagen by encoding proteins involved in the biosynthesis of type I procollagen. Cartilage-associated protein (CRTAP), LEPRE, PPIB, SERPINH1, and FKBP10 indirectly alter type I collagen synthesis, while SP7, and SERPINF1 do not [2].

Classification/Characterization

Multiple classification systems have been devised to characterize the varying degrees of phenotypic penetrance displayed by OI. Initially categorized by Looser in 1906 as whether fractures were present at birth (congenital) or after birth (tarda), Seedorff expanded on this in 1949 to include fractures within the first year of life (tarda gravis) or after the first year of life (tarda levis) [3]. In 1985, Frederic Shapiro further divided the congenital and tarda into type A and B depending on the timing of initial fracture and the radiographic appearance of the bones at initial fracture. Congenita A is classified as in utero/at birth with crumpled femurs and ribs and congenita B has normal bone contour. Tarda A is classified as fractures before walking age and tarda B is fractures after walking age [3]. The classification system of Sillence, from 1979, is still the most widely used system and was initially broken up into four types. Type I is the mildest form, is autosomal dominant and is broken up into type A (without dentinogenesis imperfecta) and type B (with dentinogenesis imperfecta). Patients will have blue sclera and a normal life expectancy. Type II is inherited in an autosomal recessive pattern and is lethal (primarily from respiratory failure, intracranial hemorrhage, or brainstem compression). Type III is a severe, autosomal dominant or recessive inheritance, and typically presents with normal sclerae and fractures around birth that can result in progressive deformity.

J.W. Lisle, M.D. (✉)
Department of Orthopedics and Rehabilitation, University of Vermont/Fletcher Allen Health Care,
192 Tilley Drive, South Burlington, VT 05445, USA
e-mail: Jennifer.lisle@med.uvm.edu

A.C. Lesiak, M.S., M.D.
Department of Orthopaedics and Rehabilitation, Fletcher Allen Health Care, University of Vermont College of Medicine,
Robert T. Stafford Hall, 4th Floor, 95 Carrigan Drive, Burlington, VT 05405-0084, USA
e-mail: alex.lesiak@vtmednet.org

L.E. Fonseca, B.A.
Department of Medicine, Fletcher Allen Health Care,
111 Colchester Avenue, Burlington, VT 05401, USA
e-mail: Lauren.Fonseca@vtmednet.org

D.R. Laub Jr. (ed.), *Congenital Anomalies of the Upper Extremity: Etiology and Management*,
DOI 10.1007/978-1-4899-7504-1_26,

Type IV is of intermediate severity, has an autosomal dominant inheritance, and has significant phenotypic variation [1, 3]. The initial Sillence classification system has since been expanded to include patients who do not have a collagen mutation. Type V is autosomal dominant, has hypertrophic callus development after fracture, and can have calcification of the interosseous membranes that can limit pronation and supination and lead to radial head dislocation. Type VI is autosomal recessive, has moderate to severe skeletal deformity and fractures and does not respond as well to bisphosphonate therapy. Type VII is autosomal recessive and has moderate to severe skeletal deformity that includes coax vara and rhizomelic limb shortening [3, 5].

Management

Operative and non-operative/medical management of OI is for symptomatic treatment only and is not curative and includes a multidisciplinary team effort to improve function, minimize disability, and maximize mobility status and quality of life [1]. Various different systemic medical therapy strategies have been attempted and include calcitonin, sodium fluoride, calcium anabolic steroids, growth hormone, magnesium oxide, vitamin C, and vitamin D, all of which have had mixed results [1]. Bisphosphonates are the only medical management option for OI that has been shown to have a beneficial effect and is now considered the standard of care [4, 5]. The nitrogen-containing bisphosphonates inhibits protein prenylation and guanosine triphosphatase formation, which results in osteoclast apoptosis [3], and this ultimately results in increased cortical thickness and bone mineral density [4]. In addition to this, decreased chronic bone pain, improved ambulation scores, decreased fracture rates, increased vertebral height, and improved grip strength (with pamidronate therapy) have also been seen in the initial 6 weeks after bisphosphonate therapy [3, 4]. Cyclical intravenous pamidronate and zoledronic acid are the bisphosphonates most frequently used in patients with OI and is limited to a few years due to the unknown long-term effects of bisphosphonates [3–5]. Osteonecrosis of the jaw is associated with bisphosphonate therapy, however, no reports of OI patients have been identified and the risk of this in OI patients is currently unknown [3].

Bone marrow transplantation is another treatment option that has so far not proven to be beneficial and requires more research to determine its true efficacy. Gene therapy and stem cell therapy are other areas of research that could be beneficial for OI patients but have yet been thoroughly investigated [3, 5].

Surgical principles and goals are designed to restore the normal bone axis by correcting deformity, minimize the incidence of fracture, avoid bone bowing, and use gentle technique to preserve muscle and minimize soft tissue injury [1, 3, 4]. Plates and screws are rarely indicated for fractures in OI patients, and the standard is use of an intramedullary device. Osteotomies are also used in conjunction with internal fixation to correct significant deformity. Multiple different rod systems have been proposed for use including double Rush rods, Bailey–Dubow and Sheffield rods, and Fassier–Duval telescoping nail with the overlying theme of selecting the largest diameter rod that will pass through the medullary canal at its narrowest point [3, 4]. The Fassier–Duval nail allows a minimally invasive technique to be used, can be used on multiple long bones during the same surgical setting, and thus far has had a lower revision rate [4].

Humeral intramedullary rods with either Rush rods or Fassier–Duval nails require the device to not impinge in the shoulder, and the patient to have full range of motion at the end of the procedure. Forearm deformity can be corrected with ulnar intramedullary wires and radial osteotomy and intramedullary fixation with the latter being much more technically challenging [4].

Marfan Syndrome

Background

Antoine Marfan, a French pediatrician, first described the skeletal characteristics of Marfan syndrome in 1896 in a 5-year-old girl who presented a tall stature and slender digits; however, this was more likely a presentation of congenital contractural arachnodactyly [6]. Marfan further characterized features of Marfan syndrome including ectopia lentis and mitral valve disease. Ultimately, it was Victor McKusick who stated that Marfan syndrome was a connective tissue disorder that encompassed abnormalities of the cardiovascular (including aortic dissections and aortic valve pathology), ocular, and skeletal systems [6].

Genetics

Harry Dietz discovered the genetic cause of Marfan syndrome in 1991 when he reported that a mutation in genes that code for fibrillin-1, an extracellular matrix protein, leads to classic Marfan syndrome, which is characterized as a clinically and phenotypically variable inherited disorder [6, 7]. Approximately 25 % of cases are thought to be from de novo mutations, primarily in genes for fibrillin-1, and the remaining cases are inherited in an autosomal dominant fashion [6]. FBN-1 gene, found on chromosome 15q21.1, is the only gene known to cause classic Marfan syndrome when mutated and is present in over 90 % of Marfan syndrome patients [6, 7].

Fibrillin-1 also interacts with transforming growth factor (TGF)-β, a cytokine that influences cell proliferation, differentiation, extracellular matrix formation, cell-cycle arrest, and apoptosis. Mutations in fibrillin-1 can lead to abnormal signaling pathways via this interaction. Mutations in TGFβR1, on chromosome 9, and TGFβR2, on chromosome 3, also alter the TGF-β signaling pathway. Mutations in TGFβR2 have been identified in patients diagnosed with Marfan syndrome (termed Marfan syndrome type II), yet these patients did not have characteristic findings of Marfan syndrome. Loeys–Dietz syndrome, which has many features similar to and unique from Marfan syndrome, is characterized by mutations in either TGFβR1 or TGFβR2 [6, 7]. Dietz states that patients with mutations in TGFβR1 and TGFβR2 tend to have a more aggressive vascular disease and risk of vessel rupture than patients with classic Marfan syndrome, and due to this Loeys–Dietz syndrome, rather than Marfan syndrome type II, in order to further individualize care, counseling, and management [7].

Multiple related disorders are also caused by mutations in the FBN-1 gene and TGF-β signaling pathway including mitral valve prolapse syndrome, MASS phenotype (Mitral valve prolapse, Aortic enlargement, Skin, and Skeletal features), Familial ectopia lentis, Shprintzen–Goldberg syndrome, Weill–Marchesani syndrome, Stiff skin syndrome (TB4 of FBN-1), geleophysic dysplasia (ADAMTSL2), acromicric dysplasia (TB5 of FBN-1), Loeys–Dietz syndrome (TGFβR1 and 2), Loeys–Dietz like syndrome (SMAD3), Myhre syndrome (SMAD4), and isolated skeletal or cardiovascular features of Marfan syndrome [6–8].

Classification/Diagnosis

The typical description of a patient with Marfan syndrome to make a clinician suspicious is a patient who is thin, tall, has long slender limbs (dolichostenomelia), arachnodactyly (long, thin, hyperextensible fingers), a pectus deformity, and scoliosis [6, 9]. The Ghent nosology, a revision from the Berlin criteria, is a stricter set of diagnostic criteria including family history, personal medical history, physical exam, slit lamp evaluation, and echocardiography, used to assist in the diagnosis and treatment of Marfan syndrome [6–8]. The nosology assesses seven systems (skeletal, ocular, cardiovascular, pulmonary, skin and integument, dura, and family history) and has major (uncommon in other diseases) and minor criteria. To consider the skeletal system involved, a patient must have at least two major criteria or one major criterion and two minor criteria. Major criteria include pectus carinatum, pectus excavatum requiring surgery, scoliosis >20° or spondylolisthesis, medial displacement of the medial malleolus causing pes planus, protrusio acetabuli, reduced upper-to-lower segment ratio or arm span-to-height ratio >1.05, positive wrist and thumb signs, and reduced extension at the elbows (<170°). A minor criterion is joint hypermobility/laxity, which can lead to contractures, particularly of the fingers and elbows [6]. While it has been shown that patients with Marfan syndrome have a decreased bone mineral density, there is no difference in their risk for fracture [6].

The wrist and thumb signs are used to evaluate arachnodactyly. The wrist sign/test (aka Walker–Murdoch) is positive when the patient wraps their fingers around their contralateral wrist and their thumb overlaps the distal phalanx of their small finger. The thumb sign/test is positive when the patient grips their thumb in their palm and the entire nail of the thumb projects beyond the ulnar border of the hand [6–9].

Management

Treatment options for patients with Marfan syndrome require a multidisciplinary team effort including geneticist, cardiologist and cardiothoracic surgeons, ophthalmologist, and an orthopedist [7]. The upper extremity manifestations usually require no treatment unless contractures become symptomatic after which time, conservative management may be initiated [10]. This includes physical therapy and bracing for elbow and finger contractures. The hyperlaxity seen in Marfan patients typically requires no treatment; however, it may predispose them to easier dislocation. In certain circumstances, capsular reconstruction has been required to reduce pain and restore function [11]. Ultimately, it is the responsibility of all providers to ensure that appropriate referrals have been made to the aforementioned specialists if there is any clinical suspicion for Marfan syndrome.

Achondroplasia

Background

Disproportionate short stature, macrocephaly, depressed nasal bridge, foramen magnum stenosis, thoracolumbar kyphosis, spinal stenosis, prominent buttocks, protuberant abdomen, genu varum, possible radial head dislocation, and trident hands characterize achondroplasia. Jules Parrot first used the term achondroplasia, which means "without cartilage formation," in 1878 to help distinguish patients with achondroplasia (disproportionate short stature) from patients with rickets (proportionate short stature), although it was the art from Egypt, Greece, and Rome that first depicted examples of achondroplastic patients [12–14].

Genetics

Achondroplasia is inherited in an autosomal dominant fashion and is part of a spectrum of disorders caused by different mutations in the genes encoding fibroblast growth factor receptor 3 (FGFR3). This gene is found on chromosome 4p16.3 and this receptor is expressed in articular chondrocytes [15]. Other disorders caused by FGFR3 mutations include hypochondroplasia, severe achondroplasia with developmental delay and acanthosis nigricans, and two types of thanatophoric dysplasia [13]. Approximately 80 % of cases are due to sporadic mutations and increased paternal age has been associated with an increased risk of new mutation [14, 15].

Classification/Characterization

Most features of achondroplasia can be traced back to the effect of increased FGFR3 signaling on endochondral bone growth [13]. These features are quite distinct, can present at different stages of life, and are typically recognized clinically or radiographically rather than via DNA analysis; however, approximately 20 % of patients go unrecognized at birth [12–14]. Third trimester prenatal ultrasound can identify short limbs in the 3rd percentile or less, head circumference greater than the 95th percentile, and a low nasal bridge [12, 14, 15]. At birth, short stature, rhizomelic limb shortening, and characteristic facial features (frontal bossing, midface hypoplasia) are evident. In addition, certain joints may be hypermobile, primarily the knees and hands, yet contractures of the elbows and hips can also be present [12–15]. In infancy, patients have normal mental development, although motor development is typically delayed secondary to muscular hypotonia. Apnea symptoms from foramen magnum stenosis and thoracolumbar kyphosis become more evident as the individual grows [12, 14, 15].

In the upper extremity, the rhizomelic shortening is the result of short humeri with the fingertips only able to reach the top of the greater trochanters and consequently, individuals may be unable to reach the top of their head [14, 15]. An elbow flexion contracture can also develop and is secondary to a flexion deformity of the distal humerus. Elbow deformities may also include radial head subluxation or dislocation [14]. The hands have equal length metacarpals and digits and have extra space between the third and fourth rays. This creates three groups of digits (thumb, index and long, and ring and small) and gives the hand a trident appearance [14, 15].

Management

A multidisciplinary team should be involved in the care of any patient with achondroplasia to improve function and positively affect their quality of life and should include but not be limited to pediatricians, pediatric and adult orthopedic surgeons (including spine surgeons), otolaryngologists, endocrinologists, and dentists. Operative and non-operative/medical management of achondroplasia is used primarily for symptomatic or cosmetic reasons. Human growth hormone has been trialed for achondroplastic children. While there is some improvement in growth rate and height, long-term follow-up results show no real benefit and it is not currently recommended worldwide for treatment of achondroplasia [12–15]. Other medical therapies that are being investigated include the use of parathyroid hormone and C-type natriuretic peptide. These could activate signaling pathways that could counteract the excessive FGFR3 signals in physes [13–15]. Physical therapy has also been suggested to assist with flexion contractures, but in general, elbow contractures and radial head subluxation/dislocations do not require any intervention since there is no functional loss [12–14].

Elective surgical limb lengthening has been used to address the short status of achondroplasia patients who average between 112 and 145 cm in height, which corresponds to 6–7 standard deviations below the average of an unaffected adult [12–15]. This process is extremely time-consuming and is still controversial. While it may have significant social and emotional effects, there is little evidence to support any functional benefit. Most of the discussion surrounding surgical limb lengthening is in reference to lower extremity lengthening. This is partially due to the fact that upper extremity length discrepancies are less common and better tolerated than lower extremity discrepancies [16]. On the other hand, there have been reports of functional limitations from upper extremity length discrepancies and treated with humeral lengthening. More recently, humeral lengthening by distraction osteogenesis with a monolateral frame has shown improved functional results when compared to circular frames [16].

Table 26.1 provides a brief description, the genetics, natural history, and treatment possibilities of these various conditions.

Table 26.1 Dysplasias, syndromes, and certain genetic conditions and their associated upper extremity skeletal anomalies

	Achondroplasia	*Hypochondroplasia*	*Pseudoachondroplasia*
Description	Rhizomelic shortening secondary to short humeri, flexion contractures from flexion deformities of distal humerus, elbow abnormalities, and trident appearance of hand [extra space between third and fourth rays]. Short stature noticeable at birth, foramen magnum stenosis, thoracolumbar kyphosis, spinal stenosis, and genu varum [14, 17]	Defective conversion of cartilage to bone. Less severe form of achondroplasia—body changes milder and often overlooked. Normal trunk length, disproportionately short arms and legs, hands and feet are broad and short. Differentiated from achondroplasia by lack of facial dysmorphism, less severe short stature, less obvious skeletal disproportion, and milder radiologic findings [17, 20]	Moderate to severe disproportionate short stature, ligamentous laxity, and progressive degenerative joint disease. Short-limb dwarfism with epiphyseal and metaphyseal involvement. Moderate brachydactyly, joint hyperextensibility in hands, restricted extension at elbows, and overall joint pain. Osteoarthritis in early adulthood [21–23]
	Radiographic findings: Rhizomelia, mesomelia, acromelia of extremities; brachydactyly, metacarpal metaphyseal cupping, phalangeal metaphyseal widening in hands; prominent deltoid insertion area in arms; third metacarpal shortening [18, 19]	Radiographic findings: Same as achondroplasia, but milder [18]	Radiographic findings: Brachydactyly proximally rounded and shortened metacarpals with small or cone-shaped epiphyses in hands, short phalanges, irregular metaphyses, and irregular carpals. Elbows may appear enlarged [18, 21]
Genetics	Autosomal dominant, fully penetrant, but 80 % of cases are sporadic. Locus—4p16.3; Gene—FGFR3; Protein—FGFR3 [14, 24]	Autosomal dominant; Locus—4p16.3; Gene—FGFR3; Protein—FGFR3 [24]	Autosomal dominant; Locus—19p12-13.1; Gene—COMP; Protein—Cartilage Oligomeric Matrix Protein (COMP) [24]
Natural History	Short stature is present at birth. Motor development may be delayed. Average height for adult male—131 cm (52 in.). Average height for adult female—124 cm (49 in.) [14, 25]	Same as achondroplasia, but milder [17, 20]	Normal length and facies at birth. Often presents at the onset of walking with a waddling gait. By 2 years of age, growth rate below the standard growth curve which leads to disproportionate short-limb short stature. Average adult heights: 116 cm for females and 120 cm for males [21]
Treatment	Growth hormone therapy. Upper extremity limb lengthening has been documented with an average arm length gain of 10.2 ± 1.25 cm. Surgical realignment may be performed as well [14, 25]	Growth hormone therapy and limb lengthening if necessary [26]	Evaluate for skeletal manifestations. Anterior/posterior radiographs of hands. Assess ligamentous laxity. Analgesics for joint pain [21]
	Thanatophoric dwarfism/dysplasia type 1	*Thanatophoric dwarfism/dysplasia type 2*	*Marfan syndrome*
Description	Underdevelopment of the entire skeleton, short-curve long bones, metaphyseal flaring, underdeveloped pelvic bones, flat acetabular roof, flat and underdeveloped vertebral bodies, cloverleaf skull may or may not be present [27, 28]	In TD2, long bones not as short as in TD1, nor are they bent and/or bowed. Metaphyses are flared and cupped. Flat vertebral bodies—but not as flat as TD1, almost all fetuses have cloverleaf skull. Overall, less severe bone involvement than TDI [27, 28]	Characterized by tall stature, thin habitus, long and slender digits, ligamentous laxity, arachnodactyly, and camptodactyly. Reduced upper-to-lower segment ratio. Bones are typically osteopenic and fracture often [6, 19]
	Radiographic findings: Generalized micromelia, long bones of extremities are short and have telephone receiver-like appearance; skeletal maturation and ossification centers are not altered on radiograph [18, 28]	Radiographic findings: Generalized micromelia, long bones of extremities are short and have telephone receiver-like appearance; skeletal maturation and ossification centers are not altered on radiograph [18, 28]	
Genetics	Autosomal dominant; Locus—4p16.3; Gene—FGFR3; Protein—FGFR3 [24]		Autosomal dominant; Locus—15q21.1; Gene—FBN1; Protein—Fibrillin-1 [24]
Natural History	Most common type of lethal neonatal skeletal dysplasia; overall association with rhizomelic limb shortening, macrocephaly, and cloverleaf skull. Difficult to differentiate from other forms of short-limb dwarfism—most important difference is that TD has severe rib shortening, restricted lung volume, and respiratory distress leading to death within a few hours of birth. Most infants do not survive past a few hours or days due to respiratory insufficiency [27–29]		Children taller than average for age. By adulthood, may reach 7 ft tall [19]

(continued)

Table 26.1 (continued)

	Achondroplasia	*Hypochondroplasia*	*Pseudoachondroplasia*
Treatment	At birth, infant may require suboccipital decompression to alleviate craniocervical junction constriction. Joint contractures or joint hypermobility should be evaluated and followed [29]		Therapy with nighttime splinting in extension is often successful for treatment of camptodactyly. More severe cases may require tendon transfer, release of volar structures and PIPJ. Surgery outcomes are unpredictable [30]
	Osteogenesis imperfecta	*Nail–Patella syndrome*	*Diastrophic dysplasia*
Description	Characterized by fragile bones, low bone mass, blue sclerae, dentinogenesis imperfecta, hearing loss, and scoliosis. Frequent fractures produce limb deformities. Bowing may occur without prior fracture. Non-accidental injury must be considered in differential diagnosis [3, 5, 31]	Abnormal development of tissue derived from mesenchyme. Nail dysplasia or absence and radial head dislocation may be seen in the upper extremity. Decreased muscle mass in proximal upper extremity [19, 32]	Endochondral ossification affected causing short stature from shortened limbs, progressive spinal deformities, foot deformities, frequent joint subluxation and dislocation, large joint contractures, ear pinnae deformities, and/or cleft palate. Hitchhiker thumb, shortened fingers, synostosis of the proximal interphalangeal joints, and ulnar deviation of fingers. Radial dislocation may also be seen clinically [33–35]
	Radiographic findings: Osteopenia, bone fractures, and bone deformities [31]	Radiographic findings: Radial head and capitellum hypoplasia, elbow dislocation [18]	Radiographic findings: Micromelia; short, thick tubular bones; epiphyseal dysplasia; metaphyseal flaring of long bones; bifid or V-shaped distal humerus, may also be pointed and hypoplastic; radial bowing; proximal radial dislocation at birth; brachydactyly and short ovoid first metacarpal; irregular carpal bones; joint dislocations [18, 33]
Genetics	*OI Types I–IV*: Autosomal dominant; Gene—COL1A1 or COL1A+G42; Protein—type 1 collagen	Autosomal dominant; Locus—9q34.1; Gene—LMX1B; Protein—LIM homeobox transcription factor 1 [24]	Autosomal recessive; Locus—5q32-33; Gene—DTDST; Protein—SLC26A2 sulfate transporter [24]
	OI Type V: Autosomal dominant; Gene—unknown		
	OI Type VI: Autosomal recessive; Gene—unknown		
	OI Type VII: Autosomal recessive; Protein—Cartilage-associated protein [CRTAP] [24]		
Natural History	More severe forms of OI may experience bone fragility and fracture in utero and/or at birth. Milder forms may remain nearly absent in adulthood. Overall, fracture incidence decreases after puberty and increases after menopause and males in their 60s [1]	Non-progressive nail dystrophy and elbow deformities. Patellae may be absent or hypoplastic [19, 32]	Diagnosis can be made through ultrasound and molecular genetic testing prenatally or clinically at birth. Normal mental status. Growth and motor capabilities greatly affected by deformities. Disproportionate dwarfism with a mean height of 130–140 cm can be seen in affected adults [36]
Treatment	Bisphosphonates may be used to decrease fracture frequency, improve vertebral bone density, and strengthen grip. Surgical goal is to minimize fracture frequency, restore bone axis, and avoid bowing. Long bone internal fixation in children is common via multilevel osteotomies and telescopic intramedullary nail fixation. Long-term rod revision surgery may be required [3, 4]	Patient may be followed and regularly assessed. Surgery is sometimes necessary [19, 32]	Focus on improving mobility through casting to maintain joint positioning, physiotherapy, and other forms of therapy. Cervical spinal surgery only indicated with clinical or neurophysiological evidence of spinal cord impingement—otherwise, cervical kyphosis typically spontaneously corrects. In cases of premature degenerative arthrosis, arthroplasty is indicated. Early physical therapy may prevent joint contractures [33, 35]

(continued)

Table 26.1 (continued)

	Kniest's dysplasia	*Cleidocranial dysostosis/dysplasia*	*Niemann-Pick disease*
Description	Damage to articular and epiphyseal cartilage leading to disproportionate dwarfism. Children present with enlarged elbow and wrist joints with restricted movement, abnormal hands with long, knobby fingers. Round faces and barrel-shaped kyphotic trunk [19, 37]	Abnormal development of membranous bones such as the clavicle. Characterized by drooping shoulders, elongated neck, and shoulder adduction anteriorly. Central clavicle may be absent and a small piece of bone articulating with the acromion [26, 38]	Lipid storage disease. Previously not known to have skeletal involvement. Joint and/or limb pain has been reported as well as decreased bone mineral density [BMD] in both affected pediatric and adult patients [39]
	Radiographic findings: Generalized ossification delay; epiphyses becoming hypoplastic/dysplastic; cloudy effect in physeal plate in late childhood; metaphyseal flare and epiphyseal fragmentation; reduced joint space in small joints of hand [18, 37]	Radiographic findings: Multiple pseudoepiphyses of metacarpals and tapered distal phalanges in hands [18]	
Genetics	Autosomal dominant; Locus—12q13.1; Gene—COL2A1; Protein—type 2 collagen [24]	Autosomal dominant; Locus—6p21; Gene—RUNX2; Protein—Run related transcription factor 2 [24]	Autosomal recessive; Gene—SMPD1; Locus—p11; Protein—Acid sphingomyelinase [24, 26]
Natural History	Bone formation in fetus and infant most affected. Slow growth. Normal milestones and intelligence [19, 37]	Mean adult height for males is 162 cm [26]	Patients with neurological involvement do not survive beyond 3 years Patients without neurodegeneration usually survive into late childhood or adulthood [39]
Treatment	UE management not well documented	Orthopedic intervention may be necessary if severe impairment or disability occurs [38]	No definitive treatment. Early intervention for low BMD such as load-bearing activities and muscle strengthening exercises. Frequent pulmonary disease and chronic fatigue must be considered [39]
	Mucopolysaccharidoses		
Description	Defective endochondral and membranous growth. Presents with dysostosis multiplex—short stature, platyspondyly with anterior beaking, 'bullet-shaped' phalanges. Joint contractures and carpal tunnel syndrome are common. Osteopenia may occur in association with pathologic fractures		
	MPS I H—Hurler syndrome: Carpal tunnel syndrome, joint contractures, and dysostosis multiplex		
	MPS I S—Scheie syndrome: Carpal tunnel syndrome, joint contractures, and dysostosis multiplex		
	MPS II—Hunter syndrome: only X-linked MPS disorder, Carpal tunnel syndrome, joint contractures, and dysostosis multiplex		
	MPS IIIA-B—Sanfilippo Types A-B: Less severe than I, II, VI, and VII		
	MPS IVA—Morquio Type A: severe skeletal dysplasia, joint hypermobility, and dysplastic odontoid process		
	MPS IVB—Morquio Type B: severe skeletal dysplasia, joint hypermobility, and dysplastic odontoid process		
	MPS VI—Maroteaux–Lamy syndrome: Carpal tunnel syndrome, joint contractures, and dysostosis multiplex		
	MPS VII—Sly syndrome: Joint contractures and dysostosis multiplex [40–42]		
	Radiographic findings: Coarsened long bones, shortened ulna, Madelung deformity of distal radius, shortened metacarpals with proximal tapering, and broad clavicles [42]		
Genetics	Autosomal recessive; Gene—varies by type of MPS [42]		
Natural History	Affected infants may appear healthy at birth. MPS presents later—timeline varies by form. Often children have short stature and some have progressive mental deterioration [19, 42]		
Treatment	Carpal tunnel release and deformity correction. Bisphosphonates may be used to help increase bone density. Palliative and supportive care such as physical and occupational therapy when indicated [40–42]		
	Hereditary multiple exostoses/multiple osteocartilaginous exostoses/diaphyseal aclasia	*Fibrodysplasia ossificans progressiva*	*Chondroectodermal dysplasia/Ellis–van Creveld syndrome*
Description	Multiple cartilage-capped boney protuberances, or osteochondromas, at metaphyses of long bones. Mild short stature and disproportionate short-limbs. Rarely, an enchondroma may undergo a malignant transformation into secondary chondrosarcoma. UE most commonly presents with length discrepancy between the radius and ulna—radial bowing, radial tilting, and radial head dislocation may occur [43]	Fibrous tissues, muscles, and periosteal regions undergo progressive ossification. Shortened and deformed thumbs [19]	Short stature, irregular bone growth ad structure. Polydactyly also occurs [19]

(continued)

Table 26.1 (continued)

	Achondroplasia	*Hypochondroplasia*	*Pseudoachondroplasia*
Genetics	*HME-1*: Autosomal dominant, Locus—8q23-24.1; Gene—EXT1; Protein—Exostosin-1 *HME-2*: Autosomal dominant, Locus—11p12-11; Gene—EXT2; Protein—Exostosin-2 *HME-3*: Autosomal dominant, Locus—19p [24]	Autosomal dominant; Locus—4q27-31, 17q21-22, or 2q23-24 [19]	Autosomal recessive; Locus—4p16 [19]
Natural History	Numerous osteochondromas develop near growth plates. During childhood and adolescence, osteochondromas create a pseudo-growth plate and cause deformity with growth [44]	At age five, patient starts developing large ectopic osseous collections in muscular regions. These osseous collections cause severe disability and limits joint movement [19]	
Treatment	Growth deformity correction and removal of symptomatic osteochondromas. To manage impending or complete radial head dislocation: Ulnar collateral carpal ligament release at the wrist and radial head resection at skeletal maturity. Ulnar wrist deviations are usually asymptomatic. If not, acute and guided-growth interventions may be successful. Malignant transformation into chondrosarcoma must be resected. Typically low grade [43]	No known effective treatment. Surgery, corticosteroids, and radiotherapy have been used. Bisphosphonates have been used to decrease ectopic osseous masses but clinical benefits are not well established [45]	Surgical excision of polydactyly [30]
	Ehlers Danlos syndrome (EDS)	*Spondyloepiphyseal DYSPLASIA*	*Multiple epiphyseal dysplasia*
Description	Connective tissue disorder characterized by congenital joint hypermobility, skin hyperextensibility, and tissue fragility. Joint dislocations due to little to no trauma are common as is chronic limb pain. Severity varies with type of EDS [46, 47]	Short stature due to growth disorder of spine and epiphyses. Short trunk [48]	Abnormal endochondral epiphyseal ossification centers lead to short stature. Early degenerative arthritis and chondral lesions may present. Progression of the disease may atrophy muscles causing muscle fatigue and pain [49–51] Radiographic findings: Small, irregular, flattened epiphyses; small, irregular carpals; proximal metacarpal rounding; Brachydactyly [18, 52]
Genetics	Autosomal recessive; Locus—15q14; Gene—CHST14; Protein—carbohydrate sulfotransferase 14, dermatan 4-sulfotransferase [24]	Autosomal dominant; Locus—12q13.1; Gene—COL2A1; Protein—type 2 collagen [24]	Autosomal dominant; mutations in five different genes have been identified: COMP, COL9A1, COL9A2, COL9A3, and MATN3. 80 % COMP mutation, 10-20 % cannot be identified [49]
Natural History	May present in the first few years of life. Joint hypermobility progression [53]	Typically normal in size and proportion at birth. Osteoarthritis with progressive joint and back pain. Normal motor and cognitive milestones [54]	May present in early childhood with knee pain and delayed ossification of femoral epiphyses [49]
Treatment	Orthopedic intervention may be necessary with symptomatic events	Joint replacement and pain management [54]	Early Childhood intervention to minimize and/or counteract joint deformity and preserve mobility [49]

(continued)

Table 26.1 (continued)

	Metaphyseal chondrodysplasia (metaphyseal dysplasia)	*Chondrodysplasia punctata*	*Enchondroma*
Description	Short stature; metaphyseal irregularity, normal epiphyses, normal vertebrae [55]	Neonatal epiphyseal stippling and decreased growth	Usually a solitary, benign lesion. Multiple enchondromas have increased rate of recurrence. Approximately 40 % of enchondromas occur in the hand. Primary enchondromas of the hand typically present as pathological fracture, deformity with or without pain, and swelling. Long bone enchondromas are usually asymptomatic [56, 57]
	Radiographic findings: Irregularity of expanded metaphyses, wide separation of epiphyses from metaphyses. Hands have shortening with metacarpal and phalangeal cupping and coning [18]	Radiographic findings: Skeletal calcifications of the epiphyses and carpals	Radiographic findings: Stippled calcifications, endosteal scalloping, cortical thinning, and medullary expansion [58, 59]
Genetics	McKusick—Autosomal recessive	Most common form—X-linked dominant	
	Schmid, Jansen, Kozlowski—Autosomal dominant [26]		
Natural History	Defects may be absent or minimal at birth and develop within months or years [55]	Most affected patients die within the first year of life [26]	Malignant transformation to chondrosarcoma possible but rare—must be considered in the differential [56, 57]
Treatment	UE management not well documented	UE management not well documented	In absence of progressive changes, annual clinical and radiographic examination. Overall goal of surgeon is to prevent pathological fracture and remove tumor. Standardized treatment protocol for hand enchondroma is lacking. Treatment options include observation, curettage, and curettage with autogenous bone grafting or bone graft substitute. Various bone graft materials may be used to fill the bony defect post-curettage. Sassoon, et al. recommend use of an allograft or no graft to avoid donor graft site morbidity. Internal fixation may be necessary for cortical thinning and/or fracture stabilization [57, 58, 60]
	Ollier's disease/enchondromatosis	*Fibrous dysplasia*	*Camurati–Engelmann disease [progressive diaphyseal dysplasia]*
Description	Development of multiple benign enchondromas located in the epiphyses of bones. Commonly seen in the phalanges. Also skeletal deformities, limb length discrepancies, pain, and the potential risk for malignant changes [61–63]	Bone-forming tissue unable to produce mature lamellar bone resulting in benign fibro-osseous lesion or lesions. Pain, swelling, deformity, and/or pathological fractures are common clinical presentations [64–66]	Sclerosing bone dysplasia causing progressive thickening of the diaphyses, bone pain, muscle weakness and atrophy
	Radiographic findings: Broadened metaphyses, long bone bowing	Radiographic findings: Intramedullary lesion causing bone expansion limited by cortical rim. Cortical thinning without periosteal reaction [64, 66]	
Genetics	SP; PTHR1 and PTPN11 mutations found in a few cases only, role still unclear [24]	SP; Locus—20q13; Gene—GNAS1; Protein—guanine nucleotide-binding protein, alpha-stimulating activity subunit 1 [24]	Autosomal dominant; Locus—19q13; Gene—*TGFB1*; Protein—transforming growth factor-β1

(continued)

Table 26.1 (continued)

	Achondroplasia	*Hypochondroplasia*	*Pseudoachondroplasia*
Natural History	As child grows, enchondroma increases in size. Enchondroma subject to pathological fracture. Bony masses cause angular deformities and asymmetrical growth [61]	Usually presents in first three decades of life. Child may present with pain, limp, and/or pathologic fracture. Though rare, lesion may transform into either a benign or malignant tumor [64]	Most cases present in the first decade of life. Progression is slow and unpredictable. Normal life span
Treatment	Limb lengthening and deformity correction often with Ilizarov fixation. Observation for possible malignant transformation. Surgical excision if chondrosarcoma occurs [61, 62]	In absence of symptoms, regular radiographs and observation are indicated until satisfied that lesion is inactive. A growing child without symptoms should be seen twice yearly for clinical evaluation of range of motion, angular deformity, and limb length discrepancy. If symptomatic lesion, "conventional surgical procedures." In cases of deformity or mechanical deficit, orthopedic intervention may be necessary to remove lesion and graft defect. Internal fixation with intramedullary rods may be used. Bisphosphonate use has been reported to have successful outcomes [45, 65, 66]	NSAIDs for bone pain and physical therapy. UE management not well documented [26]
	Osteopoikilosis	*Osteopathia striata*	*Melorheostosis*
Description	Sclerosing bone dysplasia, usually asymptomatic, but can cause soft tissue fibrosis and joint contractures	Sclerosing bone dysplasia with linear striations in bone seen on radiograph. Typically asymptomatic	Sclerosing dysplasia with painless, soft-tissue contractures. Linear hyperostosis progresses slowly
	Radiographic findings: Well defined, bilateral osteosclerotic nodules located in metaphyses and epiphyses of long bones, carpus, and scapulae	Radiographic findings: Dense linear striations seen in tubular and flat bones	Radiographic findings: Asymmetrical bands of sclerosis, described as "molten wax flowing down the side of a candle." Location varies with age—endosteal in children, extracortical, subperiosteal in adults. Hyperostosis patches seen in carpals
Genetics	Autosomal dominant	Autosomal dominant	Non-hereditary
Natural History	Presents during childhood. Children reach normal stature		Presents by age 6 with joint contractures
Treatment	UE management for joint contractures and fibrosis if necessary [26]	Treatment unnecessary [26]	NSAIDs for pain. Lengthening, realigning, and contracture correction have been carried out successfully with the Ilizarov technique but with frequent complications [26]
	Pyknodysostosis	*Gorham disease/idiopathic osteolysis/disappearing bone disease*	*Dyschondrosteosis (Leri–Weill syndrome)*
Description	Failure of bone resorption leads to mild short stature and numerous skeletal deformities including pectus excavatum	Massive osteolysis originating from one bone may progressively involve adjacent bones. Resorbed bone is replaced by fibrous tissue	Mild mesomelic short stature. Forearm deformities, notably in the distal radius causing a Madelung deformity
		Radiographic findings: Intramedullary and subcortical radiolucent foci. Foci progressively merge	Radiographic findings: Madelung deformity, humeral head hypoplasia
Genetics	Autosomal recessive	Non-hereditary	Autosomal dominant; Gene—*SHOX*
Natural History		Often presents in second and third decades of life	Short stature, forearm and/or wrist deformity, pain typically develops by 8 years of age. Adult heights range from 135 to 170 cm
Treatment	Growth hormone therapy to increase stature [26]	Surgery with or without radiation therapy has shown some success, but not consistently [26]	Growth hormone has been successful in some. If wrist pain occurs, use splint and anti-inflammatories. If wrist continue to be symptomatic, reconstruction may be necessary via double osteotomy of the distal radius and ulnar recession [26]

(continued)

Table 26.1 (continued)

	Larsen syndrome	*Gaucher's disease*	*Craniocarpotarsal dysplasia/Freeman-Sheldon/"Whistling Face" syndrome/distal arthrogryposis Type II*
Description	Hypertelorism, multiple joint dislocations, focal bone deformities. Wide distal phalanx of thumb, no distal tapering of fingers, and hypotonia may be seen Radiographic findings: Accessory ossification centers in the carpals and shortened metacarpals	Lysosomal storage disorder that causes bone pain, osteomyelitis, osteopenia, pathologic fractures, and osteonecrosis. Bone crises are common	The hands have same deformity as distal arthrogryposis. Joint contractures, elbow flexion deformities, limited range of motion in shoulder
Genetics	Both an autosomal dominant form and an autosomal recessive form	Autosomal recessive; Locus—p1; Protein—glucocerebrosidase	Typically sporadic. Some evidence of autosomal dominant and autosomal recessive inheritance patterns
Natural History		Age of presentation varies by type. Mean age at diagnosis—25 years	Presents in the first decade of life. Dysphagia and aspiration may cause death in the affected infant. Normal intelligence
Treatment	UE management not well documented [26]	Opioid analgesics for severe pain. Supportive treatment of bone crisis bearing in mind increased bleeding risk and abnormal bone [26]	Treat contractures similarly to distal arthrogryposis. Physical and occupational therapy for the hands [26]
	Cornelia de Lange's syndrome	*Klippel–Trenaunay syndrome*	
Description	Syndrome caused by a genetic mutation affecting central nervous system development. Upper extremity involvement consists of a small hand, clinodactyly of the fifth digit, proximally placed thumb, and limited range of motion in the elbow. Radial head dislocation is common. Rarely, ulnar absence and a monodigital hand may occur. Characteristic facial features: corners of mouth are down-turned, synophrys, elongated philtrum, and long eyelashes	Three major features of this developmental disorder—varicose veins, cutaneous capillary-venous malformation, and soft tissue and bone hypertrophy in affected limbs. Overgrowth of bones in girth, length, and width in affected limb. Finger deformities and carpal tunnel syndrome have both been documented	
Genetics	Gene—*NIPBL*		
Natural History	Intrauterine growth impedance. Child remains small in size. Low rates of survival in the first year of life. Mental retardation with delayed milstones	Typically presents at birth or infancy	
Treatment	Most deformities are asymptomatic limiting the utilization of surgical intervention [26]	Regular compression has shown good results in the hypertrophied limb. Surgery may be utilized only in cases of severe debilitating deformities [26]	

References

1. Kocher MS, Shapiro F. Osteogenesis imperfecta. J Am Acad Orthop Surg. 1998;6(4):225–36. PubMed PMID: 9682085.
2. van Dijk FS, Cobben JM, Kariminejad A, Maugeri A, Nikkels PGJ, van Rijn RR, et al. Osteogenesis imperfecta: a review with clinical examples. Mol Syndromol. 2011;1:1–20.
3. Burnei G, Vlad C, Georgescu I, Gavriliu TS, Dan D. Osteogenesis imperfecta: diagnosis and treatment. J Am Acad Orthop Surg. 2008;16(6):356–66. PubMed PMID: 18524987.
4. Esposito P, Plotkin H. Surgical treatment of osteogenesis imperfecta: current concepts. Curr Opin Pediatr. 2008;20(1):52–7. PubMed PMID: 18197039.
5. Cheung MS, Glorieux FH. Osteogenesis imperfecta: update on presentation and management. Rev Endocr Metab Disord. 2008;9(2):153–60. PubMed PMID: 18404382.
6. Shirley ED, Sponseller PD. Marfan syndrome. J Am Acad Orthop Surg. 2009;17(9):572–81. PubMed PMID: 19726741.
7. Dietz HC. Marfan syndrome. In: Pagon RA, Adam MP, Bird TD, Dolan CR, Fong CT, Stephens K, editors. GeneReviews. Seattle, WA: University of Washington, Seattle; 1993.

8. Bolar N, Van Laer L, Loeys BL. Marfan syndrome: from gene to therapy. Curr Opin Pediatr. 2012;24(4):498–504. PubMed PMID: 22705998.
9. Watt AJ, Chung KC. Generalized skeletal abnormalities. Hand Clin. 2009;25(2):265–76. PubMed PMID: 19380065.
10. Marie-Josee Paris P, Marie Jose Benjamin O, Gayle Lang O, Reg Wilcox P. Standard of care: Marfan syndrome. 2009.
11. Gomes N, Hardy P, Bauer T. Arthroscopic treatment of chronic anterior instability of the shoulder in Marfan's syndrome. Arthroscopy. 2007;23(1):110 e1–5. PubMed PMID: 17210441.
12. Baujat G, Legeai-Mallet L, Finidori G, Cormier-Daire V, Le Merrer M. Achondroplasia. Best Pract Res Clin Rheumatol. 2008;22(1):3–18. PubMed PMID: 18328977.
13. Horton WA, Hall JG, Hecht JT. Achondroplasia Lancet. 2007;370(9582):162–72. PubMed PMID: 17630040.
14. Shirley ED, Ain MC. Achondroplasia: manifestations and treatment. J Am Acad Orthop Surg. 2009;17(4):231–41. PubMed PMID: 19307672.
15. Amirfeyz R, Gargan M. Achondroplasia. Curr Orthop. 2005;19(6):467–70.
16. Pawar AY, McCoy Jr TH, Fragomen AT, Rozbruch SR. Does humeral lengthening with a monolateral frame improve function? Clin Orthop Relat Res. 2013;471(1):277–83. PubMed PMID: 22926491. Pubmed Central PMCID: 3528891.
17. Hanson AA. Improving mobility in a client with hypochondroplasia (dwarfism): a case report. J Bodyw Mov Ther. 2010;14(2):172–8. PubMed PMID: 20226364.
18. Alanay Y, Lachman RS. A review of the principles of radiological assessment of skeletal dysplasias. J Clin Res Pediatr Endocrinol. 2011;3(4):163–78. PubMed PMID: 22155458. Pubmed Central PMCID: 3245489.
19. Mankin HJ, Jupiter J, Trahan CA. Hand and foot abnormalities associated with genetic diseases. Hand. 2011;6(1):18–26. PubMed PMID: 22379434. Pubmed Central PMCID: 3041879.
20. Song SH, Balce GC, Agashe MV, Lee H, Hong SJ, Park YE, et al. New proposed clinico-radiologic and molecular criteria in hypochondroplasia: FGFR 3 gene mutations are not the only cause of hypochondroplasia. Am J Med Genet A. 2012;158A(10):2456–62. PubMed PMID: 22903874.
21. Briggs MD, Wright MJ. Pseudoachondroplasia. In: Pagon RA, Adam MP, Bird TD, Dolan CR, Fong CT, Stephens K, editors. GeneReviews. Seattle, WA: University of Washington, Seattle; 1993.
22. Jackson GC, Mittaz-Crettol L, Taylor JA, Mortier GR, Spranger J, Zabel B, et al. Pseudoachondroplasia and multiple epiphyseal dysplasia: a 7-year comprehensive analysis of the known disease genes identify novel and recurrent mutations and provides an accurate assessment of their relative contribution. Hum Mutat. 2012;33(1):144–57. PubMed PMID: 21922596. Pubmed Central PMCID: 3272220.
23. Li QW, Song HR, Mahajan RH, Suh SW, Lee SH. Deformity correction with external fixator in pseudoachondroplasia. Clin Orthop Relat Res. 2007;454:174–9. PubMed PMID: 16957646.
24. Warman ML, Cormier-Daire V, Hall C, Krakow D, Lachman R, LeMerrer M, et al. Nosology and classification of genetic skeletal disorders: 2010 revision. Am J Med Genet A. 2011;155A(5):943–68. PubMed PMID: 21438135. Pubmed Central PMCID: 3166781.
25. Carter EM, Davis JG, Raggio CL. Advances in understanding etiology of achondroplasia and review of management. Curr Opin Pediatr. 2007;19(1):32–7. PubMed PMID: 17224659.
26. Lovell WW, Winter RB, Morrissy RT, Weinstein SLV. Lovell and Winter's pediatric orthopaedics. 4th ed. Philadelphia, PA: Lippincott-Raven; 1996.
27. Martinez-Frias ML, Egues X, Puras A, Hualde J, de Frutos CA, Bermejo E, et al. Thanatophoric dysplasia type II with encephalocele and semilobar holoprosencephaly: insights into its pathogenesis. Am J Med Genet A. 2011;155A(1):197–202. PubMed PMID: 21204232.
28. Miller E, Blaser S, Shannon P, Widjaja E. Brain and bone abnormalities of thanatophoric dwarfism. AJR Am J Roentgenol. 2009;192(1):48–51. PubMed PMID: 19098178.
29. Karczeski B, Cutting GR. Thanatophoric dysplasia. In: Pagon RA, Adam MP, Bird TD, Dolan CR, Fong CT, Stephens K, editors. GeneReviews. Seattle, WA: University of Washington, Seattle; 1993.
30. Watson S. The principles of management of congenital anomalies of the upper limb. Arch Dis Child. 2000;83(1):10–7. PubMed PMID: 10868991. Pubmed Central PMCID: 1718383.
31. Renaud A, Aucourt J, Weill J, Bigot J, Dieux A, Devisme L, et al. Radiographic features of osteogenesis imperfecta. Insights Imaging. 2013;4(4):417–29. PubMed PMID: 23686748. Pubmed Central PMCID: 3731461.
32. Heckman DS, McCoy AJ, Spritzer CE, Garrett WE. Intercondylar synovial septum in two patients with nail-patella syndrome. J Knee Surg. 2013;26 Suppl 1:S107–11. PubMed PMID: 23288746.
33. Bonafe L, Mittaz-Crettol L, Ballhausen D, Superti-Furga A. Diastrophic Dysplasia. In: Pagon RA, Adam MP, Bird TD, Dolan CR, Fong CT, Stephens K, editors. GeneReviews. Seattle, WA: University of Washington, Seattle; 1993.
34. Crockett MM, Carten MF, Hurko O, Sponseller PD. Motor milestones in children with diastrophic dysplasia. J Pediatr Orthop. 2000;20(4):437–41. PubMed PMID: 10912597.
35. Honorio JC, Bruns RF, Grundtner LF, Raskin S, Ferrari LP, Araujo Junior E, et al. Diastrophic dysplasia: prenatal diagnosis and review of the literature. Sao Paulo Med J. 2013;131(2):127–32.
36. Kruger L, Pohjolainen T, Kaitila I, Kautiainen H, Arkela-Kautiainen M, Hurri H. Health-related quality of life and socioeconomic situation among diastrophic dysplasia patients in Finland. J Rehabil Med. 2013;45(3):308–13. PubMed PMID: 23389768.
37. Subramanian S, Gamanagatti S, Sinha A, Sampangi R. Kniest syndrome. Indian Pediatr. 2007;44(12):931–3. PubMed PMID: 18175850.
38. Campos Junior W, Cardoso RM, Fidelis R, Silva ES, Ramos R. A familial case of cleidocranial dysostosis presenting upper limb ischemia. Sao Paulo Med J. 2005;123(6):292–4.
39. Wasserstein M, Godbold J, McGovern MM. Skeletal manifestations in pediatric and adult patients with Niemann Pick disease type B. J Inherit Metab Dis. 2013;36(1):123–7. PubMed PMID: 22718274.
40. Pastores GM. Musculoskeletal complications encountered in the lysosomal storage disorders. Best Pract Res Clin Rheumatol. 2008;22(5):937–47. PubMed PMID: 19028373.
41. White KK. Orthopaedic aspects of mucopolysaccharidoses. Rheumatology. 2011;50 Suppl 5:v26–33. PubMed PMID: 22210667.
42. White KK, Sousa T. Mucopolysaccharide disorders in orthopaedic surgery. J Am Acad Orthop Surg. 2013;21(1):12–22. PubMed PMID: 23281467.
43. Jones KB. Glycobiology and the growth plate: current concepts in multiple hereditary exostoses. J Pediatr Orthop. 2011;31(5):577–86. PubMed PMID: 21654469. Pubmed Central PMCID: 3111916.
44. Jager M, Westhoff B, Portier S, Leube B, Hardt K, Royer-Pokora B, et al. Clinical outcome and genotype in patients with hereditary multiple exostoses. J Orthop Res. 2007;25(12):1541–51. PubMed PMID: 17676624.
45. Hickey J, Lemons D, Waber P, Seikaly MG. Bisphosphonate use in children with bone disease. J Am Acad Orthop Surg. 2006;14(12):638–44. PubMed PMID: 17077335.
46. Celletti C, Castori M, La Torre G, Camerota F. Evaluation of kinesiophobia and its correlations with pain and fatigue in joint hypermobility syndrome/ehlers-danlos syndrome hypermobility type. Biomed Res Int. 2013;2013:580460. PubMed PMID: 23936820. Pubmed Central PMCID: 3725998.

47. Karaa A, Stoler JM. Ehlers Danlos syndrome: an unusual presentation you need to know about. Case Rep Pediatr. 2013;2013:764659. PubMed PMID: 23762718. Pubmed Central PMCID: 3670523.
48. Miyoshi K, Nakamura K, Haga N, Mikami Y. Surgical treatment for atlantoaxial subluxation with myelopathy in spondyloepiphyseal dysplasia congenita. Spine. 2004;29(21):E488–91. PubMed PMID: 15507788.
49. Dahlqvist J, Orlen H, Matsson H, Dahl N, Lonnerholm T, Gustavson KH. Multiple epiphyseal dysplasia. Acta Orthop. 2009;80(6):711–5. PubMed PMID: 19995321. Pubmed Central PMCID: 2823319.
50. Bajuifer S, Letts M. Multiple epiphyseal dysplasia in children: beware of overtreatment! Can J Surg. 2005;48(2):106–9. PubMed PMID: 15887789. Pubmed Central PMCID: 3211600035.
51. Taketomi S, Hiraoka H, Nakagawa T, Miyamoto Y, Kuribayashi S, Fukuda A, et al. Osteochondral autograft for medial femoral condyle chondral lesions in a patient with multiple epiphyseal dysplasia: long-term result. J Orthop Sci. 2012;17(4):507–11. PubMed PMID: 21559955.
52. Lachman RS, Krakow D, Cohn DH, Rimoin DL. MED, COMP, multilayered and NEIN: an overview of multiple epiphyseal dysplasia. Pediatr Radiol. 2005;35(2):116–23. PubMed PMID: 15503005.
53. Malfait F, De Coster P, Hausser I, van Essen AJ, Franck P, Colige A, et al. The natural history, including orofacial features of three patients with Ehlers-Danlos syndrome, dermatosparaxis type (EDS type VIIC). Am J Med Genet A. 2004;131(1):18–28. PubMed PMID: 15389701.
54. Tiller GE, Hannig VL. X-linked spondyloepiphyseal dysplasia tarda. In: Pagon RA, Adam MP, Bird TD, Dolan CR, Fong CT, Stephens K, editors. GeneReviews. Seattle, WA: University of Washington Seattle; 1993.
55. Camera A, Camera G. Distinctive metaphyseal chondrodysplasia with severe distal radius and ulna involvement (upper extremity mesomelia) and normal height. Am J Med Genet A. 2003;122A(2):159–63. PubMed PMID: 12955769.
56. Bickels J, Wittig JC, Kollender Y, Kellar-Graney K, Mansour KL, Meller I, et al. Enchondromas of the hand: treatment with curettage and cemented internal fixation. J Hand Surg. 2002;27(5):870–5. PubMed PMID: 12239678.
57. Sassoon AA, Fitz-Gibbon PD, Harmsen WS, Moran SL. Enchondromas of the hand: factors affecting recurrence, healing, motion, and malignant transformation. J Hand Surg. 2012;37(6):1229–34. PubMed PMID: 22542061.
58. Marco RA, Gitelis S, Brebach GT, Healey JH. Cartilage tumors: evaluation and treatment. J Am Acad Orthop Surg. 2000;8(5):292–304. PubMed PMID: 11029557.
59. Plate AM, Lee SJ, Steiner G, Posner MA. Tumorlike lesions and benign tumors of the hand and wrist. J Am Acad Orthop Surg. 2003;11(2):129–41. PubMed PMID: 12670139.
60. Yasuda M, Masada K, Takeuchi E. Treatment of enchondroma of the hand with injectable calcium phosphate bone cement. J Hand Surg. 2006;31(1):98–102. PubMed PMID: 16443112.
61. Pannier S, Legeai-Mallet L. Hereditary multiple exostoses and enchondromatosis. Best Pract Res Clin Rheumatol. 2008;22(1):45–54. PubMed PMID: 18328980.
62. Popkov D, Journeau P, Popkov A, Haumont T, Lascombes P. Ollier's disease limb lenghtening: should intramedullary nailing be combined with circular external fixation? Orthop Traumatol Surg Res. 2010;96(4):348–53. PubMed PMID: 20472523.
63. Tomlinson PJ, Turner J, Monsell FP. The distribution of enchondromata in the hands of patients with Ollier's disease. J Hand Surg Eur Vol. 2010;35(2):154–5. PubMed PMID: 20118132.
64. Kashima TG, Gamage NM, Ye H, Amary MF, Flanagan AM, Ostlere SJ, et al. Locally aggressive fibrous dysplasia. Virchows Arch. 2013;463(1):79–84. PubMed PMID: 23760783.
65. Parekh SG, Donthineni-Rao R, Ricchetti E, Lackman RD. Fibrous dysplasia. J Am Acad Orthop Surg. 2004;12(5):305–13. PubMed PMID: 15469225.
66. Stanton RP, Ippolito E, Springfield D, Lindaman L, Wientroub S, Leet A. The surgical management of fibrous dysplasia of bone. Orphanet J Rare Dis. 2012;7 Suppl 1:S1. PubMed PMID: 22640754. Pubmed Central PMCID: 3359959.

Index

D.R. Laub Jr. (ed.), *Congenital Anomalies of the Upper Extremity: Etiology and Management*,
DOI 10.1007/978-1-4899-7504-1, © Springer Science+Business Media New York 2015

D

FSC
www.fsc.org
MIX
Papier | Fördert
gute Waldnutzung
FSC® C083411

Kolibri 360 GmbH
Ferdinand-Jühlke-Straße 7
99095 Erfurt, Deutschland
produktsicherheit@kolibri360.de